TO YOUR HEALTH

If you're serious about good eating, it's essential that you have the most up-to-date, comprehensive nutritional reference available. And whether you're under a doctor's supervision or just trying to maintain a healthy lifestyle, you can depend on Corinne T. Netzer, the bestselling expert who sets the standard against which all others are measured with the latest, most accurate nutritional information available.

With Corinne T. Netzer's help, you can find essential food counts quickly and easily in one authoritative guide. . . . Take it to the office . . . keep a copy in the kitchen . . . carry it with you on trips—it's the ultimate reference you need to answer your dietary questions!

MORE LISTINGS THAN EVER BEFORE!

THE COMPLETE BOOK OF FOOD COUNTS
5TH EDITION

CORINNE T. NETZER

Fifth Edition

THE COMPLETE
BOOK
OF
FOOD COUNTS

Corinne T. Netzer

A DELL BOOK

Published by
Dell Publishing
a division of
Random House, Inc.
1540 Broadway
New York, New York 10036

Cover photo copyright © 2000 by Steven Simpson/FPG International

Dell books may be purchased for business or promotional use or for special sales. For information please write to: Special Markets Department, Random House, Inc., 1540 Broadway, New York, NY 10036.

Dell® is a registered trademark of Random House, Inc., and the colophon is a trademark of Random House, Inc.

ISBN: 0-440-22563-9

Printed in the United States of America

Published simultaneously in Canada

January 2001

10 9

OPM

Introduction

The fifth edition of *The Complete Book of Food Counts* is the largest compilation of essential food data in this format. It contains data (calories, protein, carbohydrates, fat, cholesterol, sodium, and fiber) for basic generic foods, brand-name foods, and restaurant chains. Whether you are interested in dieting or nutrition—or both—you will find this book unique and invaluable as a reference.

Since this book is alphabetized, you should have no difficulty finding whatever you wish to look up. There are, however, times when you may have to look in more than one place. If you are searching for a particular food and cannot find it immediately, look for it under a category, such as cakes, puddings, cookies, soups. Wherever sensible, I have cross-referenced listings, but the pressure of space has made it impossible to do that for every item.

Compare only foods listed in similar measures. This rule particularly applies to the confusion between measures by capacity and measures by weight. Eight ounces is not necessarily equivalent to eight fluid ounces or one cup. Eight ounces is a measure of how much something weighs; one cup is a measure of how much space it occupies. For instance, a cup of lightweight food, such as puffed rice or popcorn, weighs about one ounce, and eight ounces of the same product would fill many cups. Naturally, you can convert a similar unit of measure into a smaller or larger amount. The following table may be useful in making such conversions.

Equivalents by Capacity
(all measures level)

1 quart	=	4 cups
1 cup	=	8 fluid ounces
	=	½ pint
	=	16 tablespoons
2 tablespoons	=	1 fluid ounce
1 tablespoon	=	3 teaspoons

Equivalents by Weight
1 pound = 16 ounces
3.57 ounces = 100 grams
1 ounce = 28.35 grams

All the material contained in *The Complete Book of Food Counts* is based on information from the United States government, from producers and processors of brand-name foods, and from food chains. The data contained herein are the most complete and accurate available as this book goes to press. Please bear in mind that seasonal and regional differences can affect the nutritional value of foods. Also, the food industry often changes recipes and sizes and may discontinue products or add new ones. In the future I will revise and update this book to keep you completely informed.

Good luck and good dieting.

CORINNE T. NETZER

Abbreviations and Symbols

cal.	calories
carbo	carbohydrates
chol.	cholesterol
cont.	container
diam.	diameter
fl.	fluid
gms	grams
″	inch
<	less than
lb(s).	pound(s)
mgs	milligrams
n.a.	not available
oz	ounce(s)
pkg.	package
pkt.	packet
pc(s).	piece(s)
prot.	protein
sod.	sodium
sq.	square(s)
tbsp.	tablespoon
tsp.	teaspoon
tr.	trace
w/	with
*	prepared according to basic package directions, except as noted

A

Food and Measure	cal.	prot. (gms)	carbo. (gms)	fat (gms)	chol. (mgs)	sod. (mgs)	fiber (gms)
Abalone, meat only; raw, 4 oz.	119	19.4	6.8	.9	96	341	0
Abruzzese sausage (*Boar's Head Cinghiale*), 1 oz.	100	8.0	<1.0	8.0	15	540	0
Acerola, fresh:							
trimmed, ½ cup	16	2	3.8	.1	0	4	<1.0
juice, 6 fl. oz.	36	.7	8.7	.5	0	6	<1.0
Acorn squash, ½ cup, except as noted:							
raw (*Frieda's*), ¾ cup, 3 oz.	35	1.0	9.0	0	0	0	2.0
baked, cubed	57	1.1	14.9	.1	0	4	2.9
boiled, mashed	41	.8	10.7	.1	0	3	3.4
Adobo, ¼ tsp.:							
(*Durkee*)	0	0	0	0	0	320	0
(*Goya*)	0	0	0	0	0	360	0
Adzuki beans:							
dry (*Arrowhead Mills*), ¼ cup	160	11.0	29.0	.5	0	0	6.0
boiled, ½ cup	147	8.7	28.5	.1	0	9	n.a.
Adzuki beans, canned, ½ cup:							
(*Eden* Organic Aduki)	110	7.0	19.0	0	0	10	5.0
sweetened	351	5.6	81.4	<.1	0	323	n.a.
Agar, see "Seaweed"							
Aioli, see "Mayonnaise"							
Alfredo sauce, canned or in jars, ¼ cup, except as noted:							
(*Classico* Di Liguria)	120	3.0	12.0	7.0	20	550	2.0

Food and Measure	cal.	prot. (gms)	carbo. (gms)	fat (gms)	chol. (mgs)	sod. (mgs)	fiber (gms)
Alfredo sauce, canned *(cont.)*							
(*Five Brothers*)	110	2.0	3.0	10.0	40	430	0
(*Progresso* Authentic),							
½ cup	200	8.0	7.0	15.0	50	850	1.0
(*Ragú*)	110	2.0	3.0	10.0	40	430	0
w/mushrooms (*Five*							
Brothers)	80	2.0	3.0	6.0	20	460	0
tomato (*Five Brothers*)	150	11.0	13.0	8.0	25	680	3.0
Alfredo sauce, refrig-							
erated, ¼ cup:							
(*Contadina*)	180	3.0	5.0	16.0	35	270	0
(*Contadina* Light)	80	4.0	5.0	5.0	20	330	0
(*Di Giorno*)	230	4.0	2.0	22.0	45	550	0
(*Di Giorno* Light Vari-							
eties)	170	5.0	16.0	10.0	30	600	0
mushroom (*Con-*							
tadina)	100	2.0	6.0	7.0	15	340	1.0
Alfredo sauce mix							
(*Knorr*), 2 tbsp. . . .	60	2.0	7.0	3.0	5	760	0
Algae, see "Seaweed"							
Allspice, 1 tsp.	5	.1	1.4	.2	0	1	.4
Almond, shelled,							
1 oz., except as							
noted:							
(*Beer Nuts* Classic) . . .	170	6.0	6.0	14.0	0	65	3.0
(*Blue Diamond*							
Smokehouse),							
3 tbsp., 1.1 oz.	180	6.0	4.0	16.0	0	170	2.0
whole (*Sonoma* Or-							
ganic), ¼ cup,							
1.1 oz.	180	6.0	6.0	15.0	0	0	4.0
barbecue (*Blue Dia-*							
mond), 3 tbsp.,							
1.1 oz.	170	6.0	5.0	15.0	0	250	4.0
dried:							
1 oz.	167	5.7	5.8	14.8	0	3	3.1
slivered, 1 cup	795	26.9	27.5	70.5	0	15	14.7
dry-roasted:							
(*Arrowhead Mills*),							
¼ cup	200	7.0	7.0	18.0	0	250	4.0

Food and Measure	cal.	prot. (gms)	carbo. (gms)	fat (gms)	chol. (mgs)	sod. (mgs)	fiber (gms)
(*River Queen* Unsalted)	160	5.0	7.0	14.0	0	0	4.0
salted	167	4.6	6.9	14.7	0	221	3.9
honey-roasted:							
(*Blue Diamond*), 3 tbsp., 1.1 oz.	170	5.0	8.0	14.0	0	35	2.0
1 oz.	168	5.2	7.9	14.2	0	37	n.a.
hot and spicy (*Blue Diamond*), 3 tbsp., 1.1 oz.	190	6.0	5.0	16.0	0	150	2.0
natural, whole (*Blue Diamond*), 1.1 oz.	180	6.0	6.0	15.0	0	0	3.0
oil-roasted, salted ...	176	5.8	4.5	16.4	0	221	3.2
roasted, salted:							
(*Blue Diamond*), 3 tbsp., 1.1 oz.	180	6.0	4.0	17.0	0	110	3.0
(*River Queen*), 3 tbsp., 1 oz. ...	160	5.0	4.0	15.0	0	140	3.0
slivered (*Paradise/ White Swan*), ¼ cup, 1.1 oz.	200	8.0	3.0	17.0	0	0	2.0
toasted	167	5.8	6.5	14.4	0	3	3.2
Almond butter (*Arrowhead Mills*), 2 tbsp.	210	5.0	7.0	20.0	0	0	2.0
Almond meal, partially defatted, 1 oz.	116	11.2	8.2	5.2	0	2	n.a.
Almond paste, 1 oz.	127	3.4	12.4	7.2	0	3	4.2
Almond syrup (*Trader Vic's* Orgeat), 1 fl. oz.	100	0	25.0	0	0	15	0
Amaranth, ½ cup:							
raw, trimmed	4	.3	.6	<.1	0	3	n.a.
boiled, drained	14	1.4	2.7	.1	0	14	n.a.
Amaranth, wholegrain, 1 oz.	106	4.1	18.8	1.8	0	6	4.3
Amaranth flour (*Arrowhead Mills*), ¼ cup	110	4.0	19.0	1.5	0	0	2.0
Amaranth seeds (*Arrowhead Mills*), ¼ cup	170	7.0	29.0	2.0	0	0	3.0

Food and Measure	cal.	prot. (gms)	carbo. (gms)	fat (gms)	chol. (mgs)	sod. (mgs)	fiber (gms)
Amaretto syrup:							
(*Ferrara*), 2 oz.	130	0	32.0	0	0	12	0
(*Watkins*), 1 tbsp. ...	40	0	18.0	0	0	0	0
Anaheim chili, see							
"Pepper, chili"							
Anasazi beans, dry							
(*Arrowhead Mills*),							
¼ cup	150	10.0	27.0	.5	0	0	9.0
Anchovy, meat only:							
fresh, European, raw,							
1 oz.	37	5.8	0	1.4	n.a.	29	0
canned, in olive oil:							
(*Duet*), 6 pcs.	25	4.0	0	1.5	n.a.	750	0
drained, 1 oz.	60	8.2	0	2.8	n.a.	1040	0
5 medium, .7 oz.	42	5.8	0	1.9	n.a.	734	0
Andouille sausage,							
see "Sausage"							
Angel hair pasta:							
dry, see "Pasta"							
refrigerated:							
(*Contadina*),							
1¼ cups	230	9.0	43.0	2.5	85	20	2.0
(*Di Giorno*), 2 oz.	160	7.0	31.0	1.0	0	190	1.0
Angel hair pasta en-							
tree, frozen, 1 pkg.:							
(*Lean Cuisine*), 10 oz.	260	9.0	46.0	4.5	0	470	2.0
(*Smart Ones*), 10 oz.	240	8.0	46.0	3.0	0	720	4.0
w/chunky tomatoes							
(*The Budget Gour-*							
met Value Classics							
Low Fat), 8 oz.	230	8.0	38.0	5.0	10	430	3.0
Angel hair pasta mix,							
1 cup*:							
chicken broccoli (*Lip-*							
ton Pasta & Sauce)	260	8.0	43.0	7.5	0	810	2.0
w/herbs (*Pasta Roni*)	320	9.0	42.0	13.0	5	710	2.0
w/lemon and butter							
(*Pasta Roni*)	360	9.0	48.0	15.0	0	980	2.0
w/Parmesan:							
(*Lipton* Pasta &							
Sauce).........	280	8.0	41.0	10.5	10	960	2.0

Food and Measure	cal.	prot. (gms)	carbo. (gms)	fat (gms)	chol. (mgs)	sod. (mgs)	fiber (gms)
(*Pasta Roni*)	320	9.0	40.0	14.0	5	890	2.0
Anise seed, 1 tsp.	7	.4	1.1	.3	0	<1	.3
Appaloosa beans, dried (*Frieda's*), ½ cup	120	7.0	22.0	0	0	0	9.0
Apple, fresh, ½ cup, except as noted:							
(*Frieda's* Lady), 5 oz.	80	0	21.0	.5	0	0	3.0
w/peel, 2¾" apple . . .	81	.3	21.1	.5	0	1	3.7
w/peel, sliced	32	.1	8.4	.2	0	<1	3.0
peeled, 2¾" apple . . .	72	.2	19.0	.4	0	<1	2.4
peeled, sliced	31	.1	8.2	.2	0	<1	1.0
cooked, peeled:							
sliced, boiled	46	.2	11.7	.3	0	1	2.1
sliced, microwaved	48	.2	12.3	.4	0	1	2.4
Apple, canned:							
diced, regular or cinnamon flavor (*Del Monte* Cup), 4 oz.	70	0	18.0	0	0	10	<1.0
rings, in heavy syrup (*Comstock/Wilderness*), 2 rings	25	0	7.0	0	0	20	0
sliced:							
(*Comstock* Original), ½ cup	30	0	7.0	0	0	10	2.0
(*Wilderness*), ⅓ cup	30	0	7.0	0	0	10	2.0
Apple, dried:							
(*Sonoma* Organic), 11 rings, 1.4 oz. . . .	110	0	29.0	0	0	0	4.0
diced, unsulfured (*AlpineAire*), 1 oz. . . .	100	0	26.0	0	0	150	2.0
flakes, unsulfured (*AlpineAire*), 1 oz. . . .	110	0	26.0	0	0	95	1.0
Apple, escalloped, frozen (*Stouffer's* Side Dish), 6 oz.	180	0	37.0	3.0	0	70	3.0
Apple butter, 1 tbsp.:							
(*Dutch Girl*)	45	0	11.0	0	0	10	0
(*Eden* Organic)	20	0	6.0	0	0	0	0
cider or spiced (*Smucker's*)	45	0	11.0	0	0	10	0

Food and Measure	cal.	prot. (gms)	carbo. (gms)	fat (gms)	chol. (mgs)	sod. (mgs)	fiber (gms)
Apple chips:							
(*Seneca*), 1 oz.	140	0	20.0	7.0	0	15	2.0
(*Weight Watchers*), ¾ oz.	70	0	18.0	0	0	125	3.0
Apple cider, see "Apple Juice"							
Apple cider mix, hot (*Swiss Miss*), 1 pkt.	85	0	21.0	0	0	65	<1.0
Apple dip, 2 tbsp., except as noted:							
candy (*Concord Farms*), mix for 1 apple	50	0	14.0	0	0	0	0
caramel:							
(*Concord Farms*), mix for 1 apple	50	0	13.0	0	0	0	0
(*Smucker's* Fat Free)	130	1.0	30.0	0	0	85	0
(*T. Marzetti's* 4 oz.)	150	1.0	24.0	6.0	4	90	0
(*T. Marzetti's* 36 oz.)	150	1.0	23.0	6.0	4	90	0
(*T. Marzetti's* Fat Free 2 oz.)	150	1.0	38.0	0	0	170	0
(*T. Marzetti's* Fat Free 18 oz.)	120	1.0	27.0	0	0	120	0
peanut butter caramel(*T. Marzetti's*)	150	3.0	21.0	6.0	0	135	1.0
Apple drink (*Snapple* Apple Crisp), 10 fl. oz.	140	0	36.0	0	0	30	0
Apple drink blends, 8 fl. oz., except as noted:							
berry burst (*Dole*) ...	120	0	31.0	0	0	20	0
berry pear (*Tropicana Twister*)	140	0	34.0	0	0	20	0
blueberry strawberry:							
(*Hood*)	120	0	30.0	0	0	5	0
(*Veryfine* Quencher)	140	0	34.0	0	0	10	0
cherry (*Snapple* Squeeze)..........	120	0	30.0	0	0	10	0

Food and Measure	cal.	prot. (gms)	carbo. (gms)	fat (gms)	chol. (mgs)	sod. (mgs)	fiber (gms)
cherry, black, white grape (*Veryfine* Quencher 30%) ...	120	0	31.0	0	0	10	0
cherryberry (*Veryfine*), 11.5 fl. oz.	190	0	47.0	0	0	35	0
cranberry:							
(*Tropicana*), 11.5 fl. oz.	200	0	49.0	0	0	45	0
(*Veryfine*)	150	0	38.0	0	0	10	0
(*Veryfine*), 10 fl. oz.	190	0	48.0	0	0	10	0
(*Veryfine*), 11.5 fl. oz.	220	0	55.0	0	0	15	0
(*Veryfine* Diet)	15	0	4.0	0	0	15	0
cranberry raspberry:							
(*Hood* 30% Juice)	130	0	32.0	0	0	5	0
(*Minute Maid*)	123	0	33.0	0	0	24	0
grape raspberry (*Veryfine* Quencher)	130	0	31.0	0	0	10	0
peach kiwi (*Veryfine* Quencher 30%) ...	140	0	34.0	0	0	25	0
peach plum (*Veryfine* Quencher 30%) ...	130	0	34.0	0	0	30	0
raspberry blackberry (*Tropicana Twister*)	120	0	31.0	0	0	20	0
raspberry cherry (*Veryfine* Quencher 30%)	130	0	33.0	0	0	30	0
strawberry banana (*Veryfine* Quencher 30%)	130	0	33.0	0	0	30	0
Apple juice, 8 fl. oz., except as noted:							
(*After the Fall* Organic/ Vermont)	90	0	22.0	0	0	20	0
(*After the Fall Vermont Harvest*)	110	1.0	27.0	0	0	5	0
(*Apple & Eve*)	110	1.0	26.0	0	0	5	0
(*Eden* Organic)	80	0	23.0	0	0	0	0
(*Hood*)	120	0	31.0	0	0	5	0
(*Minute Maid*)	112	0	28.0	0	0	28	0
(*Mott's* 100% Natural)	120	0	29.0	0	0	20	0

Food and Measure	cal.	prot. (gms)	carbo. (gms)	fat (gms)	chol. (mgs)	sod. (mgs)	fiber (gms)
Apple juice *(cont.)*							
(*Ocean Spray*)	110	0	28.0	0	0	35	0
(*R.W. Knudsen* Clear/ Aseptic)	110	0	28.0	0	0	5	0
(*R.W. Knudsen* Natural/Organic/Gravenstein)	120	0	30.0	0	0	25	0
(*Santa Cruz*)	120	0	30.0	0	0	25	0
(*Season's Best*)	120	<1.0	29.0	0	0	25	0
(*Snapple*), 12 fl. oz.	180	0	44.0	0	0	40	0
(*Tree Top*)	120	0	29.0	0	0	25	0
(*Veryfine*)	120	0	30.0	0	0	15	0
(*Veryfine*), 10 fl. oz.	150	0	38.0	0	0	20	0
(*Veryfine*), 11.5 fl. oz.	170	0	43.0	0	0	20	0
(*Veryfine* Golden/Red Delicious/Granny Smith/Macintosh/ Natural), 12 fl. oz.	180	0	45.0	0	0	20	0
(*Veryfine* Juice-Up)	120	0	30.0	0	0	35	0
frozen*:							
(*R.W. Knudsen*) . . .	120	0	30.0	0	0	25	0
(*Tree Top*)	120	0	29.0	0	0	15	0
spiced (*Apple & Eve* Cider & Spice)	110	1.0	26.0	0	0	5	0
Apple juice blends, 8 fl. oz., except as noted:							
all blends, except apricot, cherry cider, and apple-cranberry (*R.W. Knudsen*) . . .	120	0	30.0	0	0	25	0
apricot:							
(*After the Fall*)	100	1.0	26.0	0	0	20	0
(*R.W. Knudsen*) . . .	120	0	30.0	0	0	35	0
cherry:							
(*After the Fall*)	100	1.0	24.0	0	0	20	0
cider (*R.W. Knudsen*)	130	0	33.0	0	0	35	0
cranberry:							
(*Apple & Eve*)	120	1.0	30.0	0	0	20	0

Food and Measure	cal.	prot. (gms)	carbo. (gms)	fat (gms)	chol. (mgs)	sod. (mgs)	fiber (gms)
(*R.W. Knudsen* Aseptic)........	110	1.0	29.0	0	0	25	0
grape:							
(*Apple & Eve*), 8.45 fl. oz.	130	0	32.0	0	0	15	0
(*Juicy Juice*)	130	1.0	30.0	0	0	10	0
raspberry (*After the Fall*)	90	1	23.0	0	0	20	0
strawberry (*After the Fall*)	100	1.0	24.0	0	0	20	0
Apple pastry (see also specific listings), frozen, 1 pc.:							
dumpling (*Pepperidge Farm*), 3 oz.	290	3.0	44.0	11.0	0	160	3.0
fruit square (*Pepperidge Farm*), 2½ oz.	210	2.0	27.0	10.0	0	210	2.0
Applesauce, ½ cup, except as noted:							
(*Mott's*)	100	0	25.0	0	0	0	1.0
(*Mott's*), 4 oz.	90	0	22.0	0	0	0	1.0
(*Mott's* Chunky)	100	0	24.0	0	0	0	2.0
(*Seneca*)...........	100	0	24.0	0	0	0	2.0
(*Tree Top* Original) ...	100	0	24.0	0	0	150	1.0
unsweetened:							
(*Eden* Organic)	50	0	15.0	0	0	15	2.0
(*Mott's* Natural Style), 4 oz.	50	0	12.0	0	0	0	1.0
(*Santa Cruz* Natural)	45	0	15.0	0	0	5	0
(*Seneca* 100% Natural)	60	0	14.0	0	0	0	2.0
(*Tree Top*)	70	0	18.0	0	0	140	1.0
cinnamon:							
(*Mott's*)	110	0	28.0	0	0	0	1.0
(*Mott's*), 4 oz.	100	0	26.0	0	0	0	1.0
(*Seneca*)	100	0	24.0	0	0	0	3.0
golden (*Leroux Creek* 100% Natural), 4 oz.	80	0	19.0	0	0	0	2.0
golden delicious (*Seneca*)	90	0	22.0	0	0	0	3.0

Food and Measure	cal.	prot. (gms)	carbo. (gms)	fat (gms)	chol. (mgs)	sod. (mgs)	fiber (gms)
Applesauce *(cont.)*							
McIntosh (*Seneca*) . . .	100	0	24.0	0	0	0	2.0
Applesauce blends,							
1/2 cup or 4 oz.:							
all blends (*Santa Cruz*							
Natural)	45	0	15.0	0	0	5	0
apple-cherry or mango							
(*Leroux Creek*)	90	<1.0	15.0	0	0	30	2.0
berry or cherry (*Le-*							
roux Creek)	80	0	19.0	0	0	0	2.0
mango-peach (*Fruitsa-*							
tions)	70	0	19.0	0	0	0	1.0
strawberry (*Fruitsa-*							
tions)	90	0	23.0	0	0	10	1.0
Apricot, fresh:							
medium, 12 per lb.	51	1.5	11.8	.4	0	1	2.5
pitted, halves, 1/2 cup	37	1.1	8.6	.3	0	1	1.9
Apricot, canned,							
halves, 1/2 cup:							
(*Del Monte* Lite)	60	0	16.0	0	0	10	1.0
almond flavor, in light							
syrup (*Del Monte*)	90	0	22.0	0	0	10	1.0
in juice (*Libby's* Lite)	60	1.0	13.0	0	0	10	1.0
in light syrup, un-							
peeled (*Del Monte*							
Orchard Select)	80	0	21.0	0	0	10	1.0
in heavy syrup (*Del*							
Monte)	100	0	26.0	0	0	10	1.0
Apricot, dried:							
(*Sonoma* Organic),							
10 pcs., 1.4 oz. . . .	130	2.0	31.0	0	0	0	3.0
(*Sun•Maid*), 1/4 cup	110	1.0	25.0	0	0	0	2.0
sulfured, 2 oz.	135	2.1	35.0	.3	0	6	5.1
Apricot, frozen,							
sweetened, 1/2 cup	119	.9	30.4	.1	0	5	2.1
Apricot nectar,							
8 fl. oz.:							
(*Goya*)	130	1.0	31.0	0	0	15	0
(*Kern's*)	150	<1.0	36.0	0	0	5	0
(*R.W. Knudsen*)	120	0	30.0	0	0	35	0
(*Santa Cruz*)	120	0	30.0	0	0	35	0

Food and Measure	cal.	prot. (gms)	carbo. (gms)	fat (gms)	chol. (mgs)	sod. (mgs)	fiber (gms)
Apricot syrup							
(*Smucker's*), ¼ cup	210	0	52.0	0	0	0	0
Apricot-pineapple							
nectar (*Kern's*),							
11.5 oz.	220	<1.0	53.0	0	0	5	2.0
Arame, see "Sea-							
weed"							
Arby's, 1 serving:							
breakfast items:							
bacon, 2 strips	90	5.0	0	7.0	15	220	0
biscuit, plain	280	6.0	34.0	15.0	0	730	1.0
croissant, plain	220	4.0	25.0	12.0	25	230	0
danish, cinnamon							
nut	360	6.0	60.0	11.0	0	105	1.0
egg portion	95	.5	.5	8.0	180	54	0
french *Toastix,*							
6 pcs.	430	10.0	52.0	21.0	0	550	3.0
ham, 1.5 oz.	45	7.0	0	1.0	20	405	0
sausage, 1.3 oz. . . .	163	7.0	0	15.0	25	321	0
Swiss cheese, .5 oz.	45	4.0	.5	3.0	12	175	0
table syrup, 1 oz.	100	0	25.0	0	0	30	0
roast beef sandwich:							
Arby's melt							
w/cheddar	368	18.0	36.0	18.0	31	937	2.0
Arby-Q	431	20.0	48.0	18.0	37	1321	3.0
bac'n cheddar							
deluxe	539	22.0	38.0	34.0	44.0	1140	3.0
beef'n cheddar	507	25.0	40.0	28.0	50.0	1216	2.0
Big Montana	686	48.0	47.0	35.0	121	2295	3.0
giant roast beef	555	35.0	43.0	28.0	71	1561	5.0
junior roast beef . . .	324	17.0	35.0	14.0	30	779	2.0
regular roast beef	388	23.0	33.0	19.0	43	1009	3.0
super roast beef . . .	523	25.0	50.0	27.0	43	1189	5.0
chicken:							
breaded fillet	536	28.0	46.0	28.0	45	1016	5.0
Cordon Bleu	623	38.0	46.0	33.0	77	1594	5.0
chicken fingers,							
2 pcs.	290	16.0	20.0	16.0	32	677	.5
grilled BBQ	388	23.0	47.0	13.0	43	1002	2.0
grilled deluxe	430	23.0	41.0	20.0	61	848	3.0

Food and Measure	cal.	prot. (gms)	carbo. (gms)	fat (gms)	chol. (mgs)	sod. (mgs)	fiber (gms)
***Arby's*, chicken** *(cont.)*							
roast chicken:							
club	546	31.0	37.0	31.0	58	1103	2.0
deluxe	433	24.0	36.0	22.0	34	763	2.0
Santa Fe	463	29.0	38.0	22.0	54	818	1.0
sandwiches, sub roll:							
french dip	475	30.0	40.0	22.0	55	1411	3.0
hot ham'n Swiss . . .	500	30.0	43.0	23.0	68	1664	2.0
Italian sub	633	30.0	46.0	36.0	83	2089	2.0
Philly beef'n Swiss	755	39.0	48.0	47.0	91	2025	3.0
roast beef sub	700	38.0	44.0	42.0	84	2034	4.0
triple cheese melt	720	37.0	46.0	45.0	91	1797	2.0
turkey sub	550	31.0	47.0	27.0	65	2084	2.0
sandwiches, other:							
fish fillet	529	23.0	50.0	27.0	43	864	2.0
ham'n cheese	359	24.0	34.0	14.0	53	1283	2.0
ham'n cheese melt	329	20.0	34.0	13.0	40	1013	2.0
light menu:							
roast beef deluxe	296	18.0	33.0	10.0	42	826	6.0
roast chicken deluxe	276	20.0	33.0	6.0	33	777	4.0
roast turkey deluxe	260	20.0	33.0	7.0	33	1262	4.0
salad, garden	61	3.0	12.0	.5	0	40	5.0
salad, roast chicken	149	20.0	12.0	2.0	29	418	5.0
salad, side	23	1.0	4.0	.3	0	15	2.0
potato, baked:							
plain	355	7.0	82.0	.3	0	26	7.0
w/margarine and							
sour cream	578	9.0	85.0	24.0	25	209	7.0
broccoli'n cheddar	571	14.0	89.0	20.0	12	565	9.0
deluxe	736	19.0	86.0	36.0	59	499	7.0
potato cakes, 2 pcs.	204	2.0	20.0	12.0	0	397	0
fries:							
curly	300	4.0	38.0	15.0	0	853	0
curly, cheddar	333	5.0	40.0	18.0	3	1016	0
homestyle, 2.5 oz.	212	2.5	29.0	10.0	0	414	2.0
homestyle, 4 oz.	340	4.0	46.0	15.5	0	665	3.0
homestyle, 5 oz.	423	5.5	57.0	19.0	0	828	4.0
soups, 8 oz.:							
clam chowder	190	9.0	18.0	9.0	25	965	1.0
cream of broccoli	160	7.0	15.0	8.0	25	1005	

Food and Measure	cal.	prot. (gms)	carbo. (gms)	fat (gms)	chol. (mgs)	sod. (mgs)	fiber (gms)
lumberjack mixed vegetable	90	2.0	10.0	4.0	5	1150	1.0
old fashion chicken noodle	80	6.0	11.0	2.0	20	850	1.0
potato w/bacon	170	6.0	23.0	7.0	20	905	2.0
Timberline chili	220	18.0	17.0	10.0	30	1130	7.0
Wisconsin cheese	280	10.0	20.0	18.0	10	1065	2.0
sauces/condiments:							
Arby's sauce, 1/2 oz.	15	.1	4.0	.2	0	113	0
barbecue sauce, 1/2 oz.	30	0	7.0	0	0	185	0
beef au jus, 2 oz.	10	0	1.0	0	0	440	0
cheese sauce:							
cheddar, 3/4 oz.	35	1.0	1.0	3.0	4	139	0
Parmesan, 1/2 oz.	70	1.0	2.0	7.0	5	130	0
horsey sauce, 1/2 oz.	60	0	2.0	5.0	5	150	0
ketchup, 1/2 oz.	16	.3	4.0	0	0	143	0
mayonnaise, 1/2 oz.	110	0	0	12.0	5	80	0
mayonnaise, light, 1/4 oz.	12	.5	.5	1.0	0	64	.5
mustard, .16 oz.	5	0	1.0	0	0	70	0
sub sauce, Italian, 1/2 oz.	70	0	1.0	7.0	0	240	0
tartar sauce, 1 oz.	140	0	0	15.0	30	220	0
dressings, 1/2 oz.:							
blue cheese	290	2.0	2.0	31.0	50	139	0
buttermilk ranch, re- duced cal	50	0	12.0	0	0	710	0
honey french	280	0	18.0	23.0	0	400	0
honey mayonnaise, reduced cal	70	0	1.0	7.0	20	135	0
Italian, reduced cal	20	0	3.0	1.0	0	1000	0
red ranch	75	0	5.0	6.0	0	115	0
Thousand Island . . .	260	0	7.0	26.0	30	420	0
desserts/shakes:							
apple turnover	330	4.0	48.0	14.0	0	180	0
cherry turnover	320	4.0	46.0	13.0	0	190	0
cheesecake, plain	320	5.0	23.0	23.0	95	240	0
chocolate chip cookie	125	2.0	16.0	6.0	10	85	0

Food and Measure	cal.	prot. (gms)	carbo. (gms)	fat (gms)	chol. (mgs)	sod. (mgs)	fiber (gms)
Arby's, desserts/shakes *(cont.)*							
shake, 12 oz.:							
chocolate	451	15.0	76.0	12.0	36	341	0
jamocha	384	15.0	62.0	10.0	36	262	0
vanilla	360	15.0	50.0	12.0	36	281	0
swirl, polar, 11.6 oz.:							
Butterfinger.....	457	15.0	62.0	18.0	28	318	0
Heath	543	15.0	76.0	22.0	39	346	0
Oreo	482	15.0	66.0	22.0	35	521	0
peanut butter cup	517	20.0	61.0	24.0	34	385	1.0
Snickers	511	15.0	73.0	19.0	33	351	1.0
Arrowhead, raw, 2⅝″ corm	12	.6	2.4	<.1	0	3	<1.0
Arrowroot (*Durkee*), ¼ tsp.	0	0	0	0	0	0	0
Arrowroot flour, 1 cup	457	.4	112.8	.1	0	2	4.4
Artichoke, globe, fresh:							
boiled, 10.6 oz.	60	4.2	13.4	.2	0	114	6.5
hearts, boiled, drained, ½ cup	42	2.9	9.4	.1	0	80	4.5
Artichoke, canned:							
(*Progresso*), 1 pc., 2.9 oz.	30	2.0	6.0	0	0	240	1.0
bottoms (*Gourmet Award*), 3 pcs.	18	2.0	3.0	0	0	488	2.0
hearts (*Reese*), 4.5 oz., 4 quarters	50	3.0	9.0	0	0	380	2.0
Artichoke, frozen, hearts:							
(*Birds Eye*), ½ cup ...	40	3.0	8.0	0	0	45	6.0
9-oz. pkg.	96	6.7	19.8	1.1	0	120	9.9
Artichoke, Jerusalem, see "Jerusalem artichoke"							
Artichoke appetizer, marinated (*Progresso*), 2 pcs., 1.1 oz.	50	0	2.0	5.0	0	110	0

Food and Measure	cal.	prot. (gms)	carbo. (gms)	fat (gms)	chol. (mgs)	sod. (mgs)	fiber (gms)
Artichoke sauce (*Italia In Talola*), 2 tbsp.	110	0	2.0	12.0	0	360	<1.0
Arugula, trimmed, 1 oz.	7	.7	1.0	.2	0	8	n.a.
Asparagus, fresh:							
raw, 4 spears, 3.8 oz.	14	1.3	2.6	.1	0	1	1.2
boiled, 4 spears, ½"-diam. base	14	1.6	2.5	.2	0	7	1.3
boiled, drained, cuts, ½ cup	22	2.3	3.8	.3	0	10	1.9
Asparagus, canned:							
(*Seneca*), ½ cup	20	2.0	3.0	0	0	220	2.0
all styles (*Del Monte*), ½ cup	20	2.0	3.0	0	0	420	1.0
spears, 4½ oz.:							
(*Green Giant*)	20	2.0	3.0	0	0	450	1.0
extra large (*Le-Sueur*)	20	2.0	3.0	0	0	440	1.0
extra long (*Green Giant*)	20	2.0	3.0	0	0	400	1.0
cuts, ½ cup:							
(*Bush's Best*)	25	3.0	2.0	0	0	380	1.0
(*Green Giant*)	20	2.0	3.0	0	0	420	1.0
(*Green Giant* 50% Less Sodium) . . .	20	2.0	3.0	0	0	210	1.0
Asparagus, freeze-dried, diced (*AlpineAire*), ½ oz. . . .	50	6.0	6.0	0	0	0	1.0
Asparagus, frozen:							
(*Birds Eye Farm Fresh Stir Fry*), 2 cups . . .	90	5.0	16.0	.5	0	35	3.0
spears:							
(*Birds Eye*), 8 pcs.	20	3.0	4.0	0	0	5	1.0
(*Freshlike*), 7 pcs.	20	3.0	3.0	0	0	5	2.0
boiled, 4 pcs.	17	1.8	2.9	.3	0	2	1.2
cuts:							
(*Birds Eye*), ½ cup	25	3.0	4.0	0	0	5	2.0
(*Freshlike*), ¾ cup	20	3.0	3.0	0	0	5	2.0
(*Green Giant Harvest Fresh*), ⅔ cup	25	2.0	4.0	0	0	85	1.0

Food and Measure	cal.	prot. (gms)	carbo. (gms)	fat (gms)	chol. (mgs)	sod. (mgs)	fiber (gms)
Asparagus bean, see "Winged bean"							
Au jus gravy, ¼ cup:							
(*Franco-American*) . . .	10	<1.0	2.0	.5	<5	310	0
(*Heinz* Home Style Bistro)	15	1.0	3.0	.5	0	360	0
Au jus gravy mix (*Knorr* Classics), 1 tsp.	10	0	2.0	0	0	310	0
Aubergine, see "Eggplant"							
Avocado, California:							
medium, 8 oz.	306	3.6	12.0	30.0	0	21	4.7
trimmed, 1 oz.	50	.6	2.0	4.9	0	3	.8
pureed, ½ cup	204	2.4	8.0	19.9	0	14	3.1
Avocado, cocktail (*Frieda's*), 1 pc., 1.4 oz.	60	1.0	3.0	6.0	0	0	2.0
Avocado dip (see also "Guacamole"), 2 tbsp.:							
(*Kraft*)	60	1.0	4.0	4.0	0	240	0
(*Nalley*)	120	0	3.0	12.0	10	200	0
Avocado oil, see "Oil"							

B

Food and Measure	cal.	prot. (gms)	carbo. (gms)	fat (gms)	chol. (mgs)	sod. (mgs)	fiber (gms)
Babaganoush, see "Eggplant appetizer"							
Bacon, cooked, 2 slices, except as noted:							
(*Armour*)	60	4.0	0	4.0	10	280	0
(*Black Label*)	80	5.0	0	7.0	15	330	0
(*Black Label* Center Cut), 3 slices	70	5.0	0	5.5	15	340	0
(*Black Label* Low Salt)	80	5.0	0	7.0	15	230	0
(*Boar's Head*)	60	4.0	0	5.0	10	190	0
(*Hormel* Microwave), 4 slices	70	6.0	0	5.0	20	310	0
(*Jones Dairy Farm* Country Carved) . . .	90	4.0	0	8.0	15	350	0
(*Old Smokehouse*) . . .	80	5.0	0	7.0	15	280	0
(*Oscar Mayer*)	60	4.0	0	5.0	10	250	0
(*Oscar Mayer* Center Cut)	50	4.0	0	4.5	15	270	0
(*Oscar Mayer* Lower Sodium)	60	4.0	0	4.0	10	170	0
(*Range Brand*)	110	7.0	0	9.0	20	460	0
(*Red Label*)	80	5.0	0	7.0	15	330	0
thick, 1 slice:							
(*Jones Dairy Farm* Country Carved)	70	3.0	0	6.0	15	290	0
(*Oscar Mayer*)	60	4.0	0	5.0	10	250	0
turkey, see "Turkey bacon"							
Bacon, Canadian:							
(*Boar's Head*), 2 oz.	70	12.0	1.0	2.5	30	560	0
(*Hormel*), 2 oz.	70	10.0	0	3.0	30	640	0

Food and Measure	cal.	prot. (gms)	carbo. (gms)	fat (gms)	chol. (mgs)	sod. (mgs)	fiber (gms)
Bacon, Canadian *(cont.)*							
(*Oscar Mayer*),							
2 slices, 1.6 oz. . . .	50	8.0	0	1.5	25	620	0
Bacon, Irish, back,							
2 slices, 2 oz.	130	10.0	1.0	10.0	30	570	0
"Bacon," vegetarian,							
frozen, 2 slices:							
(*Morningstar Farms*							
Breakfast Strips) . . .	60	2.0	2.0	4.5	0	220	<1.0
(*Worthington Strip-*							
ples)	60	2.0	2.0	4.5	0	220	<1.0
Bacon bits:							
imitation, 1½ tbsp.:							
(*Bac'n Pieces*)	30	3.0	2.0	1.5	0	220	0
chips/bits (*Bac*Os*)	30	3.0	2.0	1.5	0	120	0
real, 1 tbsp.:							
bits (*Hormel*)	30	3.0	0	1.5	5	250	0
bits (*Oscar Mayer*)	25	3.0	0	1.5	5	220	0
pieces (*Hormel*) . . .	25	3.0	0	1.5	10	180	0
pieces (*Oscar*							
Mayer)	25	2.0	0	1.5	5	170	0
Bacon dip, 2 tbsp.:							
cheese, see "Cheese							
dip"							
horseradish:							
(*Heluva* Good)	60	1.0	2.0	5,0	20	200	0
(*Heluva* Good Fat							
Free)	25	1.0	4.0	0	0	210	0
(*Kraft*)	60	1.0	3.0	5.0	0	220	0
(*Kraft* Premium) . . .	50	1.0	2.0	5.0	15	200	0
onion:							
(*Breakstone's*)	60	1.0	2.0	5.0	20	170	0
(*Knudsen* Premium)	60	1.0	2.0	5.0	20	170	0
(*Kraft* Premium) . . .	60	1.0	2.0	5.0	15	160	0
(*Nalley*)	110	1.0	2.0	11.0	15	220	0
ranch, see "Ranch							
dip"							
Bacon dip mix, dry,							
1 tsp.:							
cheddar (*Watkins*) . . .	10	0	2.0	0	0	140	0
horseradish (*Watkins*)	10	1.0	1.0	0	0	90	0

Food and Measure	cal.	prot. (gms)	carbo. (gms)	fat (gms)	chol. (mgs)	sod. (mgs)	fiber (gms)
Bagel, 1 pc.:							
plain:							
(*Awrey's*), 2.6 oz.	200	7.0	40.0	1.0	0	340	<1.0
(*Awrey's*), 4 oz. . . .	280	10.0	56.0	1.0	0	590	3.0
(*Thomas'*), 3.7 oz.	280	10.0	56.0	1.5	0	530	2.0
(*Wonder*), 3 oz. . . .	210	8.0	43.0	1.0	0	350	2.0
mini (*Awrey's*),							
9/10 oz.	100	3.0	22.0	0	0	160	0
blueberry:							
(*Awrey's*), 4 oz. . . .	280	10.0	60.0	1.0	0	590	4.0
(*Wonder*), 3 oz. . . .	220	7.0	43.0	1.0	0	450	1.0
cinnamon raisin:							
(*Awrey's*), 2.6 oz.	200	7.0	42.0	1.0	0	250	<1.0
(*Awrey's*), 4 oz. . . .	270	10.0	58.0	1.0	0	560	4.0
(*Thomas'*), 3.7 oz.	280	10.0	59.0	1.5	0	490	3.0
(*Wonder*), 3 oz. . . .	210	8.0	42.0	1.0	0	360	2.0
onion (*Wonder*), 3 oz.	210	8.0	43.0	1.0	0	340	1.0
rye (*Wonder* Beef-							
steak), 3 oz.	220	9.0	42.0	1.0	0	520	2.0
wheat (*Wonder*), 3 oz.	210	8.0	43.0	1.0	0	350	2.0
Bagel, frozen, 1 pc.:							
plain:							
(*Amy's*)	230	8.0	48.0	1.5	0	490	2.0
(*Lender's*)	150	6.0	30.0	.5	0	320	1.0
(*Lender's* Bake at							
Home)	240	9.0	48.0	1.5	0	500	1.0
(*Sara Lee*)	210	8.0	43.0	.5	0	500	20
blueberry (*Sara Lee*)	210	8.0	41.0	1.0	0	570	2.0
cinnamon raisin:							
(*Amy's*)	240	8.0	52.0	1.5	0	480	3.0
(*Lender's*)	160	5.0	32.0	1.0	0	240	1.0
(*Lender's* Bake at							
Home)	230	7.0	48.0	1.5	0	430	2.0
(*Lender's* Big'N							
Crusty)	230	7.0	47.0	2.0	0	350	2.0
(*Sara Lee*)	220	8.0	45.0.	1.0	0	320	3.0
cinnamon swirl							
(*Lender's*)	150	5.0	32.0	.5	0	270	1.0
egg:							
(*Lender's*)	160	6.0	30.0	1.5	10	320	1.0
(*Lender's* Big'N							
Crusty)	230	8.0	47.0	1.5	25	460	1.0

Food and Measure	cal.	prot. (gms)	carbo. (gms)	fat (gms)	chol. (mgs)	sod. (mgs)	fiber (gms)
Bagel, frozen, egg *(cont.)*							
(*Sara Lee*)	210	7.0	44.0	.5	0	460	2.0
oat bran (*Sara Lee*) . . .	210	8.0	42.0	1.0	0	570	3.0
onion:							
(*Lender's*)	160	5.0	40.0	1.5	0	300	2.0
(*Lender's* Bake at							
Home)	230	8.0	48.0	1.5	0	560	1.0
(*Sara Lee*)	210	7.0	44.0	0	0	540	2.0
poppyseed:							
(*Amy's*)	230	8.0	48.0	2.0	0	480	2.0
(*Lender's*)	160	5.0	32.0	1.0	0	240	1.0
(*Sara Lee*)	210	8.0	41.0	1.0	0	570	2.0
sesame:							
(*Amy's*)	240	8.0	48.0	2.0	0	480	2.0
(*Sara Lee*)	210	8.0	420	1.5	0	530	2.0
Bagel chips:							
cheese, three (*Pepper-*							
idge Farm), 1 oz.	140	4.0	16.0	7.0	5	240	<1.0
garlic (*Christie New*							
York Style), 1¼ oz.	180	4.0	20.0	9.0	0	275	n.a.
onion and garlic,							
toasted (*Pepperidge*							
Farm), 1 oz.	110	3.0	18.0	4.5	0	280	2.0
onion multigrain (*Pep-*							
peridge Farm), 1 oz.	120	3.0	19.0	3.5	0	200	1.0
Bagel sandwich, see							
specific listings							
Bagel spread mix,							
dry, 1 tsp., except as							
noted:							
apple-cinnamon (*Wat-*							
kins)	20	0	5.0	0	0	0	0
garden vegetable							
(*Watkins*)	10	0	2.0	0	0	120	0
onion-dill (*Watkins*)	10	0	3.0	0	0	300	0
strawberry cream							
(*Watkins*), 1½ tsp.	25	0	7.0	0	0	0	0
Baked beans, canned,							
½ cup:							
(*Allens*)	150	6.0	29.0	1.0	0	350	8.0

Food and Measure	cal.	prot. (gms)	carbo. (gms)	fat (gms)	chol. (mgs)	sod. (mgs)	fiber (gms)
(*Bush's Best* Bold & Spicy)	120	6.0	24.0	1.0	0	560	5.0
(*Bush's Best* Boston Recipe)	170	6.0	32.0	1.5	0	440	6.0
(*Bush's Best* Original)	150	7.0	29.0	1.0	0	550	7.0
(*Campbell's* New England Style/Old Fashioned)	180	5.0	32.0	3.0	5	460	6.0
(*Eden* Organic)	150	8.0	27.0	0	0	130	7.0
(*Friend's* Original) . . .	170	8.0	32.0	1.0	<5	390	7.0
(*Grandma Brown's* Home Baked)	160	8.0	28.0	1.5	0	340	8.0
(*Open Range* Ranch)	125	6.0	23.0	3.0	<5	630	8.0
(*Van Camp's* Fat Free)	140	6.0	32.0	0	0	525	3.0
(*Van Camp's* Original)	145	6.0	32.0	1.0	0	560	6.0
w/bacon:							
(*Grandma Brown's*)	150	7.0	26.0	2.5	0	300	7.0
and onion (*B&M*)	190	8.0	12.0	2.0	<5	450	8.0
sweet hickory (*Van Camp's*)	140	6.0	32.0	1.0	0	470	6.0
w/bacon–brown sugar:							
(*Bush's Best* Homestyle)	150	6.0	28.0	1.5	5	480	8.0
flavor (*Campbell's*)	170	5.0	29.0	3.0	5	490	7.0
barbecue (*B&M*)	170	7.0	33.0	2.0	0	460	6.0
chili, see "Chili beans"							
honey:							
(*B&M*)	170	8.0	30.0	2.0	0	450	8.0
(*Health Valley*)	110	7.0	25.0	0	0	135	7.0
w/onion:							
(*Bush's Best*)	150	7.0	26.0	1.5	0	500	6.0
(*Van Camp's* Southern Style)	145	6.0	35.0	1.0	<5	555	8.0
w/pork:							
(*B&M*)	180	8.0	33.0	2.0	<5	430	7.0
(*Crest Top*)	130	7.0	21.0	1.0	0	330	6.0
(*Green Giant/Joan of Arc*)	120	5.0	23.0	1.0	0	490	4.0
(*Hunt's*)	130	6.0	28.0	1.0	0	515	4.0
(*Hunt's* Homestyle)	160	6.0	27.0	5.0	<5	620	7.0

Food and Measure	cal.	prot. (gms)	carbo. (gms)	fat (gms)	chol. (mgs)	sod. (mgs)	fiber (gms)
Baked beans, w/pork *(cont.)*							
(*Showboat*)	120	6.0	22.0	1.5	5	550	6.0
(*Trappey's/Wagon Master*)	110	5.0	21.0	1.0	0	710	7.0
(*Van Camp's* Bold & Spicy)	115	7.0	23.0	1.0	0	430	6.0
(*Van Camp's* Large)	100	6.0	22.0	1.5	0	425	5.0
(*Van Camp's* Small)	110	6.0	23.0	1.5	0	490	6.0
(*Van Camp's* Southwest)	125	6.0	27.0	<1.0	0	350	6.0
(*Wagon Master* 2 lb. 10 oz. can)	130	7.0	23.0	1.0	0	420	9.0
peas (*East Texas Fair* Peas 'n Pork)	110	6.0	19.0	1.5	0	540	5.0
smoked ham (*Van Camp's*)	135	n.a.	29.0	1.0	0	490	6.0
tomato sauce (*Campbell's*)	130	5.0	24.0	2.0	5	420	6.0
w/pork and jalapeños (*Trappey's*)	130	5.0	24.0	2.0	0	610	6.0
red kidney:							
(*B&M*)	170	7.0	32.0	3.0	<5	440	6.0
(*Friend's*)	170	7.0	32.0	1.0	<5	510	6.0
vegetarian:							
(*B&M*)	170	8.0	31.0	1.0	0	220	7.0
(*Bush's Best*)	130	6.0	24.0	0	0	550	6.0
(*Heinz*)	140	6.0	27.0	.5	0	480	5.0
(*Van Camp's*)	110	6.0	23.0	.5	0	400	5.0
yellow-eye (*B&M*) . . .	180	8.0	30.0	3.0	<5	450	8.0
Baking mix (see also "Biscuit mix"), all-purpose:							
(*Arrowhead Mills*), ¼ cup	140	5.0	30.0	.5	0	320	2.0
(*Bisquick*), ⅓ cup	160	3.0	30.0	5.0	0	490	<1.0
(*Bisquick* Reduced Fat), ⅓ cup	150	3.0	27.0	3.0	0	500	<1.0
sweet (*Bisquick*), ¼ cup	170	1.0	31.0	4.0	0	260	0
wheat free (*Arrowhead Mills*), ¼ cup	120	2.0	27.0	.5	0	300	1.0

Food and Measure	cal.	prot. (gms)	carbo. (gms)	fat (gms)	chol. (mgs)	sod. (mgs)	fiber (gms)
Baking powder:							
(*Calumet*), ¼ tsp. . . .	0	0	0	0	0	100	0
(*Magic*), 1 tbsp.	20	0	5.0	0	0	1000	0
(*Watkins*), ¼ tsp. . . .	0	0	0	0	0	150	0
Baking soda (*Tone's*),							
1 tsp.	0	0	0	0	0	821	0
Baklava, 1.3-oz. pc.:							
wheat (*Cedar's*)	190	3.0	20.0	11.0	0	45	<1.0
white (*Cedar's*)	210	3.0	18.0	14.0	0	45	1.0
Balsam pear, ½ cup,							
except as noted:							
(*Frieda's* Bittermelon),							
1 cup, 3 oz.	15	1.0	3.0	0	0	0	2.0
leafy tips:							
raw	7	1.3	.8	.2	0	3	.6
boiled, drained	10	1.0	2.0	.1	0	4	.6
pods, ½" pcs.:							
raw	8	.5	1.7	.1	0	3	1.3
boiled, drained	12	.5	2.7	.1	0	4	1.2
Bamboo shoots,							
fresh, ½ cup:							
raw, slices	21	2.0	4.0	.2	0	3	.7
boiled, drained,							
½" slices	8	.9	1.2	.1	0	3	<1.0
canned:							
(*Chun King/La*							
Choy), 2 tbsp. . . .	5	0	1.0	0	0	0	<1.0
drained, ½ cup	13	1.1	2.1	.3	0	5	2.0
Banana, fresh:							
(*Frieda's* Burro/Nino/							
Manzano/Red),							
5 oz.	130	1.0	33.0	.5	0	0	2.0
common:							
whole, 1 lb.	271	3.1	69.1	1.4	0	3	7.1
8¾" banana	105	1.2	26.7	.6	0	1	2.7
mashed, ½ cup	104	1.2	26.4	.5	0	1	2.7
red, 7¼" long	118	1.6	30.7	.3	0	1	n.a.
Banana, baking, see							
"Plantain"							
Banana, dried:							
(*Frieda's*), 1 pc.	130	1.0	33.0	.5	0	0	2.0

Food and Measure	cal.	prot. (gms)	carbo. (gms)	fat (gms)	chol. (mgs)	sod. (mgs)	fiber (gms)
Banana, dried *(cont.)*							
dehydrated, 1/4 cup . . .	87	1.0	22.1	.5	0	1	1.9
Banana drink (*After the Fall Casablanca*),							
8 fl. oz.	100	1.0	19.0	0	0	10	0
Banana nectar,							
(*Kern's*), 11.5 fl. oz.	190	0	47.0	0	0	35	0
Banana squash, raw (*Frieda's*),							
3/4 cup, 3 oz.	30	1.0	7.0	0	0	0	1.0
Banana-pineapple nectar (*Kern's*),							
11.5 fl. oz.	220	<1.0	52.0	0	0	5	0
Barbecue beans, see "Baked beans"							
Barbecue glaze, Polynesian (*Trader Vic's*), 2 tbsp.	45	1.0	10.0	0	0	1080	0
Barbecue pocket, frozen (*Hot Pockets*),							
4.5 oz.	330	13.0	45.0	11.0	25	790	1.0
Barbecue sauce, 2 tbsp.:							
(*Heinz* Hearty Original)	35	0	9.0	0	0	510	0
(*Heinz* Old Fashioned)	40	0	10.0	0	0	440	0
(*Hunt's* Original)	40	.5	10.0	0	0	365	<1.0
(*Hunt's* Original Bold)	45	0	11.0	0	0	315	<1.0
(*KC Masterpiece* Bold)	60	<1.0	12.0	0	0	240	0
(*KC Masterpiece* Original)	60	0	13.0	0	0	210	0
(*KC Masterpiece* Original No Salt)	60	0	13.0	0	0	40	0
(*Kraft* Char-Grill)	60	0	12.0	1.0	0	440	0
(*Kraft* Extra Rich Original)	50	0	12.0	0	0	360	0
(*Kraft* Original)	40	0	10.0	0	0	460	0
(*Kraft Thick'N Spicy* Original)	50	0	12.0	0	0	440	0
(*Open Range*)	40	<1.0	9.0	0	0	330	1.0
(*Open Range* Premier)	55	1.0	13.0	0	0	415	1.0
(*Sylvia's* Original)	40	0	9.0	0	0	290	1.0

Food and Measure	cal.	prot. (gms)	carbo. (gms)	fat (gms)	chol. (mgs)	sod. (mgs)	fiber (gms)
all varieties (*Stubb's*)	25	0	6.0	0	0	220	0
Dijon (*Hunt's*)	40	.5	9.0	0	0	400	0
garlic (*Kraft*)	40	0	9.0	0	0	420	0
hickory:							
(*Hunt's*)	50	.5	12.0	0	0	380	<1.0
(*KC Masterpiece*)	60	0	13.0	0	0	220	0
(*Kraft*)	40	0	10.0	0	0	440	0
(*Kraft Thick'N Spicy*)	50	0	12.0	0	0	440	0
and brown sugar							
(*Hunt's*)	75	.5	18.0	0	0	380	1.0
hot (*Kraft*)	40	0	9.0	0	0	360	0
w/onion bits (*Kraft*)	50	0	11.0	0	0	340	<1.0
honey:							
(*Kraft*)	50	0	13.0	0	0	320	0
(*Kraft Thick'N Spicy*)	60	0	13.0	0	0	350	0
Dijon (*KC Master-*							
piece)	50	0	10.0	1.0	0	570	0
hickory (*Hunt's*) . . .	55	1.0	12.5	0	0	410	<1.0
mustard (*Hunt's*) . . .	50	0	11.5	0	0	450	<1.0
teriyaki (*KC Master-*							
piece)	60	<1.0	13.0	1.0	0	720	0
hot:							
(*Kraft*)	40	0	9.0	0	0	540	0
and spicy (*Hunt's*)	50	0	11.5	0	0	450	<1.0
Italian seasonings							
(*Kraft*)	45	0	10.0	.5	0	280	0
Jamaican (*Helen's*							
Tropical Exotics) . . .	60	1.0	12.0	1.5	0	610	1.0
Kansas City style:							
(*Kraft*)	45	0	11.0	0	0	280	<1.0
(*Kraft Thick'N Spicy*)	60	0	13.0	0	0	280	<1.0
mesquite:							
(*Hunt's*)	40	.5	9.0	0	0	360	<1.0
(*KC Masterpiece*)	60	0	13.0	0	0	210	0
(*Kraft*)	40	0	9.0	0	0	410	0
(*Kraft Thick'N Spicy*)	50	0	12.0	0	0	440	0
onion bits (*Kraft*)	50	0	11.0	0	0	340	0
Oriental glaze (*World*							
Harbors Cheriyaki)	50	0	14.0	0	0	390	0
Polynesian (*Trader*							
Vic's)	30	0	3.0	2.0	0	400	0

Food and Measure	cal.	prot. (gms)	carbo. (gms)	fat (gms)	chol. (mgs)	sod. (mgs)	fiber (gms)
Barbecue sauce *(cont.)*							
salsa style (*Kraft*)	40	0	9.0	0	0	420	0
smoky (*Open Range*)	40	<1.0	9.0	0	0	335	1.0
spicy (*KC Master-*							
piece)	60	0	13.0	0	0	210	0
teriyaki (*Kraft*)	60	<1.0	12.0	1.0	0	430	0
tropical (*World*							
Harbors Maui							
Mountain)	50	0	11.0	0	0	270	0
Barbecue sauce con-							
centrate, 2 tsp., ex-							
cept as noted:							
(*Watkins* Original) . . .	25	0	5.0	1.0	0	300	0
Caribbean (*Watkins*)	30	0	5.0	1.0	0	200	0
honey (*Watkins*)	25	0	5.0	1.0	0	290	0
mesquite (*Watkins*)	25	0	5.0	1.0	0	300	0
Oriental (*House of*							
Tsang Hong Kong),							
1 tsp.	10	0	2.0	0	0	150	0
Barley, pearled:							
dry:							
(*Arrowhead Mills*),							
¼ cup	170	5.0	37.0	.5	0	0	6.0
(*Quaker* Scotch							
Quick), ⅓ cup . . .	170	5.0	37.0	1.0	0	0	5.0
(*Quaker* Scotch							
Regular), ¼ cup	170	5.0	37.0	1.0	0	0	5.0
1 cup	704	19.8	155.5	2.3	0	18	31.2
cooked, 1 cup	193	3.6	44.3	.7	0	5	6.0
Barley flakes (*Arrow-*							
head Mills), ⅓ cup	110	4.0	28.0	1.0	0	0	5.0
Barley flour (*Arrow-*							
head Mills), ¼ cup	93	3.0	19.0	.5	0	0	3.0
Barley malt syrup							
(*Eden* Organic),							
1 tbsp.	60	1.0	14.0	0	0	0	0
Basil:							
fresh:							
1 oz.	8	.7	1.2	.2	0	0	n.a.
5 medium leaves . . .	1	.1	.1	<.1	0	0	n.a.
chopped, 2 tbsp.	1	.1	.2	<.1	0	0	n.a.

Food and Measure	cal.	prot. (gms)	carbo. (gms)	fat (gms)	chol. (mgs)	sod. (mgs)	fiber (gms)
dried:							
ground, 1 tbsp.	11	.7	2.7	.2	0	2	.5
ground, 1 tsp.	4	.2	.9	.1	0	<1	.2
Basil oil, see "Oil"							
Baskin-Robbins,							
½ cup, except as noted:							
ice cream:							
banana strawberry	130	2.0	17.0	7.0	25	40	0
Baseball nut	160	2.0	18.0	9.0	30	55	0
black walnut	160	3.0	13.0	11.0	30	45	1.0
blackberry, Oregon	140	2.0	16.0	8.0	30	50	0
blueberry cheese-cake	150	2.0	18.0	8.0	35	70	0
butter pecan, old fashioned	160	2.0	13.0	11.0	35	50	0
cherries jubilee	140	2.0	16.0	7.0	30	40	0
chocolate	150	2.0	18.0	9.0	30	60	0
chocolate, winter white	150	2.0	18.0	9.0	25	50	0
chocolate, world class	160	2.0	18.0	9.0	30	55	0
chocolate almond	180	3.0	17.0	11.0	30	55	1.0
chocolate cake, German...........	180	3.0	20.0	10.0	25	75	0
chocolate chip	150	2.0	15.0	10.0	35	45	0
chocolate chip cookie dough ...	170	2.0	20.0	9.0	35	70	0
chocolate fudge ...	160	2.0	21.0	9.0	30	80	0
chocolate mousse royale	170	2.0	20.0	10.0	25	60	1.0
chocolate passion, triple	180	3.0	21.0	11.0	35	70	0
chocolate raspberry truffle	180	3.0	23.0	9.0	30	60	0
cookies and cream	170	2.0	16.0	11.0	30	80	0
egg nog	150	2.0	16.0	8.0	40	45	0
English toffee	160	2.0	19.0	9.0	30	70	0
espresso and cream, low fat ...	100	3.0	18.0	2.5	5	60	1.0

Food and Measure	cal.	prot. (gms)	carbo. (gms)	fat (gms)	chol. (mgs)	sod. (mgs)	fiber (gms)
Baskin-Robbins, ice cream *(cont.)*							
Everybody's Favorite							
Candy Bar	170	2.0	20.0	9.0	30	90	0
fudge brownie	170	3.0	19.0	11.0	25	75	1.0
gold medal ribbon	150	2.0	20.0	8.0	30	95	0
Heath bar, chunky	170	2.0	19.0	10.0	30	70	0
Jamoca	140	2.0	14.0	9.0	35	45	0
Jamoca almond							
fudge	160	3.0	17.0	9.0	25	40	0
lemon custard	150	2.0	16.0	8.0	45	55	0
mint chocolate chip	150	3.0	15.0	10.0	35	45	0
Mississippi Mud . . .	160	2.0	22.0	8.0	25	85	0
peanut butter,							
Reese's	180	3.0	17.0	11.0	30	70	0
peanut butter and							
chocolate	180	3.0	16.0	12.0	30	95	1.0
pistachio-almond	170	3.0	13.0	12.0	30	45	1.0
pralines 'n cream	160	2.0	19.0	9.0	30	85	0
pumpkin pie	130	2.0	16.0	7.0	30	50	0
Quarterback Crunch	160	2.0	18.0	10.0	30	75	0
rocky road	170	3.0	19.0	10.0	30	60	0
rum raisin	140	2.0	18.0	7.0	30	40	0
strawberry, very							
berry	130	1.0	16.0	7.0	25	40	0
strawberry short-							
cake	160	2.0	18.0	9.0	30	70	0
vanilla	140	3.0	14.0	8.0	40	40	0
vanilla, French	160	2.0	14.0	10.0	70	45	0
ice cream, nonfat:							
berry innocent							
cheese	110	3.0	24.0	0	0	100	0
Check-It-Out Cherry	100	3.0	22.0	0	0	90	0
chocolate van twist	100	4.0	21.0	0	0	100	0
Jamoca swirl	110	3.0	23.0	0	5	105	0
ice cream, no sugar:							
call me nuts	110	3.0	21.0	2.0	5	55	1.0
cherry cordial	100	3.0	18.0	2.0	5	55	0
mad about choco-							
late	100	3.0	19.0	2.0	5	40	0
pineapple coconut	90	3.0	16.0	1.5	5	60	0
thin mint	100	3.0	16.0	2.5	5	65	0

Food and Measure	cal.	prot. (gms)	carbo. (gms)	fat (gms)	chol. (mgs)	sod. (mgs)	fiber (gms)
ices:							
daiquiri	110	0	28.0	0	0	10	0
The Mask	120	0	29.0	0	0	10	0
neon sour apple . . .	110	0	27.0	0	0	10	0
watermelon	110	0	28.0	0	0	10	0
sherbet:							
orange or rainbow	120	1.0	26.0	1.5	5	25	0
raspberry, blue	120	1.0	25.0	1.5	5	30	0
tangerine pineapple	120	1.0	22.0	1.0	5	25	0
sorbet:							
Black Tie Bubbly . . .	120	0	31.0	0	0	15	0
lemonade, mixed							
berry	110	0	28.0	0	0	10	0
pink raspberry							
lemon	120	0	27.0	0	0	10	0
BR Blast, 8 fl. oz.:							
cappuccino, nonfat	90	3.0	20.0	0	0	60	0
cappuccino,							
w/whipped cream	160	3.0	22.0	7.0	30	60	0
chocolate, nonfat	170	4.0	40.0	0	0	105	0
chocolate,							
w/whipped cream	250	4.0	46.0	7.0	25	120	0
mocha cappuccino,							
nonfat	120	3.0	26.0	0	0	75	0
mocha cappuccino,							
w/whipped cream	180	3.0	28.0	6.0	25	70	0
Yogurt Gone Crazy:							
Maui Brownie Mad-							
ness	140	4.0	26.0	3.0	5	80	1.0
Perils of Praline . . .	140	4.0	25.0	3.0	5	105	0
raspberry cheese							
Louise	130	4.0	24.0	3.0	10	90	0
yogurt smoothie, hard							
scoop, 8 fl. oz.:							
aloha berry banana	210	4.0	46.0	0	0	85	1.0
bora berry bora	190	4.0	44.0	0	0	75	2.0
calypso berry	160	3.0	35.0	0	0	75	2.0
copa banana	170	4.0	38.0	0	0	70	1.0
sunset orange	170	4.0	38.0	0	0	75	2.0
tropical tango	190	4.0	43.0	0	0	70	1.0

Food and Measure	cal.	prot. (gms)	carbo. (gms)	fat (gms)	chol. (mgs)	sod. (mgs)	fiber (gms)
Baskin-Robbins *(cont.)*							
yogurt smoothie, soft serve, 8 fl. oz.:							
aloha berry banana	180	4.0	40.0	0	5	80	1.0
bora berry bora	170	4.0	38.0	0	5	75	2.0
calypso berry	160	3.0	35.0	0	5	75	2.0
copa banana	140	4.0	30.0	0	5	65	1.0
sunset orange	150	4.0	32.0	0	5	70	2.0
tropical tango	160	3.0	36.0	0	5	65	1.0
Bass, meat only:							
freshwater, 4 oz.:							
raw	129	21.4	0	4.2	77	79	0
baked, broiled, or microwaved	166	27.4	0	5.4	99	102	0
sea, see "Sea bass"							
striped, 4 oz.:							
raw	110	20.1	0	2.7	91	78	0
baked, broiled, or microwaved	141	25.8	0	3.4	117	100	0
Bay leaf, dried: crumbled, 1 tsp.	5	.1	.3	.1	0	<1	<1.0
Bean dip, 2 tbsp.:							
(*Chi-Chi's* Fiesta)	35	1.0	4.0	1.5	0	140	1.0
(*Fritos*)	40	2.0	6.0	1.0	0	140	0
(*Fritos* Hot)	40	2.0	5.0	1.0	0	170	1.0
black bean:							
(*Old El Paso*)	25	1.0	5.0	0	0	280	1.0
(*Vita*)	33	1.0	4.0	1.0	0	93	1.0
spicy (*Valley of Mexico*)	52	4.0	9.0	0	0	90	n.a.
Bean dishes, see specific bean listings							
Bean loaf, frozen (*Natural Touch*), 1" slice	160	8.0	13.0	8.0	<5	350	5.0
Bean salad, three-bean, in jars, ½ cup:							
(*Green Giant*)	90	3.0	20.0	0	0	490	4.0
(*Seneca*)	60	1.0	13.0	0	0	140	2.0

Food and Measure	cal.	prot. (gms)	carbo. (gms)	fat (gms)	chol. (mgs)	sod. (mgs)	fiber (gms)
Bean sauce, spicy brown (*House of Tsang*), 1 tsp.	15	0	3.0	0	0	130	0
Bean sprouts, see "Sprouts" and specific listings							
Beans, see specific listings							
Beans, baked, see "Baked beans"							
Beans, mixed, canned, pinto/great northern (*Bush's Best*), ½ cup	110	7.0	19.0	0	0	500	6.0
Beans, mixed, mix (*Marrakesh Express* Terrazza Napoli), ⅓ cup dry	200	9.0	41.0	1.0	<5	460	2.0
Beans, snap or string, see "Green bean"							
Beans and franks, 1 cup:							
(*Kid's Kitchen* Wieners)	310	13.0	37.0	13.0	45	760	8.0
(*Nalley Chili Dog Chili*)	300	20.0	27.0	12.0	20	1050	8.0
(*Van Camp's Beanee Weenee* Baked)	350	16.0	49.0	12.0	35	1210	8.0
(*Van Camp's Beanee Weenee* Micro)	260	14.0	29.0	11.0	35	1020	6.0
(*Van Camp's Beanee Weenee* Small)	360	19.0	50.0	16.0	50	1420	9.0
(*Van Camp's Beanee Weenee* Chilee)	240	14.0	27.0	12.0	35	1090	9.0
(*Van Camp's Beanee Weenee* Zestee) . . .	300	14.0	40.0	12.0	35	1030	7.0
barbecue (*Van Camp's Beanee Weenee*) . . .	290	14.0	36.0	12.0	35	970	7.0
Beans and rice, see "Rice dishes, mix"							
Béarnaise sauce mix (*Knorr* Classic Sauces), 1 tsp.	10	0	2.0	0	0	110	0

Food and Measure	cal.	prot. (gms)	carbo. (gms)	fat (gms)	chol. (mgs)	sod. (mgs)	fiber (gms)
Beechnuts, dried,							
shelled, 1 oz.	164	1.8	9.5	14.2	0	n.a.	n.a.
Beef, choice grade,							
meat only[1], 4 oz.:							
brisket, whole:							
braised, lean w/fat	437	26.6	0	35.8	107	69	0
braised, lean only	274	33.7	0	14.5	105	79	0
chuck, arm pot roast:							
braised, lean w/fat	395	30.6	0	29.2	112	67	0
braised, lean only	255	37.4	0	10.5	115	75	0
chuck, blade roast:							
braised, lean w/fat	412	29.7	0	31.5	117	73	0
braised, lean only	298	35.2	0	16.3	120	81	0
flank steak[2]:							
braised, lean only	269	31.8	0	14.7	81	82	0
broiled, lean only	256	30.0	0	14.2	77	92	0
ground, raw:							
extra lean	265	21.1	0	19.3	78	75	0
lean	298	20.0	0	23.4	85	78	0
regular	351	18.8	0	30.0	96	77	0
ground, broiled, me-							
dium:							
extra lean	290	28.8	0	18.5	95	79	0
lean	308	28.0	0	20.9	99	87	0
regular	328	27.3	0	23.5	102	94	0
porterhouse steak:							
broiled, lean w/fat	346	28.2	0	25.1	94	69	0
broiled, lean only	247	31.9	0	12.2	91	75	0
rib, whole:							
roasted, lean w/fat	426	25.1	0	35.4	96	71	0
roasted, lean only	276	30.9	0	15.9	91	82	0
rib, large end (ribs 6–9):							
roasted, lean w/fat	434	25.3	0	36.2	96	71	0
roasted, lean only	284	31.2	0	16.7	92	83	0
rib, small end (ribs 10–12):							
broiled, lean w/fat	376	26.7	0	31.3	95	70	0
broiled, lean only	264	31.8	0	14.3	91	78	0

[1] *Retail cuts trimmed to ¼" fat, except as noted.*
[2] *Trimmed to 0" fat.*

Food and Measure	cal.	prot. (gms)	carbo. (gms)	fat (gms)	chol. (mgs)	sod. (mgs)	fiber (gms)
round, bottom:							
braised, lean w/fat	322	32.5	0	20.3	109	57	0
braised, lean only	249	35.8	0	10.7	109	58	0
round, eye of:							
roasted, lean w/fat	273	30.2	0	16.0	82	67	0
roasted, lean only	198	32.9	0	6.5	78	70	0
round, full cut:							
broiled, lean w/fat	272	31.0	0	15.4	91	69	0
broiled, lean only	217	33.1	0	8.3	88	73	0
round, tip:							
roasted, lean w/fat	280	30.1	0	16.9	94	70	0
roasted, lean only	213	32.6	0	8.3	92	74	0
round, top:							
broiled, lean w/fat	254	34.2	0	12.0	96	68	0
broiled, lean only	214	35.9	0	6.7	95	69	0
fried, lean w/fat	314	36.7	0	17.4	110	77	0
fried, lean only	257	39.8	0	9.7	110	81	0
shank, crosscuts:							
braised, lean w/fat	298	34.8	0	16.6	91	69	0
braised, lean only	228	38.2	0	7.2	88	73	0
shortribs:							
braised, lean w/fat	534	24.5	0	47.6	107	57	0
braised, lean only	335	34.9	0	20.6	105	66	0
sirloin, top:							
broiled, lean w/fat	305	31.3	0	19.0	102	70	0
broiled, lean only	229	34.4	0	9.1	101	75	0
fried, lean w/fat	370	31.9	0	25.9	111	79	0
fried, lean only	270	36.8	0	12.4	112	87	0
T-bone steak:							
broiled, lean w/fat	338	28.3	0	24.0	94	69	0
broiled, lean only	243	31.9	0	11.8	91	75	0
tenderloin:							
broiled, lean w/fat	345	28.4	0	24.8	98	67	0
broiled, lean only	252	32.0	0	12.7	95	71	0
top loin:							
broiled, lean w/fat	338	28.8	0	23.8	90	71	0
broiled, lean only	243	32.5	0	11.5	86	77	0
Beef, canned, see "Beef entree, canned or packaged" and specific listings							

Food and Measure	cal.	prot. (gms)	carbo. (gms)	fat (gms)	chol. (mgs)	sod. (mgs)	fiber (gms)
Beef, corned (see also "Beef lunch meat"):							
(*Mosey's*), 4 oz.	200	14.0	1.0	15.0	55	1180	0
(*Nathan's*), 4 oz.	160	14.0	1.0	11.0	60	1310	0
brisket, cooked, 4 oz.	285	20.6	.5	21.5	111	1286	0
canned, 2 oz.:							
(*Delta*)	120	13.0	0	8.0	50	500	0
(*Hormel*)	120	15.0	0	7.0	50	490	0
(*Libby's*)	120	15.0	0	7.0	50	490	0
hash, see "Beef hash"							
Beef, dried:							
(*Hormel*), 10 slices, 1 oz.	45	8.0	0	1.0	20	1010	0
canned (*Hormel*), 10 slices, 1 oz.	50	8.0	1.0	1.5	25	1190	0
cured, 1 oz.	47	8.3	.4	1.1	n.a.	984	0
freeze-dried, diced (*AlpineAire*), ½ oz. ...	60	11.0	0	2.0	35	180	0
Beef, refrigerated:							
back ribs (*Lloyd's*), 2 ribs w/sauce, 5 oz.	360	21.0	15.0	25.0	70	940	1.0
teriyaki (*Mosey's Time for Dinner*), 5 oz.	200	29.0	5.0	7.0	75	520	0
"Beef," vegetarian:							
canned:							
(*Worthington* Savory Slices), 3 slices	150	10.0	6.0	9.0	0	540	3.0
(*Worthington* Vegetable Steaks), 2 pcs.	80	15.0	3.0	1.5	0	300	3.0
(*Worthington Prime Stakes*), 1 pc. ...	120	10.0	4.0	7.0	0	440	4.0
stew (*Worthington* Country), 1 cup	210	13.0	20.0	9.0	0	830	5.0
frozen:							
(*Worthington* Meatless), ⅜" slice ...	110	9.0	4.0	7.0	0	620	3.0

Food and Measure	cal.	prot. (gms)	carbo. (gms)	fat (gms)	chol. (mgs)	sod. (mgs)	fiber (gms)
corned (*Worthington* Slices), 4 slices	140	10.0	5.0	9.0	0	520	2.0
smoked (*Worthington*), 6 slices	120	11.0	6.0	6.0	0	730	3.0
"hamburger," see "Burger, vegetarian"							
Beef dinner, frozen, 1 pkg.:							
broccoli:							
(*Swanson*), 10 oz.	350	11.0	53.0	10.0	30	830	4.0
Beijing (*Healthy Choice*), 12 oz.	300	21.0	45.0	4.5	25	420	6.0
mesquite w/barbecue sauce (*Healthy Choice*), 11 oz.	320	21.0	38.0	9.0	55	490	5.0
patty, charbroiled (*Healthy Choice*), 11 oz.	310	16.0	40.0	9.0	45	550	4.0
and peppers, Cantonese (*Healthy Choice*), 11½ oz.	270	22.0	32.0	6.0	55	480	5.0
pot roast, Yankee:							
(*Banquet Extra Helping*), 14½ oz.	410	25.0	33.0	20.0	50	1680	3.0
(*Healthy Choice*), 11 oz.	290	19.0	38.0	7.0	55	460	4.0
(*Swanson*), 11½ oz.	250	12.0	39.0	4.5	20	850	5.0
(*Swanson Hungry Man*), 16 oz.	350	25.0	48.0	6.0	45	1080	5.0
Salisbury steak:							
(*Banquet Extra Helping*), 16½ oz.	780	27.0	47.0	54.0	130	2200	7.0
(*Healthy Choice*), 11½ oz.	330	18.0	48.0	7.0	50	470	6.0
(*Swanson*), 11 oz.	360	16.0	35.0	16.0	30	920	6.0
(*Swanson Hungry Man*), 16¼ oz.	590	29.0	47.0	33.0	70	1450	7.0
sirloin steak, chopped (*Swanson*), 10½ oz.	380	19.0	37.0	14.0	40	730	5.0

Food and Measure	cal.	prot. (gms)	carbo. (gms)	fat (gms)	chol. (mgs)	sod. (mgs)	fiber (gms)
Beef dinner *(cont.)*							
sirloin tips (*Swanson Hungry Man*),							
15¾ oz.	440	25.0	49.0	16.0	55	960	6.0
steak, chicken-fried (*Banquet Extra Helping*), 16 oz.	820	29.0	63.0	50.0	60	2260	6.0
Stroganoff (*Healthy Choice*), 11 oz.	310	19.0	44.0	7.0	60	440	3.0
tips (*Healthy Choice*), 11¼ oz.	260	20.0	32.0	6.0	40	390	6.0
Beef entree, canned or packaged, 1 cup, except as noted:							
chow mein:							
(*Chun King* Bi-Pack)	105	9.0	15.0	2.0	10	750	3.0
(*La Choy* Bi-Pack)	85	10.0	9.0	1.5	10	830	2.5
fajita (*Nalley* Superba)	230	15.0	30.0	6.0	15	720	12.0
hash, see "Beef hash"							
pepper, Oriental:							
(*Chun King* Bi-Pack)	105	11.0	11.0	3.0	20	1060	3.0
(*La Choy* Bi-Pack) . . .	100	12.0	10.0	2.0	15	1025	2.0
pepper steak (*Chun King/La Choy* Skillet Dinner)	75	4.0	15.0	<1.0	0	1920	3.0
pot roast (*Dinty Moore American Classics*), 1 bowl	200	24.0	19.0	3.0	45	730	2.0
roast:							
w/gravy (*Hormel*), ½ cup	150	25.0	3.0	4.0	75	640	0
w/potatoes (*Dinty Moore American Classics*), 1 bowl	240	24.0	24.0	5.0	45	870	2.0
Salisbury steak (*Dinty Moore American Classics*), 1 bowl	300	22.0	24.0	13.0	60	1060	3.0
stew:							
(*Dinty Moore* Can)	180	10.0	18.0	8.0	30	920	2.0
(*Dinty Moore* Microwave Cup)	160	8.0	16.0	7.0	30	900	2.0

Food and Measure	cal.	prot. (gms)	carbo. (gms)	fat (gms)	chol. (mgs)	sod. (mgs)	fiber (gms)
(*Dinty Moore American Classics*),							
1 bowl	250	15.0	22.0	11.0	45	1170	2.0
(*Hormel* Microwave)	150	11.0	13.0	6.0	30	890	2.0
(*Hunt's*)	155	14.0	20.0	4.0	20	1140	5.0
(*Nalley* Homestyle)	210	17.0	18.0	8.0	35	990	2.0
(*Nalley Big Chunk*)	260	13.0	25.0	12.0	25	1140	4.0
burger (*Dinty Moore* Microwave Cup)	240	12.0	19.0	13.0	40	930	3.0
Beef entree, dried,							
1 serving:							
casserole, bean and							
(*AlpineAire*)	280	23.0	31.0	7.0	35	770	11.0
pilaf (*AlpineAire*)	320	19.0	55.0	3.0	40	660	3.0
rotini (*AlpineAire*)	330	21.0	53.0	4.0	40	510	2.0
stew with, hearty							
(*Mountain House*)	150	10.0	24.0	2.0	20	920	3.0
Stroganoff w/noodles:							
(*AlpineAire*)	310	20.0	37.0	9.0	55	950	1.0
(*Mountain House*)	240	10.0	28.0	10.0	15	800	1.0
tamale pie (*AlpineAire* Western)	370	23.0	47.0	10.0	55	960	7.0
teriyaki w/rice (*Mountain House*)	250	12.0	42.0	4.0	15	850	2.0
and turkey, barbecue, w/beans (*AlpineAire*)	320	20.0	53.0	3.0	40	660	7.0
Beef entree, frozen							
(see also "Beef, refrigerated"), 1 pkg., except as noted:							
broccoli and							
(*Stouffer's Skillet Sensations*), ½ of 25-oz. pkg.	310	18.0	52.0	3.0	25	1350	3.0
cheddar:							
(*Stouffer's Skillet Sensations*), ½ of 25-oz. pkg.	600	26.0	58.0	29.0	55	1340	5.0
melt (*The Budget Gourmet*), 8½ oz.	310	16.0	29.0	16.0	35	600	2.0

Food and Measure	cal.	prot. (gms)	carbo. (gms)	fat (gms)	chol. (mgs)	sod. (mgs)	fiber (gms)
Beef entree, frozen *(cont.)*							
chipped, creamed:							
(*Freezer Queen* Cook-in-Pouch), 4 oz.	100	6.0	8.0	5.0	15	360	1.0
(*Stouffer's*), ½ cup	160	10.0	3.0	15.0	35	620	0
chunky, and tomatoes (*Stouffer's* Home-style), 10 oz.	280	16.0	33.0	9.0	45	1480	1.0
enchilada, see "Enchi-lada entree"							
fajita (*Lean Cuisine Skillet Sensations*), ½ of 24-oz. pkg.	300	19.0	48.0	3.5	25	760	6.0
home style (*Stouffer's Skillet Sensations*), ½ of 25-oz. pkg.	360	30.0	34.0	11.0	70	1090	4.0
macaroni, see "Maca-roni entree, frozen"							
w/mushroom gravy (*Banquet* Family), 1 patty w/gravy	230	11.0	6.0	18.0	30	700	11.0
w/noodles, gravy (*Banquet* Family), 1 cup	150	11.0	16.0	5.0	35	1120	2.0
w/onion gravy (*Ban-quet* Family), 1 patty w/gravy...........	180	8.0	7.0	14.0	20	630	2.0
Oriental:							
(*The Budget Gour-met* Low Fat), 8 oz.	210	9.0	31.0	6.0	15	870	2.0
(*Lean Cuisine Cafe Classics*), 9¼ oz.	240	17.0	35.0	3.5	30	590	2.0
pepper (*La Choy*), 1 cup..........	150	8.0	30.0	<1.0	10	715	2.0
patty:							
charbroiled, mush-room gravy and (*Freezer Queen* Family), 1 patty w/gravy	170	9.0	7.0	12.0	15	600	2.0

Food and Measure	cal.	prot. (gms)	carbo. (gms)	fat (gms)	chol. (mgs)	sod. (mgs)	fiber (gms)
charbroiled, w/potatoes, peas, carrots (*Freezer Queen*), 9½ oz.	230	16.0	17.0	11.0	20	1120	5.0
grilled peppercorn (*Healthy Choice*), 9 oz.	220	16.0	26.0	6.0	30	470	5.0
onion gravy and (*Freezer Queen Family*), 1 patty w/gravy	170	10.0	7.0	11.0	55	720	0
w/vegetables (*Banquet*), 9½ oz. . . .	310	11.0	22.0	20.0	40	1090	3.0
Western style (*Banquet*), 9½ oz. . . .	380	14.0	28.0	23.0	40	1400	5.0
pepper steak:							
(*Weight Watchers Main Street Bistro*), 10 oz.	240	17.0	32.0	5.0	20	690	4.0
green (*Stouffer's*), 10½ oz.	330	17.0	45.0	9.0	35	680	3.0
Oriental (*Healthy Choice*), 9½ oz.	250	19.0	34.0	4.0	35	470	3.0
w/rice (*The Budget Gourmet*), 8½ oz.	230	10.0	32.0	6.0	20	840	2.0
and peppers, w/rice (*Freezer Queen*), 8½ oz.	210	14.0	35.0	1.5	20	710	1.0
peppercorn (*Lean Cuisine Cafe Classics*), 8¾ oz.	220	15.0	23.0	7.0	35	580	2.0
pie/pot pie:							
(*Banquet*), 7 oz. . . .	400	9.0	38.0	23.0	30	1000	1.0
(*Stouffer's*), 10 oz.	440	18.0	36.0	25.0	55	1140	4.0
(*Swanson*), 7 oz.	420	13.0	42.0	22.0	25	730	2.0
(*Swanson Hungry Man*), 14 oz.	660	24.0	70.0	31.0	50	1590	6.0
Yankee (*Marie Callender's*), ½ of 16½-oz. pie	640	17.0	62.0	36.0	15	1450	4.0

Food and Measure	cal.	prot. (gms)	carbo. (gms)	fat (gms)	chol. (mgs)	sod. (mgs)	fiber (gms)
Beef entree, frozen, pie/pot pie (cont.)							
Yankee (*Marie Cal-* *lender's*), 9½ oz.	560	16.0	53.0	31.0	5	1430	3.0
portobello (*Lean Cuisine Cafe Classics*), 9 oz.	220	15.0	23.0	7.0	35	590	2.0
pot roast:							
(*Freezer Queen*), 9¼ oz.	140	9.0	20.0	2.5	15	560	5.0
(*Freezer Queen* Family), 1 cup	210	22.0	24.0	3.0	50	360	3.0
(*Lean Cuisine American Favorites*), 9 oz.	210	13.0	25.0	6.0	30	570	6.0
(*Marie Callender's*), 1 cup	260	17.0	31.0	7.0	45	790	3.0
(*Stouffer's Hearty Portions*), 16 oz.	370	23.0	44.0	11.0	45	1410	8.0
w/potato, carrots (*Freezer Queen Homestyle*), 9 oz.	160	15.0	19.0	3.0	40	470	4.0
and potatoes (*Stouffer's* Homestyle), 8⅞ oz. . . .	250	16.0	29.0	8.0	35	780	4.0
Yankee (*Banquet*), 9.4 oz.	230	14.0	20.0	10.0	60	1130	4.0
roasted:							
oven (*Lean Cuisine American Favorites*), 9¼ oz.	260	18.0	28.0	8.0	50	590	4.0
and potatoes (*Lean Cuisine Skillet Sensations*), ½ of 24-oz. pkg.	290	18.0	38.0	7.0	35	760	9.0
Salisbury steak:							
(*Banquet*), 9½ oz.	380	12.0	28.0	24.0	60	1140	4.0
(*Banquet* Family), 1 patty w/gravy	230	11.0	7.0	17.0	30	630	1.0
(*The Budget Gourmet* Low Fat), 8½ oz.	240	16.0	27.0	7.0	40	550	2.0

Food and Measure	cal.	prot. (gms)	carbo. (gms)	fat (gms)	chol. (mgs)	sod. (mgs)	fiber (gms)
(*Lean Cuisine American Favorites*), 9½ oz.	280	24.0	29.0	8.0	60	590	4.0
(*Lean Cuisine Hearty Portions*), 15½ oz.	340	28.0	40.0	7.0	50	850	10.0
(*Stouffer's* Homestyle), 9 oz.	380	26.0	28.0	18.0	60	1170	1.0
gravy and (*Freezer Queen* Cook-in-Pouch), 5 oz. . . .	150	8.0	8.0	10.0	20	680	2.0
gravy and (*Freezer Queen* Family), 1 patty w/gravy	160	9.0	6.0	11.0	20	810	3.0
gravy and, w/potatoes, corn (*Freezer Queen*), 9½ oz.	260	14.0	19.0	14.0	20	980	5.0
and gravy, w/whipped potatoes (*Freezer Queen*), 8½ oz.	300	18.0	26.0	14.0	30	840	5.0
grilled, and gravy (*Smart Ones*), 9½ oz.	290	22.0	29.0	8.0	50	770	4.0
and macaroni and cheese (*Stouffer's*), ⅙ of 68-oz. pkg.	420	23.0	37.0	20.0	55	1250	2.0
w/pasta shells (*Stouffer's Hearty Portions*), 16 oz.	570	41.0	47.0	24.0	100	1640	4.0
sirloin (*Marie Callender's*), 14 oz.	550	30.0	51.0	25.0	85	1680	6.0
sandwich, see "Beef sandwich"							
sirloin, roast (*The Budget Gourmet* Supreme), 8 oz.	270	12.0	34.0	10.0	40	740	3.0
sliced:							
(*Banquet*), 9 oz.	270	26.0	19.0	10.0	70	740	4.0

Food and Measure	cal.	prot. (gms)	carbo. (gms)	fat (gms)	chol. (mgs)	sod. (mgs)	fiber (gms)
Beef entree, frozen, sliced *(cont.)*							
barbecue sauce and (*Stouffer's* Home-style), 10 oz.	370	21.0	32.0	18.0	70	1230	7.0
gravy and (*Freezer Queen* Cook-in Pouch), 4 oz. . . .	60	9.0	5.0	1.0	20	400	<1.0
gravy and (*Freezer Queen* Deluxe Family), ²/₃ cup	80	11.0	6.0	1.5	35	690	0
gravy and, w/potatoes, carrots (*Freezer Queen*), 9 oz. . . .	140	14.0	17.0	2.0	25	840	3.0
w/gravy (*Banquet* Family), 2 slices w/gravy	100	13.0	7.0	3.0	40	850	<1.0
steak, chicken-fried:							
w/gravy (*Marie Callender's*), 15 oz.	650	23.0	69.0	31.0	50	2260	7.0
and mashed potato (*Marie Callender's* Family), 1 patty and ½ cup potato	600	20.0	48.0	36.0	75	1960	4.0
steak, country-fried (*Stouffer's Hearty Portions*), 16 oz.	560	22.0	61.0	25.0	50	1750	7.0
steak, Philly (*Healthy Choice* Hearty Handfuls), 6.1 oz.	290	16.0	47.0	5.0	25	550	5.0
stew, 1 cup:							
(*Banquet* Family)	160	14.0	17.0	4.0	25	1120	4.0
(*Freezer Queen* Family)	130	11.0	8.0	7.0	20	560	2.0
Stroganoff:							
(*The Budget Gourmet* Low Fat), 8 oz.	220	13.0	29.0	6.0	20	620	3.0
(*Lean Cuisine Hearty Portions*), 14¼ oz.	350	23.0	44.0	9.0	30	890	9.0

Food and Measure	cal.	prot. (gms)	carbo. (gms)	fat (gms)	chol. (mgs)	sod. (mgs)	fiber (gms)
(*Stouffer's*), 9¾ oz.	390	23.0	30.0	20.0	85	1100	2.0
w/noodles (*Marie Callender's*), 1 cup	600	30.0	59.0	27.0	70	1140	5.0
teriyaki (*Lean Cuisine Skillet Sensations*), ½ of 24-oz. pkg.	280	14.0	48.0	3.0	25	700	5.0
tips:							
Français (*Healthy Choice*), 9½ oz.	280	20.0	40.0	5.0	30	520	4.0
in mushroom sauce (*Marie Callender's*), 13.6 oz.	430	25.0	39.0	19.0	50	1620	6.0
Southern (*Lean Cuisine American Favorites*), 8¾ oz.	290	13.0	47.0	6.0	30	560	7.0
vegetables, and (*Lean Cuisine American Favorites*), 9 oz.	210	11.0	33.0	4.0	25	590	3.0
Beef gravy, ¼ cup:							
(*Franco-American*) . . .	30	1.0	4.0	2.0	<5	300	0
(*Franco-American* Fat Free)	20	0	5.0	0	<5	310	0
(*Franco-American* Slow Roasted)	25	1.0	4.0	.5	<5	330	0
(*Franco-American* Slow Roasted Fat Free)	20	1.0	4.0	0	<5	360	0
(*Heinz* Home Style Savory)	25	2.0	2.0	1.0	0	350	0
Beef hash, canned, 1 cup, except as noted:							
corned:							
(*Broadcast*), 7½ oz.	440	15.0	21.0	32.0	65	1220	7.0
(*Jones Dairy Farm*), 2 oz.	100	6.0	5.0	6.0	20	290	n.a.
(*Libby's*)	490	18.0	25.0	38.0	75	1510	8.0
(*Mary Kitchen*)	390	21.0	22.0	24.0	80	1000	2.0

Food and Measure	cal.	prot. (gms)	carbo. (gms)	fat (gms)	chol. (mgs)	sod. (mgs)	fiber (gms)
Beef hash, canned, corned *(cont.)*							
(*Mary Kitchen* 50% Less Fat)	280	19.0	25.0	12.0	65	1070	3.0
(*Nalley*)	490	22.0	26.0	34.0	65	1110	4.0
roast (*Mary Kitchen*)	390	21.0	22.0	24.0	70	790	2.0
Beef hash, dried (*AlpineAire* All American), 2 oz.	220	18.0	24.0	3.5	50	1120	0
Beef jerky, see "Sausage stick"							
Beef lunch meat (see also "Bologna," etc.), 2 oz., except as noted:							
cooked (*Boar's Head* Custom Cut No Salt)	90	14.0	0	3.5	35	40	0
corned:							
(*Black Bear*)	60	10.0	2.0	1.5	30	550	0
(*Boar's Head* Cap-Off Top Round)	80	14.0	0	2.5	30	360	0
(*Boar's Head* First Cut)	80	12.0	0	3.0	40	460	0
(*Boar's Head* Round)	80	12.0	0	3.0	30	510	0
(*Healthy Choice* Deli Zesty)	60	10.0	0	1.5	10	400	0
(*Healthy Choice* Hearty Deli Zesty), 4 slices, 1.8 oz.	60	10.0	1.0	2.0	25	450	0
(*Healthy Deli*)	80	11.0	2.0	3.0	30	480	0
pepper, eye round (*Boar's Head*)	90	14.0	0	3.0	40	130	0
roast:							
(*Hansel 'n Gretel*)	70	11.0	2.0	1.5	30	310	0
(*Healthy Deli*)	70	12.0	0	2.0	30	320	0
Cajun (*Boar's Head*)	80	14.0	0	2.5	35	200	0
Cajun (*Healthy Choice*)	60	11.0	1.0	1.0	25	360	0
chopped (*Healthy Choice*), 1-oz. slice	30	5.0	1.0	1.0	10	240	0

Food and Measure	cal.	prot. (gms)	carbo. (gms)	fat (gms)	chol. (mgs)	sod. (mgs)	fiber (gms)
chopped (*Healthy Choice* Deli-Thin), 6 slices, 1.9 oz.	60	10.0	1.0	1.5	20	470	0
Italian style (*Healthy Choice*)	60	11.0	1.0	1.0	20	360	0
Italian style (*Healthy Deli*)	70	11.0	1.0	1.5	30	320	0
medium (*Healthy Choice* Deli)	60	10.0	2.0	1.0	20	470	0
medium rare (*Healthy Choice*)	60	11.0	1.0	1.5	25	470	0
top round (*Boar's Head* No Salt) ...	90	14.0	0	3.0	30	40	0
top round:							
(*Boar's Head*)	90	14.0	0	3.0	30	80	0
(*Boar's Head* Cap-Off)	70	14.0	0	2.0	30	80	0
Beef pie, see "Beef entree, frozen"							
Beef pocket (see also "Beef sandwich"), frozen, 4½-oz. pc., except as noted:							
and cheddar (*Hot Pockets*)	350	15.0	36.0	16.0	45	610	3.0
cheese steak:							
(*Big Stuffs*), 5.4 oz.	440	18.0	48.0	19.0	60	900	1.0
(*Deli Stuffs*)	350	15.0	40.0	14.0	45	680	3.0
Philly steak w/cheese:							
(*Croissant Pockets*)	350	15.0	37.0	16.0	50	790	2.0
(*Lean Pockets*)	260	15.0	35.0	7.0	30	560	1.0
melt (*Hot Pockets Toaster Breaks*), 2.1 oz.	190	5.0	20.0	10.0	10	370	1.0
Beef sandwich, frozen, 1 pc., except as noted:							
barbecued (*Hormel Quick Meal*)	370	15.0	38.0	17.0	45	560	1.0
w/cheese (*Kid Cuisine* Buckaroo), 8½ oz.	410	12.0	58.0	15.0	30	600	4.0

Food and Measure	cal.	prot. (gms)	carbo. (gms)	fat (gms)	chol. (mgs)	sod. (mgs)	fiber (gms)
Beef sandwich *(cont.)*							
cheeseburger:							
(*Hormel Quick Meal*)	400	19.0	36.0	20.0	55	600	1.0
(*White Castle*),							
2 pcs.	310	15.0	23.0	17.0	30	480	6.0
bacon (*Hormel*							
Quick Meal)	420	22.0	34.0	22.0	65	800	1.0
hamburger:							
(*Hormel Quick Meal*)	350	17.0	34.0	16.0	45	400	1.0
(*White Castle*),							
2 pcs.	270	12.0	23.0	14.0	20	270	5.0
Beef sauce, see							
"Steak sauce" and							
specific listings							
Beef sausage, see							
"Sausage"							
Beef seasoning mix,							
see specific listings							
Beef spread:							
roast beef (*Under-*							
wood), ¼ cup, 2 oz.	140	9.0	0	11.0	45	390	0
Beef stew, see "Beef							
entree"							
Beef stew base, see							
"Soup base mix"							
Beef stew seasoning,							
see "Goulash sea-							
soning mix"							
Beefalo, meat only,							
roasted, 4 oz.	213	34.8	0	7.2	66	93	0
Beer, 12 fl. oz.:							
regular	146	.9	13.2	0	0	19	0
light	100	.7	4.8	0	0	10	0
Beet, fresh:							
raw:							
2 medium, 2″ diam.	70	2.6	15.6	.3	0	126	4.6
trimmed, sliced,							
½ cup	29	1.1	6.5	.1	0	53	1.9
boiled, drained:							
2 medium, 2″ diam.	44	1.7	10.0	.2	0	77	1.7
sliced, ½ cup	38	1.4	8.5	.2	0	65	1.4

Food and Measure	cal.	prot. (gms)	carbo. (gms)	fat (gms)	chol. (mgs)	sod. (mgs)	fiber (gms)
Beet, canned, ½ cup, except as noted:							
whole or sliced:							
(*Del Monte*)	35	1.0	8.0	0	0	290	2.0
(*Green Giant*)	35	1.0	8.0	0	0	260	2.0
(*Green Giant* No Salt)	35	1.0	8.0	0	0	60	2.0
(*Seneca*)	35	<1.0	7.0	0	0	240	2.0
(*Seneca* No Salt) . . .	40	<1.0	7.0	0	0	20	2.0
baby (*LeSueur*) . . .	35	1.0	8.0	0	0	260	2.0
w/liquid	36	1.0	8.3	.1	0	324	1.4
Harvard:							
(*Green Giant*)	60	<1.0	15.0	0	0	270	2.0
(*Greenwood* Sweet & Tangy)	100	1.0	27.0	0	0	370	1.0
(*Seneca*)	90	<1.0	21.0	0	0	180	2.0
w/liquid	89	1.0	22.4	.1	0	199	1.0
pickled:							
(*Seneca*), 1 oz.	15	0	45	0	0	45	0
whole or sliced (*Greenwood* Sweet & Tangy)	100	1.0	24.0	0	0	420	1.0
crinkle (*Del Monte*)	80	1.0	19.0	0	0	380	2.0
sliced, w/onions (*Greenwood* Sweet & Tangy)	100	1.0	24.0	0	0	420	1.0
Beet greens, ½ cup:							
raw, 1″ pcs.	4	.4	.8	<.1	0	38	.7
boiled, drained, 1″ pcs.	20	1.9	3.9	.1	0	173	2.1
Berliner, pork and beef, 1 oz.	65	4.3	.7	4.9	13	368	0
Berries, mixed, frozen (*Cascadian Farm Harvest Berries*), 1 cup	65	1.0	16.0	1.0	0	0	5.0
Berry drink blends, 8 fl. oz., except as noted:							
(*R.W. Knudsen* Razzleberry)	130	0	33.0	0	0	35	0

Food and Measure	cal.	prot. (gms)	carbo. (gms)	fat (gms)	chol. (mgs)	sod. (mgs)	fiber (gms)
Berry drink blends *(cont.)*							
(*R.W. Knudsen* Razzleberry Aseptic) . . .	110	1.0	29.0	0	0	25	0
(*Tropicana*)	130	0	32.0	0	0	15	0
(*V8 Splash*)	110	0	28.0	0	0	40	0
(*Whipper Snapple* Power Smoothie), 10 fl. oz.	160	0	40.0	0	0	60	0
nectar (*Santa Cruz* Organic)	110	0	27.0	0	0	25	0
Berry juice, 8 fl. oz.:							
(*After the Fall* Oregon)	100	0	25.0	0	0	25	0
(*Juicy Juice*)	130	1.0	31.0	0	0	15	0
(*Veryfine* Juice-Up)	140	0	34.0	0	0	15	0
Biryani paste (*Patak's*), 2 tbsp.	160	1.0	4.0	16.0	0	990	2.0
Biscuit, 1 pc.:							
(*Awrey's* Country), 2 oz.	140	3.0	21.0	5.0	0	490	<1.0
(*Awrey's* Round), 1 oz.	70	2.0	10.0	3.0	0	230	0
(*Awrey's* Round), 2 oz.	150	3.0	22.0	5.0	0	480	<1.0
(*Awrey's* Round Sliced), 3 oz.	230	5.0	35.0	8.0	0	720	1.0
Biscuit, refrigerated, 1 pc., except as noted:							
(*Big Country Butter Tastin'*)	100	2.0	13.0	4.0	0	360	0
(*Grands!* Extra Rich)	220	4.0	25.0	12.0	0	580	<1.0
(*Grands!* Homestyle)	210	4.0	25.0	10.0	0	620	<1.0
(*Grands! Butter Tastin'*)	200	4.0	24.0	10.0	0	620	<1.0
(*Pillsbury* Country), 3 pcs.	150	4.0	29.0	2.0	0	540	<1.0
blueberry (*Grands!*)	210	4.0	29.0	9.0	0	510	<1.0
buttermilk:							
(*Big Country*)	100	2.0	14.0	4.0	0	360	0
(*1869* Brand)	100	2.0	12.0	5.0	0	320	0
(*Grands!*)	200	4.0	24.0	10.0	0	620	<1.0

Food and Measure	cal.	prot. (gms)	carbo. (gms)	fat (gms)	chol. (mgs)	sod. (mgs)	fiber (gms)
(*Grands!* Reduced Fat)	190	4.0	27.0	7.0	0	620	<1.0
(*Pillsbury*), 3 pcs.	150	4.0	29.0	2.0	0	540	<1.0
(*Pillsbury* Tender Layer), 3 pcs.	160	4.0	22.0	4.5	0	520	<1.0
flaky (*Hungry Jack*)	100	2.0	14.0	4.5	0	360	0
cinnamon and sugar (*Hungry Jack*)	110	2.0	17.0	4.0	0	280	<1.0
corn, golden (*Grands!*)	210	4.0	26.0	10.0	0	600	<1.0
flaky:							
(*Grands!*)	200	4.0	25.0	9.0	0	580	<1.0
(*Hungry Jack*)	100	2.0	14.0	4.5	0	360	0
(*Hungry Jack Butter Tastin'*)	100	2.0	14.0	4.5	0	350	0
Southern style:							
(*Big Country*)	100	2.0	14.0	4.0	0	360	0
(*Grands!*)	200	4.0	24.0	10.0	0	620	<1.0
flaky (*Hungry Jack*)	100	2.0	14.0	4.5	0	360	0
wheat (*Grands!*)	200	4.0	27.0	8.0	0	600	2.0
Biscuit mix, dry:							
(*Arrowhead Mills*), ¼ cup	120	5.0	23.0	1.0	0	200	3.0
(*Gladiola*), ⅓ cup	160	3.0	23.0	6.0	0	480	<1.0
Bitter melon, see "Balsam pear"							
Black bean, dried, ½ cup, except as noted:							
(*Frieda's*), ⅓ cup, 3 oz.	120	8.0	20.0	0	0	n.a.	11.0
boiled	113	7.6	20.4	.5	0	1	7.5
turtle soup:							
boiled	120	7.5	22.4	.3	0	3	4.9
dried (*Arrowhead Mills*), ¼ cup	150	10.0	28.0	.5	0	10	9.0
dried	312	19.6	58.2	.8	0	8	22.9
Black bean, canned, (see also "Refried beans"), ½ cup:							
(*Eden* Organic)	100	7.0	18.0	0	0	15	6.0

Food and Measure	cal.	prot. (gms)	carbo. (gms)	fat (gms)	chol. (mgs)	sod. (mgs)	fiber (gms)
Black bean, canned *(cont.)*							
(*Green Giant/Joan of Arc*)	100	6.0	18.0	0	0	400	5.0
(*Old El Paso*)	110	7.0	17.0	1.0	0	400	7.0
(*Progresso*)	110	7.0	17.0	1.0	0	400	7.0
w/ginger and lemon (*Eden* Organic)	120	7.0	21.0	0	0	200	7.0
seasoned (*Allens/Trappey's*)	120	7.0	20.0	1.5	0	410	7.0
Black bean, dehydrated (*AlpineAire*), ½ cup	100	6.0	18.0	.5	0	0	9.0
Black bean dip, see "Bean dip"							
Black bean dishes, mix, dry:							
instant (*Fantastic Foods* International), ⅓ cup	160	10.0	29.0	1.5	0	310	7.0
and penne (*Marrakesh Express* Terrazza), ⅓ cup	180	8.0	36.0	.5	0	480	2.0
Black bean sauce, 1 tbsp.:							
(*Ka•Me*)	20	1.0	3.0	.5	0	280	0
garlic (*Lee Kum Kee*)	25	1.0	3.0	1.0	0	1270	<1.0
Blackberry, fresh, ½ cup	37	.5	9.2	.3	0	tr.	3.6
Blackberry, canned, ½ cup:							
(*Allen-Wolco*)	60	2.0	13.0	.5	0	20	9.0
in light syrup (*Oregon*)	120	1.0	29.0	0	0	10	6.0
in heavy syrup (*Comstock/Wilderness*)	110	1.0	26.0	0	0	50	1.0
in heavy syrup	118	1.7	29.6	.2	0	3	4.4
Blackberry, frozen:							
(*Cascadian Farm*), 1 cup	80	1.0	20.0	.5	0	10	3.0
unsweetened, ½ cup	49	.9	11.8	.3	0	1	3.8

Food and Measure	cal.	prot. (gms)	carbo. (gms)	fat (gms)	chol. (mgs)	sod. (mgs)	fiber (gms)
Blackberry syrup							
(*Knott's Berry Farm*),							
1 fl. oz.	120	0	30.0	0	0	0	0
(*Smucker's*), ¼ cup	210	0	52.0	0	0	0	0
Black-eyed peas:							
fresh or frozen, see							
"Cowpeas"							
mature:							
dry (*Frieda's*),							
⅓ cup, 3 oz.	130	8.0	21.0	1.0	0	250	11.0
boiled, ½ cup	100	6.7	17.9	.5	0	3	5.6
Black-eyed peas,							
canned, ½ cup:							
(*Eden* Organic)	90	6.0	16.0	1.0	0	25	4.0
fresh shell:							
(*Allens/East Texas*							
Fair/Homefolks/							
Dorman)	120	7.0	21.0	1.0	0	350	6.0
(*Bush's Best*)	110	7.0	18.0	1.0	0	500	5.0
w/jalapeño							
(*Homefolks*)	120	7.0	20.0	1.0	0	580	5.0
w/jalapeño (*Stubb's*)	120	7.0	20.0	.5	0	580	5.0
w/snaps (*Allens/*							
East Texas Fair/							
Homefolks)	120	8.0	20.0	1.0	0	420	5.0
dry:							
(*Allens/East Texas*							
Fair)	110	7.0	18.0	1.0	0	340	4.0
(*Bush's Best*)	100	5.0	19.0	0	0	410	4.0
(*Bush's Showboat*)	100	5.0	19.0	0	0	410	4.0
(*Green Giant/Joan of*							
Arc)	90	6.0	16.0	0	0	250	3.0
w/bacon (*Allens/*							
Sunshine)	105	7.0	20.0	1.5	0	390	5.0
w/bacon (*Bush's*							
Best)	110	6.0	18.0	1.0	5	630	5.0
w/bacon (*Trappey's*)	120	7.0	19.0	2.0	0	350	5.0
w/bacon and jalape-							
ños (*Bush's Best*)	120	6.0	16.0	2.5	5	660	5.0
w/bacon and jalape-							
ños (*Trappey's*)	110	6.0	19.0	1.5	0	470	5.0

Food and Measure	cal.	prot. (gms)	carbo. (gms)	fat (gms)	chol. (mgs)	sod. (mgs)	fiber (gms)
Black-eyed peas, canned, dry *(cont.)*							
w/snaps (*Bush's Best*)	110	7.0	17.0	.5	0	550	5.0
Black-eyed peas, frozen (*Birds Eye*), ½ cup	110	7.0	21.0	.5	0	10	4.0
Blimpie:							
6″ sub:							
Blimpie Best	410	26.0	47.0	13.0	50	1480	4.0
cheese trio	510	26.0	51.0	23.0	60	1060	2.0
club	450	30.0	53.0	13.0	40	1350	3.0
ham, salami, provolone	590	32.0	52.0	28.0	70	1880	3.0
ham and Swiss	400	25.0	47.0	13.0	35	970	5.0
roast beef	340	27.0	47.0	4.5	20	870	2.0
tuna	570	21.0	50.0	32.0	50	790	2.0
turkey	320	19.0	51.0	4.5	10	890	3.0
grilled chicken salad	350	47.0	13.0	12.0	140	1190	0
Blintz, frozen, 1 pc.:							
apple (*King Kold*)	110	7.0	19.0	1.0	35	135	0
blueberry (*King Kold*)	130	7.0	23.0	1.0	35	150	0
blueberry or cherry (*Ratner's*)	100	3.0	20.0	.5	15	15	<1.0
cheese:							
(*Golden*)	80	6.0	13.0	2.0	13	135	2.0
(*King Kold*)	110	10.0	14.0	1.5	35	260	0
(*Ratner's*)	90	7.0	15.0	.5	15	15	<1.0
cherry (*King Kold*) . . .	110	7.0	18.0	1.0	35	140	0
potato:							
(*Golden*)	90	3.0	15.0	4.0	5	170	2.0
(*King Kold*)	110	7.0	12.0	3.0	35	210	<1.0
strawberry (*King Kold*)	120	7.0	20.0	1.0	35	135	0
Blood sausage, 1 oz.	107	4.1	.4	9.8	34	n.a.	0
Bloody Mary mixer, 8 fl. oz., except as noted:							
(*Mr & Mrs T*)	40	1.0	9.0	0	0	1440	0
(*Tabasco*)	60	2.0	11.0	0	0	1550	<1.0
extra spicy (*Tabasco*)	60	3.0	11.0	0	0	1640	2.0
spicy (*Trader Vic's*), 4 fl. oz.	20	1.0	6.0	0	0	690	0

Food and Measure	cal.	prot. (gms)	carbo. (gms)	fat (gms)	chol. (mgs)	sod. (mgs)	fiber (gms)
Blue squash, Australian (*Frieda's*), ³/₄ cup, 3 oz.	30	1.0	7.0	0	0	0	1.0
Blueberry, fresh, ¹/₂ cup	41	.5	10.2	.3	0	5	2.0
Blueberry, canned, ¹/₂ cup:							
in light syrup (*Oregon*)	110	<1.0	26.0	0	0	5	2.0
in heavy syrup (*Comstock/Wilderness*)	110	1.0	26.0	0	0	15	2.0
Blueberry, dried:							
(*Frieda's*), ¹/₄ cup, 1.4 oz.	140	1.0	33.0	0	0	0	4.0
(*Sonoma*), ¹/₄ cup, 1.4 oz.	140	1.0	33.0	0	0	0	5.0
freeze-dried (*AlpineAire*), ²/₃ oz. . . .	80	1.0	17.0	1.0	0	0	4.0
Blueberry, frozen:							
(*Cascadian Farm*), 1 cup	90	1.0	22.0	.5	0	10	2.0
sweetened, ¹/₂ cup . . .	94	.5	25.2	.2	0	2	2.4
Blueberry juice (*After the Fall* Maine Coast), 8 fl. oz.	100	0	25.0	0	0	20	0
Blueberry syrup, ¹/₄ cup, except as noted:							
(*Knott's Berry Farm*), 1 fl. oz.	120	0	30.0	0	0	0	0
(*Maple Grove Farms*)	250	0	62.0	0	0	0	0
(*Smucker's*)	210	0	52.0	0	0	0	0
(*Smucker's Light*) . . .	130	0	33.0	0	0	0	0
Bluefish, meat only:							
raw, 4 oz.	141	22.7	0	4.8	67	68	0
baked, broiled, or microwaved, 4 oz. . . .	180	29.1	0	6.2	86	87	0
Boar, wild, meat only, roasted, 4 oz.	181	32.1	0	5.0	n.a.	n.a.	0
Bockwurst, raw, 1 oz.	87	3.8	.1	7.8	n.a.	n.a.	0
Bok choy, see "Cabbage, Chinese"							

Food and Measure	cal.	prot. (gms)	carbo. (gms)	fat (gms)	chol. (mgs)	sod. (mgs)	fiber (gms)
Bologna (see also "Turkey bologna"), 2 oz., except as noted:							
(*Black Bear* German)	160	7.0	1.0	14.0	30	450	0
(*Boar's Head*)	150	7.0	<1.0	13.0	35	530	0
(*Boar's Head* Lower Sodium)	150	8.0	0	13.0	30	410	0
(*Diet Delight*)	130	8.0	4.0	8.0	25	400	0
(*Hansel 'n Gretel* Classic/German)	150	8.0	3.0	12.0	30	670	0
(*Healthy Choice*), 1-oz. slice	30	4.0	3.0	2.0	15	240	0
(*Healthy Choice* Deli-Thin), 4 slices, 1.9 oz.	80	7.0	2.0	4.0	10	480	0
(*Oscar Mayer*), 1 oz.	90	3.0	1.0	8.0	30	290	0
(*Oscar Mayer* Fat Free), 1 oz.	25	3.0	2.0	0	10	250	0
(*Russer Light*)	120	8.0	3.0	8.0	30	400	0
beef:							
(*Boar's Head*)	150	7.0	0	13.0	35	520	0
(*Diet Delight*)	150	8.0	4.0	11.0	30	400	0
(*Hansel 'n Gretel*)	160	7.0	4.0	13.0	30	710	0
(*Healthy Choice*), 1-oz. slice	35	4.0	3.0	1.0	10	240	0
(*Hebrew National*), 3 slices, 2 oz. . . .	160	7.0	0	15.0	30	380	0
(*Hebrew National* Chub)	180	7.0	0	16.0	40	440	0
(*Oscar Mayer*), 1 oz.	90	3.0	1.0	8.0	20	310	0
(*Russer Light*)	120	8.0	3.0	8.0	30	400	0
garlic:							
(*Boar's Head*)	150	7.0	1.0	13.0	35	530	0
(*Oscar Mayer*), 1.4-oz. slice	130	4.0	1.0	12.0	30	420	0
ring (*Oscar Mayer* Wisconsin)	180	6.0	2.0	16.0	35	460	0
"Bologna," vegetarian, frozen (*Worthington Bolòno*), 3 slices	80	10.0	2.0	3.5	0	720	2.0

Food and Measure	cal.	prot. (gms)	carbo. (gms)	fat (gms)	chol. (mgs)	sod. (mgs)	fiber (gms)
Bonito, meat only,							
raw, 4 oz.	146	29.3	.5	2.3	n.a.	50	0
Borage:							
raw, 1″ pcs., ½ cup	9	.8	1.4	.3	0	35	<1.0
boiled, drained, 4 oz.	28	2.4	4.0	.9	0	98	<2.0
Bouillabaisse season-							
ing mix (*Knorr*),							
1 tbsp.	20	1.0	3.0	.5	<5	550	0
Bouillon (see also							
"Bouillon, concen-							
trate"):							
beef:							
(*Herb-Ox*), *1 cube*	5	0	<1.0	0	0	900	0
(*Herb-Ox* Instant),							
1 tsp. or pkt.	5	0	<1.0	0	0	1020	0
(*Herb-Ox* Instant							
Low Sodium),							
1 pkt.	10	0	2.0	0	0	5	0
(*Maggi*), 1 cube . . .	5	0	0	0	0	1120	0
(*Maggi*), ½ tablet	15	<1.0	1.0	.5	0	1220	0
(*Maggi* Instant),							
1 tsp.	5	0	1.0	0	0	570	0
(*MBT/Wyler's*),							
1 pkt.	15	1.0	2.0	0	0	810	0
(*MBT/Wyler's* Very							
Low Sodium),							
1 pkt.	15	<1.0	3.0	0	0	5	0
(*Wyler's*), 1 tsp. . . .	5	0	1.0	0	0	900	0
(*Wyler's* Reduced							
Sodium), 1 tsp.	5	0	1.0	0	0	600	0
(*Wyler's/Steero* Very							
Low Sodium),							
1 tsp.	10	0	2.0	0	0	10	0
chicken:							
(*Herb-Ox/Herb-Ox*							
Instant), 1 cube,							
1 tsp., or 1 pkt.	5	0	<1.0	0	0	1100	0
(*Herb-Ox* Instant							
Low Sodium),							
1 pkt.	10	0	2.0	0	0	5	0
(*Maggi*), 1 cube . . .	5	0	0	0	0	1060	0

Food and Measure	cal.	prot. (gms)	carbo. (gms)	fat (gms)	chol. (mgs)	sod. (mgs)	fiber (gms)
Bouillon, chicken *(cont.)*							
(*Maggi* 2.5 oz.),							
½ tablet	15	<1.0	1.0	1.0	0	1350	0
(*Maggi* 3.5 oz.),							
1 tsp.	5	0	<1.0	0	0	1060	0
(*Maggi* 8 oz.), 1 tsp.	5	0	<1.0	0	0	600	0
(*Maggi* Dominican),							
½ tablet	20	0	1.0	1.5	0	1100	0
(*Maggi* Instant),							
1 tsp.	5	0	1.0	0	0	640	0
(*MBT/Wyler's*),							
1 pkt.	15	<1.0	2.0	0	0	860	0
(*MBT/Wyler's* Very							
Low Sodium),							
1 pkt.	15	0	3.0	0	0	10	0
(*Wyler's*), 1 tsp. . . .	5	0	1.0	0	0	900	0
(*Wyler's* Reduced							
Sodium), 1 tsp.	5	0	1.0	0	0	600	0
(*Wyler's/Steero* Very							
Low Sodium),							
1 tsp.	10	0	2.0	0	0	0	0
chicken and tomato:							
(*Maggi*), ½ tablet	15	0	<1.0	1.0	0	1130	0
(*Maggi*), 1 tsp. . . .	5	0	<1.0	0	0	620	0
onion (*MBT* Instant),							
1 pkt.	15	0	3.0	0	0	800	0
vegetable:							
(*Herb-Ox*), 1 cube	5	0	<1.0	0	0	980	0
(*Maggi* Vegetarian),							
1 cube	5	0	1.0	0	0	820	0
(*MBT*), 1 pkt.	10	0	2.0	0	0	860	0
(*Wyler's*), 1 tsp. . . .	5	0	1.0	0	0	870	0
Bouillon concentrate,							
liquid, 2 tsp.:							
beef:							
(*Herb-Ox*)	20	2.0	2.0	0	0	570	0
(*Knorr*).	15	2.0	1.0	0	0	850	0
chicken:							
(*Herb-Ox*)	15	1.0	1.0	0	0	620	0
(*Knorr*)	5	<1.0	<1.0	0	0	740	0

Food and Measure	cal.	prot. (gms)	carbo. (gms)	fat (gms)	chol. (mgs)	sod. (mgs)	fiber (gms)
Bourguignonne seasoning mix (*Knorr*), 1 tbsp.	35	<1.0	6.0	1.0	0	410	0
Bowtie pasta, see "Pasta, dry"							
Bowtie pasta dishes, mix:							
chicken primavera (*Lipton* Pasta & Sauce), 1 cup*	290	9.0	43.0	10.0	10	820	2.0
w/creamy mushroom sauce (*DeBoles*), 2.4 oz.	240	9.0	48.0	1.5	5	520	3.0
Florentine beans (*Bean Cuisine* Pasta & Beans), 1.5 oz.	160	7.0	29.0	1.5	0	10	4.0
w/herb sauce, savory (*Knorr*), 2/3 cup	260	12.0	47.0	2.0	<5	790	6.0
Italian cheese (*Lipton* Pasta & Sauce), 1 cup*	300	10.0	41.0	11.5	15	900	<1.0
Bowtie pasta entree, frozen, 1 pkg., except as noted:							
Alfredo (*Marie Callender's*), 13 oz. . . .	620	20.0	40.0	42.0	80	1080	8.0
and chicken (*Lean Cuisine Cafe Classics*), 9½ oz.	250	16.0	34.0	5.0	45	530	3.0
creamy tomato sauce (*Lean Cuisine*), 10 oz.	260	9.0	43.0	6.0	35	550	6.0
and kasha (*Cohen's Famous*), ¾ cup . . .	160	4.0	22.0	6.0	25	220	2.0
marinara (*Marie Callender's*), 13 oz. . . .	430	18.0	48.0	19.0	30	930	6.0
and meat sauce (*Marie Callender's*), 13 oz.	480	25.0	44.0	22.0	45	970	3.0
and mushrooms marsala (*Smart Ones*), 9.6 oz.	270	11.0	40.0	7.0	40	520	4.0

Food and Measure	cal.	prot. (gms)	carbo. (gms)	fat (gms)	chol. (mgs)	sod. (mgs)	fiber (gms)
Boysenberry, fresh, see "Blackberry"							
Boysenberry, canned, ½ cup:							
in light syrup (*Oregon*)	120	<1.0	27.0	0	0	10	3.0
in heavy syrup (*Comstock/Wilderness*)	120	1.0	28.0	0	0	90	2.0
in heavy syrup	113	1.3	28.6	.2	0	4	3.3
Boysenberry, frozen, unsweetened, ½ cup	33	.7	8.1	.1	0	1	2.6
Boysenberry syrup:							
(*Knott's Berry Farm*), 1 fl. oz.	120	0	30.0	0	0	0	0
(*Maple Grove Farms*), ¼ cup	250	0	61.0	0	0	0	<1.0
(*Smucker's*), ¼ cup	210	0	52.0	0	0	0	0
Brains, 4 oz.:							
beef, fried	222	14.3	0	18.0	2262	179	0
lamb, fried	310	19.2	0	25.2	2840	178	0
pork, braised	156	13.8	0	10.8	2894	103	0
veal, fried	242	16.4	0	19.0	2404	200	0
Bran, see "Cereal, ready-to-eat" and specific grains							
Bratwurst, 1 link:							
(*Ball Park*), 2 oz.	190	11.0	2.0	17.0	45	740	0
(*Boar's Head*), 4 oz.	300	19.0	0	27.0	50	950	0
(*Hillshire Farm*), 2.7 oz.	230	9.0	2.0	21.0	45	460	0
pork, cooked, 1 oz.	85	4.0	.6	7.3	17	158	0
Braunschweiger (see also "Liverwurst"), 2 oz., except as noted:							
(*Black Bear*)	180	9.0	2.0	15.0	55	460	0
(*Boar's Head* Lite) . . .	120	9.0	1.0	8.0	50	450	0
(*Hansel 'n Gretel*)	170	9.0	4.0	13.0	95	730	0
(*Russer Light*)	120	8.0	3.0	8.0	60	400	0
chub:							
(*Jones Dairy Farm* Light)	100	10.0	1.0	6.0	140	500	0

Food and Measure	cal.	prot. (gms)	carbo. (gms)	fat (gms)	chol. (mgs)	sod. (mgs)	fiber (gms)
(*Jones Dairy Farm* Original 8 oz.) ...	160	8.0	1.0	14.0	115	520	0
(*Jones Dairy Farm* Original 16 oz.)	150	9.0	1.0	12.0	130	520	0
bacon, 20% (*Jones Dairy Farm*)	150	9.0	1.0	12.0	120	560	0
w/onion (*Jones Dairy Farm*)	160	8.0	2.0	13.0	110	560	0
chunk:							
(*Jones Dairy Farm* Light)	90	10.0	1.0	5.0	125	430	0
(*Jones Dairy Farm* Original)	180	8.0	1.0	16.0	110	460	0
sliced:							
(*Jones Dairy Farm* 8 oz.), 2 slices, 1.6 oz.	150	6.0	1.0	13.0	90	370	0
(*Jones Dairy Farm* 12 oz.), 1.2-oz slice	110	5.0	1.0	10.0	70	280	0
(*Oscar Mayer*), 1-oz. slice	100	4.0	1.0	9.0	50	320	0
spread (*Oscar Mayer*)	190	8.0	1.0	17.0	90	630	0
Brazil nut, shelled, 1 oz., 6 large or 8 medium kernels ...	186	4.1	3.6	18.8	0	<1	1.6
Bread, 1 slice, except as noted:							
apple walnut (*Pepperidge Farm*)	80	2.0	14.0	2.0	0	120	1.0
bran:							
(*Arnold Branola*) ...	100	4.0	19.0	1.5	0	160	3.0
honey (*Pepperidge Farm*)	90	3.0	17.0	1.0	0	160	2.0
butter (*Wonder*)	80	2.0	15.0	1.5	0	170	0
buttermilk:							
(*Arnold*)	110	4.0	20.0	1.5	0	190	<1.0
(*Wonder*)	70	2.0	13.0	1.0	0	170	0
cinnamon:							
(*Arnold*)	90	2.0	14.0	3.0	<5	95	<1.0
(*Pepperidge Farm*)	80	3.0	14.0	2.5	0	115	2.0

Food and Measure	cal.	prot. (gms)	carbo. (gms)	fat (gms)	chol. (mgs)	sod. (mgs)	fiber (gms)
Bread *(cont.)*							
cinnamon raisin:							
(*Arnold*)	90	2.0	15.0	2.5	<5	95	<1.0
(*Wonder*)	70	1.0	13.0	1.0	0	120	0
French:							
(*Bread du Jour* Twin), 3″ slice . . .	140	5.0	16.0	.5	0	190	0
(*Pepperidge Farm*), ⅑ loaf	130	4.0	25.0	1.5	0	280	1.0
(*Pepperidge Farm* Sliced), ⅑ loaf . . .	120	4.0	24.0	1.5	0	260	1.0
(*Pepperidge Farm* Twin), ⅑ of 2 loaves	130	4.0	26.0	1.5	0	270	1.0
(*Wonder*), 2″ slice	140	4.0	27.0	1.5	0	350	1.0
golden swirl (*Pepper- idge Farm* Vermont Maple)	90	2.0	15.0	2.5	0	100	<1.0
grain:							
crunchy (*Pepper- idge Farm*)	90	4.0	15.0	1.5	0	130	2.0
whole (*Pepperidge Farm* 100%)	90	4.0	15.0	1.0	0	160	2.0
hazelnut (*Monk's*) . . .	70	2.0	12.0	1.5	0	110	2.0
Italian:							
(*Arnold Bakery Light*), 2 slices	80	4.0	21.0	1.0	0	150	5.0
(*Wonder*), 2 slices	120	3.0	21.0	1.5	0	290	1.0
(*Wonder Light*), 2 slices	80	4.0	19.0	1.0	0	230	5.0
brown and serve (*Pepperidge Farm*), ⅑ loaf . . .	130	4.0	24.0	2.0	0	260	1.0
kamut, sprouted (*Shi- loh Farms* Egyptian)	90	6.0	18.0	1.0	0	115	5.0
mountain bread, 2.4-oz. pc.:							
grain (*Cedar's*)	200	7.0	35.0	4.0	0	380	4.0
wheat (*Cedar's*) . . .	180	7.0	34.0	1.5	0	340	4.0
white (*Cedar's*)	180	7.0	35.0	1.0	0	290	1.0

Food and Measure	cal.	prot. (gms)	carbo. (gms)	fat (gms)	chol. (mgs)	sod. (mgs)	fiber (gms)
multigrain:							
(*Wonder* Fat Free)	70	2.0	13.0	0	0	160	1.0
(*Wonder Good Hearth*)	70	2.0	12.0	1.5	0	140	1.0
5-grain, sprouted (*Shiloh Farms*)	90	5.0	19.0	.5	0	110	4.0
5-grain, sprouted (*Shiloh Farms* No Salt)	90	5.0	19.0	.5	0	0	4.0
7-grain (*Pepperidge Farm* Light Style), 3 slices	140	6.0	28.0	1.0	0	320	5.0
7-grain, hearty (*Pepperidge Farm*)	100	3.0	18.0	1.5	0	180	2.0
7-grain, sprouted (*Shiloh Farms*)	90	5.0	19.0	.5	0	130	3.0
7-grain, sprouted (*Shiloh Farms* No Salt)	90	5.0	19.0	.5	0	0	3.0
7-grain, sprouted (*Shiloh Farms* Breads for Life*)	90	5.0	19.0	.5	0	130	3.0
9-grain (*Pepperidge Farm*) . . . .*.	90	4.0	16.0	1.0	0	170	2.0
10-grain, sprouted (*Shiloh Farms*), 2 slices	140	9.0	26.0	1.5	0	120	5.0
sprouted (*Shiloh Farms* Sandwich)	80	4.0	17.0	.5	0	100	3.0
three-seed (*Arnold's Best*)	100	4.0	12.0	3.5	0	120	2.0
oat:							
bran (*Shiloh Farms*)	90	5.0	18.0	1.0	0	130	3.0
and bran (*Wonder Oatmeal Goodness*)	80	3.0	15.0	1.0	0	250	1.0
bran/fiber (*Wonder Good Hearth*) . . .	100	3.0	19.0	1.0	0	160	2.0

Food and Measure	cal.	prot. (gms)	carbo. (gms)	fat (gms)	chol. (mgs)	sod. (mgs)	fiber (gms)
Bread, oat *(cont.)*							
crunchy, hearty (*Pepperidge Farm*)	100	4.0	17.0	2.0	0	180	2.0
honey and (*Wonder Good Hearth*) ...	80	3.0	15.0	1.5	0	170	1.0
nut (*Arnold* Oatnut)	110	4.0	19.0	2.0	0	160	4.0
and sunflower (*Wonder Oatmeal Goodness*)	90	3.0	14.0	1.5	0	150	1.0
oatmeal:							
(*Pepperidge Farm*)	80	3.0	15.0	1.0	0	200	1.0
(*Pepperidge Farm Light*), 3 slices...	140	7.0	27.0	1.0	0	310	5.0
soft (*Pepperidge Farm*)	60	2.0	12.0	.5	0	150	0
thin-sliced (*Pepperidge Farm*)	60	2.0	11.0	1.0	0	160	1.0
pita:							
(*Thomas' Sahara*), 2-oz. pc.	150	5.0	29.0	1.5	0	330	1.0
onion (*Thomas' Sahara*), 2-oz. pc.	160	5.0	32.0	1.5	0	320	2.0
6-grain (*Cedar's*), ½ pc., 1.5 oz. ...	94	5.0	18.0	0	0	115	2.0
wheat, whole (*Cedar's*), ½ pc., 1.5 oz.	129	4.0	25.0	1.0	0	160	4.0
white (*Cedar's*), ½ pc., 1.5 oz. ...	122	4.0	23.0	1.0	0	150	1.0
potato:							
(*Arnold* Country)	100	3.0	20.0	1.0	0	180	<1.0
(*Wonder*)	70	2.0	13.0	1.0	0	140	0
(*Wonder* Fat Free)	70	2.0	13.0	0	0	200	1.0
hearty (*Pepperidge Farm* Russet) ...	90	4.0	18.0	1.5	<5	260	3.0
pumpernickel:							
(*Arnold*)	80	3.0	15.0	1.0	0	200	<1.0
(*Rubschlager* Russian)	90	3.0	17.0	1.5	0	210	2.0

Food and Measure	cal.	prot. (gms)	carbo. (gms)	fat (gms)	chol. (mgs)	sod. (mgs)	fiber (gms)
(*Wonder Good Hearth*)	80	3.0	13.0	1.5	0	230	1.0
dark (*Pepperidge Farm* Classic)	80	3.0	15.0	1.0	0	230	1.0
party (*Pepperidge Farm*), 8 slices...	110	6.0	22.0	1.5	0	320	4.0
raisin:							
(*Monk's*)	80	2.0	16.0	1.0	0	110	2.0
w/cinnamon (*Pepperidge Farm*) ...	80	3.0	14.0	1.5	0	105	1.0
whole wheat (*Shiloh Farms*), 2 slices	140	7.0	30.0	1.0	0	160	3.0
rye:							
(*Rubschlager* Jewish Style Deli) ...	70	2.0	13.0	1.0	0	135	2.0
(*Wonder Good Hearth* Jewish)	80	3.0	14.0	1.5	0	230	1.0
Dijon, thin sliced (*Pepperidge Farm*), 2 slices ...	100	4.0	18.0	1.5	0	340	2.0
dill (*Arnold*)	80	3.0	15.0	1.0	0	180	<1.0
hearty (*Wonder Beefsteak*)	70	2.0	13.0	1.0	0	180	1.0
onion (*Pepperidge Farm*)	80	3.0	15.0	1.0	0	210	1.0
party (*Pepperidge Farm*), 8 slices...	110	6.0	22.0	1.5	0	410	3.0
seeded (*Arnold* Real Jewish)	80	3.0	15.0	1.0	0	220	<1.0
seeded, thin-sliced (*Arnold* Real Jewish Melba Thin), 2 slices	110	3.0	21.0	1.5	0	300	1.0
seeded or seedless (*Levy's* Real Jewish)	90	3.0	16.0	1.5	0	230	<1.0
seeded or seedless (*Pepperidge Farm* Jewish)	80	3.0	15.0	1.0	0	210	1.0
seedless (*Arnold* Real Jewish)	80	3.0	15.0	1.5	0	220	<1.0

Food and Measure	cal.	prot. (gms)	carbo. (gms)	fat (gms)	chol. (mgs)	sod. (mgs)	fiber (gms)
Bread, rye *(cont.)*							
soft (*Wonder* Beef-steak)	70	2.0	14.0	1.0	0	200	0
soft (*Wonder* Beef-steak Light), 2 slices	80	5.0	17.0	1.0	0	260	5.0
sourdough:							
(*Pepperidge Farm* Light Style), 3 slices	130	6.0	27.0	1.0	0	320	4.0
(*Pepperidge Farm* Twin), 1/9 of 2 loaves	130	4.0	26.0	1.5	0	270	1.0
(*Wonder*)	60	2.0	11.0	.5	0	140	0
(*Wonder* Light), 2 slices	80	4.0	18.0	1.0	0	260	5.0
spelt (*Shiloh Farms*)	100	4.0	21.0	1.0	0	140	2.0
sunflower seed:							
and bran (*Monk's*)	70	3.0	14.0	1.5	0	120	2.0
whole wheat (*Shiloh Farms*), 2 slices	160	9.0	23.0	4.5	5	250	4.0
Vienna:							
light (*Pepperidge Farm*), 3 slices ...	130	6.0	28.0	1.0	0	300	5.0
thick-sliced (*Pepperidge Farm*) ...	70	3.0	12.0	1.0	0	150	<1.0
wheat:							
(*Arnold Bakery Light*), 2 slices	80	4.0	20.0	.5	0	135	4.0
(*Arnold* Country)	100	4.0	19.0	1.5	0	190	1.0
(*Home Pride*)	80	2.0	14.0	1.0	0	190	0
(*Monk's* 100% Stoneground) ...	70	3.0	13.0	1.0	0	125	2.0
(*Pepperidge Farm* 1.5 lb.)	90	3.0	16.0	1.5	0	190	1.0
(*Pepperidge Farm* Family 2 lb.)	70	2.0	13.0	1.0	0	135	1.0
(*Pepperidge Farm* Light), 3 slices ...	130	7.0	28.0	1.0	0	290	5.0
(*Pepperidge Farm* Natural)	90	4.0	16.0	1.5	0	170	1.0

Food and Measure	cal.	prot. (gms)	carbo. (gms)	fat (gms)	chol. (mgs)	sod. (mgs)	fiber (gms)
(*Shiloh Farms* Homestyle), 2 slices	160	7.0	29.0	1.5	<5	115	<1.0
(*Wonder* Family) ...	70	2.0	13.0	1.0	0	160	1.0
(*Wonder* Light), 2 slices	80	5.0	18.0	.5	0	240	5.0
(*Wonder* Split Top)	70	2.0	13.0	1.0	0	170	1.0
cracked, thin-sliced (*Pepperidge Farm*)	70	2.0	12.0	1.0	0	140	<1.0
honey (*Butternut*)	70	2.0	12.0	1.0	0	150	1.0
sesame, hearty (*Pepperidge Farm*)	100	4.0	18.0	1.5	0	190	2.0
very thin-sliced (*Pepperidge Farm*), 3 slices...	110	4.0	22.0	2.0	0	230	4.0
whole (*Arnold* 100%)	90	5.0	17.0	1.0	0	190	2.0
whole (*Arnold* Stoneground 100%)	60	3.0	12.0	.5	0	135	2.0
whole (*Arnold Brick Oven* 8 oz.), 2 slices	110	5.0	20.0	2.5	0	190	3.0
whole (*Arnold Brick Oven* 1 lb.), 2 slices	120	5.0	22.0	2.5	0	200	3.0
whole (*Arnold Brick Oven* 2 lb.)	80	4.0	13.0	1.5	0	125	2.0
whole (*Wonder* 100% Stone Ground)	70	3.0	12.0	1.0	0	160	1.0
whole, soft (*Pepperidge Farm* 100%)	60	2.0	11.0	.5	0	95	1.0
whole, thin-sliced (*Pepperidge Farm*)	60	3.0	11.0	1.0	0	120	<1.0
winter (*Arnold's Best*)	90	4.0	13.0	3.5	0	105	2.0

Food and Measure	cal.	prot. (gms)	carbo. (gms)	fat (gms)	chol. (mgs)	sod. (mgs)	fiber (gms)
Bread *(cont.)*							
wheat and rye, sprouted, w/onions (*Shiloh Farms* Zesty), 2 slices	140	9.0	26.0	2.0	0	160	5.0
wheatberry, honey:							
(*Wonder Good Hearth*)	70	2.0	14.0	1.0	0	160	0
hearty (*Pepperidge Farm*)	100	3.0	18.0	1.5	0	200	2.0
white:							
(*Arnold* Country)	110	3.0	20.0	1.5	0	240	<1.0
(*Arnold Brick Oven* 1 lb.), 2 slices ...	130	4.0	25.0	2.0	0	150	<1.0
(*Arnold Brick Oven* 2 lb.)	90	2.0	16.0	1.5	0	160	<1.0
(*Home Pride*)	80	2.0	14.0	1.0	0	200	0
(*Monk's*)	70	3.0	14.0	1.0	0	110	2.0
(*Pepperidge Farm* Sandwich), 2 slices	130	4.0	23.0	2.0	0	260	<1.0
(*Pepperidge Farm* Toasting)	90	3.0	16.0	3.0	0	200	0
(*Wonder*), .9 oz. ...	70	2.0	12.0	1.0	0	160	0
(*Wonder*), 1.1 oz.	80	2.0	15.0	1.0	0	160	0
(*Wonder*), 1.3 oz.	100	3.0	18.0	1.5	0	200	0
(*Wonder*), 2 slices, 1.6 oz.	120	3.0	22.0	1.5	0	240	1.0
(*Wonder* Light), 2 slices	80	4.0	19.0	.5	0	260	5.0
(*Wonder* Old Fashioned)	70	2.0	12.0	1.0	0	130	0
(*Wonder* Texas Toast)	120	3.0	22.0	1.5	0	240	1.0
hearty (*Pepperidge Farm*)	90	3.0	19.0	1.0	0	190	2.0
honey (*Wonder* Fat Free)	70	2.0	13.0	0	0	180	1.0
thin-sliced (*Pepperidge Farm*)	80	2.0	13.0	1.5	0	135	0

Food and Measure	cal.	prot. (gms)	carbo. (gms)	fat (gms)	chol. (mgs)	sod. (mgs)	fiber (gms)
thin-sliced (*Pepperidge Farm* Large Family)	80	2.0	14.0	1.5	0	160	0
very thin-sliced (*Pepperidge Farm*), 3 slices...	110	4.0	23.0	1.5	0	270	2.0
Bread, brown, canned, 1/2" slice:							
(*B&M*)	130	3.0	29.0	.5	0	390	2.0
raisin (*B&M*)	130	3.0	29.0	.5	0	360	2.0
Bread, frozen and refrigerated:							
cheddar, two (*Pepperidge Farm*), 1/6 loaf	210	5.0	21.0	11.0	50	280	1.0
French loaf, crusty (*Pillsbury*), 1/5 loaf	150	5.0	27.0	2.0	0	390	<1.0
garlic loaf:							
(*New York*), 2 slices, 1", 2 oz.	190	4.0	28.0	7.0	0	390	1.0
(*New York* Reduced Fat), 2 slices, 1", 2 oz.	160	4.0	29.0	3.0	0	340	1.0
(*Pepperidge Farm*), 1/6 loaf	160	5.0	14.0	10.0	30	250	1.0
mozzarella (*Pepperidge Farm*), 1/6 loaf	200	6.0	21.0	10.0	40	280	1.0
Parmesan (*Pepperidge Farm*), 1/6 loaf	160	6.0	19.0	7.0	10	260	2.0
sourdough (*Pepperidge Farm*), 1/6 loaf	180	5.0	20.0	9.0	10	220	2.0
garlic toast:							
(*New York* Texas), 1 slice, 1.4 oz.	170	2.0	16.0	10.0	0	260	1.0
w/cheese (*New York* Texas), 1 slice, 1.7 oz.	190	4.0	17.0	11.0	5	330	1.0
Monterey jack and jalapeño (*Pepperidge Farm*), 1/6 loaf	200	5.0	22.0	10.0	40	280	1.0

Food and Measure	cal.	prot. (gms)	carbo. (gms)	fat (gms)	chol. (mgs)	sod. (mgs)	fiber (gms)
Bread, mix (see also "Bread mix, sweet"):							
cracked wheat (*Pillsbury* Bread Machine), 1/12 loaf* . . .	130	4.0	25.0	2.0	0	260	2.0
Italian herb (*Fleischmann's* Bread Machine), 1/8 loaf*	160	5.0	29.0	2.0	0	310	2.0
multigrain (*Arrowhead Mills*), 1/3 cup	160	7.0	31.0	1.0	0	200	3.0
oatmeal, honey (*Fleischmann's* Bread Machine), 1/8 loaf*	160	5.0	33.0	1.0	0	270	3.0
rye (*Arrowhead Mills*), 1/3 cup	160	5.0	33.0	.5	0	190	3.0
seitan (*Arrowhead Mills* Quick), 1/3 cup	160	23.0	11.0	.5	0	60	2.0
sourdough (*Fleischmann's* Bread Machine), 1/8 loaf*	150	5.0	29.0	1.5	0	160	2.0
spelt (*Arrowhead Mills*), 1/3 cup	150	6.0	31.0	1.0	0	190	5.0
wheat:							
stoneground (*Fleischmann's* Bread Machine), 1/8 loaf*	160	5.0	32.0	1.0	0	180	3.0
whole (*Arrowhead Mills*), 1/3 cup	150	7.0	31.0	1.0	0	190	5.0
white:							
(*Arrowhead Mills*), 1/3 cup	150	4.0	31.0	.5	0	170	2.0
country (*Fleischmann's* Bread Machine), 1/8 loaf*	170	6.0	31.0	2.5	0	170	2.0
crusty (*Pillsbury* Bread Machine), 1/12 loaf*	130	4.0	25.0	2.0	0	250	<1.0

Food and Measure	cal.	prot. (gms)	carbo. (gms)	fat (gms)	chol. (mgs)	sod. (mgs)	fiber (gms)
Bread, mix*, sweet:							
apple cinnamon:							
(*Fleischmann's*							
Bread Machine),							
⅛ loaf	160	5.0	32.0	1.0	0	160	2.0
(*Pillsbury*), ¹/₁₂ loaf	190	2.0	31.0	6.0	20	170	1.0
banana:							
(*Betty Crocker*							
Quick-bread),							
¹/₁₁ loaf	180	3.0	27.0	7.0	40	220	0
(*Pillsbury*), ¹/₁₂ loaf	170	3.0	26.0	6.0	35	200	<1.0
blueberry (*Pillsbury*),							
¹/₁₂ loaf	160	2.0	29.0	6.0	20	160	<1.0
carrot (*Pillsbury*),							
¹/₁₆ loaf	140	2.0	22.0	5.0	25	150	<1.0
cinnamon raisin:							
(*Betty Crocker*							
Quick-bread),							
¹/₁₃ loaf	190	2.0	29.0	7.0	35	190	0
(*Fleischmann's*							
Bread Machine),							
⅛ loaf	160	5.0	33.0	1.0	0	170	2.0
cinnamon swirl (*Pillsbury*), ¹/₁₂ loaf	220	2.0	32.0	9.0	35	170	0
corn bread, see "Corn bread"							
cranberry (*Pillsbury*),							
¹/₁₂ loaf	160	2.0	30.0	4.0	20	160	<1.0
cranberry orange							
(*Fleischmann's*							
Bread Machine),							
⅛ loaf	150	2.0	33.0	1.5	0	150	2.0
date (*Pillsbury*),							
¹/₁₂ loaf	180	3.0	32.0	4.0	20	160	1.0
gingerbread (*Pillsbury*), ⅛ loaf	220	3.0	40.0	5.0	0	340	<1.0
lemon poppyseed							
(*Pillsbury*), ¹/₁₂ loaf	180	3.0	27.0	7.0	20	160	<1.0
nut (*Pillsbury*), ¹/₁₂ loaf	170	3.0	27.0	6.0	20	190	1.0
pumpkin (*Pillsbury*),							
¹/₁₂ loaf	170	3.0	27.0	6.0	20	200	<1.0

Food and Measure	cal.	prot. (gms)	carbo. (gms)	fat (gms)	chol. (mgs)	sod. (mgs)	fiber (gms)
Bread crisps, 1 oz.:							
cinnamon raisin swirl							
(*Pepperidge Farm*)	130	2.0	19.0	5.0	0	100	3.0
garlic butter swirl							
(*Pepperidge Farm*)	140	3.0	16.0	8.0	5	230	<1.0
Bread crumbs, ¼ cup							
or 1 oz.:							
plain (*Progresso*)	110	4.0	19.0	1.5	0	210	1.0
garlic-herb							
(*Progresso*)	100	4.0	18.0	1.5	0	530	1.0
Italian (*Progresso*)	110	4.0	20.0	1.5	0	430	1.0
Parmesan (*Progresso*)	100	4.0	17.0	1.5	0	870	1.0
Bread cubes, see "Stuffing"							
Bread dough, see "Bread, frozen and refrigerated"							
Breadfruit seeds:							
boiled, shelled, 1 oz.	48	1.5	9.1	.7	0	n.a.	n.a.
roasted, shelled, 1 oz.	59	1.8	11.4	.8	0	n.a.	n.a.
Breadstick:							
plain:							
(*Bread du Jour* Original), 1 pc.	130	5.0	25.0	1.0	0	290	1.0
(*Stella D'oro*), 1 pc.	40	1.0	7.0	1.0	0	40	0
(*Stella D'oro* Deli Style Free), 5 pcs.	60	2.0	12.0	0	0	130	<1.0
(*Stella D'oro* Fat Free), 2 pcs.	70	2.0	15.0	0	0	150	1.0
(*Stella D'oro* Grissini Style Fat Free), 3 pcs.	60	2.0	12.0	0	0	130	1.0
(*Stella D'oro* Sodium Free), 1 pc.	45	1.0	7.0	1.0	0	0	0
brown and serve (*Pepperidge Farm*), 1 pc.	150	7.0	28.0	1.5	0	290	1.0
buttery (*Awrey's Deli Stix*), 2 pcs.	130	3.0	16.0	6.0	0	140	<1.0
cheddar, thin (*Pepperidge Farm*), 7 pcs.	70	2.0	10.0	2.5	5	120	<1.0

Food and Measure	cal.	prot. (gms)	carbo. (gms)	fat (gms)	chol. (mgs)	sod. (mgs)	fiber (gms)
w/cheese (*Handi-Snacks*), 1 pc.	130	4.0	11.0	7.0	15	340	0
dill onion (*Awrey's Deli Stix*), 2 pcs.	130	3.0	16.0	6.0	0	170	<1.0
garlic:							
(*Stella D'oro*), 1 pc.	40	1.0	7.0	1.0	0	60	0
(*Stella D'oro* Deli Fat Free), 5 pcs.	60	2.0	12.0	0	0	120	<1.0
(*Stella D'oro* Fat Free), 2 pcs.	70	2.0	14.0	0	0	150	1.0
(*Stella D'oro* Grissini Style Fat Free), 3 pcs.	60	2.0	12.0	0	0	120	<1.0
garlic and pepper (*Awrey's Deli Stix*), 2 pcs.	140	3.0	16.0	6.0	0	180	<1.0
Italian spice (*Awrey's Deli Stix*), 2 pcs.	140	3.0	16.0	6.0	0	230	<1.0
onion:							
(*Stella D'oro*), 1 pc.	40	1.0	6.0	1.0	0	35	0
thin (*Pepperidge Farm*), 7 pcs. ...	70	2.0	11.0	2.0	0	115	<1.0
pepper, cracked (*Stella D'oro*), 4 pcs.	70	2.0	11.0	2.0	0	290	<1.0
potato onion (*Stella D'oro*), 4 pcs.	70	2.0	11.0	2.0	0	300	0
salsa (*Stella D'oro*), 4 pcs.	70	2.0	11.0	1.5	0	250	<1.0
salted (*Stella D'oro*), 4 pcs.	70	2.0	11.0	2.0	0	290	<1.0
sesame:							
(*Stella D'oro*), 1 pc.	50	1.0	7.0	2.5	0	45	<1.0
(*Stella D'oro* Low-fat), 2 pcs.	70	2.0	14.0	1.0	0	90	1.0
thin (*Pepperidge Farm*), 7 pcs. ...	60	2.0	11.0	1.5	5	125	<1.0
sourdough (*Bread du Jour*), 1 pc.	130	3.0	17.0	1.0	0	280	1.0
wheat (*Stella D'oro*), 1 pc.	40	1.0	6.0	1.0	0	20	0

Food and Measure	cal.	prot. (gms)	carbo. (gms)	fat (gms)	chol. (mgs)	sod. (mgs)	fiber (gms)
Breadstick, frozen or refrigerated:							
(*Pillsbury*), 1 pc.	110	3.0	19.0	2.0	0	290	<1.0
garlic (*New York*), 1 pc.	130	3.0	22.0	4.0	0	270	1.0
garlic and herb (*Pillsbury*), 2 pcs.	180	4.0	25.0	7.0	0	580	<1.0
Breakfast bar, see "Granola and cereal bar"							
Breakfast dishes, see specific listings							
Breakfast sandwich, frozen (see also "Burrito, breakfast"), 1 pc.:							
Canadian bacon and cheese on muffin (*Swanson Great Starts*)	290	14.0	25.0	15.0	95	750	2.0
egg pocket, w/sausage and cheese (*Croissant Pockets*)	340	13.0	39.0	15.0	95	740	2.0
English muffin (*Weight Watchers*)	210	13.0	28.0	5.0	20	420	2.0
sausage, egg, and cheese, on biscuit (*Swanson Great Starts*)	460	16.0	37.0	28.0	115	1060	3.0
vegetarian:							
bagel (*Morningstar Farms Scramblers*)	320	28.0	40.0	4.5	10	900	4.0
English muffin (*Morningstar Farms Scramblers*)	240	22.0	32.0	2.5	5	700	5.0
English muffin, cheese (*Morningstar Farms Scramblers*)	280	28.0	35.0	3.0	10	1000	5.0

Food and Measure	cal.	prot. (gms)	carbo. (gms)	fat (gms)	chol. (mgs)	sod. (mgs)	fiber (gms)
Broad beans:							
raw, ½ cup	40	3.1	6.4	.4	0	28	2.3
boiled, drained, 4 oz.	64	5.4	11.5	.6	0	47	<3.0
Broad beans, mature:							
boiled, ½ cup	93	6.5	16.7	.3	0	4	4.6
canned, ½ cup:							
(*Progresso* Fava)	110	6.0	20.0	.5	0	250	5.0
w/liquid	91	7.0	15.9	.3	0	580	n.a.
Broccoli, fresh:							
raw:							
8.7-oz. stalk	42	4.5	7.9	.5	0	40	4.5
chopped, ½ cup . . .	12	1.3	2.3	.2	0	12	1.3
boiled, drained:							
stalk, 6.3 oz.	51	5.4	9.1	.6	0	46	5.2
chopped, ½ cup . . .	22	2.3	3.9	.2	0	20	2.3
Broccoli, freeze-dried							
(*AlpineAire*), ¼ oz.	25	2.0	4.0	0	0	20	2.0
Broccoli, frozen,							
1 cup, except as							
noted:							
(*Birds Eye/Freshlike*							
Stir Fry)	30	2.0	5.0	0	0	30	2.0
(*Seneca*)	25	2.0	4.0	0	0	25	3.0
(*Seneca* Normandy)	30	1.0	5.0	0	0	20	3.0
(*Seneca* Stir Fry)	30	1.0	6.0	0	0	15	3.0
spears:							
(*Birds Eye*), 3 pcs.	25	3.0	4.0	0	0	20	2.0
(*Freshlike*), 2 pcs.	25	3.0	4.0	0	0	25	2.0
(*Green Giant* Se-							
lect), 3 oz.	25	2.0	4.0	0	0	20	2.0
(*Green Giant Har-							
vest Fresh*),							
3.5 oz.	25	2.0	4.0	0	0	125	2.0
baby (*Birds Eye*),							
3 pcs.	25	3.0	4.0	0	0	10	3.0
10-oz. pkg.	84	8.7	15.2	1.0	0	49	8.5
florets:							
(*Birds Eye*), 3 oz.	25	3.0	5.0	0	0	30	3.0
(*Green Giant* Se-							
lect), 1⅓ cups . . .	25	2.0	4.0	0	0	20	2.0
(*Seabrook*)	25	2.0	4.0	0	0	20	2.0

Food and Measure	cal.	prot. (gms)	carbo. (gms)	fat (gms)	chol. (mgs)	sod. (mgs)	fiber (gms)
Broccoli, frozen, florets *(cont.)*							
baby (*Birds Eye Farm Fresh*)	25	2.0	4.0	0	0	20	2.0
cuts:							
(*Birds Eye*), ½ cup	25	2.0	5.0	0	0	30	3.0
(*Cascadian Farm*), ½ cup	24	3.0	4.0	0	0	20	3.0
(*Freshlike*)	25	2.0	4.0	0	0	20	2.0
(*Green Giant*)	25	2.0	4.0	0	0	25	2.0
(*Green Giant Harvest Fresh*), ⅔ cup	25	2.0	4.0	0	0	150	2.0
chopped:							
(*Birds Eye*), ½ cup	25	2.0	5.0	0	0	15	2.0
(*Freshlike*), ½ cup	25	2.0	4.0	0	0	20	2.0
(*Green Giant*), ¾ cup	25	2.0	4.0	0	0	25	2.0
10-oz. pkg.	75	8.0	13.6	.8	0	68	8.5
in butter sauce, spears (*Green Giant*), 4 oz.	50	2.0	7.0	1.5	<5	330	2.0
in cheese sauce:							
(*Birds Eye Side Orders*), ½ cup	70	3.0	7.0	4.0	5	500	2.0
(*Freezer Queen* Family), ⅔ cup	50	2.0	6.0	2.0	5	340	2.0
(*Green Giant*), ⅔ cup	70	3.0	9.0	2.5	<5	520	2.0
cheddar (*Cascadian Farm*), ½ cup . . .	60	5.0	7.0	2.5	5	290	3.0
Broccoli combinations, frozen:							
baby:							
(*Birds Eye* Blend), ¾ cup	70	4.0	8.0	1.5	0	30	3.0
(*Freshlike* Blend), ⅔ cup	70	4.0	8.0	1.5	0	30	3.0
beans, onion, red pepper (*Birds Eye Farm Fresh*), ½ cup	25	2.0	6.0	0	0	15	2.0

Food and Measure	cal.	prot. (gms)	carbo. (gms)	fat (gms)	chol. (mgs)	sod. (mgs)	fiber (gms)
carrots:							
cauliflower (*Green Giant* Select Skillet), ⅔ cup	25	2.0	4.0	0	0	30	2.0
water chestnuts (*Birds Eye Farm Fresh*), ½ cup . . .	30	2.0	7.0	0	0	30	3.0
water chestnuts (*Green Giant* Select Stir-fry), ⅔ cup	25	1.0	5.0	0	0	30	2.0
cauliflower:							
(*Birds Eye* Florets), 3 oz.	25	2.0	4.0	0	0	30	2.0
(*Birds Eye Farm Fresh*), ½ cup . . .	20	2.0	4.0	0	0	20	2.0
red pepper (*Birds Eye Farm Fresh*), ½ cup	20	2.0	5.0	0	0	20	2.0
cauliflower, carrots:							
(*Birds Eye Farm Fresh*), ½ cup . . .	25	2.0	5.0	0	0	30	2.0
(*Green Giant Harvest Fresh*), 1 cup	30	2.0	5.0	0	0	125	3.0
in cheese sauce (*Birds Eye Side Orders*), ½ cup	70	3.0	7.0	4.0	5	460	2.0
in cheese sauce (*Green Giant*), ⅔ cup	80	3.0	11.0	2.5	<5	560	2.0
corn, sweet pepper, in butter sauce (*Green Giant*), ¾ cup	60	2.0	8.0	2.0	<5	300	2.0
corn, red pepper (*Birds Eye Farm Fresh*), ½ cup	50	3.0	12.0	0	0	15	3.0

Food and Measure	cal.	prot. (gms)	carbo. (gms)	fat (gms)	chol. (mgs)	sod. (mgs)	fiber (gms)
Broccoli combinations *(cont.)*							
w/pasta:							
and cauliflower, carrots, in cheese sauce (*Freezer Queen* Family), 1 cup	70	3.0	10.0	2.0	<5	290	2.0
and peas, corn, red pepper, in butter Sauce (*Green Giant*), ¾ cup	70	3.0	11.0	2.0	<5	280	2.0
red pepper, onion, mushrooms (*Birds Eye Farm Fresh*), ½ cup	25	2.0	5.0	0	0	20	2.0
Broccoli dishes, frozen:							
au gratin (*Stouffer's*), ½ cup	100	5.0	8.0	5.0	10	370	3.0
pie (*Amy's*), 7½ oz.	430	11.0	46.0	22.0	45	630	4.0
soufflé (*Melrose*), ⅓ cup	80	4.0	9.0	3.0	45	260	2.0
Broccoli rabe, fresh (*Frieda's* Rapini), ¾ cup, 3 oz.	15	2.0	3.0	0	0	15	0
Broccoli-cheese in pastry, frozen, 1 pc.:							
(*Pepperidge Farm*) . . .	240	6.0	24.0	14.0	50	430	3.0
croissant (*Sara Lee*)	280	11.0	30.0	13.0	30	430	2.0
Broccoli-cheese pocket, frozen, 1 pc.:							
(*Amy's*)	270	8.0	37.0	10.0	15	560	3.0
cheddar (*Ken & Robert's Veggie Pockets*)	250	9.0	38.0	8.0	0	460	4.0
Broiling sauce, see "Grilling sauce" and specific listings							

Food and Measure	cal.	prot. (gms)	carbo. (gms)	fat (gms)	chol. (mgs)	sod. (mgs)	fiber (gms)
Broth, see "Bouillon" and "Soup"							
Broth concentrate, see "Bouillon concentrate"							
Brown gravy, in jars, w/onions (*Franco-American*), ¼ cup	25	0	4.0	1.0	<5	340	0
Brown gravy mix:							
(*Knorr*), 2 tsp.	20	<1.0	3.0	.5	0	420	0
(*Knorr* Classic), 2 tsp.	20	<1.0	3.0	.5	0	420	0
(*Loma Linda Gravy Quik*), ¼ cup*.	20	<1.0	4.0	0	0	370	0
(*Pillsbury*), ¼ cup*	15	0	3.0	0	0	270	0
Brownie, 1 pc., except as noted:							
(*Hostess* Light)	140	1.0	28.0	2.5	10	80	1.0
chocolate:							
Bavarian (*Awrey's*)	250	3.0	29.0	15.0	60	110	1.0
decadent (*Awrey's*)	230	2.0	30.0	12.0	30	120	1.0
peanut (*Awrey's* Sensation)	230	3.0	27.0	13.0	30	135	1.0
fudge:							
(*Dolly Madison/ Hostess*)	330	3.0	54.0	11.0	45	190	1.0
(*Entenmann's*), ½ pc., 1½ oz. . . .	200	3.0	23.0	11.0	45	50	1.0
nut (*Awrey's*)	190	2.0	23.0	11.0	25	130	<1.0
nut, chewy (*Awrey's*)	210	2.0	28.0	11.0	25	115	1.0
w/out nuts (*Awrey's*)	200	2.0	30.0	9.0	30	120	1.0
mini (*Hostess* Bites), 3 pcs., 1.3 oz. . . .	170	2.0	21.0	9.0	30	80	1.0
Brownie, mix, 1 pc.*, except as noted:							
(*Arrowhead Mills*) . . .	110	2.0	27.0	0	0	100	2.0
(*Arrowhead Mills* Fat Free)	120	2.0	28.0	0	0	110	2.0
(*Betty Crocker* Original Supreme)	160	2.0	27.0	6.0	20	110	0

Food and Measure	cal.	prot. (gms)	carbo. (gms)	fat (gms)	chol. (mgs)	sod. (mgs)	fiber (gms)
Brownie, mix *(cont.)*							
(*Betty Crocker* Pouch)	190	2.0	27.0	8.0	25	130	1.0
(*Betty Crocker* T-Rex Fossils)	180	2.0	24.0	8.0	25	100	0
(*Betty Crocker* Turtle)	170	2.0	23.0	8.0	20	100	0
(*Duncan Hines* Dark 'N Chunky)	160	2.0	26.0	7.0	10	100	1.0
blonde, w/white chocolate chunks (*Duncan Hines*)	170	2.0	25.0	8.0	20	100	0
caramel (*Betty Crocker* Supreme)	190	2.0	27.0	9.0	25	120	0
cheesecake swirl (*Pillsbury* Thick 'n Fudgy)	170	2.0	21.0	9.0	30	90	<1.0
chocolate:							
chunk (*Betty Crocker* Supreme)	180	2.0	24.0	9.0	20	100	0
chunk (*Pillsbury* Thick 'n Fudgy)	160	1.0	22.0	7.0	15	90	<1.0
dark, w/*Hershey's* syrup (*Betty Crocker* Supreme)	170	2.0	25.0	7.0	20	110	0
double (*Pillsbury* Thick 'n Fudgy)	150	1.0	23.0	6.0	15	95	<1.0
German (*Betty Crocker* Supreme)	220	2.0	29.0	8.0	20	130	1.0
milk, chunk (*Duncan Hines*)	170	2.0	26.0	7.0	20	110	0
devil's food (*SnackWell's*)	140	2.0	28.0	2.5	0	205	<1.0
frosted (*Betty Crocker* Supreme)	210	2.0	31.0	9.0	20	125	1.0
fudge:							
(*Betty Crocker* Supreme)	190	2.0	30.0	7.0	20	125	1.0
(*Betty Crocker* Supreme Family) . . .	170	2.0	23.0	7.0	20	105	0
(*Duncan Hines* Dark 'N Fudgy)	170	2.0	25.0	8.0	15	110	1.0

Food and Measure	cal.	prot. (gms)	carbo. (gms)	fat (gms)	chol. (mgs)	sod. (mgs)	fiber (gms)
(*Martha White* Moist 'n Fudgy)	170	2.0	24.0	7.0	10	130	<1.0
(*Pillsbury* 15 oz.)	150	2.0	22.0	6.0	15	80	<1.0
(*Pillsbury* 21.5 oz.)	190	2.0	24.0	9.0	10	90	1.0
(*SnackWell's*)	150	2.0	29.0	2.5	0	115	1.0
(*Sweet Rewards* Low Fat)	130	2.0	27.0	2.5	0	115	1.0
(*Sweet Rewards* Reduced Fat)	140	2.0	27.0	3.5	20	110	1.0
chewy (*Duncan Hines*)	160	1.0	25.0	7.0	10	110	0
chewy (*Martha White*)	150	2.0	23.0	6.0	20	140	<1.0
chewy (*Martha White* Pan Size), 1/20 pan*	140	2.0	25.0	3.5	0	120	1.0
chocolate, dark (*Betty Crocker* Supreme)	170	2.0	24.0	7.0	20	110	0
double (*Duncan Hines*)	170	2.0	29.0	7.0	20	130	1.0
hot (*Betty Crocker* Supreme)	170	2.0	23.0	8.0	20	110	0
Mississippi mud (*Duncan Hines*)	160	1.0	27.0	6.0	10	105	0
peanut butter candy (*Betty Crocker* w/*Reese's Pieces*)	180	3.0	23.0	9.0	20	105	0
raspberry dark chocolate (*Duncan Hines*)	150	1.0	23.0	7.0	10	200	0
walnut:							
(*Betty Crocker* Supreme)	180	2.0	22.0	9.0	20	95	0
(*Duncan Hines*)	170	2.0	24.0	8.0	10	105	0
(*Martha White*)	170	2.0	23.0	8.0	10	125	1.0
(*Pillsbury* Thick 'n Fudgy)	190	2.0	24.0	10.0	20	100	1.0
wheat free (*Arrowhead Mills*)	120	3.0	26.0	2.0	0	110	2.0

Food and Measure	cal.	prot. (gms)	carbo. (gms)	fat (gms)	chol. (mgs)	sod. (mgs)	fiber (gms)
Brownie à la mode, frozen (*Weight Watchers*), 3.1 oz.	190	5.0	33.0	4.0	30	190	2.0
Browning sauce:							
(*Gravy Master*), ¼ tsp.	10	0	2.0	0	0	110	0
(*Maggi*), 1 tsp.	15	1.0	2.0	0	0	270	0
Brussels sprouts, fresh:							
raw, ½ cup	19	1.5	3.9	.1	0	11	1.8
boiled, .7-oz. sprout	8	.5	1.8	.1	0	4	.9
boiled, drained, ½ cup	30	2.0	6.8	.4	0	17	3.4
Brussels sprouts, frozen:							
(*Birds Eye* Deluxe), 11 pcs.	35	3.0	7.0	0	0	15	3.0
(*Birds Eye* Southern), 6 pcs.	35	3.0	7.0	0	0	15	3.0
(*Freshlike*), 6 pcs. ...	35	3.0	5.0	0	0	25	3.0
boiled, drained, ½ cup	33	2.8	6.5	.3	0	18	1.4
baby, in butter sauce (*Green Giant*), ⅔ cup	60	3.0	9.0	1.5	<5	270	4.0
w/cauliflower and carrots (*Birds Eye Farm Fresh*), ½ cup	30	2.0	7.0	0	0	20	3.0
Buckwheat:							
whole-grain, 1 oz. ...	97	3.8	20.3	1.0	0	<1	2.8
whole-grain, 1 cup ...	584	22.5	121.6	5.8	0	1	17.0
Buckwheat flour:							
(*Arrowhead Mills*), ¼ cup	100	4.0	21.0	1.0	0	0	3.0
1 oz.	95	3.6	20.0	.9	0	n.a.	11.4
1 cup	402	15.1	84.7	3.7	0	n.a.	12.0
Buckwheat groats, dry, except as noted:							
(*Wolff's* Kasha), ¼ cup	170	6.0	35.0	1.0	0	10	2.0
brown (*Arrowhead Mills*), ¼ cup	140	5.0	30.0	1.0	0	0	3.0
roasted:							
dry, 1 oz.	98	3.3	21.2	.8	0	3	n.a.

Food and Measure	cal.	prot. (gms)	carbo. (gms)	fat (gms)	chol. (mgs)	sod. (mgs)	fiber (gms)
cooked, 1 cup	182	6.7	39.5	1.2	0	8	n.a.
Buffalo "wing," vegetarian, frozen (*Morningstar Farms*), 5 pcs.	200	13.0	16.0	9.0	0	730	3.0
Buffalo wing sauce, 2 tbsp., except as noted:							
(*Heinz*)	15	0	4.0	0	0	750	1.0
(*Stubb's*), 1 tbsp. ...	10	0	2.0	0	0	65	0
(*World Harbors* After Glow Hot Zings) ...	30	0	7.0	0	0	390	0
hot (*Nance's* Chicken Wing)	15	0	3.0	0	0	650	0
mild (*Nance's* Chicken Wing)	20	0	4.0	0	0	630	0
Bulgur:							
dry:							
(*Arrowhead Mills*), ¼ cup	150	5.0	33.0	.5	0	0	4.0
1 oz.	97	3.5	21.5	.4	0	5	5.2
1 cup	479	17.2	106.2	1.9	0	23	25.6
cooked, 1 cup	152	5.6	33.8	.4	0	9	8.2
salad, see "Tabouli"							
Bulgur pilaf mix (*Casbah*), ¾ cup	240	10.0	36.0	1.0	0	460	4.0
Bun, see "Roll"							
Bun, sweet, 1 pc.:							
(*Dolly Madison Bear Claw*)	270	5.0	40.0	10.0	25	330	1.0
apple (*Dolly Madison* Sweet Roll)	200	3.0	33.0	6.0	5	240	0
cheese (*Entenmann's*)	300	6.0	37.0	15.0	55	300	1.0
cherry (*Dolly Madison/ Hostess* Sweet Roll)	210	3.0	34.0	6.0	10	180	1.0
cinnamon:							
(*Entenmann's Light*)	160	3.0	32.0	3.0	0	240	1.0
(*Dolly Madison* Texas)	440	7.0	69.0	15.0	25	410	1.0

Food and Measure	cal.	prot. (gms)	carbo. (gms)	fat (gms)	chol. (mgs)	sod. (mgs)	fiber (gms)
Bun, sweet, cinnamon *(cont.)*							
(*Dolly Madison/* *Hostess* Sweet Roll)	230	3.0	36.0	7.0	10	200	1.0
(*Krispy Kreme*)	220	5.0	26.0	11.0	0	160	4.0
honey:							
(*Dolly Madison*) ...	440	6.0	49.0	25.0	15	260	1.0
glazed (*Hostess*) ...	320	4.0	34.0	19.0	15	210	1.0
iced/frosted (*Hostess*)	410	5.0	42.0	24.0	20	270	1.0
sticky (*Entenmann's*)	260	4.0	39.0	10.0	40	240	1.0
Bun, sweet, frozen or refrigerated, 1 pc.:							
apple cinnamon, iced (*Pillsbury*)	150	2.0	23.0	6.0	0	320	<1.0
caramel (*Pillsbury*) ...	170	2.0	24.0	7.0	0	330	<1.0
cinnamon:							
(*Sara Lee*)	370	5.0	410	15.0	40	300	1.0
iced (*Pillsbury*)	150	2.0	23.0	6.0	0	340	<1.0
iced (*Pillsbury* Reduced Fat)	140	2.0	24.0	4.0	0	340	<1.0
cinnamon raisin, iced (*Pillsbury*)	170	2.0	26.0	6.0	0	320	<1.0
orange, iced (*Pillsbury*)	170	2.0	25.0	7.0	0	340	<1.0
Burbot, meat only:							
raw, 4 oz.	102	21.9	0	.9	68	110	0
baked, broiled, or microwaved, 4 oz. ...	130	28.1	0	1.2	87	141	0
Burdock root:							
(*Frieda's* Gobo Root), ¾ cup, 3 oz.	60	1.0	15.0	0	0	0	3.0
raw, 7.3-oz. pc.	112	1.3	13.6	.1	0	4	5.1
raw, pieces, ½ cup ...	43	.9	10.3	.1	0	3	1.9
boiled, 1" pcs., ½ cup	55	1.3	13.2	.1	0	3	1.1
Burger, vegetarian:							
canned:							
(*LaLoma* Redi-Burger), ⅝" slice	120	18.0	7.0	2.5	0	450	4.0
(*LaLoma* Vege-Burger), ¼ cup	70	11.0	2.0	1.5	0	115	1.0

Food and Measure	cal.	prot. (gms)	carbo. (gms)	fat (gms)	chol. (mgs)	sod. (mgs)	fiber (gms)
(*Worthington*),							
¼ cup	60	9.0	1.0	2.0	0	270	1.0
frozen, crumbles:							
(*Green Giant Harvest Burger* for							
Recipes), ⅔ cup	90	15.0	7.0	0	0	370	3.0
(*Morningstar Farms* Recipe Crumbles),							
⅔ cup	90	10.0	4.0	3.0	0	260	2.0
(*Natural Touch* Crumbles), ½ cup	60	10.0	4.0	0	0	260	2.0
frozen patties, see "Burger, vegetarian, patty, frozen"							
mix, dry:							
(*Fantastic Nature's Burger* Original),							
¼ cup or 1 patty*	170	8.0	30.0	3.0	0	320	5.0
(*Loma Linda*), ¼ cup chunks or							
3 tbsp. granules	70	10.0	6.0	1.0	0	350	3.0
(*Natural Touch* Burger Kit),							
¼ pkg.	80	14.0	6.0	0	0	360	4.0
(*Worthington Granburger*),							
3 tbsp.	60	10.0	3.0	.5	0	410	1.0
barbecue (*Fantastic Nature's Burger*),							
cup or 1 patty*	170	7.0	34.0	1.5	0	580	5.0
southwestern (*Natural Touch* Burger Kit), ¼ pkg.	90	12.0	9.0	0	0	360	4.0
refrigerated:							
(*Morningstar Farms* Quarter Prime),							
3.4 oz.	140	24.0	6.0	2.0	0	370	3.0
garden vegetable (*Morningstar Farms*), 3.5 oz.	150	17.0	12.0	3.5	0	390	5.0

Food and Measure	cal.	prot. (gms)	carbo. (gms)	fat (gms)	chol. (mgs)	sod. (mgs)	fiber (gms)
Burger, vegetarian, patty, frozen, 2½-oz. pc., except as noted:							
(*Fantastic Nature's Burger* Classic)	110	18.0	4.0	3.0	0	340	4.0
(*Fantastic Nature's Burger* Original) ...	140	7.0	23.0	3.0	0	440	4.0
(*Gardenburger* Original)	130	8.0	18.0	3.0	15	290	5.0
(*Gardenburger* Veggie Medley)	100	6.0	17.0	0	0	280	3.0
(*Green Giant Harvest Burger* Original), 3.2 oz.	140	18.0	8.0	4.0	0	370	5.0
(*Ken & Robert's Veggie Burger*)	130	5.0	26.0	1.0	0	260	3.0
(*Morningstar Farms Hard Rock Cafe*), 3 oz.	170	6.0	18.0	8.0	0	340	3.0
(*Morningstar Farms Prime*), 3.4 oz.	140	24.0	6.0	2.0	0	370	3.0
(*Morningstar Farms Better'n Burger*), 2.8 oz.	70	11.0	6.0	0	0	360	3.0
(*Morningstar Farms Grillers*)	140	14.0	5.0	6.0	0	260	3.0
(*Natural Touch* Vegan Burger), 2¾ oz. ...	70	11.0	6.0	0	0	370	3.0
(*VegiBurger*), 3 oz.	110	13.0	12.0	1.0	0	320	1.0
bean, zesty (*Gardenburger*) ...	120	7.0	19.0	2.5	10	290	5.0
black bean: Southwestern (*Fantastic Nature's Burger*)	150	7.0	20.0	2.0	0	290	4.0
spicy (*Morningstar Farms*), 2¾ oz.	110	11.0	16.0	2.0	0	470	5.0
spicy (*Natural Touch*), 2¾ oz.	100	11.0	15.0	1.0	0	330	5.0

Food and Measure	cal.	prot. (gms)	carbo. (gms)	fat (gms)	chol. (mgs)	sod. (mgs)	fiber (gms)
California (*Amy's* Veggie Burger)	100	4.0	17.0	3.0	0	290	3.0
Chicago (*Amy's* Veggie Burger)	100	6.0	9.0	4.0	5	190	2.0
fire-roasted vegetable (*Gardenburger*) . . .	120	7.0	17.0	3.0	10	270	2.0
garden grill (*Morningstar Farms*)	120	6.0	18.0	2.5	0	280	4.0
garden vegetable: (*Morningstar Farms*), 2.4 oz.	100	10.0	9.0	2.5	0	350	4.0
(*Natural Touch*), 2³/₄ oz.	110	10.0	8.0	2.5	0	280	3.0
Greek, classic (*Gardenburger*) . . .	120	6.0	17.0	3.0	10	310	2.0
hamburger style: (*Gardenburger* Fat Free)	100	16.0	7.0	0	0	370	3.0
(*Gardenburger* Low Fat)	110	16.0	7.0	2.5	5	380	3.0
Italian (*Green Giant Harvest Burger*), 3.2 oz.	140	17.0	8.0	4.5	0	370	5.0
mushroom, savory (*Gardenburger*) . . .	120	6.0	18.0	3.0	10	270	4.0
roasted red pepper and garlic (*Fantastic Nature's Burger*) . . .	130	6.0	20.0	2.5	0	350	3.0
Southwestern (*Green Giant Harvest Burger*), 3.2 oz. . . .	140	16.0	9.0	4.0	0	370	5.0
Texas (*Amy's* Veggie Burger)	130	12.0	15.0	2.5	0	270	3.0
tofu (*Natural Touch* Okara), 2¹/₄ oz.	110	11.0	4.0	5.0	0	360	3.0
Burger King, 1 serving:							
breakfast dishes:							
biscuit	300	6.0	35.0	15.0	0	830	1.0
biscuit w/egg	380	11.0	37.0	21.0	140	1010	<1.0

Food and Measure	cal.	prot. (gms)	carbo. (gms)	fat (gms)	Chol. (mgs)	sod. (mgs)	fiber (gms)
Burger King, breakfast dishes *(cont.)*							
biscuit w/sausage and egg	490	13.0	36.0	33.0	35	1240	1.0
biscuit w/sausage, egg, and cheese	620	20.0	37.0	43.0	185	1650	1.0
cini-minis, w/out vanilla icing, 4 pcs.	440	6.0	51.0	23.0	25	710	1.0
Croissan'wich, w/sausage, cheese	450	13.0	21.0	35.0	45	940	1.0
Croissan'wich, w/sausage, egg, and cheese	530	18.0	23.0	41.0	185	1120	1.0
french toast sticks, 5 pcs.	440	7.0	51.0	23.0	2	490	3.0
hash browns, large	410	3.0	42.0	26.0	0	750	4.0
hash brown, small	240	2.0	25.0	15.0	0	440	2.0
breakfast components:							
bacon, 3 pcs.	40	3.0	0	3.0	10	170	0
ham	35	6.0	0	1.0	15	770	0
A.M. Express jam:							
grape..........	30	0	7.0	0	0	0	0
strawberry	30	0	8.0	0	0	0	0
vanilla icing, 1 oz.	110	0	20.0	3.0	0	40	0
whipped classic blend	65	0	0	7.0	1	75	0
sandwiches:							
bacon cheeseburger	400	24.0	27.0	22.0	70	940	1.0
bacon double cheeseburger ...	620	41.0	28.0	38.0	125	1230	1.0
Big King	640	38.0	28.0	42.0	125	980	1.0
BK Big Fish	720	23.0	59.0	43.0	80	1180	3.0
BK Broiler chicken	530	29.0	45.0	26.0	105	1060	2.0
BK Broiler chicken, w/out mayo	370	29.0	45.0	9.0	105	1060	2.0
cheeseburger	360	21.0	27.0	19.0	60	760	1.0
chicken	710	26.0	54.0	43.0	60	1400	2.0
chicken, w/out mayo	500	26.0	54.0	20.0	60	1400	2.0
Chick'N Crisp	460	16.0	37.0	27.0	35	890	3.0
Chick'N Crisp, w/out mayo..........	360	16.0	37.0	16.0	35	890	3.0

Food and Measure	cal.	prot. (gms)	carbo. (gms)	fat (gms)	chol. (mgs)	sod. (mgs)	fiber (gms)
double cheese-burger	580	38.0	27.0	36.0	120	1060	1.0
Double Whopper	920	49.0	47.0	59.0	155	980	3.0
Double Whopper, w/out mayo	760	49.0	47.0	42.0	155	980	3.0
Double Whopper, w/cheese	1010	55.0	47.0	67.0	180	1460	3.0
Double Whopper, w/cheese, w/out mayo	850	55.0	47.0	50.0	180	1460	3.0
hamburger	320	19.0	27.0	15.0	50	520	1.0
Whopper	660	29.0	47.0	40.0	85	900	3.0
Whopper, w/out mayo	510	29.0	47.0	23.0	85	900	3.0
Whopper, w/cheese	760	35.0	47.0	48.0	110	1380	3.0
Whopper, w/cheese, w/out mayo	600	35.0	47.0	31.0	110	1380	3.0
Whopper Jr.	400	19.0	28.0	24.0	55	530	2.0
Whopper Jr., w/out mayo	320	19.0	28.0	15.0	55	530	2.0
Whopper Jr., w/cheese	450	22.0	28.0	28.0	65	770	2.0
Whopper Jr., w/cheese, w/out mayo	370	22.0	28.0	19.0	65	770	2.0
sandwich condiments:							
Bull's Eye barbecue Sauce, 1/2 oz.	20	0	5.0	0	0	140	0
ketchup, 1/2 oz.	15	0	4.0	0	0	180	0
King sauce, 1/2 oz.	70	0	2.0	7.0	4	70	0
tartar sauce, 1 1/2 oz.	260	0	0	29.0	20	330	0
Chicken Tenders:							
4 pcs.	180	11.0	9.0	11.0	30	470	0
5 pcs.	230	14.0	11.0	14.0	40	590	<1.0
8 pcs.	350	22.0	17.0	22.0	65	940	1.0
dipping sauces, 1 oz.:							
barbecue	35	0	9.0	0	0	400	0
honey flavored	90	0	23.0	0	0	10	0
honey mustard	90	0	10.0	6.0	1	150	0
ranch	170	0	2.0	17.0	3	200	0
sweet and sour	45	0	11.0	0	0	50	0

Food and Measure	cal.	prot. (gms)	carbo. (gms)	fat (gms)	chol. (mgs)	sod. (mgs)	fiber (gms)
Burger King (cont.)							
side orders:							
french fries:							
small	250	2.0	32.0	13.0	0	550	2.0
medium	400	3.0	50.0	21.0	0	820	4.0
king size	590	5.0	74.0	30.0	0	1180	5.0
french fries, w/out salt added:							
small	250	2.0	32.0	13.0	0	480	2.0
medium	400	3.0	50.0	21.0	0	760	4.0
king size	590	5.0	74.0	30.0	0	1110	5.0
onion rings:							
medium	380	5.0	46.0	19.0	2	550	4.0
king size	600	8.0	74.0	30.0	4	880	6.0
dessert/shakes:							
Dutch apple pie	300	3.0	39.0	15.0	0	230	2.0
shakes:							
chocolate, small	330	9.0	58.0	7.0	25	250	3.0
chocolate, medium	440	12.0	75.0	10.0	30	330	4.0
vanilla, small	330	10.0	56.0	7.0	20	250	1.0
vanilla, medium	430	13.0	73.0	9.0	30	350	2.0
shakes, syrup added:							
chocolate, small	390	10.0	72.0	7.0	20	350	2.0
chocolate, medium	570	14.0	105.0	10.0	30	520	3.0
strawberry, small	390	10.0	72.0	7.0	20	260	1.0
strawberry, medium	550	13.0	104.0	9.0	30	350	2.0
Burrito, frozen, 1 pc.:							
bean, black, vegetable (*Amy's*)	320	9.0	54.0	8.0	0	480	4.0
bean and cheese:							
(*Amy's*)	280	10.0	43.0	8.0	10	460	6.0
(*Old El Paso*)	300	12.0	44.0	9.0	15	840	3.0
(*Patio*)	300	9.0	46.0	9.0	15	590	4.0
bean and rice (*Amy's*)	250	9.0	44.0	5.0	0	450	6.0
beef and bean:							
(*Hormel Quick Meal*)	300	9.0	37.0	13.0	40	550	3.0

Food and Measure	cal.	prot. (gms)	carbo. (gms)	fat (gms)	chol. (mgs)	sod. (mgs)	fiber (gms)
hot (*Old El Paso*) . . .	320	12.0	45.0	10.0	15	850	3.0
hot (*Patio*)	320	10.0	43.0	12.0	25	840	4.0
hot, red chili peppers (*Patio*)	320	10.0	42.0	12.0	20	850	4.0
medium (*Old El Paso*)	320	12.0	46.0	10.0	15	800	3.0
medium (*Patio*)	310	10.0	45.0	10.0	20	860	4.0
mild (*Old El Paso*)	320	12.0	48.0	9.0	15	690	4.0
mild (*Patio*)	330	10.0	45.0	12.0	20	890	4.0
cheese (*Hormel Quick Meal*)	250	9.0	41.0	6.0	30	640	4.0
chicken (*Patio*)	290	11.0	44.0	8.0	20	740	2.0
chili, red (*Hormel Quick Meal*)	280	9.0	37.0	11.0	35	560	3.0
pizza:							
cheese (*Old El Paso*)	240	13.0	27.0	9.0	20	430	0
pepperoni (*Old El Paso*)	260	12.0	31.0	10.0	20	510	0
sausage (*Old El Paso*)	250	11.0	32.0	9.0	15	420	0
Burrito, breakfast, frozen, 1 pkg.:							
(*Amy's*)	230	9.0	38.0	5.0	0	480	5.0
bacon (*Swanson Great Starts*)	250	0	27.0	11.0	90	540	1.0
Burrito dinner, frozen, 16 oz.:							
beef (*Chi-Chi's* Burro)	590	27.0	76.0	19.0	55	2060	11.0
chicken (*Chi-Chi's* Burro)	540	26.0	77.0	14.0	55	2110	10.0
Burrito dinner mix: (*Chi-Chi's* Kit),							
2 shells, seasoning	300	7.0	52.0	7.0	0	1180	2.0
(*Old El Paso* Kit), 1 pc.*	290	15.0	26.0	14.0	40	780	1.0
Burrito seasoning mix:							
(*Lawry's*), 1 tbsp. . . .	30	1.0	6.0	0	0	700	0
(*Old El Paso*), 2 tsp.	20	<1.0	4.0	0	0	340	<1.0

Food and Measure	cal.	prot. (gms)	carbo. (gms)	fat (gms)	chol. (mgs)	sod. (mgs)	fiber (gms)
Butter:							
regular, unsalted:							
(*Land O Lakes*),							
1 tbsp.	100	0	0	11.0	30	0	0
stick or 4 oz.	813	1.0	0	92.0	248	12	0
1 tbsp.	100	.1	0	11.4	31	1	0
1 tsp.	34	<.1	0	3.8	10	<1	0
regular, salted:							
(*Land O Lakes*),							
1 tbsp.	100	0	0	11.0	30	80	0
1 stick or 4 oz. . . .	813	1.0	0	92.0	248	937	0
1 tbsp.	100	.1	0	11.4	31	115	0
1 tsp.	34	<.1	0	3.8	10	39	0
whipped, unsalted:							
(*Land O Lakes*),							
1 tbsp.	70	0	0	7.0	20	50	0
½ cup or 1 stick . . .	542	.6	<.1	61.3	165	8	0
1 tbsp.	67	.1	tr.	7.6	20	1	0
1 tsp.	23	tr.	tr.	2.6	7	<1	0
whipped, salted:							
(*Land O Lakes*),							
1 tbsp.	70	0	0	7.0	20	0	0
½ cup or 1 stick . . .	542	.6	<.1	61.3	165	625	0
1 tbsp.	67	.1	tr.	7.6	20	78	0
1 tsp.	23	tr.	tr.	2.6	7	26	0
light (see also "Margarine"), 1 tbsp.:							
salted:							
(*Land O Lakes*)	50	0	0	6.0	20	70	0
whipped (*Land O Lakes*)	35	0	0	3.5	10	45	0
unsalted (*Land O Lakes*)	50	0	0	6.0	20	0	0
Butter, flavored,							
1 tbsp.:							
honey:							
(*Downey's*)	60	0	8.0	1.0	<5	10	0
(*Land O Lakes*)	90	0	4.0	8.0	15	35	0
roasted garlic (*Land O Lakes*)	100	0	0	11.0	20	95	0

Food and Measure	cal.	prot. (gms)	carbo. (gms)	fat (gms)	chol. (mgs)	sod. (mgs)	fiber (gms)
Butter flavor sprinkles, 1 tsp.:							
(*Molly McButter*)	5	0	1.0	0	0	180	0
garlic-herb (*Molly McButter*)	5	0	1.0	0	0	125	0
Butter oil, see "Oil"							
Butter salt (*Durkee*), ½ tsp.	0	0	0	0	0	340	0
Butterbeans, see "Lima beans"							
Butterbur:							
fresh:							
raw, .2-oz. stalk . . .	1	<.1	.2	<.1	0	<1	<1.0
boiled, drained, 4 oz.	9	.3	2.4	<.1	0	5	n.a.
canned, chopped, ½ cup	2	.1	.2	.1	0	3	n.a.
Buttercup squash (*Frieda's*), ¾ cup, 3 oz.	30	1.0	7.0	0	0	0	1.0
Butterfish, meat only:							
raw, 4 oz.	166	19.6	0	9.1	74	100	0
baked, broiled, or microwaved, 4 oz. . . .	212	25.1	0	11.7	94	129	0
Buttermilk, see "Milk"							
Butternut, dried:							
in shell, 1 lb.	750	30.5	14.8	69.8	0	1	5.8
shelled, 1 oz.	174	7.1	3.4	16.2	0	<1	1.3
Butternut squash, fresh:							
(*Frieda's*), ¾ cup, 3 oz.	40	1.0	10.0	0	0	0	2.0
raw, cubed, ½ cup . . .	32	.7	8.1	.1	0	3	1.1
baked, cubed, ½ cup	41	.9	10.7	.1	0	4	2.9
Butternut squash, frozen:							
12-oz. pkg.	192	6.0	49.0	.3	0	8	4.4
boiled, drained, mashed, ½ cup	47	1.5	12.1	.1	0	2	n.a.

Food and Measure	cal.	prot. (gms)	carbo. (gms)	fat (gms)	chol. (mgs)	sod. (mgs)	fiber (gms)
Butterscotch baking chips, 1 tbsp.:							
(*Hershey's*)	80	<1.0	10.0	4.0	0	10	0
(*Nestlé*)	80	0	9.0	4.0	0	15	0
Butterscotch caramel topping, see "Butterscotch topping"							
Butterscotch syrup (*Smucker's* Sundae), 2 tbsp.	110	0	27.0	0	0	70	0
Butterscotch topping, 2 tbsp.:							
(*Kraft*)	130	<1.0	28.0	1.5	<5	150	0
(*Mrs. Richardson's*)	130	<1.0	30.0	1.0	0	200	0
(*Smucker's* Fat Free)	130	0	31.0	0	0	0	<1.0
caramel: (*Smucker's* Special Recipe)	130	1.0	30.0	1.0	<5	70	<1.0
fudge (*Mrs. Richardson's*)	130	<1.0	30.0	1.5	<5	60	0

C

Food and Measure	cal.	prot. (gms)	carbo. (gms)	fat (gms)	chol. (mgs)	sod. (mgs)	fiber (gms)
Cabbage:							
raw:							
5¾″ head, 2½ lbs.	228	13.1	49.3	2.4	0	164	20.9
shredded, ½ cup ...	9	.5	1.9	.1	0	6	.8
boiled, drained, shred-							
ded, ½ cup	17	.8	3.4	.3	0	6	2.1
Cabbage, Chinese,							
½ cup, except as							
noted:							
bok choy:							
(*Frieda's*), 1 cup,							
3 oz.	10	1.0	2.0	0	0	55	1.0
raw, whole, 1 lb.	52	6.0	8.7	.8	0	257	4.0
raw, shredded	5	.5	.8	.1	0	23	.4
boiled, drained,							
shredded	10	1.3	1.5	.1	0	29	1.4
pe-tsai:							
raw, whole, 1 lb.	68	5.1	13.6	.8	0	38	4.2
raw, shredded	6	.5	1.2	.1	0	3	.4
boiled, drained,							
shredded	8	.9	1.4	.1	0	6	1.0
Cabbage, dehydrated,							
diced (*AlpineAire*),							
.7 oz.	70	3.0	13.0	.5	0	40	5.0
Cabbage, marinated,							
see "Kim chee"							
Cabbage, mustard							
(*Frieda's*), 1 cup,							
3 oz.	20	2.0	4.0	0	0	20	2.0
Cabbage, napa							
(*Frieda's*), 1 cup,							
3 oz.	15	1.0	3.0	0	0	10	1.0

Food and Measure	cal.	prot. (gms)	carbo. (gms)	fat (gms)	chol. (mgs)	sod. (mgs)	fiber (gms)
Cabbage, red, fresh:							
raw, whole, 1 lb.	100	5.0	22.2	.9	0	38	7.3
raw, shredded, ½ cup	10	.5	2.1	.1	0	4	.7
boiled, drained, shred-							
ded, ½ cup	16	.8	3.5	.2	0	6	1.5
Cabbage, red, in jars,							
sweet and sour							
(*Greenwood*),							
½ cup	100	1.0	24.0	0	0	380	0
Cabbage, savoy:							
raw, whole, 1 lb.	100	7.3	22.1	.4	0	102	11.2
raw, shredded, ½ cup	10	.7	2.1	<.1	0	10	1.1
boiled, drained, shred-							
ded, ½ cup	18	1.3	4.0	.1	0	17	n.a.
Cabbage entree, fro-							
zen, stuffed,							
w/whipped potato							
(*Lean Cuisine*),							
9½ oz.	170	8.0	24.0	5.0	15	380	5.0
Cactus pads							
(*Frieda's*), ¾ cup,							
3 oz.	20	1.0	4.0	0	0	5	1.0
Cactus pear, see							
"Prickly pear"							
Cake, ⅛ cake, except							
as noted:							
almond-topped (*En-*							
tenmann's)	180	4.0	23.0	8.0	25	120	<1.0
angel food:							
(*Dolly Madison*),							
⅕ cake	160	3.0	34.0	1.5	0	190	1.0
(*Hostess*)	160	3.0	33.0	1.5	0	180	1.0
apple, crumb-topped							
(*Entenmann's*							
Orchard Delight) ...	260	3.0	40.0	10	15	140	1.0
banana:							
chocolate chip (*Aw-*							
rey's Marquise),							
1/16 cake	310	2.0	40.0	17.0	30	190	<1.0
crunch (*En-*							
tenmann's)	220	2.0	32.0	9.0	40	280	<1.0

Food and Measure	cal.	prot. (gms)	carbo. (gms)	fat (gms)	chol. (mgs)	sod. (mgs)	fiber (gms)
frosted (*Entenmann's*), ⅙ cake	370	3.0	50.0	19.0	55	290	<1.0
loaf (*Entenmann's Light*)	140	2.0	33.0	0	0	260	<1.0
sheet (*Awrey's*), 1/24 cake	350	3.0	40.0	20.0	55	290	<1.0
Black Forest torte (*Awrey's*), 1/12 cake	350	3.0	38.0	22.0	45	330	1.0
blueberry crumb (*Entenmann's* Orchard Delight)	250	2.0	38.0	10.0	20	190	1.0
Boston cream (*Awrey's*), 1/16 cake	190	2.0	30.0	7.0	25	230	0
butter (*Entenmann's* Sunshine), ⅙ cake	310	4.0	43.0	14.0	100	350	<1.0
carrot, iced:							
cream cheese (*Awrey's* 2-Layer), 1/16 cake	390	4.0	44.0	22.0	40	300	1.0
sheet (*Awrey's* Supreme), 1/24 cake	400	5.0	47.0	23.0	50	350	2.0
cheesecake, pineapple (*Entenmann's*), ⅕ cake	350	7.0	37.0	19.0	85	300	<1.0
cherry cordial (*Awrey's* Marquise), 1/16 cake	240	2.0	30.0	14.0	25	190	<1.0
chocolate:							
chip crumb (*Entenmann's*)	370	3.0	45.0	20.0	35	180	<1.0
crunch (*Entenmann's*), ⅑ cake	300	3.0	46.0	12.0	25	360	1.0
double, butter cream (*Awrey's* 3-Layer), 1/16 cake	310	3.0	48.0	13.0	40	320	2.0
double, butter cream (*Awrey's* 2-Layer), 1/16 cake	250	3.0	38.0	11.0	35	280	1.0

Food and Measure	cal.	prot. (gms)	carbo. (gms)	fat (gms)	chol. (mgs)	sod. (mgs)	fiber (gms)
Cake, chocolate *(cont.)*							
double, sheet (*Awrey's*), 1/24 cake	310	4.0	48.0	13.0	40	330	2.0
double, torte (*Awrey's*), 1/12 cake	340	3.0	52.0	15.0	35	320	2.0
German, butter cream (*Awrey's* 3-Layer), 1/16 cake	360	4.0	46.0	19.0	40	290	<1.0
German, sheet (*Awrey's*), 1/24 cake	340	4.0	41.0	19.0	45	290	0
peanut (*Awrey's* Marquise Fantasy), 1/16 cake ...	330	5.0	38.0	19.0	25	270	<1.0
tropical (*Awrey's* Marquise), 1/16 cake	230	3.0	34.0	11.0	25	210	<1.0
white iced (*Awrey's* 2-Layer), 1/16 cake	270	3.0	34.0	15.0	40	290	1.0
coconut, butter cream:							
sheet (*Awrey's*), 1/24 cake	380	3.0	43.0	22.0	55	360	0
yellow (*Awrey's* 3-Layer), 1/16 cake	360	3.0	41.0	21.0	45	320	0
coffee cake:							
(*Awrey's* Long John), 1/12 cake	190	2.0	21.0	12.0	10	75	0
cheese (*Entenmann's*)	160	3.0	21.0	7.0	25	140	<1.0
Danish ring (*Entenmann's*), 1/5 cake	250	4.0	27.0	14.0	30	200	<1.0
Danish twist:							
cheese (*Entenmann's*)	230	3.0	28.0	12.0	30	200	<1.0
cinnamon apple (*Entenmann's Light*)	140	2.0	34.0	0	0	160	1.0
lemon (*Entenmann's Light*)	130	2.0	29.0	0	0	190	1.0
raspberry (*Entenmann's Light*)	140	2.0	32.0	0	0	180	1.0
(*Entenmann's* Louisiana Crunch), 1/9 cake	330	3.0	47.0	14.0	47	290	<1.0

Food and Measure	cal.	prot. (gms)	carbo. (gms)	fat (gms)	chol. (mgs)	sod. (mgs)	fiber (gms)
(*Entenmann's* Metropolitan), ⅙ cake ...	340	3.0	46.0	16.0	45	270	<1.0
espresso, French (*Awrey's* Marquise), 1/16 cake	320	2.0	30.0	22.0	30	210	<1.0
fruit (*Benson's* Old Home), 4 slices, 4.6 oz.	470	6.0	78.0	16.0	20	240	4.0
golden:							
loaf (*Entenmann's Light*)	130	2.0	28.0	0	0	190	<1.0
fudge iced (*Entenmann's*), ⅙ cake	340	3.0	48.0	16.0	50	260	1.0
lemon:							
butter cream (*Awrey's* 3-Layer), 1/16 cake	320	2.0	38.0	19.0	45	320	0
butter cream (*Awrey's* 2-Layer), 1/16 cake	290	2.0	34.0	17.0	40	300	0
coconut (*Entenmann's*), ⅙ cake	380	3.0	44.0	22.0	50	300	<1.0
crunch (*Entenmann's*), ⅑ cake	320	3.0	48.0	13.0	50	280	<1.0
marble loaf (*Entenmann's Light*)	130	2.0	28.0	0	0	210	<1.0
Neapolitan torte (*Awrey's*), 1/12 cake	360	3.0	41.0	21.0	45	330	0
old fashioned loaf (*Entenmann's*)	200	2.0	27.0	9.0	40	200	<1.0
orange:							
butter cream (*Awrey's* 3-Layer), 1/16 cake	330	2.0	41.0	18.0	35	280	0
sheet (*Awrey's* Frosty), 1/24 cake	350	3.0	43.0	18.0	45	340	0
peach, Georgia (*Awrey's* Marquise), 1/16 cake..........	260	2.0	34.0	14.0	30	240	0

Food and Measure	cal.	prot. (gms)	carbo. (gms)	fat (gms)	chol. (mgs)	sod. (mgs)	fiber (gms)
Cake *(cont.)*							
pineapple loaf (*Entenmann's*)	220	3.0	30.0	11.0	45	210	0
pound, golden (*Awrey's*), 1/6 cake	130	1.0	20.0	5.0	10	85	<1.0
raisin loaf (*Entenmann's*)	220	3.0	33.0	8.0	45	200	1.0
raspberry and cream (*Awrey's* Marquise), 1/16 cake	260	2.0	34.0	14.0	25	210	0
raspberry nut (*Awrey's* Marquise), 1/16 cake	310	3.0	38.0	17.0	30	180	0
rocky road (*Entenmann's*)	260	3.0	39.0	12.0	15	220	2.0
sour cream loaf (*Entenmann's*)	220	1.0	24.0	12.0	50	150	<1.0
sponge, no icing, sheet (*Awrey's*), 1/24 cake	190	3.0	28.0	8.0	28	320	0
strawberry:							
(*Awrey's* Supreme Marquise), 1/16 cake	240	2.0	36.0	11.0	5	290	<1.0
torte (*Awrey's*), 1/12 cake	270	3.0	37.0	12.0	40	290	<1.0
yellow, white iced, sheet (*Awrey's*), 1/24 cake	360	3.0	42.0	21.0	55	370	0
Cake, frozen, 1/8 cake, except as noted:							
Boston cream:							
(*Mrs. Smith's*)	180	2.0	27.0	7.0	20	170	0
(*Pepperidge Farm*)	260	3.0	42.0	9.0	45	120	<1.0
cappuccino (*Manzoni*), 1/5 cake	220	2.0	27.0	11.0	45	45	<1.0
carrot (*Pepperidge Farm* Deluxe)	310	2.0	39.0	16.0	40	320	1.0
cheesecake, 1/4 cake, except as noted:							
(*Sara Lee* Original)	350	7.0	39.0	18.0	50	320	1.0
(*Sara Lee* Lowfat)	310	9.0	40.0	13.0	70	310	2.0

Food and Measure	cal.	prot. (gms)	carbo. (gms)	fat (gms)	chol. (mgs)	sod. (mgs)	fiber (gms)
cherry cream (*Sara Lee*)...........	350	6.0	55.0	12.0	35	310	2.0
chocolate chip (*Sara Lee*)...........	410	8.0	47.0	21.0	65	300	2.0
chocolate mousse (*Sara Lee*), 1/5 cake	400	5.0	370	25.0	30	190	2.0
French (*Sara Lee*), 1/6 cake	350	5.0	24.0	21.0	20	280	1.0
French (*Weight Watchers*), 3.9 oz.	170	7.0	28.0	4.0	15	230	2.0
New York (*Weight Watchers*), 2½ oz.	150	6.0	21.0	5.0	15	140	1.0
strawberry cream (*Sara Lee*)	330	6.0	49.0	12.0	40	310	2.0
strawberry French (*Sara Lee*), 1/6 cake	320	4.0	43.0	14.0	20	230	1.0
chocolate layer:							
double (*Sara Lee*)	260	3.0	33.0	13.0	25	180	2.0
fudge (*Pepperidge Farm*), 1/6 cake ...	300	2.0	38.0	16.0	35	230	2.0
fudge stripe (*Pepperidge Farm*), 1/6 cake	290	2.0	38.0	14.0	35	150	2.0
German (*Pepperidge Farm*), 1/6 cake ...	300	2.0	37.0	16.0	35	280	2.0
German (*Sara Lee*)	280	4.0	34.0	15.0	30	160	2.0
chocolate mousse (*Pepperidge Farm*)	250	2.0	35.0	10.0	25	120	2.0
coconut, layer:							
(*Pepperidge Farm*), 1/6 cake	300	2.0	41.0	14.0	40	200	1.0
(*Sara Lee*)	280	3.0	34.0	14.0	30	170	2.0
coffee cake:							
butter streusel (*Sara Lee*), 1/6 cake	220	4.0	25.0	12.0	35	240	<1.0
cheese (*Sara Lee* Lowfat), 1/6 cake	180	3.0	28.0	6.0	20	230	0

Food and Measure	cal.	prot. (gms)	carbo. (gms)	fat (gms)	chol. (mgs)	sod. (mgs)	fiber (gms)
Cake, frozen, coffee cake *(cont.)*							
crumb (*Sara Lee*)	220	3.0	32.0	9.0	15	210	<1.0
pecan (*Sara Lee*), 1/6							
cake	230	4.0	24.0	12.0	25	170	<1.0
raspberry (*Sara*							
Lee), 1/6 cake	220	3.0	27.0	8.0	15	220	<1.0
devil's food layer (*Pep-*							
peridge Farm),							
1/6 cake	290	2.0	40.0	14.0	35	220	2.0
fudge, double (*Weight*							
Watchers), 2.7 oz.	190	4.0	36.0	4.0	25	200	2.0
golden layer:							
(*Pepperidge Farm*),							
1/6 cake	290	3.0	40.0	14.0	50	230	2.0
fudge (*Sara Lee*) . . .	270	3.0	34.0	13.0	25	130	1.0
lemon mousse (*Pep-*							
peridge Farm)	250	2.0	34.0	12.0	40	100	<1.0
pineapple cream (*Pep-*							
peridge Farm),							
1/9 cake	240	2.0	38.0	10.0	30	120	<1.0
pound, 1/4 cake, except							
as noted:							
(*Pepperidge Farm*							
Butter), 1/5 cake	290	5.0	39.0	13.0	110	280	<1.0
(*Sara Lee* Butter)	320	4.0	38.0	16.0	85	280	<1.0
(*Sara Lee* Butter							
Family), 1/6 cake	310	4.0	36.0	17.0	75	360	<1.0
(*Sara Lee* Lowfat)	280	4.0	42.0	11.0	65	350	<1.0
chocolate swirl							
(*Sara Lee*)	330	5.0	42.0	16.0	75	350	<1.0
strawberry swirl							
(*Sara Lee*)	290	4.0	44.0	11.0	60	140	<1.0
strawberry:							
cream (*Pepperidge*							
Farm), 1/9 cake . . .	230	2.0	38.0	9.0	30	115	1.0
layer, stripe (*Pep-*							
peridge Farm),							
1/6 cake	310	2.0	47.0	13.0	65	150	<1.0
shortcake (*Sara Lee*)	180	2.0	27.0	7.0	15	140	<1.0
tiramisu:							
(*Manzoni*), 1/5 cake	230	2.0	65.0	11.0	65	65	0

Food and Measure	cal.	prot. (gms)	carbo. (gms)	fat (gms)	chol. (mgs)	sod. (mgs)	fiber (gms)
(*Manzoni* Individual), 3½ oz.	290	3.0	39.0	13.0	95	80	1.0
vanilla layer:							
(*Pepperidge Farm*), ⅙ cake	290	2.0	41.0	13.0	45	190	<1.0
(*Sara Lee*)	250	2.0	31.0	13.0	35	140	0
zabaglione (*Manzoni*), ⅕ cake	240	2.0	28.0	12.0	65	65	0
Cake, mix, 1/12 cake*, except as noted:							
angel food:							
(*Duncan Hines*)	130	3.0	30.0	0	0	320	0
(*Pillsbury Moist Supreme*)	140	3.0	31.0	0	0	330	0
(*SuperMoist* Easy), ¼ pkg.	170	3.0	37.0	0	0	330	0
(*SuperMoist* Traditional)	130	3.0	30.0	0	0	150	0
chocolate swirl (*SuperMoist*) ...	150	3.0	34.0	0	0	310	0
confetti (*SuperMoist*) ...	150	3.0	34.0	0	0	320	0
white (*SuperMoist* One Step)	140	3.0	32.0	0	0	320	0
banana:							
(*Duncan Hines* Supreme)	250	3.0	36.0	11.0	55	270	0
(*Pillsbury Moist Supreme*)	250	3.0	35.0	11.0	55	280	0
brownie, w/mini kisses (*Betty Crocker Stir 'n Bake*), ⅙ pkg.	220	3.0	36.0	7.0	0	170	1.0
butter pecan (*SuperMoist*)	240	3.0	35.0	10.0	55	280	0
butter recipe (*Pillsbury Moist Supreme*) ...	260	3.0	36.0	12.0	75	360	0
butterscotch (*Duncan Hines*)	250	3.0	36.0	11.0	55	270	0
caramel (*Duncan Hines*)	250	3.0	36.0	11.0	55	270	0

Food and Measure	cal.	prot. (gms)	carbo. (gms)	fat (gms)	chol. (mgs)	sod. (mgs)	fiber (gms)
Cake, mix *(cont.)*							
carrot:							
(*Pillsbury Moist Supreme*)	250	3.0	34.0	11.0	55	280	<1.0
(*SuperMoist*), 1/10 cake*	320	4.0	42.0	15.0	65	340	0
w/cream cheese (*Betty Crocker Stir 'n Bake*), 1/6 pkg.	250	2.0	46.0	7.0	0	290	0
cheesecake, 1/6 cake*:							
(*Jell-O No Bake*) ...	350	7.0	46.0	16.0	5	510	1.0
(*Jell-O* Homestyle No Bake)	360	7.0	49.0	15.0	5	550	<1.0
blueberry (*Jell-O* No Bake)	320	5.0	49.0	12.0	5	390	<1.0
cherry (*Jell-O* No Bake)	330	5.0	51.0	12.0	5	390	<1.0
strawberry (*Jell-O* No Bake)	340	5.0	52.0	12.0	5	400	<1.0
cherry, wild, vanilla (*Duncan Hines*)	250	3.0	36.0	11.0	55	270	0
cherry chip (*SuperMoist*), 1/10 cake*	290	4.0	42.0	12.0	65	360	0
chocolate:							
(*Manischewitz*), 6 tbsp. mix	230	5.0	44.0	6.0	0	550	6.0
(*Pillsbury Moist Supreme*)	250	3.0	35.0	11.0	35	280	<1.0
butter (*SuperMoist*)	250	4.0	35.0	11.0	75	420	1.0
butter recipe (*Pillsbury Moist Supreme*)	270	4.0	33.0	13.0	75	420	1.0
chip (*SuperMoist*)	250	3.0	35.0	11.0	55	270	0
dark (*Pillsbury Moist Supreme*)	250	3.0	34.0	11.0	55	340	1.0
fudge (*SuperMoist*)	270	3.0	35.0	12.0	55	340	1.0
German (*Pillsbury Moist Supreme*)	230	3.0	34.0	9.0	0	290	<1.0
German (*SuperMoist*) ...	270	3.0	365.0	13.0	55	330	0

Food and Measure	cal.	prot. (gms)	carbo. (gms)	fat (gms)	chol. (mgs)	sod. (mgs)	fiber (gms)
milk (*SuperMoist*)	240	4.0	34.0	10.0	55	300	1.0
mocha (*Duncan Hines*)	290	4.0	34.0	15.0	55	390	1.0
swirl, double (*SuperMoist*) ...	270	4.0	35.0	13.0	55	330	1.0
Swiss (*Duncan Hines*)	290	4.0	34.0	15.0	55	390	1.0
chocolate caramel nut (*Pillsbury Bundt*), 1/16 cake*	290	3.0	28.0	18.0	40	210	<1.0
coffee cake:							
(*Aunt Jemima Easy*), 1/8 pkg. mix	160	2.0	27.0	5.0	0	240	<1.0
chocolate chip (*Pillsbury Streusel*), 1/16 cake*	270	3.0	38.0	12.0	40	210	<1.0
cinnamon (*Pillsbury Streusel*), 1/16 cake*	260	3.0	36.0	11.0	40	210	0
devil's food:							
(*Duncan Hines*)	290	4.0	34.0	15.0	55	390	1.0
(*Pillsbury Moist Supreme*)	270	4.0	33.0	14.0	55	340	1.0
(*SnackWell's*), 1/6 cake*	200	3.0	13.0	4.0	35	380	2.0
(*SuperMoist*)	270	3.0	35.0	13.0	55	340	0
(*Sweet Rewards*)	200	4.0	36.0	5.0	55	380	1.0
w/chocolate (*Betty Crocker Stir 'n Bake*), 1/6 pkg. ...	240	2.0	42.0	8.0	0	270	1.0
fudge:							
butter (*Duncan Hines*), 1/10 cake*	320	3.0	40.0	17.0	80	300	2.0
Dutch dark (*Duncan Hines*)	290	4.0	34.0	15.0	55	390	1.0
hot (*Pillsbury Bundt*)	350	4.0	39.0	20.0	55	280	1.0
marble (*Duncan Hines*)	250	3.0	36.0	11.0	55	270	0

Food and Measure	cal.	prot. (gms)	carbo. (gms)	fat (gms)	chol. (mgs)	sod. (mgs)	fiber (gms)
Cake, mix, fudge *(cont.)*							
marble							
(*SuperMoist*),							
1/10 cake*	290	4.0	43.0	12.0	65	330	0
swirl (*Pillsbury*							
Moist Supreme)	250	3.0	37.0	10.0	55	290	1.0
Funfetti:							
(*Pillsbury Moist Su-*							
preme)	240	3.0	36.0	9.0	0	290	<1.0
(*Pillsbury Moist Su-*							
preme Halloween)	230	3.0	34.0	9.0	0	290	<1.0
(*Pillsbury Moist Su-*							
preme Valentine)	240	3.0	35.0	10.0	35	280	<1.0
gingerbread (*Betty*							
Crocker Cake/Cookie							
Mix), 1/8 cake*	230	3.0	39.0	6.0	25	350	0
lemon:							
(*Duncan Hines* Su-							
. preme)	250	3.0	36.0	11.0	55	270	0
(*Pillsbury Moist Su-*							
preme), 1/10 cake*	300	4.0	42.0	13.0	65	350	1.0
(*SuperMoist*)	240	3.0	36.0	10.0	55	290	0
lime, key (*Duncan*							
Hines)	250	3.0	36.0	11.0	55	270	0
marble (*Manische-*							
witz), 1/4 cup mix . . .	230	2.0	48.0	4.0	0	710	2.0
orange (*Duncan Hines*							
Supreme)	250	3.0	36.0	11.0	55	270	0
party swirl							
(*SuperMoist*)	250	3.0	35.0	10.0	55	300	0
peanut butter choco-							
late swirl							
(*SuperMoist*)	240	4.0	34.0	10.0	55	320	0
pineapple:							
(*Duncan Hines* Su-							
preme)	250	3.0	36.0	11.0	55	270	0
(*SuperMoist*)	250	3.0	35.0	10.0	55	290	0
upside down (*Betty*							
Crocker), 1/6 cake*	400	3.0	63.0	15.0	35	350	0

Food and Measure	cal.	prot. (gms)	carbo. (gms)	fat (gms)	chol. (mgs)	sod. (mgs)	fiber (gms)
pound:							
(*Betty Crocker*),							
⅛ cake*	260	4.0	45.0	8.0	55	210	0
(*Martha White*),							
¼ cup mix	270	2.0	44.0	9.0	0	320	<1.0
rainbow chip							
(*SuperMoist*),							
1/10 cake*	280	3.0	41.0	12.0	0	360	0
sour cream white							
(*SuperMoist*),							
1/10 cake*	280	3.0	41.0	11.0	0	390	0
spice:							
(*Duncan Hines*)	250	3.0	36.0	11.0	55	270	0
(*SuperMoist*)	240	3.0	35.0	10.0	55	290	0
strawberry:							
(*Duncan Hines* Supreme)	250	3.0	36.0	11.0	55	270	0
(*Pillsbury Moist Supreme*)	250	3.0	35.0	11.0	55	290	<1.0
(*SuperMoist*)	250	3.0	35.0	10.0	55	280	0
cream cheese (*Pillsbury Bundt*),							
1/16 cake*	300	3.0	34.0	17.0	60	200	0
swirl (*SuperMoist*),							
1/10 cake*	290	4.0	42.0	12.0	65	370	0
vanilla, French:							
(*Duncan Hines*)	250	3.0	36.0	11.0	55	270	0
(*Pillsbury Moist Supreme*)	250	3.0	34.0	11.0	35	290	<1.0
(*SuperMoist*)	240	3.0	35.0	10.0	55	290	0
vanilla, golden							
(*SuperMoist*)	240	3.0	35.0	10.0	55	290	0
white:							
(*Duncan Hines*)	250	3.0	35.0	12.0	45	220	0
(*Pillsbury Moist Supreme*), 1/10 cake*	270	3.0	41.0	10.0	0	340	<1.0
(*SnackWell's*),							
⅙ cake*	200	3.0	13.0	4.5	35	320	1.0
(*SuperMoist*)	250	4.0	34.0	11.0	55	310	0
(*Sweet Rewards*)	190	3.0	36.0	4.0	0	310	0

Food and Measure	cal.	prot. (gms)	carbo. (gms)	fat (gms)	chol. (mgs)	sod. (mgs)	fiber (gms)
Cake, mix *(cont.)*							
white 'n fudge swirl (*Pillsbury Moist Supreme*)	250	3.0	37.0	10.0	35	290	<1.0
yellow:							
(*Duncan Hines*)	250	3.0	36.0	11.0	55	270	0
(*Manischewitz*), ¼ cup mix	240	1.0	47.0	6.0	0	290	1.0
(*Pillsbury Moist Supreme*)	240	3.0	35.0	10.0	55	290	<1.0
(*SnackWell's*), ⅙ cake*	210	3.0	13.0	4.5	35	320	1.0
(*SuperMoist*)	250	3.0	35.0	10.0	55	290	0
(*Sweet Rewards*) ·	200	3.0	37.0	4.5	55	300	0
butter (*SuperMoist*)	260	3.0	36.0	11.0	75	370	0
Cake, snack (see also specific listings), 1 pc., except as noted:							
angel (*Dolly Madison Frosty*), 3½ oz. ...	330	4.0	65.0	6.0	0	270	1.0
apple crumb (*Dolly Madison*), 1.6 oz.	160	2.0	28.0	5.0	15	160	0
banana (*Dolly Madison Dream Flip*), 3½ oz.	390	3.0	59.0	16.0	30	240	1.0
butter (*Entenmann's*), 3 oz.	320	4.0	45.0	13.0	110	400	<1.0
carrot (*Dolly Madison*), 4 oz.	230	4.0	67.0	8.0	0	500	1.0
cheese puffs:							
(*Entenmann's*), 3 oz.	330	5.0	30.0	21.0	30	310	<1.0
guava (*Entenmann's*), 2.8 oz.	290	4.0	33.0	17.0	15	250	1.0
cheesecake, New York (*Carousel*), 3 oz.	250	4.0	16.0	19.0	95	180	1.0
chocolate:							
(*Devil Dogs*), 1.6 oz.	170	2.0	30.0	7.0	0	180	1.0

Food and Measure	cal.	prot. (gms)	carbo. (gms)	fat (gms)	chol. (mgs)	sod. (mgs)	fiber (gms)
(*Dolly Madison* Squares), 1.6 oz.	210	2.0	28.0	10.0	10	150	0
(*Funny Bones*), 2 pcs., 2½ oz.	300	5.0	42.0	12.0	0	220	4.0
(*Hostess Chocodiles*), 2 oz.	240	2.0	33.0	11.0	20	180	1.0
(*Hostess Chocolicious*), 1.7 oz.	190	1.0	30.0	7.0	10	210	1.0
(*Hostess Ding Dongs/King Dons*), 2 pcs., 2.8 oz.	360	3.0	44.0	19.0	15	240	2.0
(*Hostess Ho-Hos*), 2 pcs., 2 oz.	250	2.0	34.0	12.0	20	150	1.0
(*Hostess Suzy Q's*), 2 oz.	230	2.0	35.0	9.0	10	270	1.0
(*Ring Dings*), 2 pcs., 2.7 oz.	330	2.0	43.0	18.0	0	210	2.0
(*Ring Dings* Mini), 4 pcs., 2.6 oz.	310	3.0	45.0	13.0	0	220	4.0
(*Tastykake* Junior), 3.3 oz.	360	4.0	57.0	13.0	70	270	2.0
(*Yodels*), 2 pcs., 2.2 oz.	280	2.0	35.0	16.0	0	150	2.0
creme-filled (*Entenmann's Mini Cakes*), 2 oz.	220	2.0	31.0	10.0	15	250	<1.0
cinnamon butter-crumb:							
(*Dolly Madison*), 1.6 oz.	170	2.0	28.0	6.0	15	170	0
(*Dolly Madison* Low Fat), 1½ oz.	140	1.0	29.0	1.5	0	150	0
coconut:							
(*Tastykake* Juniors), 3.3 oz.	320	4.0	59.0	8.0	65	260	1.0
covered (*Hostess Sno Balls*), 1.8 oz.	180	1.0	31.0	5.0	5	190	1.0

Food and Measure	cal.	prot. (gms)	carbo. (gms)	fat (gms)	chol. (mgs)	sod. (mgs)	fiber (gms)
Cake, snack, coconut *(cont.)*							
loaf (*Dolly Madison Mini*), 3½ oz. . . .	350	3.0	62.0	10.0	5	350	1.0
coffee cake:							
(*Drake's*), 1.1 oz.	130	1.0	18.0	6.0	5	80	1.0
crumb (*Hostess*), 1.1 oz.	130	1.0	19.0	5.0	10	110	0
crumb, chocolate (*Drake's*), 1.1 oz.	170	2.0	23.0	7.0	0	110	1.0
mini (*Drake's*), 4 pcs., 1¾ oz. . . .	210	2.0	32.0	8.0	15	130	1.0
creme cakes (*Dolly Madison*), 2 pcs., 1.9 oz.	210	1.0	32.0	8.0	25	230	0
crumb cake:							
(*Hostess* Light), 1 oz.	90	1.0	19.0	.5	0	100	0
French (*Entenmann's*), 3 oz.	360	4.0	49.0	16.0	85	340	<1.0
cupcake:							
apple-filled (*Tastykake* Low Fat), 2 pcs., 2 oz.	160	2.0	33.0	2.0	0	220	0
butter cream iced (*Tastykake*), 2 pcs., 2¼ oz. . . .	250	3.0	42.0	8.0	10	280	2.0
holiday (*Dolly Madison*), 1.9 oz.	180	1.0	35.0	3.0	5	190	0
lemon-filled (*Tastykake* Low Fat), 2 pcs., 2 oz.	160	3.0	34.0	2.0	5	230	0
orange (*Hostess*), 1½ oz.	160	1.0	27.0	5.0	10	160	0
raspberry-filled (*Tastykake* Low Fat), 2 pcs., 2 oz.	160	2.0	34.0	2.0	0	220	0
spice (*Dolly Madison*), 2 oz.	230	2.0	33.0	10.0	20	160	0
vanilla (*Tastykake* Low Fat), 2 pcs., 2¼ oz.	210	2.0	44.0	3.0	0	260	1.0

Food and Measure	cal.	prot. (gms)	carbo. (gms)	fat (gms)	chol. (mgs)	sod. (mgs)	fiber (gms)
cupcake, chocolate:							
(*Dolly Madison*),							
2 oz.	210	2.0	35.0	7.0	5	330	1.0
(*Hostess*), 1.8 oz.	180	2.0	30.0	6.0	5	290	1.0
(*Hostess* Light),							
1.6 oz.	140	2.0	29.0	1.5	0	190	1.0
(*Tastykake*), 2 pcs.,							
2.1 oz.	220	3.0	39.0	6.0	10	270	2.0
creme-filled (*En-*							
tenmann's Light							
Fat Free), 2 oz.	160	1.0	39.0	0	0	150	1.0
creme-filled (*Tas-*							
tykake Low Fat),							
2 pcs., 2¼ oz. . . .	200	3.0	42.0	2.5	0	250	1.0
creme-filled (*Yankee*							
Doodles), 2 pcs.,							
2 oz.	220	2.0	32.0	9.0	0	200	2.0
cream-filled, mini							
(*Yankee Doodles*),							
4 pcs., 1.8 oz. . . .	190	2.0	30.0	7.0	0	180	1.0
iced (*Tastykake*),							
2 pcs., 2¼ oz. . . .	250	3.0	41.0	8.0	10	270	2.0
iced (*Tastykake*							
Mini), 2 pcs.,							
1 oz.	110	1.0	18.0	4.0	5	115	1.0
date-nut pastry (*Aw-*							
rey's), 1.2 oz.	130	1.0	20.0	5.0	10	85	<1.0
devil's food:							
(*Dolly Madison*							
Zingers), 2 pcs.,							
2.6 oz.	270	2.0	46.0	8.0	5	230	1.0
(*Dolly Madison Koo*							
Koos), 1.8 oz. . . .	200	1.0	29.0	9.0	5	190	0
golden, cream-filled:							
(*Hostess Twinkies*),							
1½ oz.	150	1.0	25.0	5.0	20	200	0
(*Hostess Twinkies*							
Light), 1½ oz. . . .	130	1.0	27.0	1.5	10	190	0
lemon (*Dolly Madison*							
Zingers), 1.4 oz. . . .	150	1.0	22.0	6.0	5	90	0

Food and Measure	cal.	prot. (gms)	carbo. (gms)	fat (gms)	chol. (mgs)	sod. (mgs)	fiber (gms)
Cake, snack *(cont.)*							
marble (*Entenmann's*),							
3 oz.	320	1.0	45.0	14.0	105	400	<1.0
pound:							
(*Awrey's*), 2¼ oz.	210	3.0	31.0	8.0	40	230	<1.0
(*Dolly Madison*							
Mini), 3.2 oz. . . .	310	5.0	48.0	11.0	15	390	1.0
raspberry:							
(*Dolly Madison*							
Squares), 1.8 oz.	190	1.0	28.0	8.0	5	110	0
(*Dolly Madison*							
Zingers), 1.4 oz.	150	1.0	22.0	6.0	5	90	0
shortcake (*Hostess*							
Dessert cups), 1 oz.	100	1.0	17.0	2.0	15	120	0
yellow (*Dolly Madison*							
Zingers), 2½ oz.	280	2.0	50.0	8.0	5	160	1.0
Cake, snack, mix (see							
also specific list-							
ings), 1 pc.*, except							
as noted:							
(*Duncan Hines* Double							
Decker Cookie Bar)	130	1.0	18.0	7.0	15	85	0
(*Pillsbury M&M's*) . . .	170	2.0	27.0	6.0	10	140	<1.0
(*Pillsbury Oreo*)	180	2.0	26.0	7.0	10	160	<1.0
apple cinnamon:							
(*Duncan Hines* Fruit							
Crisp), ⅛ cake*	260	3.0	47.0	8.0	0	320	2.0
(*Sweet Rewards*),							
⅛ cake*	170	2.0	39.0	0	0	270	0
banana (*Sweet Re-*							
wards), ⅛ cake* . . .	170	3.0	39.0	0	0	290	0
bar, all varieties							
(*Weight Watchers*),							
1.2 oz.	130	1.0	27.0	2.0	0	85	2.0
chocolate:							
(*Sweet Rewards*),							
⅛ cake*	170	3.0	38.0	0	0	330	1.0
bar (*Betty Crocker*							
Hershey)	150	1.0	21.0	6.0	15	120	0
chip (*Pillsbury Chips*							
Ahoy!)	150	2.0	25.0	5.0	10	125	<1.0

Food and Measure	cal.	prot. (gms)	carbo. (gms)	fat (gms)	chol. (mgs)	sod. (mgs)	fiber (gms)
milk, chunk, bar (*Duncan Hines*)	140	2.0	18.0	7.0	15	85	0
chocolate peanut butter bar (*Betty Crocker* Supreme)	200	3.0	25.0	9.0	20	190	0
cupcake:							
angel food (*Duncan Hines* Polka Dot), 1/8 pkg.*	160	3.0	35.0	0	0	290	0
dirt (*Duncan Hines*), 1/6 pkg.*	300	3.0	35.0	17.0	35	310	1.0
date bar (*Betty Crocker* Classic), 1/12 pkg.*	150	1.0	23.0	6.0	0	90	1.0
dessert bar, easy layer (*Betty Crocker* Supreme)	140	1.0	21.0	4.0	0	85	0
lemon:							
(*Sweet Rewards*), 1/8 cake*	170	3.0	39.0	0	0	290	0
bar (*Betty Crocker* Sunkist)	140	2.0	24.0	4.5	40	90	0
lemon cheesecake (*Pillsbury*)	190	2.0	22.0	10.0	15	105	0
peach pecan (*Duncan Hines* Fruit Crisp), 1/8 cake*	250	2.0	44.0	8.0	0	200	1.0
Calamari, see "Squid"							
Calamari dishes, frozen:							
crisps, breaded (*Acadian Gourmet*), 12 pcs., 3.1 oz. . . .	230	9.0	19.0	13.0	100	580	2.0
in tomato sauce (*Plumpy*), 1 cup . . .	160-	23.0	12.0	2.5	325	1030	1.0
Calves' liver, see "Liver"							
Candy:							
almond, candy-coated (*Blue Diamond* Jordan), 13 pcs., 1.4 oz.	190	4.0	28.0	7.0	0	0	1.0

Food and Measure	cal.	prot. (gms)	carbo. (gms)	fat (gms)	chol. (mgs)	sod. (mgs)	fiber (gms)
Candy *(cont.)*							
almond bar:							
(*Mars*), 1.8 oz.	240	3.0	31.0	13.0	5	70	1.0
(*Mars* Fun Size),							
2 bars	190	3.0	24.0	10.0	5	65	1.0
(*Baby Ruth*), 2.1 oz.	270	4.0	36.0	13.0	0	130	2.0
(*Baby Ruth* Fun Size),							
1 bar	100	2.0	12.0	5.0	0	45	<1.0
(*Bittyfinger*), 2 bars	170	2.0	27.0	7.0	0	85	<1.0
(*Buncha Crunch*),							
1.4 oz.	200	2.0	26.0	10.0	10	60	<1.0
butter rum (*Pearson*							
Nips), 2 pcs.	60	0	11.0	1.5	0	0	400
(*Butterfinger*), 2.1 oz.	270	3.0	42.0	11.0	0	130	1.0
(*Butterfinger* Fun							
Size), 2 bars	100	1.0	15.0	3.5	0	45	0
(*Butterfinger BB's*),							
1.7 oz.	230	2.0	33.0	9.0	0	95	1.0
candy cane, 1 pc.:							
(*Spangler*), ½ oz.	55	0	14.0	0	0	0	0
(*Starburst*), .7 oz.	70	0	1.0	0	0	5	0
candy corn, 1 oz.	110	0	27.0	0	0	40	0
caramel:							
(*Kraft*), 5 pcs.	170	2.0	32.0	3.0	<5	110	0
(*Pearson Nips*),							
2 pcs.	60	0	11.0	1.5	0	40	0
(*Rolo*), 1.9 oz.	220	3.0	28.0	11.0	10	95	0
chocolate (*Kraft*							
Fudgies), 5 pcs.	180	1.0	32.0	5.0	0	90	0
chocolate coated							
(*Milk Duds*),							
13 pcs., 1.4 oz.	170	1.0	29.0	5.0	0	90	0
chocolate coated							
(*Pom Poms*),							
1.6 oz.	200	1.0	35.0	6.0	<5	70	2.0
caramel cookie bar:							
(*Twix* Family), 1 oz.	140	1.0	19.0	7.0	0	60	0
(*Twix* Fun Size),							
1 pc.	80	1.0	10.0	4.0	0	30	0
(*Twix* Miniatures),							
3 pcs., 1.1 oz. ...	150	1.0	19.0	7.0	0	60	0

Food and Measure	cal.	prot. (gms)	carbo. (gms)	fat (gms)	chol. (mgs)	sod. (mgs)	fiber (gms)
(*Twix* Single), 2 oz.	280	3.0	37.0	14.0	5	115	1.0
caramel and peanut butter (*Hershey's Sweet Escapes*), 1.4 oz.	150	2.0	25.0	5.0	<5	125	<1.0
cherries, chocolate covered:							
(*Perugina*), 3 pcs.	140	<1.0	23.0	6.0	0	0	1.0
bing, dried, 5 pcs., 1.4 oz.	190	2.0	26.0	9.0	<5	25	3.0
dark (*Cella*), 2 pcs.	110	<1.0	18.0	4.0	0	10	1.0
milk (*Cella*), 2 pcs.	110	<1.0	18.0	4.0	0	15	1.0
chocolate, assorted:							
(*Godiva*), 1½ oz.	210	2.0	27.0	11.0	5	20	0
(*Lindt* Swiss Tradition Deluxe), 1½ oz.	230	3.0	21.0	15.0	5	30	1.0
(*Perugina*), 3 pcs.	170	2.0	21.0	10.0	<5	30	1.0
chocolate, bittersweet:							
(*Lindt* Surfin Swiss), 14 pcs., 1.4 oz.	210	2.0	21.0	13.5	0	5	0
(*Perugina*), ½ bar	220	3.0	23.0	15.0	<5	0	4.0
hazelnut (*Lindt*), 14 pcs., 1.4 oz.	220	3.0	18.0	15.0	5	5	0
hazelnut (*Perugina Baci*), 3 pcs.	250	3.0	21.0	18.0	<5	0	2.0
chocolate, candy coated:							
(*M&M's*), ½ oz.	210	2.0	30.0	9.0	5	25	1.0
(*M&M's*), 1.7 oz.	240	2.0	34.0	10.0	5	30	1.0
(*M&M's* Fun Size), 1 bag	100	1.0	15.0	4.5	5	15	1.0
(*M&M's* King Size), ½ bag	220	2.0	32.0	9.0	5	25	1.0
almond (*M&M's*), ½ oz.	230	4.0	25.0	13.0	5	20	2.0
almond (*M&M's*), 1.3 oz.	200	3.0	21.0	11.0	5	15	2.0
crispy (*M&M's*), ¼ cup, 1½ oz.	200	2.0	30.0	9.0	5	65	1.0

Food and Measure	cal.	prot. (gms)	carbo. (gms)	fat (gms)	chol. (mgs)	sod. (mgs)	fiber (gms)
Candy, chocolate, candy coated *(cont.)*							
mini (*M&M's*), 3 boxes	210	2.0	29.0	10.0	5	30	1.0
mini (*M&M's*), 1.2-oz. tube	170	2.0	24.0	8.0	5	25	1.0
peanut (*M&M's*), ½ oz.	220	4.0	26.0	11.0	5	20	1.0
peanut (*M&M's*), 1.7 oz.	250	5.0	30.0	13.0	5	25	2.0
peanut (*M&M's* Fun Size), 1 bag	110	2.0	13.0	5.0	0	10	1.0
peanut (*M&M's* King Size), ½ bag	240	4.0	28.0	18.0	5	20	2.0
peanut butter (*M&M's*), ½ oz.	220	4.0	24.0	18.0	5	90	2.0
peanut butter (*M&M's*), 1.6 oz.	240	5.0	27.0	20.0	5	95	2.0
peanut butter (*M&M's* Fun Size), 1 bag	110	2.0	12.0	6.0	0	45	1.0
chocolate, dark:							
(*Dove*), ¼ of 6-oz. bar	230	2.0	26.0	14.0	5	0	3.0
(*Dove*), 1.3-oz. bar	200	2.0	22.0	14.0	5	0	2.0
(*Dove* Miniatures), 7 pcs.	220	2.0	22.0	14.0	5	0	2.0
(*Ghirardelli*), 1¼ oz.	180	2.0	22.0	11.0	0	0	0
(*Ghirardelli*), 1½ oz.	210	2.0	26.0	14.0	0	0	0
(*Hershey's Special Dark*), 1.45 oz.	230	2.0	25.0	13.0	0	0	2.0
(*Lindt* Lindor Truffle), 7 pcs., 1.4 oz.	220	1.0	16.0	19.0	<5	10	1.0
(*Perugina*), ½ bar	230	2.0	26.0	14.0	<5	0	2.0
almond (*Ghirardelli*), 1½ oz.	220	3.0	23.0	15.0	0	0	1.0
almond (*Perugina*), ½ bar	240	3.0	23.0	15.0	<5	0	3.0

Food and Measure	cal.	prot. (gms)	carbo. (gms)	fat (gms)	chol. (mgs)	sod. (mgs)	fiber (gms)
hazelnut (*Perugina*), ½ bar	240	2.0	23.0	16.0	<5	0	2.0
w/raspberries (*Ghirardelli*), 1½ oz.	210	2.0	26.0	13.0	0	0	1.0
chocolate, milk:							
(*Dove*), ¼ of 6-oz. bar	230	3.0	25.0	14.0	10	25	1.0
(*Dove*), 1.3 oz.	200	2.0	22.0	12.0	5	25	1.0
(*Dove* Miniatures), 7 pcs.	230	2.0	25.0	13.0	10	25	1.0
(*Ghirardelli*), 1¼ oz.	190	2.0	21.0	11.0	5	25	0
(*Ghirardelli*), 1½ oz.	220	3.0	25.0	14.0	10	30	0
(*Hershey's*), 1.55 oz.	230	3.0	25.0	13.0	10	40	1.0
(*Hershey's* Nuggets), 4 pcs.	210	3.0	23.0	12.0	10	35	1.0
(*Hershey's Hugs*), 8 pcs.	210	3.0	22.0	12.0	10	35	0
(*Hershey's Kisses*), 8 pcs.	210	3.0	23.0	12.0	10	35	1.0
(*Hershey's Miniatures*), 5 pcs. . . .	230	3.0	25.0	13.0	5	30	1.0
(*Lindt* Chocoletti), 7 pcs., 1.4 oz. . . .	220	2.0	19.0	16.0	5	35	<1.0
(*Lindt* Gourmet Truffle), 2 balls, 1.2 oz.	190	2.0	16.0	14.0	<5	20	<1.0
(*Lindt* Mocca), 14 pcs., 1.4 oz.	210	2.0	21.0	13.0	5	35	0
(*Lindt* Swiss), 14 pcs., 1.4 oz.	210	3.0	22.0	12.0	5	60	0
(*Nestlé*), 1.45 oz.	220	2.0	26.0	13.0	10	25	<1.0
(*Perugina*), ½ bar	230	3.0	25.0	13.0	10	30	<1.0
(*Symphony*), 1½ oz.	230	3.0	24.0	14.0	10	40	<1.0
almond (*Cadbury*), 9 blocks	220	4.0	21.0	13.0	10	80	1.0

Food and Measure	cal.	prot. (gms)	carbo. (gms)	fat (gms)	chol. (mgs)	sod. (mgs)	fiber (gms)
Candy, chocolate, milk *(cont.)*							
almond (*Ghirardelli*), 1¼ oz.	170	3.0	19.0	12.0	5	25	0
almond (*Ghirardelli*), 1½ oz.	230	4.0	22.0	15.0	5	25	1.0
almond (*Ghirardelli*), 2.1 oz.	320	5.0	32.0	21.0	10	85	1.0
almond (*Hershey's*), 1.45 oz.	230	5.0	20.0	14.0	5	35	1.0
almond (*Hershey's* Golden), 2.8 oz.	450	10.0	36.0	30.0	10	50	3.0
almond (*Hershey's* Golden Solitaire), 2.8 oz.	450	9.0	37.0	29.0	10	45	3.0
almond (*Hershey's* Nuggets), 4 pcs.	210	4.0	20.0	13.0	5	30	1.0
almond (*Hershey's* Hugs), 9 pcs. . . .	230	4.0	23.0	13.0	10	35	<1.0
almond (*Hershey's* Kisses), 8 pcs.	210	4.0	19.0	13.0	5	25	1.0
almond (*Lindt* Alba), 5 pcs., 1½ oz. . . .	220	3.0	19.0	15.0	5	45	0
almond (*Lindt* Swiss), 12 pcs., 1.4 oz.	220	4.0	18.0	14.0	5	50	1.0
almond (*Perugina*), ½ bar	240	4.0	23.0	15.0	10	25	1.0
almond-toffee (*Symphony*), 1½ oz.	240	4.0	22.0	15.0	10	60	1.0
cappuccino filling (*Perugina*), ⅓ bar	170	2.0	17.0	10.0	10	40	<1.0
caramel (*Caramello*), 1.6 oz.	220	3.0	29.0	10.0	10	60	<1.0
caramel (*Lindt*), 6 pcs., 1.4 oz. . . .	220	2.0	23.0	13.5	5	40	0

Food and Measure	cal.	prot. (gms)	carbo. (gms)	fat (gms)	chol. (mgs)	sod. (mgs)	fiber (gms)
cherry (*Lindt*), 6 pcs., 1.4 oz. . . .	180	2.0	24.0	9.0	5	40	0
cookies and cream (*Ghirardelli*), 1.3 oz.	190	2.0	22.0	11.0	5	65	0
cookies and cream (*Hershey's* Nuggets), 4 pcs.	200	4.0	22.0	11.0	5	75	0
crisps (*Cadbury's Krisp*), 9 blocks	200	3.0	25.0	10.0	10	80	<1.0
crisps (*Crunch*), 1.55 oz.	230	2.0	29.0	12.0	10	65	<1.0
crisps (*Crunch* Fun Size), 4 bars	210	2.0	26.0	11.0	10	60	<1.0
crisps (*Ghirardelli*), 1¼ oz.	180	2.0	22.0	10.0	5	25	0
crisps (*Ghirardelli*), 2.1 oz.	300	4.0	37.0	17.0	10	95	0
crisps (*Ghirardelli*), 2½ oz.	360	5.0	44.0	20.0	10	115	0
crisps (*Krackel*), 1.45 oz.	220	3.0	25.0	12.0	10	55	1.0
fruit, nuts (*Chunky*), 1.4 oz.	210	3.0	24.0	11.0	5	20	1.0
fruit, nuts (*Perugina*), ½ bar	230	3.0	25.0	13.0	10	40	1.0
hazelnut (*Lindt* Swiss), 14 pcs., 1.4 oz.	220	3.0	18.0	15.0	5	50	0
hazelnut (*Perugina*), ½ bar	240	3.0	23.0	15.0	10	25	1.0
macadamia (*Ghirardelli*), 1¼ oz.	190	2.0	19.0	13.0	5	25	0
macadamia (*Ghirardelli*), 2½ oz.	380	5.0	38.0	26.0	10	50	1.0
macadamia (*Hershey's Golden*), 2.4 oz.	380	6.0	35.0	24.0	15	60	2.0

Food and Measure	cal.	prot. (gms)	carbo. (gms)	fat (gms)	chol. (mgs)	sod. (mgs)	fiber (gms)
Candy, chocolate, milk *(cont.)*							
macadamia (*Perugina*), ½ bar	240	3.0	23.0	16.0	10	25	1.0
mint (*Lindt* Lindor Truffle), 7 pcs., 1.4 oz.	170	<1.0	25.0	9.0	5	25	1.0
orange (*Lindt*), 6 pcs., 1.4 oz. . . .	190	2.0	24.0	10.0	5	40	0
peanut (*Mr. Goodbar*), 1¾ oz.	270	5.0	25.0	17.0	5	20	2.0
pecan (*Ghirardelli*), 1½ oz.	230	3.0	22.0	16.0	5	25	1.0
pistachio (*Lindt* Pistache), 5 pcs., 1½ oz.	230	2.0	19.0	16.0	5	50	0
raspberry (*Lindt*), 6 pcs., 1.4 oz. . . .	180	2.0	24.0	9.0	5	60	0
raspberry (*Perugina*), bar	150	1.0	20.0	7.0	<5	15	<1.0
strawberry (*Lindt*), 6 pcs., 1.4 oz. . . .	180	2.0	24.0	9.0	5	40	0
toffee (*Ghirardelli*), 1½ oz.	220	2.0	26.0	13.0	10	45	0
wafers (*Ghirardelli*), 11 pcs.	210	3.0	29.0	12.0	10	30	0
chocolate, mint:							
(*Cadbury's* Mint), 5 blocks	190	2.0	27.0	8.0	<5	5	1.0
(*Ghirardelli*), 1¼ oz.	180	2.0	22.0	12.0	5	10	0
(*Ghirardelli*), 1½ oz.	220	2.0	26.0	14.0	5	15	0
(*Ghirardelli*), 2.1 oz.	310	3.0	37.0	19.0	5	20	0
(*Pearson Nips*), 2 pcs.	60	0	11.0	1.5	0	40	0
cookies and (*Hershey's*), 1.55 oz.	230	3.0	27.0	12.0	10	80	1.0
cookies and (*Hershey's* Nuggets), 4 pcs.	200	3.0	24.0	10.0	5	70	1.0

Food and Measure	cal.	prot. (gms)	carbo. (gms)	fat (gms)	chol. (mgs)	sod. (mgs)	fiber (gms)
wafers (*Ghirardelli*), 11 pcs.	210	2.0	27.0	12.0	5	15	0
chocolate, white:							
(*Lindt* Swiss), 14 pcs., 1.4 oz.	220	2.0	22.0	14.0	5	50	0
(*Lindt* White Lindor Truffle), 7 pcs., 1.4 oz.	240	2.0	17.0	19.0	5	25	0
(*Perugina*), 1½ oz.	250	3.0	22.0	17.0	10	45	0
and cookie (*Hershey's Cookies n' Creme*), 1½ oz.	230	4.0	24.0	13.0	5	85	0
w/crisps (*Nestlé White Crunch*), 1.4 oz.	220	3.0	23.0	13.0	10	70	0
raspberry (*Ghirardelli*), 1.3 oz.	200	2.0	21.0	12.0	5	35	0
chocolate parfait (*Pearson Nips*), 2 pcs.	60	0	10.0	2.0	0	30	0
chocolate sticks, 11 pcs., 1.3 oz.:							
cappuccino (*Rademaker*)	190	2.0	21.0	11.0	5	20	3.0
milk (*Rademaker*)	190	3.0	22.0	11.0	5	30	1.0
mint (*Rademaker*)	195	1.0	25.0	12.0	0	0	2.0
raspberry (*Rademaker*)	190	2.0	23.0	10.0	5	25	1.0
chocolate truffles (*Godiva*), 1½ oz.	220	2.0	24.0	13.0	10	15	0
coconut, chocolate coated:							
(*Lindt* Chocoletti Coconut), 7 pcs., 1.4 oz.	240	2.0	16.0	20.0	5	30	<1.0
(*Mounds*), 1.9 oz.	250	2.0	31.0	13.0	0	80	3.0
w/almonds (*Almond Joy*), 1.76 oz. ...	240	2.0	28.0	13.0	0	65	2.0
coffee (*Pearson Nips*), 2 pcs.	50	0	10.0	1.5	0	40	0

Food and Measure	cal.	prot. (gms)	carbo. (gms)	fat (gms)	chol. (mgs)	sod. (mgs)	fiber (gms)
Candy *(cont.)*							
fruit flavor:							
(*Frooties*), 12 pcs.,							
1¼ oz.	150	0	31.0	2.5	0	25	0
(*Skittles* Original),							
1½ oz.	170	0	39.0	2.0	0	5	0
(*Skittles* Original),							
2.2 oz.	240	0	54.0	2.5	0	10	0
(*Skittles* Original							
Fun Size), 3 bags	180	0	41.0	2.0	0	5	0
(*Skittles* Original							
King Size), bag	150	0	34.0	1.5	0	5	0
tropical (*Skittles*),							
1½ oz.	170	0	37.0	2.0	0	5	0
tropical (*Skittles*),							
2.2 oz.	250	0	56.0	2.5	0	10	0
tropical (*Skittles* Fun							
Size), 2 bags	160	0	36.0	1.5	0	5	0
twists (*Starburst*),							
4 pcs., 1½ oz. . . .	140	0	34.0	.5	0	10	0
twists (*Starburst*),							
2 oz.	190	0	45.0	1.0	0	15	0
wild berry (*Skittles*),							
1½ oz.	170	0	37.0	1.5	0	5	0
wild berry (*Skittles*),							
2.2 oz.	250	0	56.0	2.5	0	10	0
wild berry (*Skittles*							
Fun Size), 2 bags	160	0	36.0	1.5	0	5	0
fruit flavor, chews:							
(*Starburst* Original),							
8 pcs., 1.4 oz. . . .	160	0	33.0	3.5	0	0	0
(*Starburst* Original),							
½ of 3-oz. box . . .	170	0	35.0	3.5	0	0	0
(*Starburst* Original),							
2.1 oz.	240	0	48.0	4.5	0	0	0
(*Starburst* Original							
Fun Size), 4 packs	160	0	33.0	3.5	0	0	0
California							
(*Starburst*),							
2.1 oz.	240	0	48.0	4.5	0	0	0

Food and Measure	cal.	prot. (gms)	carbo. (gms)	fat (gms)	chol. (mgs)	sod. (mgs)	fiber (gms)
California or tropical (*Starburst*), 8 pcs., 1.4 oz., 4 fun packs	160	0	33.0	3.0	0	0	0
tropical (*Starburst*), 2.1 oz.	240	0	48.0	5.0	0	0	0
fruit flavor, gummed:							
(*Amazin' Fruit*), 1.9 oz.	180	3.0	41.0	0	0	60	0
(*Dots* Mini), ¾ oz.	80	0	20.0	0	0	10	0
(*Dots* Original/Tropi-Cal), 12 pcs., 1½ oz.	150	0	37.0	0	0	20	0
(*Heide Gummie Bears*), 1 oz.	90	0	21.0	0	0	0	0
(*Jolly Rancher* Gummis), 10 pcs. . . .	120	2.0	29.0	0	0	10	0
(*Jolly Rancher Jolly Jellies*), 6 pcs.	120	<1.0	30.0	0	0	50	0
(*Jolly Rancher Jolly Jellies* Tart n' Tangy), 6 pcs. . . .	120	<1.0	29.0	0	0	80	0
(*Jujubes*), 1 oz. . . .	110	0	26.0	0	0	10	0
(*Jujyfruits*), 1 oz.	100	0	25.0	0	0	0	0
(*Red Hot Dollars*), 1 oz.	100	0	25.0	0	0	0	0
gum, chewing, 1 stick:							
(*Doublemint/Juicy Fruit/Big Red/Winterfresh/Wrigley's Spearmint*)	10	0	2.0	0	0	0	0
(*Freedent*)	10	0	2.0	0	0	0	0
sugar free (*Extra*)	5	0	2.0	0	0	0	0
hard:							
all flavors (*Charms*), 2 pcs., .2 oz.	25	0	6.0	0	0	0	0
all flavors (*Jolly Rancher*), 3 pcs.	70	0	17.0	0	0	10	0
all flavors (*Jolly Rancher* Mini-Stix), 1 pc.	35	0	9.0	0	0	0	0

Food and Measure	cal.	prot. (gms)	carbo. (gms)	fat (gms)	chol. (mgs)	sod. (mgs)	fiber (gms)
Candy, hard *(cont.)*							
butterscotch or car-amel (*Hershey's Tastetations*), 3 pcs.	60	0	12.0	1.5	<5	85	0
chocolate or choco-late mint (*Her-shey's Tasteta-tions*), 3 pcs. . . .	60	0	12.0	1.5	<5	30	0
peppermint (*Her-shey's Tasteta-tions*), 3 pcs. . . .	60	0	15.0	0	0	15	0
jelly beans:							
(*Jolly Rancher Jelly Beans*), 25 pcs.	140	0	36.0	0	0	15	0
(*Starburst*), 1½ oz.	150	0	38.0	0	0	15	0
(*Starburst*), 1.24 oz.	130	0	32.0	0	0	15	0
(*Starburst* Egg), 2 oz.	200	0	51.0	0	0	20	0
licorice:							
(*Crows*), 12 pcs., 1½ oz.	150	0	37.0	0	0	20	0
(*Nibs*), 22 pcs.	140	1.0	31.0	1.0	0	220	0
(*Pearson Nips*), 2 pcs.	60	0	11.0	1.5	0	40	0
(*Twizzlers*), 4 pcs.	140	1.0	33.0	.5	0	230	0
cherry (*Nibs*), 22 pcs.	140	1.0	31.0	1.0	0	85	0
cherry (*Twizzlers*), 4 pcs.	150	1.0	33.0	10	0	125	0
cherry (*Twizzlers Pull 'n' Peel*), 2.2 oz.	190	2.0	43.0	1.5	0	160	2.0
chocolate (*Twiz-zlers*), 5 pcs.	140	1.0	31.0	1.0	0	160	0
strawberry (*Twiz-zlers*), 4 pcs.	140	1.0	33.0	.5	0	105	0
lollipop, all flavors, 1 pop:							
(*Astro Pops*), 1 oz.	108	0	27.0	0	0	0	0

Food and Measure	cal.	prot. (gms)	carbo. (gms)	fat (gms)	chol. (mgs)	sod. (mgs)	fiber (gms)
(*Charms*), .6 oz. . . .	70	0	18.0	0	0	0	0
(*Charms Blow Pop*), .9 oz.	100	0	24.0	0	0	0	<1.0
(*Dum-Dums*), .2 oz.	20	0	5.0	0	0	0	0
(*Dum-Dums* Double Dip/Super), .6 oz.	71	0	18.0	0	0	0	0
(*Fiesta*), .7 oz.	80	0	19.0	0	0	0	0
(*Saf-T-Pops*), .4 oz.	43	0	11.0	0	0	0	0
(*Sugar Daddy*), 1.7 oz.	200	1.0	43.0	2.5	<5	100	0
(*Tootsie Bunch Pops*), 1/2 oz.	50	0	12.0	0	0	10	0
(*Tootsie Pops*), .6 oz.	60	0	16.0	0	0	10	0
macadamias:							
butter or coconut candy glazed (*Mauna Loa*), 1 oz.	190	2.0	10.0	15.0	<5	55	1.0
coffee glazed (*Mauna Loa*), 1 oz.	190	2.0	10.0	15.0	<5	55	1.0
macadamias, chocolate coated:							
(*Mauna Loa*), 4 pcs., 1.3 oz.	220	2.0	17.0	16.0	10	15	1.0
(*Mauna Loa* Deluxe), 4 pcs., 1.3 oz. . . .	240	2.0	17.0	17.0	10	15	1.0
(*Mauna Loa* Ghirardelli*), 9 pcs., 1.3 oz. . . .	230	2.0	19.0	17.0	10	15	1.0
malted milk balls (*Whoppers*), 1 3/4-oz. box	230	2.0	36.0	9.0	0	125	<1.0
marshmallow:							
(*Kraft* Miniature), 1/2 cup	100	<1.0	25.0	0	0	30	0
(*Kraft Funmallows*), 4 pcs.	110	<1.0	26.0	0	0	20	0
(*Kraft Funmallows* Miniature), 1/2 cup	100	<1.0	25.0	0	0	20	0

Food and Measure	cal.	prot. (gms)	carbo. (gms)	fat (gms)	chol. (mgs)	sod. (mgs)	fiber (gms)
Candy, marshmallow *(cont.)*							
(*Kraft Jet-Puffed*),							
5 pcs.	110	<1.0	27.0	0	0	40	0
cocoa (*Kraft* Teddy							
Bear), ½ cup	100	1.0	23.0	0	0	25	0
peanut (*Spangler*),							
6 pcs.	163	0	41.0	0	0	0	0
(*Milky Way*), 2-oz. bar	270	2.0	41.0	10.0	5	95	1.0
(*Milky Way* Creme							
Egg), 1.2-oz. pc.	190	2.0	18.0	13.0	5	30	0
(*Milky Way* Dark),							
1.8-oz. bar	220	1.0	36.0	8.0	5	85	1.0
(*Milky Way* Dark Fun							
Size), 2 bars	170	1.0	28.0	7.0	5	65	1.0
(*Milky Way* Dark Mini-							
iatures), 5 pcs.	180	1.0	30.0	7.0	5	70	1.0
(*Milky Way* Fun Size),							
2 bars	10	2.0	28.0	7.0	5	65	0
(*Milky Way* Lite),							
1½ oz.	170	1.0	34.0	5.0	5	80	0
(*Milky Way* Lite Minia-							
tures), 5 pcs.	150	1.0	29.0	4.5	0	70	0
(*Milky Way* Minia-							
tures), 5 pcs.	190	2.0	30.0	7.0	5	65	0
mint:							
(*Kraft* Party), 7 pcs.	60	0	14.0	0	0	35	0
butter (*Kraft*),							
7 pcs.	60	0	14.0	0	0	25	0
chocolate coated							
(*Junior Mints*),							
1.6 oz.	180	<1.0	38.0	3.0	0	10	<1.0
chocolate coated							
(*York* Peppermint							
Pattie), 1½ oz.	150	<1.0	34.0	3.0	0	10	0
(*Nestlé Turtles*),							
2 pcs.	160	2.0	19.0	9.0	<5	40	1.0
nonpareils:							
(*Ghirardelli*),							
1.4 oz.	190	2.0	29.0	9.0	0	0	0
(*Sno-Caps*), 2.3 oz.	300	2.0	48.0	13.0	0	0	3.0

Food and Measure	cal.	prot. (gms)	carbo. (gms)	fat (gms)	chol. (mgs)	sod. (mgs)	fiber (gms)
nougat, chocolate coated, 1.9 oz.:							
chocolate (*Charleston Chew*)	230	1.0	42.0	6.0	0	40	<1.0
strawberry (*Charleston Chew*)	230	1.0	42.0	6.0	0	60	<1.0
vanilla (*Charleston Chew*)	230	2.0	40.0	7.0	0	50	1.0
(*Nutrageous*), 1.6 oz.	240	7.0	22.0	14.0	<5	85	1.0
(*Oh Henry!*), .9 oz.	120	2.0	16.0	5.0	<5	60	0
(*100 Grand*), 1½ oz.	200	2.0	30.0	8.0	10	75	<1.0
peanut, chocolate coated (*Goobers*), 1.38 oz.	210	5.0	19.0	13.0	<5	20	3.0
peanut bar (*Planters*), 1.6 oz.	230	6.0	22.0	14.0	0	70	2.0
peanut brittle (*Kraft*), 5 pcs.	170	3.0	29.0	5.0	0	310	1.0
peanut butter (*Pearson Nips*), 2 pcs.	60	<1.0	10.0	2.0	0	45	0
peanut butter, chocolate:							
(*5th Avenue*), 2 oz.	280	5.0	38.0	12.0	<5	95	1.0
candy coated (*Reese's Pieces*), 1.6 oz.	230	6.0	28.0	10.0	0	75	1.0
cup (*Reese's*), 1.6 oz.	240	5.0	24.0	14.0	<5	150	1.0
cup (*Reese's Crunchy*), 1.6 oz.	250	6.0	21.0	16.0	<5	75	2.0
peanut butter cookie:							
(*Twix*), .9 oz.	130	3.0	13.0	8.0	0	70	1.0
(*Twix* Singles), 2 bars, 1.7 oz.	260	5.0	26.0	16.0	5	130	2.0
(*Perugina After Eight*), bar	150	1.0	24.0	6.0	0	0	2.0
pretzel, chocolate:							
milk (*Flipz*), 1 oz.	130	2.0	20.0	6.0	<5	130	<1.0
white (*Flipz*), 1 oz.	130	2.0	19.0	6.0	0	130	0
raisins, chocolate coated (*Raisinets*), 1.58 oz.	200	2.0	31.0	8.0	<5	15	1.0

Food and Measure	cal.	prot. (gms)	carbo. (gms)	fat (gms)	chol. (mgs)	sod. (mgs)	fiber (gms)
Candy *(cont.)*							
(*Snickers*), 1.2 oz. . . .	280	4.0	35.0	14.0	5	140	1.0
(*Snickers* Creme Egg), 1.2 oz.	170	3.0	19.0	10.0	5	70	1.0
(*Snickers* Fun Size), 2 bars	190	3.0	24.0	10.0	5	100	1.0
(*Snickers* King Size), of 3.7-oz. bar	170	3.0	21.0	8.0	5	85	1.0
(*Snickers* Miniatures), 4 pcs.	170	3.0	22.0	9.0	5	90	1.0
(*Snickers* Munch), 1.4 oz.	230	6.0	17.0	15.0	10	140	2.0
(*Sugar Babies*), 30 pcs., 1.6 oz. . . .	180	<1.0	39.0	2.0	0	70	0
(*Sugar Daddy* Nuggets), 5 pcs., 1.4 oz.	170	<1.0	37.0	2.0	<5	95	0
(*3 Musketeers*), 2.1 oz.	260	2.0	46.0	8.0	5	110	1.0
(*3 Musketeers* Fun Size), 2 bars	140	1.0	26.0	4.5	5	60	0
(*3 Musketeers* Miniatures), 7 pcs.	170	1.0	32.0	5.0	5	80	1.0
toffee:							
(*Heath*), 1.4 oz. . . .	210	1.0	24.0	12.0	10	135	<1.0
(*Skor*), 1.4 oz.	220	2.0	23.0	13.0	20	110	1.0
bits (*Heath*), ½ oz.	80	<1.0	9.0	4.5	<5	60	0
bits (*Heath Bits O' Brickle*), ½ oz.	80	<1.0	9.0	5.0	5	80	0
toffee crisp, chocolate coated (*Hershey's Sweet Escapes*), 1.4 oz.	190	3.0	27.0	8.0	<5	90	<1.0
(*Tootsie Roll* Midges), 6 pcs., 1.4 oz. . . .	160	<1.0	33.0	3.0	0	40	<1.0
(*Tootsie Roll* Snack Bar), 2 bars, 1 oz.	110	<1.0	23.0	2.0	0	30	<1.0
wafer, chocolate coated:							
(*Hershey's Sweet Escapes*), 1.4 oz.	160	1.0	27.0	5.0	0	55	0
(*Kit Kat*), 1½ oz. . . .	220	3.0	26.0	12.0	5	35	<1.0

Food and Measure	cal.	prot. (gms)	carbo. (gms)	fat (gms)	chol. (mgs)	sod. (mgs)	fiber (gms)
(*Whatchamacallit*), 1.7 oz.	250	4.0	29.0	13.0	5	125	1.0
(*White Rabbit*), 8 pcs., 1.4 oz.	160	2.0	32.0	2.5	6	52	0
Cane syrup, 1 tbsp.	52	0	13.4	0	0	<1	0
Cannellini beans, see "Kidney beans"							
Cannelloni dinner, frozen (*Amy's*), 9 oz.	330	16.0	34.0	12.0	35	390	6.0
Cannelloni entree, frozen (*Lean Cuisine*), 9 oz.	230	20.0	28.0	4.0	15	570	3.0
Cantaloupe:							
½ of 5″ melon	94	2.3	22.3	.7	0	23	2.1
pulp, cubed, ½ cup	29	.7	6.7	.2	0	7	.6
Cantaloupe drink, cocktail (*Snapple*), 8 fl. oz.	120	0	31.0	0	0	10	0
Caper berries (*Haddon House*), 2 tbsp., ½ oz.	0	0	1.0	0	0	410	0
Capers, 1 tbsp.:							
(*Crosse & Blackwell*)	5	0	1.0	0	0	350	0
(*Italica*).............	0	0	<1.0	0	0	460	0
Capon, see "Chicken"							
Caponata, see "Eggplant appetizer"							
Cappicola, see "Ham lunch meat"							
Cappuccino (see also "Coffee, flavored, mix"), iced, 8 fl. oz., except as noted:							
all flavors (*Starbucks Frappuccino*), 9.5 fl. oz.	190	6.0	39.0	3.0	12	110	0
coffee (*Maxwell House Cappio*)	130	2.0	24.0	2.5	5	120	0
mocha (*Maxwell House Cappio*)	140	2.0	27.0	2.5	5	115	0

Food and Measure	cal.	prot. (gms)	carbo. (gms)	fat (gms)	chol. (mgs)	sod. (mgs)	fiber (gms)
Cappuccino *(cont.)*							
vanilla *(Maxwell House Cappio)*	140	2.0	27.0	2.5	5	110	0
Carambola:							
(Frieda's Starfruit*),* 5 oz.	45	1.0	11.0	0	0	0	4.0
1 medium, 4.7 oz.	42	.7	9.9	.4	0	2	3.4
Carambola, dried *(Frieda's Starfruit),* 1/3 cup, 1.4 oz.	120	2.0	29.0	0	0	5	10.0
Caramel, see "Candy"							
Caramel dip, see "Apple dip" and "Fruit dip mix"							
Caramel syrup *(Smucker's* Sundae*),* 2 tbsp.	110	0	27.0	0	0	70	0
Caramel topping, 2 tbsp.:							
(Kraft)	120	2.0	28.0	0	0	90	0
(Mrs. Richardson's Fat Free*)*	130	<1.0	32.0	0	0	55	0
(Smucker's Fat Free*)*	130	0	31.0	0	0	110	<1.0
(Smucker's Microwave*)*	110	0	28.0	0	0	122	0
butterscotch, see "Butterscotch topping"							
hot *(Smucker's)*	120	1.0	29.0	.5	0	60	0
Caraway seed, 1 tsp.	7	.4	1.1	.3	0	<1	<1.0
Carbonara sauce mix *(Knorr* Pasta Sauces*),* 2 tbsp.	70	4.0	5.0	3.5	10	880	0
Cardamom, 1 tsp.:							
ground *(Tone's)*	6	.2	1.3	.1	0	<1	.2
seed *(Spice Islands)*	6	.2	1.3	.1	0	<1	.2
Cardoon:							
raw, shredded, 1/2 cup	18	.6	4.4	.1	0	151	1.4
boiled, drained, 4 oz.	25	.9	6.0	.1	0	200	n.a.
Carissa:							
1 medium, .8 oz.	12	.1	2.7	.3	0	1	n.a.

Food and Measure	cal.	prot. (gms)	carbo. (gms)	fat (gms)	chol. (mgs)	sod. (mgs)	fiber (gms)
sliced, ½ cup	46	.4	10.2	1.0	0	2	n.a.
Carl's Jr., 1 serving:							
breakfast items:							
bacon, 2 strips	50	3.0	0	4.0	10	140	0
burrito	480	27.0	26.0	30.0	465	750	2.0
eggs, scrambled ...	160	13.0	1.0	11.0	425	125	0
English muffin							
w/margarine	210	5.0	27.0	9.0	0	300	2.0
French Toast Dips,							
w/out syrup	370	11.0	42.0	20.0	0	430	1.0
quesadilla	310	14.0	27.0	16.0	230	670	2.0
sausage, 1 patty ...	200	8.0	2.0	19.0	30	480	1.0
Sunrise Sandwich,							
w/out bacon or							
sausage........	360	14.0	28.0	21.0	27	700	2.0
sandwiches:							
Carl's bacon Swiss							
crispy chicken ...	720	32.0	66.0	36.0	75	1610	3.0
Carl's Catch Fish							
Sandwich	510	18.0	50.0	27.0	80	1030	1.0
Carl's ranch crispy							
chicken	620	25.0	65.0	29.0	50	1220	3.0
Charbroiled BBQ							
Chicken Sandwich	280	25.0	37.0	3.0	60	830	2.0
Charbroiled Chicken							
Club Sandwich	460	32.0	33.0	22.0	90	1110	2.0
Charbroiled Santa Fe							
Chicken Sandwich	510	28.0	32.0	31.0	95	1240	2.0
charbroiled sirloin							
steak	580	33.0	50.0	26.0	85	1110	2.0
Double Western Ba-							
con Cheeseburger	900	51.0	64.0	49.0	155	1770	2.0
hamburger, *Carl's*							
Famous Star	580	25.0	49.0	32.0	70	910	2.0
hamburger, *Super*							
Star	790	42.0	50.0	46.0	130	970	2.0
hamburger Jr.	330	18.0	34.0	13.0	45	480	1.0
Western Bacon							
Cheeseburger ...	650	32.0	63.0	30.0	80	1430	2.0
sandwich cheese:							
American	60	3.0	0	5.0	15	280	0

Food and Measure	cal.	prot. (gms)	carbo. (gms)	fat (gms)	chol. (mgs)	sod. (mgs)	fiber (gms)
Carl's Jr., sandwich cheese (cont.)							
Swiss style	50	4.0	0	3.5	10	250	0
side dishes:							
chicken stars,							
6 pcs.	280	12.0	15.0	19.0	40	330	0
CrissCut Fries	410	5.0	43.0	24.0	0	950	4.0
french fries	290	5.0	37.0	14.0	0	170	3.0
hash brown nuggets	330	3.0	32.0	21.0	0	470	3.0
onion rings	430	7.0	53.0	21.0	0	700	3.0
zucchini	340	5.0	37.0	19.0	0	860	2.0
Great Stuff potatoes:							
plain, no margarine	290	6.0	68.0	0	0	20	6.0
bacon/cheese	630	20.0	76.0	29.0	35	1700	6.0
broccoli/cheese . . .	530	11.0	74.0	21.0	15	950	7.0
sour cream/chives	430	7.0	70.0	14.0	10	135	6.0
salads:							
Charbroiled Chicken							
Salad-to-Go	200	25.0	12.0	7.0	75	440	3.0
Garden Salad-to-Go	50	3.0	4.0	2.5	10	60	2.0
salad dressings, 2 oz.:							
blue cheese	320	2.0	1.0	35.0	25	370	0
French, fat free	60	0	16.0	0	0	660	<1.0
house	220	1.0	3.0	22.0	20	440	0
Italian, fat free	15	0	4.0	0	0	770	0
Thousand Island . . .	230	1.0	5.0	23.0	20	420	0
breads/sauces:							
breadsticks	35	1.0	7.0	.5	0	60	1.0
croutons	35	<1.0	5.0	1.0	0	65	0
BBQ sauce	50	1.0	11.0	0	0	270	0
grape jelly or straw-							
berry jam	36	0	9.0	0	0	0	0
honey sauce	90	0	22.0	0	0	0	0
mustard sauce	50	0	11.0	0	0	210	0
salsa	10	0	2.0	0	0	160	0
sweet n' sour sauce	50	0	12.0	0	0	80	0
table syrup	90	0	21.0	0	0	0	0
bakery/desserts:							
blueberry muffin . . .	340	5.0	49.0	14.0	40	340	1.0
bran raisin muffin	370	7.0	61.0	13.0	45	410	6.0
cheese danish	400	5.0	49.0	22.0	15	390	1.0
chocolate cake	300	3.0	49.0	10.0	23	260	4.0

Food and Measure	cal.	prot. (gms)	carbo. (gms)	fat (gms)	chol. (mgs)	sod. (mgs)	fiber (gms)
chocolate chip cookie	370	3.0	49.0	19.0	25	350	1.0
strawberry swirl cheesecake	290	6.0	30.0	17.0	55	230	0
shakes, small:							
chocolate	390	9.0	74.0	7.0	30	280	0
strawberry	400	9.0	77.0	7.0	30	240	0
vanilla	330	11.0	54.0	8.0	35	250	0
Carnival squash (*Frieda's*), ¾ cup, 3 oz.	30	1.0	7.0	0	0	0	1.0
Carob drink mix, powder, 3 tsp.	45	.2	11.2	tr.	0	12	<1.0
Carob flour, 1 cup ...	395	4.8	91.6	.7	0	36	41.0
Carp, meat only:							
raw, 4 oz.	144	20.2	0	6.4	75	58	0
baked, broiled, or microwaved, 4 oz. ...	184	25.9	0	8.1	95	71	0
Carrot, fresh:							
raw:							
whole, 7½″ long, 2.8 oz.	31	.7	7.3	.1	0	25	2.2
shredded, ½ cup ...	24	.6	5.6	.1	0	19	1.7
baby, 1 medium, 2¾″ long	4	.1	.8	.1	0	3	n.a.
boiled, drained, sliced, ½ cup	35	.9	8.2	.1	0	52	2.6
Carrot, canned, ½ cup, sliced, except as noted:							
(*Allens/Crest Top*) ...	35	0	8.0	.5	0	230	3.0
(*Del Monte*)	35	0	8.0	0	0	300	3.0
(*Green Giant*)	25	<1.0	6.0	0	0	380	2.0
(*Seneca*)	25	<1.0	6.0	0	0	250	2.0
(*Seneca* No Salt)	25	<1.0	6.0	0	0	30	2.0
baby, whole (*LeSueur*)	35	<1.0	8.0	0	0	410	3.0
w/liquid	28	.8	6.2	.2	0	297	1.1
drained	17	.5	4.0	.1	0	176	1.1
Carrot, dehydrated, diced (*AlpineAire*), ¾ oz.	80	2.0	17.0	0	0	55	2.0

Food and Measure	cal.	prot. (gms)	carbo. (gms)	fat (gms)	chol. (mgs)	sod. (mgs)	fiber (gms)
Carrot, frozen:							
(*Seneca*), ¾ cup	25	<1.0	6.0	0	0	180	2.0
boiled, drained, sliced,							
½ cup	26	.9	6.0	.1	0	43	2.6
baby:							
(*Birds Eye*), 3 oz.	40	1.0	9.0	0	0	45	2.0
(*Birds Eye* Deluxe),							
½ cup	40	1.0	9.0	0	0	45	2.0
(*Birds Eye Farm*							
Fresh), ⅔ cup . . .	35	<1.0	6.0	0	0	45	2.0
(*Cascadian Farm*),							
1 cup	60	1.0	14.0	0	0	160	3.0
(*Freshlike*), cup	35	1.0	6.0	0	0	45	2.0
baby, cut:							
(*Green Giant*),							
¾ cup	30	<1.0	7.0	0	0	40	3.0
(*Green Giant Har-*							
vest Fresh),							
⅔ cup	20	0	5.0	0	0	70	2.0
honey-glazed (*Green*							
Giant), 1 cup	90	<1.0	13.0	3.5	0	140	2.0
sliced:							
(*Birds Eye*), ½ cup	35	1.0	9.0	0	0	45	3.0
(*Freshlike*), ⅔ cup	35	1.0	6.0	0	0	45	2.0
Carrot juice, canned,							
8 fl. oz.	98	2.3	22.8	.4	0	72	2.0
Carvel:							
Fizzler, regular, 16 oz.	340	2.0	75.0	4.5	10	105	1.0
ice cream, ½ cup:							
chocolate	190	4.0	22.0	10.0	25	100	0
chocolate, no-fat . . .	120	2.0	28.0	0	0	40	0
vanilla	200	5.0	21.0	10.0	40	110	0
vanilla, no-fat	120	4.0	25.0	0	0	55	0
ice cream cake, 4 oz.,							
except as noted:							
cookies & cream . . .	270	5.0	32.0	14.0	35	160	<1.0
8″ round, ¹⁄₁₅ cake	200	4.0	24.0	10.0	25	115	<1.0
8″ round, reduced							
fat, ¹⁄₁₅ cake	170	3.0	30.0	4.0	0	80	0
sheet cake, large,							
¹⁄₂₆ cake, 3.3 oz.	220	4.0	26.0	11.0	25	120	<1.0

Food and Measure	cal.	prot. (gms)	carbo. (gms)	fat (gms)	chol. (mgs)	sod. (mgs)	fiber (gms)
sheet cake, reduced fat, 3.5 oz.	180	3.0	32.0	4.5	0	80	0
Sinfully chocolate	280	5.0	34.0	14.0	25	150	1.0
ice cream cone, 1 pc.:							
chocolate, small ...	240	5.0	34.0	10.0	25	130	<1.0
chocolate, large ...	410	9.0	53.0	18.0	50	220	2.0
vanilla, small......	250	6.0	33.0	10.0	40	140	0
vanilla, large	430	10.0	52.0	19.0	75	240	0
vanilla Brown Bonnet............	380	6.0	43.0	21.0	40	150	<1.0
vanilla Brown Bonnet, reduced fat	300	5.0	47.0	11.0	0	95	0
sandwiches:							
Chipster	380	6.0	50.0	18.0	30	240	4.0
Chipster, reduced calorie	320	5.0	53.0	11.0	0	200	4.0
Flying Saucer, chocolate or vanilla ...	240	5.0	33.0	10.0	30	180	<1.0
Flying Saucer, chocolate or vanilla, reduced calorie	180	4.0	36.0	2.5	0	140	<1.0
shakes, 16 fl. oz.:							
chocolate, low fat	490	16.0	108.0	1.0	15	330	<1.0
chocolate, thick ...	720	18.0	96.0	31.0	115	420	0
strawberry, low fat	460	15.0	96.0	1.0	15	290	<1.0
strawberry, thick...	650	17.0	77.0	30.0	115	360	0
vanilla, low fat	460	15.0	98.0	1.0	15	280	<1.0
vanilla, thick	660	17.0	79.0	30.0	115	350	0
sherbet, 1/2 cup	140	2.0	31.0	1.0	5	45	0
Sinful Love Bar, 1 bar	460	8.0	48.0	29.0	20	240	3.0
sundaes, 8 oz.:							
butterscotch	500	7.0	80.0	17.0	60	340	1.0
chocolate	470	8.0	71.0	19.0	55	280	1.0
strawberry	420	7.0	64.0	15.0	55	230	2.0
Casaba:							
1/10 of 73/4" melon	43	1.5	10.2	.2	0	20	1.3
pulp, cubed, 1/2 cup	23	.8	5.3	.1	0	10	.7
Cashew, 1 oz., except as noted:							
(*Beer Nuts* Classic)...	170	5.0	8.0	13.0	0	80	1.0
(*Frito-Lay*)	180	5.0	7.0	15.0	0	190	1.0

Food and Measure	cal.	prot. (gms)	carbo. (gms)	fat (gms)	chol. (mgs)	sod. (mgs)	fiber (gms)
Cashew *(cont.)*							
(Paradise/White Swan Whole), ¼ cup, 1.2 oz.	210	8.0	8.0	17.0	0	90	5.0
(Planters Fancy)	170	5.0	8.0	14.0	0	120	1.0
(Planters Halves)	170	6.0	7.0	14.0	0	120	1.0
(River Queen Fancy), ¼ cup, 1.2 oz.	190	5.0	10.0	16.0	0	180	1.0
(River Queen Fancy Unsalted)*, ¼ cup, 1.2 oz.	200	6.0	10.0	16.0	0	0	1.0
(River Queen Halves), ¼ cup, 1.2 oz.	190	5.0	9.0	16.0	0	170	1.0
(River Queen Halves Unsalted)*, ¼ cup, 1.2 oz.	190	5.0	9.0	16.0	0	5	1.0
dry-roasted:							
(River Queen Unsalted)	160	4.0	9.0	13.0	0	0	1.0
18 medium, 1 oz. whole or halves,	163	4.4	9.3	13.2	0	4	.9
1 cup	787	21.0	44.8	63.5	0	21	4.1
honey-roasted *(River Queen* Halves), ¼ cup, 1.2 oz.	180	5.0	12.0	14.0	0	100	1.0
oil-roasted:							
1 oz. or 18 medium whole or halves,	163	4.6	8.1	13.7	0	5	1.1
1 cup	748	21.0	37.1	62.7	0	22	4.9
Cashew butter:							
(Arrowhead Mills), 2 tbsp.	160	5.0	8.0	14.0	0	0	1.0
(Roaster Fresh), 1 oz.	165	4.0	9.0	14.0	0	4	0
Cassava, 1 oz.	34	.9	7.6	.1	0	2	<.1
Catfish, channel:							
farmed, meat only:							
raw, 4 oz.	153	17.7	0	8.6	15	60	0
baked, broiled, or microwaved,							
4 oz.	172	21.2	0	9.1	73	91	0

Food and Measure	cal.	prot. (gms)	carbo. (gms)	fat (gms)	chol. (mgs)	sod. (mgs)	fiber (gms)
wild, meat only:							
raw, 4 oz.	108	18.6	0	3.2	66	49	0
baked, broiled, or microwaved, 4 oz.	119	20.9	0	3.2	82	57	0
Catjang, boiled, ½ cup	100	7.0	17.5	.6	0	16	n.a.
Catsup, see "Ketchup"							
Cauliflower, fresh:							
raw:							
3 florets	14	1.1	2.9	.1	0	17	1.4
1″ pcs., ½ cup	13	1.0	2.6	.1	0	15	1.3
florets (*Dole*), 3 oz.	20	2.0	2.0	.5	0	35	2.0
boiled, drained, 1″ pcs., ½ cup	14	1.1	2.6	.3	0	9	1.7
green:							
raw, ⅕ head	28	2.7	5.7	.3	0	22	3.0
raw, 1″ pcs., ½ cup	16	1.5	3.0	.2	0	12	1.6
boiled, drained, 1″ pcs., ½ cup . . .	20	1.9	3.9	.2	0	14	2.0
Cauliflower, frozen:							
(*Birds Eye*), ½ cup . . .	20	2.0	4.0	0	0	15	2.0
(*Seneca*), 1 cup	20	1.0	3.0	0	0	15	2.0
boiled, drained, 1″ pcs., ½ cup	17	1.5	3.4	.2	0	16	2.0
florets:							
(*Birds Eye*), 3 oz.	20	2.0	4.0	0	0	25	2.0
(*Freshlike*), 4 pcs.	20	2.0	3.0	0	0	25	2.0
(*Green Giant*), 1 cup	25	2.0	4.0	0	0	25	2.0
w/carrots and snow peas (*Birds Eye Farm Fresh*), ½ cup	30	2.0	6.0	0	0	25	2.0
in cheese sauce:							
(*Birds Eye Side Orders*), ½ cup	80	3.0	7.0	5.0	5	630	1.0
(*Green Giant*), ½ cup	60	2.0	8.0	2.5	<5	510	1.0
Caviar (see also "Roe"), 1 tbsp.:							
black or red	40	3.9	.6	2.9	94	240	0
carp roe (*Krinos Tarama*)	20	3.0	0	.5	50	700	0

Food and Measure	cal.	prot. (gms)	carbo. (gms)	fat (gms)	chol. (mgs)	sod. (mgs)	fiber (gms)
Caviar *(cont.)*							
lumpfish, black or red							
(*Romanoff*)	15	1.0	0	1.0	50	380	0
salmon (*Romanoff*)	35	3.0	0	1.5	55	310	0
whitefish, black (*Romanoff*)	25	1.0	1.0	1.5	45	300	0
Caviar spread, 1 tbsp.:							
(*Krinos* Taramosalata)	90	1.0	0	10.0	15	115	0
(*Krinos* Taramosalata Lite)	40	<1.0	1.0	4.0	5	110	0
Cayenne, see "Pepper"							
Ceci, see "Garbanzo beans"							
Celeriac, fresh, raw:							
(*Frieda's* Celery Root), ¾ cup, 3 oz.	35	1.0	8.0	0	0	85	2.0
trimmed, 4 oz.	44	1.7	10.4	.3	0	113	2.0
trimmed, ½ cup	31	1.2	7.2	.2	0	78	1.4
Celery:							
raw:							
7½″-stalk, 1.6 oz.	6	.3	1.5	.1	0	35	.7
diced, ½ cup	10	.5	2.2	.1	0	52	1.0
boiled, drained, diced, ½ cup	13	.6	3.0	.1	0	68	1.2
Celery, Chinese (*Frieda's* Kun Choy), 1 cup, 3 oz.	15	1.0	3.0	0	0	75	1.0
Celery, dehydrated, diced (*AlpineAire*), .3 oz.	25	1.0	5.0	0	0	125	1.0
Celery, dried, flake/ seed (*Tone's*), 1 tsp.	9	.4	.9	.5	0	4	.3
Celery, frozen (*Seneca*), ¾ cup	10	0	3.0	0	0	10	2.0
Celery root, see "Celeriac"							
Celery salt (*Tone's*), 1 tsp.	6	.3	.6	.4	0	1584	.2

Food and Measure	cal.	prot. (gms)	carbo. (gms)	fat (gms)	chol. (mgs)	sod. (mgs)	fiber (gms)
Cellophane noodle, see "Noodle, Chinese"							
Celtus, raw, trimmed, 1 oz.	6	.2	1.0	.1	0	3	<1.0
Cereal, ready-to-eat (see also specific grains), 1 cup, except as noted:							
all varieties (*Health Valley* Healthy Crunchies & Flakes), ¾ cup	130	3.0	31.0	0	0	35	4.0
amaranth flakes:							
(*Arrowhead Mills*)	128	3.0	23.0	1.0	0	0	2.0
(*Health Valley*), ¾ cup	100	3.0	24.0	0	0	35	4.0
(*Boo Berry*)	120	1.0	27.0	1.0	0	220	0
bran:							
(*Kellogg's All-Bran/ Bran Buds*), cup	80	3.0	24.0	.5	0	210	13.0
(*Multi-Bran Chex*)	200	4.0	49.0	1.5	0	360	7.0
(*Nabisco 100% Bran*), ⅓ cup	80	4.0	23.0	.5	0	120	8.0
(*Post Bran'nola*), ½ cup	200	4.0	43.0	3.0	0	240	5.0
apple/cinnamon (*Health Valley*), ¾ cup	160	5.0	41.0	0	0	10	7.0
extra fiber (*Kellogg's All-Bran*), ½ cup	50	3.0	20.0	1.0	0	120	13.0
flakes (*Arrowhead Mills*)	90	4.0	18.0	1.0	0	80	5.0
flakes (*Kellogg's All-Bran*), ½ cup	80	4.0	24.0	1.0	0	65	10.0
flakes (*Post*), ⅔ cup	90	3.0	22.0	.5	0	210	6.0
bran w/raisins:							
(*Arrowhead Mills*)	190	6.0	41.0	1.5	0	300	10.0
(*Erewhon*)	170	5.0	40.0	1.0	0	100	6.0
(*Health Valley*), ¾ cup	160	5.0	40.0	0	0	10	6.0

Food and Measure	cal.	prot. (gms)	carbo. (gms)	fat (gms)	chol. (mgs)	sod. (mgs)	fiber (gms)
Cereal, ready-to-eat, bran w/raisins *(cont.)*							
(*Kellogg's*)	200	6.0	47.0	1.5	0	370	8.0
(*Malt-O-Meal*)	200	6.0	47.0	1.5	0	390	8.0
(*Post*)	190	4.0	46.0	1.0	0	300	8.0
(*Post Bran'nola*), ½ cup	200	4.0	44.0	3.0	0	220	5.0
(*Skinner's*)	170	6.0	41.0	1.0	0	85	7.0
(*Total*)	180	4.0	43.0	1.0	0	240	5.0
flakes (*Health Valley*), 1¼ cups . . .	190	5.0	47.0	0	0	90	6.0
and nuts (*Raisin Nut Bran*), ¾ cup	200	4.0	41.0	4.0	0	250	5.0
buckwheat flakes, maple (*Arrowhead Mills*)	160	4.0	35.0	1.0	0	210	3.0
corn:							
(*Barbara's Puffins*), ¾ cup	90	2.0	23.0	1.0	0	190	5.0
(*Cap'n Crunch*), ¾ cup	110	1.0	23.0	1.5	0	205	1.0
(*Corn Bursts*)	120	1.0	29.0	0	0	120	0
(*Corn Chex*)	110	2.0	26.0	0	0	300	0
(*Erewhon Aztec*) . . .	110	2.0	26.0	0	0	70	1.0
(*Post Toasties*)	100	2.0	24.0	0	0	270	1.0
chocolate flavor (*Cocoa Puffs*) . . .	120	1.0	27.0	1.0	0	190	0
cinnamon (*Barbara's Puffins*), ¾ cup	100	2.0	26.0	1.0	0	150	6.0
maple (*Arrowhead Mills*)	190	5.0	43.0	3.0	0	140	6.0
peanut butter (*Cap'n Crunch*), ¾ cup	115	2.0	22.0	2.5	0	200	1.0
puffed (*Arrowhead Mills*)	60	2.0	11.0	.5	0	0	0
puffed (*Body Buddies*)	120	2.0	26.0	1.0	0	290	0
puffed, honey sweetened (*Health Valley*)	110	2.0	28.0	0	0	0	2.0

Food and Measure	cal.	prot. (gms)	carbo. (gms)	fat (gms)	chol. (mgs)	sod. (mgs)	fiber (gms)
puffed, sweetened (*Kellogg's Corn Pops*)	120	1.0	28.0	0	0	120	0
cornflakes:							
(*Arrowhead Mills*)	120	2.0	27.0	0	0	210	4.0
(*Barbara's Frosted*)	110	2.0	27.0	0	0	100	4.0
(*Country*)	120	2.0	26.0	0	0	270	0
(*Erewhon*), 1¼ cups	210	5.0	45.0	2.5	0	100	3.0
(*Kellogg's*)	100	2.0	24.0	0	0	300	1.0
(*Kellogg's Frosted Flakes*), ¾ cup ...	120	1.0	28.0	0	0	200	1.0
(*Kellogg's Honey Crunch Corn Flakes*), ¾ cup ...	120	2.0	26.0	1.0	0	210	1.0
(*Malt-O-Meal*)	110	2.0	26.0	0	0	320	1.0
(*New Morning*)	120	2.0	25.0	1.0	0	60	1.0
(*New Morning Fruiteo's*)	120	2.0	25.0	1.0	0	60	2.0
(*Total*), 1⅓ cups ...	110	2.0	26.0	0	0	200	0
blue bran (*Health Valley*), ¾ cup ...	100	3.0	24.0	0	0	10	4.0
chocolate flavor (*Kellogg's Cocoa Frosted Flakes*), ¾ cup	120	1.0	28.0	0	0	210	0
w/flax (*New Morning*)	120	2.0	26.0	1.0	0	60	1.0
w/ginseng (*New Morning*), ¾ cup	110	2.0	22.0	2.0	0	60	3.0
juice sweetened (*Barbara's*)	110	2.0	26.0	0	0	130	3.0
sweetened (*Arrowhead Mills*)	130	3.0	30.0	0	0	65	2.0
sweetened (*Malt-O-Meal*), ¾ cup ...	110	1.0	27.0	0	0	200	<1.0
corn and rice (*Kellogg's Crispix*)	110	2.0	25.0	0	0	210	1.0
flax, golden (*Health Valley*), ½ cup	190	6.0	38.0	3.0	0	30	6.0
granola:							
(*C.W. Post*), ⅔ cup	280	5.0	45.0	9.0	0	150	4.0

Food and Measure	cal.	prot. (gms)	carbo. (gms)	fat (gms)	chol. (mgs)	sod. (mgs)	fiber (gms)
Cereal, ready-to-eat, granola *(cont.)*							
(*Heartland*), 1/2 cup	300	9.0	41.0	11.0	0	160	4.0
(*Heartland Low Fat*), 1/2 cup	210	5.0	40.0	3.0	0	50	3.0
(*Kellogg's Lowfat*), 1/2 cup	190	4.0	39.0	3.0	0	120	3.0
all varieties (*Health Valley* 98% Fat Free), 2/3 cup	180	5.0	43.0	1.0	0	90	6.0
all varieties (*Health Valley Granola O's*), 3/4 cup	120	3.0	26.0	0	0	90	3.0
w/fruit (*Nature Valley* Lowfat), 2/3 cup	210	4.0	44.0	2.5	0	210	3.0
w/honey (*New Morning*), 3/4 cup	200	5.0	42.0	2.0	0	60	3.0
oats, honey, raisins (*Quaker* 100% Natural), 1/2 cup	225	5.0	34.0	9.0	0	20	3.0
oats and honey (*Quaker* 100% Natural), 1/2 cup	220	5.0	31.0	9.0	0	20	3.0
w/raisins (*Heartland*), 1/2 cup	290	8.0	42.0	10.0	0	140	4.0
w/raisins (*Kellogg's* Lowfat), 2/3 cup	220	5.0	47.0	3.0	0	150	3.0
w/raisins (*Quaker* 100% Natural), 2/3 cup	210	5.0	44.0	3.0	0	145	3.0
kamut:							
(*New Morning Kamutios*)	120	5.0	23.0	1.0	0	90	1.0
flakes (*Arrowhead Mills*)	110	4.0	25.0	1.0	0	75	3.0
flakes (*Erewhon*), 2/3 cup	110	5.0	25.0	0	0	75	4.0
puffed (*Arrowhead Mills*)	50	2.0	11.0	0	0	0	1.0
millet, puffed (*Arrowhead Mills*)	60	2.0	12.0	.5	0	0	0

Food and Measure	cal.	prot. (gms)	carbo. (gms)	fat (gms)	chol. (mgs)	sod. (mgs)	fiber (gms)
multigrain (see also "granola," above):							
(*Apple Jacks*)	120	2.0	30.0	0	0	150	1.0
(*Barbara's Shredded Spoonfuls*), ¾ cup	120	5.0	23.0	1.5	0	200	4.0
(*Basic 4*)	200	4.0	43.0	3.0	0	320	3.0
(*Berry Berry Kix*), ¾ cup	120	1.0	26.0	1.5	0	170	0
(*Berry Colossal Crunch*), ¾ cup	120	1.0	26.0	1.5	0	220	1.0
(*Cinnamon Grahams*), ¾ cup	120	1.0	26.0	1.0	0	230	1.0
(*Cinnamon Toast Crunch*), ¾ cup	130	1.0	24.0	3.5	0	210	1.0
(*Coco-Roos*), ¾ cup	120	1.0	27.0	1.0	0	190	<1.0
(Cocoa *Pebbles*), ¾ cup	120	1.0	25.0	1.0	0	160	<1.0
(*Colossal Crunch*), ¾ cup	120	1.0	26.0	1.5	0	230	1.0
(*Erewhon Apple Stroodles*), ¾ cup	110	3.0	25.0	.5	0	15	1.0
(*Erewhon Banana-O's*), ¾ cup	110	2.0	26.0	0	0	15	2.0
(*Erewhon Galaxy Grahams*), ¾ cup	100	3.0	23.0	.5	0	60	2.0
(*Fiber One*), ½ cup	60	2.0	24.0	1.0	0	140	13.0
(*French Toast Crunch*), ¾ cup	120	1.0	26.0	1.0	0	180	0
(*Frosted Mini-Spooners*)	190	5.0	45.0	1.0	0	0	6.0
(*Fruit Loops*)	120	2.0	28.0	1.0	0	150	1.0
(Fruity *Pebbles*), ¾ cup	110	1.0	24.0	1.0	0	150	0
(*Golden Crisp*), ¾ cup	110	1.0	25.0	0	0	40	0
(*Golden Grahams*), ¾ cup	120	1.0	26.0	1.0	0	280	1.0
(*Golden Puffs*), ¾ cup	100	2.0	25.0	0	0	40	1.0
(*Grape-Nuts*), ½ cup	200	6.0	47.0	1.0	0	350	5.0

Food and Measure	cal.	prot. (gms)	carbo. (gms)	fat (gms)	chol. (mgs)	sod. (mgs)	fiber (gms)
Cereal, ready-to-eat, multigrain *(cont.)*							
(*Honey Nut Chex*), ¾ cup	120	2.0	26.0	.5	0	220	0
(*Honey Nut Clusters*)	210	4.0	46.0	2.5	0	270	3.0
(*Honeycomb*), 1⅓ cups	110	2.0	35.0	0	0	190	<1.0
(*Kaboom*), 1¼ cups	120	2.0	24.0	1.5	0	290	1.0
(*Kellogg's Healthy Choice* Squares)	190	5.0	44.0	1.0	0	210	5.0
(*Kellogg's Just Right*)	210	4.0	46.0	1.5	0	320	3.0
(*Kellogg's Nutri-Grain*), 1¼ cups	180	4.0	38.0	2.5	0	170	4.0
(*Kellogg's Product 19*)	100	2.0	25.0	0	0	210	1.0
(*Kix*), 1⅓ cups	120	2.0	26.0	.5	0	270	1.0
(*Marshmallow Mateys*)	120	2.0	25.0	1.0	0	210	1.0
(*Multi-Grain Cheerios* Plus)	110	3.0	24.0	1.0	0	200	3.0
(*Nabisco Team Flakes*), 1¼ cups	220	4.0	49.0	0	0	360	1.0
(*Quaker Life*), ¾ cup	120	3.0	25.0	1.5	0	170	2.0
(*Team Cheerios*) ...	120	2.0	25.0	1.0	0	220	1.0
(*Tootie Fruities*) ...	120	1.0	26.0	1.0	0	140	<1.0
(*Total* Whole Grain), ¾ cup	110	3.0	24.0	1.0	0	190	3.0
(*Trix*)	120	1.0	26.0	1.5	0	200	1.0
(*Uncle Sam*)	190	7.0	38.0	5.0	0	135	10.0
w/almonds, raisins (*Kellogg's Healthy Choice*)	210	5.0	46.0	2.5	0	230	5.0
w/apples, almonds (*Kellogg's Mues-lix*), ¾ cup	200	5.0	39.0	5.0	0	260	5.0
w/blueberries (*Blueberry Morning*), 1¼ cups	230	4.0	45.0	3.5	0	250	2.0
dates, raisins, walnuts (*Fruit & Fibre*)	210	4.0	46.0	3.0	0	260	6.0

Food and Measure	cal.	prot. (gms)	carbo. (gms)	fat (gms)	chol. (mgs)	sod. (mgs)	fiber (gms)
flakes (*Arrowhead Mills*)	140	3.0	29.0	1.5	0	130	3.0
flakes (*Grape-Nuts*), ¾ cup	100	3.0	24.0	1.0	0	140	3.0
flakes (*Health Valley* Fiber 7), ¾ cup	100	3.0	24.0	0	0	15	4.0
flakes (*Health Valley* Healthy Fiber), ¾ cup	100	3.0	23.0	0	0	10	4.0
flakes (*Kellogg's Healthy Choice*), ¾ cup	110	3.0	26.0	0	0	180	3.0
w/fruit, nuts (*Banana Nut Crunch*)	250	5.0	43.0	6.0	0	200	4.0
w/fruit, nuts (*Kellogg's Just Right*)	220	4.0	49.0	2.0	0	280	3.0
peaches, raisins, almonds (*Fruit & Fibre*)	210	4.0	46.0	3.0	0	270	6.0
w/pecans (*Great Grains*), ⅔ cup	220	5.0	38.0	6.0	0	150	4.0
w/raisins, almonds, dates (*Kellogg's Mueslix*), ⅔ cup	200	5.0	41.0	3.0	0	160	4.0
raisins, dates, pecans (*Great Grains*), ⅔ cup	210	4.0	39.0	5.0	0	150	4.0
oat:							
(*Arrowhead Mills Nature O's*)	130	4.0	24.0	2.0	0	5	3.0
(*Barbara's Breakfast O's*)	120	5.0	22.0	2.0	0	115	3.0
(*Cheerios*)	110	3.0	22.0	2.0	0	280	3.0
(*Frosted Cheerios*)	120	2.0	25.0	1.0	0	210	1.0
(*Frosted Toasty O's*)	120	2.0	25.0	1.0	0	210	1.0
(*Honey Bunches of Oats*), ¾ cup	120	2.0	25.0	1.5	0	190	1.0
(*Honey Nut Cheerios*)	120	3.0	24.0	1.5	0	270	2.0
(*Honey Nut Toasty O's*)	110	3.0	24.0	1.0	0	270	2.0

Food and Measure	cal.	prot. (gms)	carbo. (gms)	fat (gms)	chol. (mgs)	sod. (mgs)	fiber (gms)
Cereal, ready-to-eat, oat *(cont.)*							
(*New Morning Oatios*)	120	4.0	21.0	1.0	0	60	2.0
(*Quaker* Oatmeal Squares)	220	7.0	44.0	3.0	0	260	4.0
(*Quaker* Toasted Oatmeal Original)	190	5.0	40.0	2.5	0	215	4.0
(*Toasty O's*)	110	3.0	22.0	2.0	0	280	3.0
w/almond (*Honey Bunches of Oats*), ¾ cup	130	3.0	24.0	3.0	0	180	1.0
w/almond (*New Morning Oatios*)	100	3.0	22.0	1.0	0	60	3.0
w/almond (*Oatmeal Crisp*)	220	6.0	41.0	5.0	0	240	4.0
apple cinnamon (*Barbara's* Toasted O's), ¾ cup	110	3.0	24.0	1.0	0	90	2.0
apple cinnamon (*Cheerios*), ¾ cup	120	2.0	25.0	2.0	0	160	1.0
apple cinnamon (*New Morning Oatios*)	90	2.0	21.0	1.5	0	60	5.0
apple cinnamon (*Oatmeal Crisp*)	210	4.0	46.0	2.0	0	270	4.0
apple cinnamon (*Toasty O's*), ¾ cup	120	2.0	25.0	1.5	0	160	1.0
w/blueberries (*New Morning Oatiola*)	200	5.0	41.0	1.5	0	60	4.0
cinnamon (*Quaker* Oatmeal Squares)	230	8.0	47.0	2.5	0	265	5.0
cinnamon (*Quaker Life*), ¾ cup	120	3.0	25.0	1.0	0	145	2.0
cocoa (*Arrowhead Mills* Cocoa O's)	130	3.0	27.0	.5	0	115	6.0
cocoa (*New Morning Oatios*)	170	6.0	37.0	1.5	0	60	4.0

Food and Measure	cal.	prot. (gms)	carbo. (gms)	fat (gms)	chol. (mgs)	sod. (mgs)	fiber (gms)
honey nut (*Barbara's* Toasty O's), ¾ cup	120	3.0	23.0	2.0	0	90	2.0
honey nut (*Quaker* Toasted Oatmeal)	190	4.0	40.0	3.0	0	185	4.0
w/marshmallow (*Alpha-Bits*)	120	2.0	25.0	10	0	160	1.0
w/marshmallows (*Lucky Charms*)	120	2.0	25.0	1.0	0	210	1.0
w/raisin (*Oatmeal Crisp*)	210	4.0	44.0	2.5	0	210	4.0
shredded (*Barbara's* Bite Size), 1¼ cups	220	6.0	46.0	2.5	0	260	6.0
sweetened (*Alpha-Bits*)	130	3.0	27.0	1.0	0	210	1.0
sweetened (*Arrowhead Mills* Nature O's)	160	8.0	31.0	2.5	0	110	3.0
oat bran:							
(*Health Valley* O's), ¾ cup	100	3.0	23.0	0	0	90	3.0
(*Health Valley* Real), ½ cup	200	6.0	34.0	3.0	0	90	5.0
(*Kellogg's Cracklin' Oat Bran*), ¾ cup	190	4.0	35.0	7.0	0	170	6.0
(*Quaker*), 1¼ cups	210	7.0	43.0	3.0	0	205	6.0
apple cinnamon (*Health Valley 10 Bran O's*), ¾ cup	100	3.0	23.0	0	0	90	3.0
flakes (*Arrowhead Mills*)	140	6.0	24.0	2.5	0	80	4.0
flakes (*Health Valley*), ¾ cup	100	3.0	24.0	0	0	90	4.0
flakes (*Kellogg's Complete*), ¾ cup	110	4.0	23.0	1.0	0	270	4.0
flakes (*New Morning*)	110	4.0	21.0	1.0	0	60	5.0
flakes, w/raisins (*Health Valley*), ¾ cup	110	3.0	26.0	0	0	15	4.0

Food and Measure	cal.	prot. (gms)	carbo. (gms)	fat (gms)	chol. (mgs)	sod. (mgs)	fiber (gms)
Cereal, ready-to-eat, oat bran *(cont.)*							
w/ginkgo (*New Morning GinkgO's*)	120	4.0	21.0	1.0	0	60	2.0
rice:							
(*Kellogg's Razzle Dazzle*), ³/₄ cup	110	1.0	25.0	0	0	170	0
(*Kellogg's Rice Krispies*), 1¹/₄ cups	120	2.0	29.0	0	0	350	0
(*Kellogg's Rice Krispies Treats*), ³/₄ cup	120	1.0	26.0	1.5	0	190	0
(*Kellogg's Smart Start*)	180	3.0	43.0	.5	0	310	2.0
(*Malt-O-Meal*)	110	2.0	26.0	0	0	320	<1.0
(*Rice Chex*), 1¹/₄ cups	120	2.0	27.0	0	0	290	0
brown (*Barbara's Rice Crisps*)	120	2.0	25.0	1.0	0	125	1.0
cocoa flavor (*Kellogg's Cocoa Krispies*), ³/₄ cup	120	1.0	27.0	1.0	0	220	0
flakes (*Arrowhead Mills*)	80	3.0	19.0	1.0	0	210	2.0
flakes (*Kellogg's Special K*)	110	6.0	23.0	0	0	220	1.0
puffed (*Arrowhead Mills*)	60	1.0	14.0	.5	0	0	0
puffed (*Malt-O-Meal*)	60	1.0	13.0	0	0	20	<1.0
puffed, crisp, honey sweetened (*Health Valley*)	110	1.0	28.0	0	0	0	2.0
rice, brown:							
(*Erewhon Poppets*)	120	2.0	25.0	1.0	0	10	<1.0
(*Erewhon Rice Twice*), ³/₄ cup ...	120	2.0	26.0	0	0	60	0
(*New Morning Crispy*)	110	2.0	23.0	1.0	0	0	1.0
crispy (*Erewhon*) *	110	2.0	25.0	0	0	180	1.0

Food and Measure	cal.	prot. (gms)	carbo. (gms)	fat (gms)	chol. (mgs)	sod. (mgs)	fiber (gms)
crispy (*Erewhon* No Salt)	110	2.0	25.0	0	0	10	1.0
frosted (*New Morning* Crispy)	210	6.0	45.0	1.5	0	60	6.0
spelt flakes (*Arrowhead Mills*)	100	4.0	23.0	.5	0	100	4.0
wheat:							
(*Erewhon* Fruit 'n Wheat), ¾ cup	170	5.0	39.0	1.5	0	105	5.0
(*Kellogg's Frosted Mini-Wheats*), 5 pcs.	180	5.0	41.0	1.0	0	170	5.0
(*Kellogg's Frosted Mini-Wheats Bite-Size*), 24 pcs. ...	200	6.0	48.0	1.0	0	200	6.0
(*Kellogg's Nutri-Grain*), ¾ cup ...	100	3.0	23.0	1.0	0	210	4.0
(*Nabisco Frosted Wheat Bites*)	190	4.0	44.0	1.0	0	10	5.0
(*Wheat Chex*)	180	5.0	41.0	1.0	0	420	5.0
apple cinnamon (*Kellogg's Mini-Wheats*), ¾ cup	180	4.0	44.0	1.0	0	20	5.0
blueberry (*Kellogg's Mini-Wheats*), ¾ cup	180	4.0	43.0	1.0	0	20	5.0
blueberry (*Nabisco Fruit Wheats*), ¾ cup	170	4.0	41.0	.5	0	15	4.0
chocolate graham (*New Morning*), 2 pcs.	120	3.0	21.0	3.0	0	120	1.0
cinnamon graham (*New Morning*), 2 pcs.	100	2.0	20.0	2.0	0	125	1.0
cinnamon graham (*New Morning Mini-Bites*), 15 pcs.	120	2.0	24.0	2.5	0	135	1.0
flakes (*Arrowhead Mills*)	160	5.0	37.0	.5	0	200	6.0

Food and Measure	cal.	prot. (gms)	carbo. (gms)	fat (gms)	chol. (mgs)	sod. (mgs)	fiber (gms)
Cereal, ready-to-eat, wheat *(cont.)*							
flakes (*Erewhon*) . . .	180	6.0	42.0	1.0	0	135	6.0
flakes (*Wheaties*)	110	3.0	24.0	1.0	0	220	3.0
germ, see "Wheat germ"							
ginger graham (*New Morning*), 2 pcs.	140	2.0	26.0	4.5	0	180	1.0
honey graham (*New Morning*), 2 pcs.	110	2.0	21.0	2.0	0	135	1.0
honey graham (*New Morning Mini-Bites*), 15 pcs.	120	2.0	24.0	2.5	0	135	1.0
lemon graham (*New Morning* Mini-Bites), 15 pcs.	120	2.0	23.0	2.5	0	130	1.0
puffed (*Arrowhead Mills*)	60	2.0	13.0	.5	0	0	1.0
puffed (*Kellogg's Smacks*), ¾ cup	100	2.0	24.0	.5	0	50	1.0
puffed (*Malt-O-Meal*)	50	2.0	11.0	0	0	60	1.0
w/raisins (*Crispy Wheaties 'n Raisins*)	190	4.0	45.0	1.0	0	270	4.0
w/raisins (*Kellogg's Raisin Squares*), ¾ cup	180	5.0	42.0	1.0	0	5	5.0
raspberry (*Nabisco Fruit Wheats*), ¾ cup	160	4.0	40.0	.5	0	15	4.0
strawberry (*Kellogg's Mini-Wheats*), ¾ cup	170	4.0	40.0	1.0	0	15	5.0
strawberry (*Nabisco Fruit Wheats*), ¾ cup	170	4.0	41.0	.5	0	15	4.0
sweetened (*Honey Frosted Wheaties*), ¾ cup	110	1.0	27.0	0	0	200	0
wheat, shredded: (*Arrowhead Mills*)	180	5.0	41.0	.5	0	0	6.0

Food and Measure	cal.	prot. (gms)	carbo. (gms)	fat (gms)	chol. (mgs)	sod. (mgs)	fiber (gms)
(*Barbara's*), 2 pcs.	140	4.0	31.0	1.0	0	0	5.0
(*Barbara's* Ultra Minis Frosted), ¾ cup	190	4.0	46.0	1.0	0	200	7.0
(*Barbara's* Ultra Minis Original), ¾ cup	190	5.0	45.0	1.0	0	240	8.0
(*Nabisco*), 2 pcs.	160	5.0	38.0	.5	0	0	5.0
(*Nabisco Spoon Size*)	170	5.0	41.0	.5	0	0	5.0
(*Quaker*), 3 pcs.	220	7.0	50.0	1.5	0	0	7.0
w/bran (*Nabisco*), 1¼ cups	200	7.0	47.0	1.0	0	250	0
sweetened (*Arrowhead Mills*)	200	5.0	44.0	1.0	0	0	6.0
wheat bran:							
flakes (*Kellogg's Complete*), ¾ cup	90	3.0	23.0	.5	0	220	5.0
flakes (*New Morning*)	110	4.0	21.0	1.0	0	5	5.0
w/raisins (*New Morning*)	90	3.0	22.0	.5	0	60	6.0
Cereal, cooking/hot (see also specific grains), uncooked, 1 pkt., except as noted:							
barley:							
(*Arrowhead Mills Bits O Barley*), ⅓ cup	140	5.0	33.0	1.0	0	0	6.0
(*Erewhon Barley Plus*), ¼ cup	170	5.0	37.0	1.0	0	0	4.0
banana nut (*Fantastic Foods* cup) ...	170	4.0	39.0	2.5	0	240	6.0
buckwheat, cream of (*Wolff's*), ⅓ cup ...	90	1.0	21.0	0	0	0	0
farina, see "wheat," below							
grits, see "Corn grits"							

Food and Measure	cal.	prot. (gms)	carbo. (gms)	fat (gms)	chol. (mgs)	sod. (mgs)	fiber (gms)
Cereal, cooking/hot *(cont.)*							
multigrain:							
(*Arrowhead Mills* Instant)	100	3.0	22.0	1.0	0	0	3.0
(*Quaker*), ½ cup . . .	130	5.0	30.0	1.0	0	0	5.0
3-grain, maple raisin (*Fantastic Foods* cup)	180	5.0	42.0	1.0	0	240	5.0
4-grain w/flax (*Arrowhead Mills*), ¼ cup	150	6.0	28.0	2.0	0	0	6.0
5-grain (*Alpineaire*)	260	13.0	35.0	2.0	0	650	11.0
5-grain, fruit-nut (*AlpineAire*)	240	8.0	45.0	3.5	0	45	5.0
7-grain (*Arrowhead Mills*), ¼ cup	140	6.0	25.0	1.5	0	0	5.0
7-grain, wheat free (*Arrowhead Mills*), ¼ cup	120	4.0	25.0	1.5	0	0	2.0
all varieties (*U.S. Mills Naturals Wafflers*), ⅔ cup	110	2.0	26.0	1.0	0	65	2.0
apple (*Health Valley* Amazing Apple!)	220	9.0	43.0	2.0	0	230	4.0
banana nut (*Arrowhead Mills* Instant)	150	4.0	31.0	1.5	0	200	4.0
banana nut (*Health Valley* Banana Gone Nuts!)	240	10.0	45.0	3.0	0	240	4.0
hearty (*Fantastic Foods* Cup)	260	9.0	52.0	2.5	0	240	4.0
hearty, w/apricot (*Fantastic Foods* Cup)	240	8.0	50.0	2.5	0	260	4.0
maple (*Health Valley* Maple Madness!)	240	9.0	47.0	2.0	0	290	4.0
oat bran:							
(*Quaker*), ½ cup . . .	150	7.0	25.0	3.0	0	230	6.0

Food and Measure	cal.	prot. (gms)	carbo. (gms)	fat (gms)	chol. (mgs)	sod. (mgs)	fiber (gms)
w/toasted wheat germ (*Erewhon*), ⅓ cup	170	10.0	31.0	2.5	0	0	5.0
oats/oatmeal:							
(*H-O* Instant), ½ cup	150	5.0	27.0	3.0	0	0	4.0
(*H-O* Regular)	110	4.0	18.0	2.5	0	220	3.0
(*H-O* Oats n Fiber)	100	4.0	19.0	2.0	0	140	3.0
(*H-O* Power Oats)	160	4.0	32.0	2.0	0	220	3.0
(*H-O* Quick), ½ cup	150	5.0	27.0	3.0	0	0	4.0
(*Quaker* Instant Oatmeal Low Sodium)	100	4.0	20.0	2.0	0	75	2.5
(*Quaker* Old Fashioned/Quick Oats), ½ cup	150	5.0	27.0	3.0	0	140	4.0
(*U.S. Mills Naturals Oats Plus*), ½ cup	200	8.0	37.0	3.0	0	90	8.0
w/added oat bran (*Erewhon* Instant)	130	6.0	25.0	2.5	0	0	4.0
apple cinnamon:							
(*Erewhon*Instant)	130	5.0	24.0	2.0	0	100	3.0
(*Fantastic Foods* Cup) . . .	170	6.0	37.0	2.0	0	240	4.0
(*H-O*)	130	3.0	26.0	3.0	0	100	3.0
(*Quaker* Instant Oatmeal)	130	3.0	30.0	1.5	0	110	3.0
apple raisin (*Erewhon* Instant) . . .	140	5.0	26.0	2.0	0	100	3.0
banana and cream (*Quaker* Instant Oatmeal)	130	3.0	25.0	3.0	0	165	2.0
blueberry and cream(*Quaker* Instant Oatmeal) . . .	130	3.0	25.0	3.0	0	175	2.0
cinnamon, raisin, almond (*Arrowhead Mills* Instant)	130	5.0	24.0	2.0	0	0	2.0
cinnamon spice (*Quaker* Instant Oatmeal)	170	4.0	35.0	2.0	0	110	3.0

Food and Measure	cal.	prot. (gms)	carbo. (gms)	fat (gms)	chol. (mgs)	sod. (mgs)	fiber (gms)
Cereal, cooking/hot, oats/oatmeal *(cont.)*							
cookies 'n cream (*Quaker* Instant Oatmeal)	160	4.0	30.0	3.0	0	200	2.0
cranberry orange (*Fantastic Foods* Cup)	180	6.0	38.0	2.0	0	210	4.0
maple, apple, spice (*Arrowhead Mills* Instant)	130	4.0	25.0	2.0	0	40	2.0
maple brown sugar:							
(*H-O*)	160	4.0	32.0	2.0	0	220	3.0
(*Quaker* Instant Oatmeal)	160	4.0	35.0	2.0	0	240	3.0
maple spice (*Erewhon* Instant) ...	130	5.0	25.0	2.0	0	100	3.0
peaches or strawberries and cream (*Quaker* Instant Oatmeal)	130	3.0	25.0	3.0	0	100	2.0
raisin, dates, walnut:							
(*Erewhon* Instant)	130	4.0	24.0	2.5	0	40	3.0
(*Quaker* Instant Oatmeal)	130	3.0	27.0	2.5	0	240	3.0
raisin spice:							
(*H-O*)	160	5.0	32.0	2.0	0	250	3.0
(*Quaker* Instant Oatmeal)	150	4.0	32.0	2.0	0	250	3.0
sweet and mellow (*H-O*)	150	4.0	30.0	2.0	0	200	2.0
rice:							
(*Arrowhead Mills* Instant)	100	2.0	22.0	.5	0	0	1.0
(*Arrowhead Mills* Rice & Shine), 1/4 cup	150	3.0	32.0	1.0	0	0	2.0
(*Lundberg* Amber Grain Hot 'n Creamy), 1/3 cup	190	3.0	44.0	1.5	0	0	2.0

Food and Measure	cal.	prot. (gms)	carbo. (gms)	fat (gms)	chol. (mgs)	sod. (mgs)	fiber (gms)
(*Lundberg* Organic Hot 'n Creamy), ⅓ cup	190	4.0	43.0	2.0	0	0	3.0
almond, sweet (*Lundberg* Hot 'n Creamy), ⅓ cup	200	3.0	40.0	3.5	0	0	4.0
apple spice (*Arrowhead Mills* Instant)	150	2.0	33.0	.5	0	0	1.0
brown (*Erewhon* Cream), ¼ cup	170	5.0	36.0	1.0	0	30	1.0
cinnamon raisin (*Lundberg* Hot 'n Creamy), ⅓ cup	190	3.0	42.0	1.5	0	0	4.0
wheat:							
(*Arrowhead Mills Bear Mush*), ¼ cup	160	5.0	33.0	1.0	0	0	2.0
(*Malt-O-Meal* Quick), 3 tbsp.	120	4.0	26.0	0	0	0	1.0
(*Wheat Hearts*), ¼ cup	130	5.0	26.0	1.0	0	0	2.0
apple cinnamon (*Malt-O-Meal*), 3 tbsp.	120	3.0	28.0	0	0	0	1.0
and berries (*Fantastic Foods* Cup) ...	170	5.0	40.0	1.0	0	230	5.0
chocolate (*Malt-O-Meal*), 3 tbsp.	120	3.0	28.0	0	0	0	1.0
cracked (*Arrowhead Mills*), ¼ cup	140	5.0	29.0	.5	0	0	6.0
farina (*H-O* Cream), 3 tbsp.	120	3.0	26.0	0	0	0	1.0
farina (*Quaker* Creamy Wheat), ¼ cup	150	5.0	35.0	.5	0	0	1.0
maple brown sugar (*Malt-O-Meal*), 3 tbsp.	120	3.0	26.0	0	0	0	1.0
whole (*Quaker* Natural), ½ cup	130	5.0	30.0	1.0	0	0	4.0

Food and Measure	cal.	prot. (gms)	carbo. (gms)	fat (gms)	chol. (mgs)	sod. (mgs)	fiber (gms)
Cereal, cooking/hot *(cont.)*							
wheat and oats, peach-berry *(Fantastic Foods* Cup)	190	5.0	42.0	1.5	0	260	5.0
Cereal bar, see "Granola and cereal bar"							
Cereal beverage, see "Coffee substitute"							
Cereal crumbs, see "Corn flake crumbs"							
Cervelat, see "Summer sausage"							
Chayote:							
raw:							
(Frieda's), ⅔ cup, 3 oz.	20	1.0	5.0	0	0	0	3.0
1 medium, 7.2 oz.	49	1.8	11.0	.6	0	8	6.1
1″ pcs., ½ cup	16	.6	3.6	.2	0	3	2.0
boiled, drained, 1″ pcs., ½ cup	19	.5	4.1	.4	0	1	n.a.
Cheese (see also "Cheese food," and "Cheese spread"), 1 oz., except as noted:							
American, processed:							
(Alpine Lace Reduced Fat/Sodium)	80	6.0	2.0	6.0	20	200	0
(Black Bear Slice), ⅔ oz.	70	4.0	0	6.0	25	240	0
(Boar's Head)	100	6.0	1.0	9.0	25	380	0
(Harvest Moon Slice), ⅔ oz.	70	4.0	0	6.0	20	320	0
(Heluva Good)	70	4.0	1.0	5.0	15	250	0
(Kraft Deluxe Loaf)	100	6.0	<1.0	9.0	25	430	0
(Kraft Deluxe Slice), ⅔ oz.	70	4.0	<1.0	6.0	15	310	0
(Kraft Deluxe Slice)	110	5.0	<1.0	9.0	25	460	0
(Kraft Deluxe Slice), ¾ oz.	80	4.0	<1.0	7.0	20	340	0

Food and Measure	cal.	prot. (gms)	carbo. (gms)	fat (gms)	chol. (mgs)	sod. (mgs)	fiber (gms)
(*Land O Lakes*), ¾-oz. slice	80	4.0	1.0	6.0	20	320	0
(*Land O Lakes*), ⅔-oz. slice	70	3.0	1.0	6.0	15	320	0
(*Land O Lakes* 50% Reduced Fat)	70	7.0	2.0	4.5	20	400	0
(*Land O Lakes* Loaf)	110	5.0	<1.0	9.0	30	430	0
(*Land O Lakes* Re- duced Salt)	110	6.0	<1.0	9.0	30	270	0
sharp (*Land O Lakes*), 2 slices, 1 oz.	100	5.0	1.0	9.0	25	420	0
sharp (*Land O Lakes* Loaf)	100	6.0	<1.0	9.0	30	360	0
sharp (*Old English* Loaf)	100	6.0	<1.0	9.0	25	440	0
sharp (*Old English* Slice)..........	110	6.0	<1.0	9.0	30	460	0
shredded (*Kraft*), ¼ cup	110	6.0	<1.0	9.0	30	440	0
hot pepper (*Alpine Lace* Loaf)	110	6.0	1.0	9.0	25	410	0
hot pepper (*Alpine Lace* Reduced Fat Loaf)	80	6.0	2.0	6.0	20	260	0
jalapeño (*Land O Lakes* 50% Re- duced Fat)	70	7.0	1.0	4.0	15	400	0
American/Swiss: (*Land O Lakes*), ⅔-oz. slice	70	4.0	1.0	5.0	15	310	0
(*Land O Lakes* Loaf)	100	6.0	0	8.0	35	380	0
blue, ¼ cup, 1 oz.: (*Kraft*)	100	6.0	<1.0	8.0	30	390	0
crumbled (*Sargento*)	100	6.0	1.0	8.0	20	380	0
brick: (*Kraft*)	110	6.0	0	9.0	30	190	0
(*Land O Lakes*)	100	7.0	<1.0	8.0	30	160	0
Brie	95	5.9	.1	7.9	20	229	0
Camembert	85	5.6	.1	6.9	20	239	0

Food and Measure	cal.	prot. (gms)	carbo. (gms)	fat (gms)	chol. (mgs)	sod. (mgs)	fiber (gms)
Cheese *(cont.)*							
(*Chedarella*)	100	7.0	0	8.0	25	200	0
cheddar:							
(*Alpine Lace* Fat Free							
Slices)	45	8.0	2.0	0	5	280	0
(*Alpine Lace* Re-							
duced Fat)	70	8.0	1.0	4.5	15	170	0
(*Boar's Head*)	110	7.0	<1.0	9.0	30	190	0
(*Boar's Head* Cana-							
dian)	110	7.0	0	10.0	35	170	0
(*Heluva* Good Low							
Sodium)	110	7.0	<1.0	9.0	25	10	0
(*Kraft*)	110	7.0	<1.0	9.0	30	180	0
(*Land O Lakes*)	110	6.0	<1.0	9.0	30	180	0
(*Sargento MooTown*							
Snackers),							
.8-oz. pc.	100	5.0	1.0	8.0	25	130	0
(*Sargento MooTown*							
Snackers Light),							
.8-oz. pc.	60	7.0	<1.0	4.0	10	170	0
curds (*Heluva* Good)	113	7.0	1.0	9.0	28	179	0
extra sharp (*Cabot*)	110	7.0	1.0	9.0	30	180	0
extra sharp (*Heluva*							
Good Father Time)	110	7.0	1.0	9.0	30	180	0
extra sharp (*Land O*							
Lakes)	110	6.0	<1.0	9.0	30	360	0
mild (*Kraft* Less Fat)	80	9.0	0	5.0	20	220	0
mild, sharp, or extra							
sharp (*Heluva*							
Good)	110	7.0	1.0	9.0	30	180	0
nacho blend							
w/peppers (*Kraft*)	110	7.0	0	9.0	30	250	0
sharp (*Cracker Bar-*							
rel/Kraft 1/3 Less							
Fat) . . . . . . , ...	80	9.0	<1.0	5.0	20	220	0
sharp (*Sargento*)	110	6.0	1.0	9.0	30	160	0
cheddar, shredded,							
1/4 cup:							
(*Kraft*)	120	7.0	<1.0	10.0	30	190	0
(*Kraft Healthy Favor-*							
ites Fat Free)	45	8.0	1.0	0	<5	220	0

Food and Measure	cal.	prot. (gms)	carbo. (gms)	fat (gms)	chol. (mgs)	sod. (mgs)	fiber (gms)
(Sargento Classic/ Fancy Supreme)	110	6.0	1.0	9.0	30	160	0
fine *(Kraft)*	90	5.0	<1.0	8.0	25	150	0
mild *(Heluva* Good Reduced Fat)	80	7.0	1.0	6.0	15	200	0
mild *(Kraft* 1/3 Less Fat)	90	10.0	<1.0	6.0	20	230	0
mild or sharp *(Heluva* Good) . . .	110	7.0	1.0	9.0	30	180	0
sharp *(Cracker Barrel* 1/3 Less Fat)	80	8.0	<1.0	5.0	20	200	0
cheddar horseradish *(Yancey's Fancy)*	100	6.0	2.0	7.0	25	370	0
Cheshire	110	6.6	1.4	8.7	29	198	0
chèvre, see "goat," below							
Colby:							
(Alpine Lace Longhorn Reduced Fat)	80	9.0	1.0	5.0	15	115	0
(Boar's Head Longhorn)	110	7.0	<1.0	9.0	30	170	0
(Heluva Good Half Moon)	117	7.0	0	9.0	30	186	0
(Heluva Good Longhorn)	110	7.0	1.0	9.0	30	170	0
(Kraft)	110	7.0	<1.0	9.0	30	180	0
(Kraft 1/3 Less Fat)	80	9.0	0	5.0	20	220	0
(Land O Lakes)	110	7.0	<1.0	9.0	30	160	0
(Sargento Slices)	110	6.0	0	9.0	30	190	0
Colby jack:							
(Heluva Good)	90	6.0	4.0	6.0	20	180	0
(Heluva Good Stick)	110	6.0	0	9.0	30	200	0
(Kraft)	110	7.0	0	9.0	30	190	0
(Land O Lakes)	110	6.0	<1.0	9.0	30	180	0
(Sargento MooTown Snackers), .8-oz. pc.	90	5.0	<1.0	8.0	20	160	0
Colby jack, shredded, 1/4 cup or 1 oz.:							
(Heluva Good)	110	6.0	1.0	9.0	30	200	0
(Kraft)	120	7.0	<1.0	10.0	30	200	0

Food and Measure	cal.	prot. (gms)	carbo. (gms)	fat (gms)	chol. (mgs)	sod. (mgs)	fiber (gms)
Cheese, Colby jack, shredded *(cont.)*							
(*Sargento Fancy Supreme*)	110	6.0	<1.0	9.0	25	190	0
cottage, 4%, 1/2 cup:							
(*Breakstone's*)	120	14.0	4.0	5.0	25	400	0
(*Friendship*)	110	12.0	4.0	5.0	25	430	0
(*Friendship* California Style)	115	15.0	3.0	5.0	25	380	0
(*Hood*)	110	13.0	5.0	4.5	25	390	0
(*Knudsen* Large Curd)	130	16.0	3.0	5.0	30	340	0
(*Knudsen* Small Curd)	120	15.0	2.0	5.0	25	400	0
(*Sealtest*)	120	14.0	4.0	5.0	25	400	0
w/chive (*Hood*)	110	13.0	5.0	4.5	25	390	0
w/pineapple (*Friendship*)	140	12.0	14.0	2.5	15	300	0
w/pineapple (*Hood*)	130	10.0	15.0	3.5	15	290	0
cottage, 2%, 1/2 cup, except as noted:							
(*Breakstone's*)	90	14.0	4.0	2.5	15	380	0
(*Friendship* Pot Style)	90	15.0	3.0	1.5	10	400	0
(*Knudsen*)........	100	16.0	3.0	2.5	15	400	0
(*Sealtest*)	90	14.0	4.0	2.5	15	380	0
w/apple, raisin, walnut (*Hood Fruit Stirs*), 6 oz.	240	11.0	39.0	5.0	10	250	1.0
w/peach (*Hood Fruit Stirs*), 6 oz.	200	11.0	33.0	2.5	10	240	0
w/strawberry (*Hood Fruit Stirs*), 6 oz.	190	11.0	32.0	2.5	10	240	<1.0
triple berry (*Hood Fruit Stirs*), 6 oz.	200	11.0	33.0	2.5	10	240	<1.0
cottage, 1.5%, 4 oz.:							
w/peach (*Knudsen*)	110	11.0	12.0	1.5	10	290	0
w/pineapple (*Knudsen*)	110	11.0	11.0	1.5	10	290	0
w/strawberry (*Knudsen*)	110	11.0	12.0	1.5	10	280	0

Food and Measure	cal.	prot. (gms)	carbo. (gms)	fat (gms)	chol. (mgs)	sod. (mgs)	fiber (gms)
w/tropical fruit (*Knudsen*)	120	11.0	15.0	2.0	10	300	0
cottage, 1%, 1/2 cup:							
(*Friendship* Low Fat)	90	16.0	3.0	1.0	10	360	0
(*Friendship* Low Fat No Salt)	90	16.0	4.0	1.0	10	50	0
(*Hood* Low Fat)	80	13.0	6.0	1.0	10	380	0
(*Hood* Low Fat No Salt)	80	13.0	6.0	1.0	10	60	0
(*Light n' Lively*)	80	14.0	4.0	1.5	15	380	0
w/black pepper and herb (*Hood*)	80	13.0	6.0	1.0	10	430	0
w/chive and toasted onion (*Hood*)	80	13.0	6.0	1.0	10	380	0
w/garden salad (*Light n' Lively*)	90	13.0	5.0	1.5	15	410	0
w/peach and pineapple (*Light n' Lively*)	120	12.0	14.0	1.0	10	350	0
w/pineapple (*Friendship* Low Fat)	120	12.0	16.0	1.0	5	290	0
w/pineapple and cherries (*Hood*)	110	10.0	16.0	1.0	10	290	0
cottage, nonfat, 1/2 cup:							
(*Friendship*)	80	15.0	4.0	0	0	380	0
(*Hood*)	80	13.0	7.0	0	5	320	0
(*Knudsen Free*)	80	15.0	4.0	0	10	370	0
(*Light n' Lively Free*)	80	14.0	5.0	0	10	440	0
w/peach (*Friendship*)	110	12.0	15.0	0	0	300	0
w/pineapple (*Friendship*)	110	12.0	16.0	0	0	300	0
w/pineapple (*Hood*)	100	10.0	16.0	0	<5	240	0
cottage, dry curd (*Breakstone's*), 1/4 cup	45	8.0	3.0	0	0	25	0
cream cheese:							
(*Friendship*), 2 tbsp.	100	2.0	1.0	10.0	35	120	0
(*Philadelphia Brand*)	100	2.0	<1.0	10.0	30	90	0

Food and Measure	cal.	prot. (gms)	carbo. (gms)	fat (gms)	chol. (mgs)	sod. (mgs)	fiber (gms)
Cheese, cream cheese *(cont.)*							
(Philadelphia Brand Free)	25	4.0	2.0	0	5	135	0
w/chives (*Philadelphia Brand*)	90	2.0	<1.0	9.0	30	150	0
w/pimiento (*Philadelphia Brand*) ...	90	2.0	<1.0	9.0	30	150	0
cream cheese, soft, 2 tbsp.:							
(*Friendship*)	100	2.0	1.0	10.0	35	120	0
(*Philadelphia Brand*)	100	2.0	1.0	10.0	30	100	0
(*Philadelphia Brand Free*)	30	5.0	2.0	0	<5	160	0
(*Philadelphia Brand Light*)	70	3.0	2.0	5	15	150	0
w/chives and onion (*Philadelphia Brand*)	110	2.0	2.0	10.0	30	110	0
w/herb and garlic (*Philadelphia Brand*)	110	1.0	2.0	10.0	30	180	0
w/olive and pimiento (*Philadelphia Brand*)	100	2.0	2.0	9.0	30	170	0
w/pineapple (*Philadelphia Brand*) ...	100	2.0	4.0	9.0	30	100	0
w/smoked salmon (*Philadelphia Brand*)	100	2.0	1.0	9.0	30	200	0
w/strawberries (*Philadelphia Brand*)	100	1.0	5.0	9.0	30	65	0
cream cheese, whipped, 3 tbsp.:							
(*Breakstone's Temp-Tee*)	110	3.0	1.0	10.0	30	115	0
(*Philadelphia Brand*)	110	2.0	1.0	11.0	35	95	0
w/smoked salmon (*Philadelphia Brand*)	100	2.0	2.0	9.0	30	200	0

Food and Measure	cal.	prot. (gms)	carbo. (gms)	fat (gms)	chol. (mgs)	sod. (mgs)	fiber (gms)
curd:							
(*Heluva* Good)	113	7.0	1.0	9.0	28	179	0
washed (*Heluva* Good)	110	7.0	1.0	9.0	30	180	0
Edam	90	7.0	0	7.0	25	280	0
farmer:							
(*Friendship*)	50	5.0	0	2.5	10	120	0
(*Friendship* No Salt)	50	5.0	0	1.5	10	10	0
(*Kraft*)	100	6.0	<1.0	8.0	25	190	0
feta:							
(*Alpine Lace* Reduced Fat)	60	5.0	1.0	4.0	10	370	0
(*Athenos*)	80	5.0	<1.0	6.0	20	320	0
(*Krinos*)	90	5.0	0	8.0	24	430	0
tomato-basil (*Alpine Lace* Reduced Fat)	50	5.0	1.0	3.0	10	370	0
fontina:							
(*Classica*)	110	7.0	<1.0	8.5	25	160	0
(*Denmark's Finest*)	90	7.0	0	7.0	15	160	0
(*Gjetost*)	130	3.0	11.0	9.0	30	90	0
Gloucester, double							
(*Boar's Head*)	110	7.0	0	10.0	35	200	0
goat:							
(*Alpine Lace* Reduced Fat)	40	2.0	<1.0	3.0	5	130	0
(*Laura Chenel Select* Chèvre)	80	4.0	1.0	7.0	25	120	0
(*Snofrisk*)	70	2.0	2.0	8.0	15	170	0
hard type	128	8.7	.6	10.1	30	98	0
semisoft type	103	6.1	.7	8.5	22	146	0
soft type	76	5.3	.3	6.0	13	104	0
Gorgonzola (*Galbani Dolcelatte*)	93	5.0	<1.0	8.0	22	234	0
Gouda (*Kraft*)	110	7.0	<1.0	9.0	25	160	0
Gruyère	117	8.5	.1	9.2	31	95	0
Havarti:							
(*Kraft*)	120	6.0	0	11.0	35	240	0
all varieties (*Boar's Head*)	110	6.0	0	10.0	35	210	0
hoop (*Friendship*)....	20	5.0	0	0	0	10	0

Food and Measure	cal.	prot. (gms)	carbo. (gms)	fat (gms)	chol. (mgs)	sod. (mgs)	fiber (gms)
Cheese *(cont.)*							
Italian blend, shredded:							
(*Heluva* Good),							
¼ cup	90	8.0	0	7.0	20	210	0
6-cheese (*Sargento Recipe Blend*),							
¼ cup	90	7.0	0	7.0	20	180	0
grated (*Kraft*),							
2 tsp.	25	3.0	0	1.5	<5	95	0
grated (*Kraft ⅓ Less Fat*), 2 tsp.	25	2.0	1.0	1.0	<5	115	0
jack, wild morel and leek (*Great Midwest*)	100	8.0	0	8.0	25	180	0
jalapeño jack (*Land O Lakes*)	100	5.0	<1.0	8.0	25	460	0
(*Jarlsberg*):							
plain	100	7.0	0	8.0	20	180	0
lite	70	9.0	0	3.5	10	130	0
hickory smoked ...	100	7.0	1.0	8.0	20	220	0
Limburger (*Kraft*) ...	90	6.0	0	8.0	25	240	0
Mexican, 4-cheese, shredded (*Sargento Recipe Blend*),							
¼ cup, 1 oz.	110	6.0	<1.0	9.0	25	200	0
Monterey jack:							
(*Heluva* Good)	100	7.0	1.0	8.0	30	170	0
(*Heluva* Good Stick)	100	6.0	0	8.0	25	180	0
(*Kraft*)	110	6.0	0	9.0	30	190	0
(*Kraft ⅓ Less Fat*)	80	9.0	0	5.0	20	220	0
(*Land O Lakes*)	110	6.0	<1.0	8.0	30	170	0
(*Sargento* Sliced)	100	6.0	0	9.0	30	190	0
hot pepper (*Land O Lakes*)	110	6.0	<1.0	8.0	30	140	0
w/jalapeño (*Heluva* Good)	110	7.0	<1.0	9.0	25	180	0
w/jalapeño (*Heluva* Good Stick)	100	7.0	0	8.0	25	180	0
w/jalapeño (*Kraft*)	110	7.0	<1.0	9.0	30	190	0
w/peppers (*Kraft ⅓ Less Fat*)	80	8.0	<1.0	5.0	20	220	0

Food and Measure	cal.	prot. (gms)	carbo. (gms)	fat (gms)	chol. (mgs)	sod. (mgs)	fiber (gms)
plain or w/jalapeño (*Boar's Head*) ...	100	6.0	0	9.0	25	170	0
Monterey jack, shredded, ¼ cup or 1 oz.:							
(*Heluva* Good)	100	7.0	1.0	8.0	30	170	0
(*Kraft*)	110	7.0	<1.0	9.0	30	200	0
(*Sargento/Fancy Supreme*)	100	6.0	0	9.0	30	190	0
mozzarella:							
(*Alpine Lace* Reduced Fat)	70	8.0	1.0	3.0	10	200	0
(*Boar's Head*)	90	6.0	<1.0	7.0	25	140	0
(*Sargento* Slices)	130	11.0	2.0	9.0	25	230	0
(*Sargento Preferred* Light Slices)	90	11.0	0	5.0	15	230	0
whole milk (*Heluva* Good)	100	7.0	<1.0	7.0	25	210	0
whole milk (*Sorrento*)	90	6.0	1.0	6.0	20	160	0
part skim (*Heluva* Good)	80	7.0	1.0	5.0	20	190	0
part skim (*Kraft*) ...	80	8.0	<1.0	5.0	15	200	0
part skim (*Land O Lakes*)	80	7.0	<1.0	6.0	15	190	0
part skim, string (*Heluva* Good) ...	90	7.0	1.0	6.0	20	230	0
mozzarella, shredded, ¼ cup or 1 oz.:							
(*Heluva* Good Reduced Fat)	70	9.0	<1.0	4.0	15	135	0
(*Kraft Healthy Favorites* Fat Free)	50	9.0	2.0	0	<5	280	<1.0
(*Sargento Classic/ Fancy Supreme*)	80	7.0	1.0	6.0	15	150	0
(*Sargento Preferred Light*)	70	8.0	<1.0	3.0	10	140	0
whole milk (*Kraft*)	90	6.0	<1.0	7.0	25	210	0
part skim (*Heluva* Good Low Moisture)	80	8.0	1.0	6.0	15	170	0
part skim (*Kraft*)	90	8.0	<1.0	6.0	20	210	0

Food and Measure	cal.	prot. (gms)	carbo. (gms)	fat (gms)	chol. (mgs)	sod. (mgs)	fiber (gms)
Cheese, mozzarella, shredded *(cont.)*							
part skim (*Kraft* 1/3 Less Fat)	80	9.0	<1.0	5.0	15	210	0
part skim, fine (*Kraft*)	70	6.0	<1.0	4.5	15	160	0
Muenster:							
(*Alpine Lace* Reduced Sodium)	100	7.0	1.0	9.0	25	85	0
(*Boar's Head*)	100	6.0	0	8.0	25	180	0
(*Boar's Head* Low Sodium)	100	6.0	0	8.0	20	75	0
(*Heluva* Good)	110	7.0	<1.0	9.0	25	180	0
(*Heluva* Good Stick)	100	6.0	0	8.0	25	180	0
(*Kraft*)	110	6.0	0	9.0	30	190	0
(*Land O Lakes*)	100	6.0	0	8.0	25	220	0
(*Sargento* Slices)	100	6.0	<1.0	9.0	25	200	0
Neufchâtel (*Philadelphia Brand*)	70	3.0	<1.0	6.0	20	120	0
(*Nokkelost*)	100	7.0	2.0	8.0	20	135	0
Parmesan, grated:							
(*Alpine Lace* cups), 2 tsp.	10	1.0	0	0	0	65	0
(*Di Giorno*), 2 tsp.	20	2.0	0	1.0	5	55	0
(*Di Giorno* 100%), 2 tsp.	20	2.0	0	1.5	5	85	0
(*Kraft* 100%), 2 tsp.	20	2.0	0	1.5	5	85	0
(*Land O Lakes*), 1 tbsp.	35	3.0	0	2.5	10	95	0
(*Sargento*), 1 tbsp.	25	2.0	0	1.5	<5	75	0
Parmesan, shredded:							
(*Di Giorno* 100%), 2 tsp.	20	2.0	0	1.5	<5	75	0
(*Kraft* 100%), 2 tsp.	20	2.0	0	1.5	<5	75	0
(*Sargento Fancy Supreme*), 1/4 cup, 1 oz.	110	9.0	1.0	7.0	25	300	0
Parmesan/Romano:							
grated (*Sargento*), 1 tbsp.	25	2.0	0	1.5	<5	70	0
shredded (*Sargento Fancy Supreme*), 1/4 cup, 1 oz.	110	9.0	1.0	7.0	25	340	0

Food and Measure	cal.	prot. (gms)	carbo. (gms)	fat (gms)	chol. (mgs)	sod. (mgs)	fiber (gms)
pimiento, processed							
(*Kraft* Deluxe)	100	6.0	<1.0	8.0	25	430	0
pizza blend, shredded,							
1/4 cup or 1 oz.:							
(*Heluva* Good)	90	7.0	1.0	7.0	20	210	0
(*Heluva* Good Reduced Fat)	70	8.0	0	4.5	15	160	0
(*Sargento Classic Supreme*)	90	7.0	0	6.0	20	210	0
(*Sargento Fancy Supreme Pizza Double Cheese*)	90	7.0	1.0	6.0	20	150	0
cheddar, mild, and mozzarella (*Kraft*)	90	6.0	<1.0	7.0	20	170	0
four cheese (*Kraft*)	90	7.0	<1.0	7.0	20	230	0
mozzarella and cheddar (*Kraft*)	100	6.0	<1.0	8.0	25	190	0
mozzarella and smoke provolone (*Kraft*)	90	6.0	<1.0	7.0	20	210	0
Port du Salut	100	6.7	.2	8.0	35	151	0
provolone:							
(*Alpine Lace* Reduced Fat/Sodium)	70	9.0	1.0	5.0	15	120	0
(*Boar's Head* Picante/Sharp)	100	7.0	1.0	8.0	25	250	0
(*Land O Lakes*)	100	7.0	<1.0	8.0	20	240	0
(*Sargento* Slices)	100	7.0	0	8.0	25	190	0
smoke flavor (*Kraft*)	100	7.0	<1.0	7.0	25	240	0
ricotta, 1/4 cup:							
(*Breakstone's*)	110	7.0	3.0	8.0	25	90	0
(*Sargento* Light) ...	60	5.0	3.0	2.5	15	55	0
(*Sargento* Old Fashioned)	90	7.0	3.0	6.0	25	75	0
whole milk	108	7.0	1.9	8.0	32	52	0
part skim (*Sargento*)	80	7.0	2.0	5.0	20	75	0
Romano, grated:							
(*Di Giorno*), 2 tsp.	20	2.0	0	1.5	5	75	0
(*Di Giorno* 100%), 2 tsp.	25	2.0	0	1.5	5	90	0

Food and Measure	cal.	prot. (gms)	carbo. (gms)	fat (gms)	chol. (mgs)	sod. (mgs)	fiber (gms)
Cheese, Romano, grated *(cont.)*							
(*Kraft* 100%), 2 tsp.	25	2.0	0	1.5	5	90	0
Romano, shredded:							
(*Di Giorno* 100%),							
2 tsp.	20	2.0	0	1.5	5	70	0
Roquefort	105	6.1	.6	8.7	26	513	0
Stilchester (*Anco*) . . .	110	7.0	0	10.0	30	170	0
string:							
(*Kraft Handi-*							
Snacks), 1 pc.	80	7.0	<1.0	6.0	20	240	0
(*Sargento MooTown*							
Snackers),							
.8-oz. pc.	70	6.0	<1.0	5.0	15	170	0
(*Sargento MooTown*							
Snackers Light),							
.8-oz. pc.	60	7.0	<1.0	3.0	10	200	0
Swiss:							
(*Alpine Lace* Re-							
duced Fat/So-							
dium)	90	8.0	1.0	6.0	20	35	0
(*Alpine Lace* Re-							
duced Fat/Sodium							
Deli)	110	10.0	0	8.0	25	45	0
(*Boar's Head* Gold							
Label Imported)	110	8.0	<1.0	8.0	20	65	0
(*Boar's Head* No							
Salt)	110	8.0	<1.0	8.0	25	10	0
(*Heluva* Good)	110	7.0	0	8.0	30	30	0
(*Kraft*)	110	8.0	0	9.0	30	50	0
(*Land O Lakes*)	110	8.0	<1.0	8.0	25	75	0
(*Sargento* Slices),							
¾-oz. slice	80	6.0	0	6.0	20	30	0
(*Sargento Preferred*							
Light Wafer Thin							
Slices)	80	9.0	<1.0	4.0	15	50	0
(*Sargento Wafer*							
Thin), 2 slices,							
1 oz.	110	8.0	0	9.0	25	40	0
baby (*Boar's Head*)	110	7.0	<1.0	9.0	25	135	0
baby (*Kraft*)	110	7.0	0	9.0	25	110	0

Food and Measure	cal.	prot. (gms)	carbo. (gms)	fat (gms)	chol. (mgs)	sod. (mgs)	fiber (gms)
baby (*Land O Lakes* Loaf)	110	6.0	0	9.0	25	125	0
baby (*Land O Lakes* Wheel)	110	8.0	<1.0	8.0	25	75	0
light (*Land O Lakes* 50% Reduced Fat)	80	9.0	<1.0	4.0	15	60	0
processed (*Kraft* Deluxe), ¾-oz. slice	70	5.0	0	5.0	20	310	0
processed (*Kraft* Deluxe), 1-oz. slice	90	7.0	<1.0	7.0	25	420	0
Swiss, shredded, ¼ cup or 1 oz.:							
(*Kraft*)	110	8.0	<1.0	9.0	30	45	0
(*Sargento Fancy Supreme*)	110	8.0	0	8.0	30	40	0
taco blend, shredded, ¼ cup or 1 oz.:							
(*Heluva* Good)	110	7.0	1.0	9.0	30	200	0
(*Sargento Classic Supreme*)	110	6.0	1.0	9.0	25	220	0
(*Sargento Preferred Light*)	70	8.0	<1.0	4.5	15	240	0
cheddar–Monterey Jack (*Kraft*)	100	6.0	<1.0	8.0	25	180	0
nacho-taco (*Sargento Fancy Supreme*)	110	6.0	1.0	9.0	25	240	0
"Cheese," substitute and nondairy:							
(*Smart Beat* Lactose Free), ⅔-oz. slice	25	4.0	3.0	0	0	180	0
American, slices:							
(*Lunchwagon*), ⅔ oz.	60	3.0	<1.0	5.0	0	210	0
(*Lunchwagon*), ¾ oz.	70	4.0	1.0	5.0	0	230	0
(*Smart Beat*), ⅔ oz.	25	4.0	3.0	0	0	180	0
American, shredded (*Harvest Moon*), ¼ cup	120	6.0	3.0	9.0	0	500	0

Food and Measure	cal.	prot. (gms)	carbo. (gms)	fat (gms)	chol. (mgs)	sod. (mgs)	fiber (gms)
"Cheese," substitute and nondairy *(cont.)*							
cheddar:							
mellow (*Smart Beat*), ⅔-oz. slice	25	4.0	3.0	0	0	180	0
sharp (*Smart Beat*), ⅔-oz. slice	25	4.0	3.0	0	0	220	0
shredded (*Harvest Moon*), ¼ cup . . .	120	6.0	3.0	9.0	0	480	0
shredded (*Sargento Fancy Supreme*), ¼ cup, 1 oz.	90	5.0	2.0	7.0	0	420	0
mozzarella, shredded, ¼ cup or 1 oz.:							
(*Harvest Moon*) . . .	110	8.0	1.0	8.0	0	430	0
(*Sargento Classic Supreme*)	80	6.0	<1.0	6.0	0	320	0
Cheese dip (see also "Cheese sauce" and "Cream cheese dip"), 2 tbsp., except as noted:							
(*Chi-Chi's* Fiesta)	40	1.0	3.0	3.0	10	270	0
and bacon (*Nalley*) . . .	110	1.0	3.0	11.0	10	240	0
blue:							
(*Kraft* Premium) . . .	45	1.0	2.0	4.0	10	200	0
(*T. Marzetti's* Veggie Dip)	180	1.0	1.0	19.0	20	220	0
chunky (*T. Marzetti's* Dip & Dressing)	150	1.0	1.0	16.0	20	310	0
cheddar:							
mild (*Frito-Lay*)	60	1.0	3.0	4.0	5	330	0
jalapeño (*Breakstone's*)	60	1.0	2.0	4.0	15	170	0
w/jalapeño (*Frito-Lay*)	50	1.0	4.0	4.0	5	300	0
and mustard (*Heluva* Good Pretzel)	80	2.0	2.0	6.0	20	230	0
w/chili (*Fritos*)	45	1.0	3.0	3.0	<5	310	0

Food and Measure	cal.	prot. (gms)	carbo. (gms)	fat (gms)	chol. (mgs)	sod. (mgs)	fiber (gms)
jalapeño (*Kraft* Premium)	60	2.0	1.0	5.0	15	250	0
nacho:							
(*Frito-Lay*)	45	2.0	4.0	3.0	5	280	0
(*Knudsen*)	60	2.0	3.0	4.0	15	200	0
(*Kraft* Premium) . . .	60	2.0	2.0	5.0	15	270	0
(*Nalley*)	120	1.0	3.0	12.0	15	290	0
w/beef (*Tostitos*), 4 tbsp.	120	4.0	6.0	8.0	10	500	<2.0
salsa:							
(*Chi-Chi's* Con Queso)	90	3.0	4.0	7.0	15	480	0
(*Heluva* Good Cheese 'N Salsa)	80	3.0	3.0	5.5	10	210	0
(*Old El Paso*)	40	<1.0	3.0	3.0	<5	300	0
(*Old El Paso* Chunky)	30	1.0	2.0	0	0	230	<1.0
(*Old El Paso* Low Fat)	30	<1.0	3.0	1.5	<5	240	0
(*Tostitos*), 4 tbsp.	80	2.0	10.0	5.0	<10	560	<2.0
(*Tostitos* Lowfat), 4 tbsp.	80	2.0	8.0	3.0	<10	560	<2.0
Cheese dip mix, nacho (*Knorr*), ½ tsp.	5	0	<1.0	.5	0	160	0
Cheese food (see also "Cheese" and "Cheese spread"), 1 oz., except as noted:							
American:							
(*Golden Image*), ¾ oz.	70	5.0	1.0	5.0	5	270	0
(*Heluva* Good), ¾-oz. slice	70	4.0	1.0	5.0	15	250	0
(*Kraft* Singles), ⅔ oz.	60	4.0	2.0	4.5	15	260	0
(*Kraft* Singles), ¾ oz.	70	4.0	2.0	5.0	15	290	0
(*Kraft* Singles), 1.2 oz.	110	6.0	3.0	8.0	30	460	0

Food and Measure	cal.	prot. (gms)	carbo. (gms)	fat (gms)	chol. (mgs)	sod. (mgs)	fiber (gms)
Cheese food, American *(cont.)*							
(*Land O Lakes*), ²/₃-oz. slice	60	3.0	2.0	4.5	15	230	0
(*Land O Lakes*), ³/₄-oz. slice	70	4.0	2.0	5.0	15	250	0
grated (*Kraft*), 1 tbsp.	25	1.0	1.0	1.5	<5	135	0
cheddar, 2 tbsp.:							
extra sharp (*Cracker Barrel*)	100	5.0	3.0	8.0	25	290	0
sharp (*Cracker Barrel*)	100	5.0	4.0	8.0	25	290	0
w/garlic (*Kraft*)	90	5.0	2.0	7.0	20	370	0
herb, Italian (*Land O Lakes*)	90	5.0	2.0	7.0	20	420	0
w/jalapeño:							
(*Kraft*)	90	5.0	2.0	7.0	20	370	0
(*Kraft* Mexican Singles), ³/₄ oz.	70	4.0	2.0	5.0	15	330	0
(*Land O Lakes*)	90	5.0	2.0	6.0	20	390	0
shredded, hot (*Velveeta*), ¹/₄ cup	130	8.0	3.0	9.0	30	540	0
shredded, mild (*Velveeta*), ¹/₄ cup	130	8.0	3.0	9.0	30	520	0
Monterey (*Kraft* Singles), ³/₄ oz.	70	4.0	2.0	5.0	15	290	0
onion (*Land O Lakes*)	90	5.0	2.0	7.0	20	450	0
pepperoni (*Land O Lakes*)	90	6.0	1.0	7.0	25	430	0
w/pimiento (*Kraft* Singles), ²/₃ oz.	60	4.0	1.0	4.5	15	260	0
w/pimiento (*Kraft* Singles), ³/₄ oz.	70	4.0	2.0	5.0	15	290	0
salami (*Land O Lakes*)	90	5.0	2.0	7.0	30	410	0
sharp (*Kraft* Singles), ³/₄ oz.	70	4.0	<1.0	6.0	20	300	0
shredded (*Velveeta*), ¹/₄ cup	130	8.0	3.0	9.0	30	100	0
Swiss (*Kraft* Singles), ³/₄ oz.	70	4.0	1.0	5.0	15	320	0

Food and Measure	cal.	prot. (gms)	carbo. (gms)	fat (gms)	chol. (mgs)	sod. (mgs)	fiber (gms)
Cheese nut casserole, dried (*AlpineAire*), 3¼ oz.	380	17.0	40.0	17.0	25	750	6.0
Cheese pastry, see "Danish"							
Cheese pocket, grilled, frozen (*Hot Pockets Toaster Breaks*), 2.1-oz. pc.	210	5.0	24.0	10.0	15	300	1.0
Cheese and pretzels, see "Pretzel"							
Cheese product (see also "Cheese food"), ¾-oz. slice, except as noted:							
(*Kraft Free* Singles), ⅔ oz.	30	4.0	3.0	0	<5	290	0
(*Kraft Free* Singles)	30	5.0	3.0	0	<5	320	0
(*Velveeta Light*), 1 oz.	60	6.0	3.0	3.0	10	420	0
American flavor:							
(*Kraft* Deluxe 25% Less Fat)	70	4.0	1.0	5	15	350	0
(*Kraft* Singles ⅓ Less Fat)	50	5.0	2.0	3.0	10	330	0
(*Light n' Lively* 50% Less Fat)	50	5.0	2.0	2.5	10	280	0
white (*Light n' Lively* 50% Less Fat) . . .	50	5.0	2.0	2.5	10	300	0
cheddar flavor:							
(*Alpine Lace* Fat Free Loaf)	45	8.0	2.0	0	5	280	0
sharp (*Kraft* Singles ⅓ Less Fat)	50	5.0	2.0	3.0	10	300	0
sharp (*Kraft Free* Singles)	30	5.0	3.0	0	<5	290	0
mozzarella flavor: (*Alpine Lace* Fat Free Loaf)	45	8.0	2.0	0	5	280	0
Swiss:							
(*Kraft* Singles ⅓ Less Fat)	50	5.0	2.0	2.5	10	270	0

Food and Measure	cal.	prot. (gms)	carbo. (gms)	fat (gms)	chol. (mgs)	sod. (mgs)	fiber (gms)
Cheese product, Swiss *(cont.)*							
(*Kraft Free* Singles)	30	5.0	3.0	0	<5	290	0
Cheese puffs, see "Cake, snack"							
Cheese sauce (see also "Cheese dip"), 2 tbsp., except as noted:							
(*Cheez Whiz Zap-A-Pack*)	90	3.0	3.0	8.0	20	580	0
nacho, ¼ cup:							
jalapeño or medium (*Gracias*)	90	3.0	7.0	6.0	5	550	1.0
mild (*Gracias*)	100	3.0	7.0	8.0	5	270	1.0
picante (*Pace* Con Queso)	90	2.0	6.0	7.0	5	380	0
w/salsa (*Cheez Whiz Zap-A-Pack*)	90	3.0	3.0	8.0	25	580	0
Cheese sauce, cooking, in jars, ¼ cup:							
Alfredo:							
(*Ragú Cheese Creations!* Classic)	120	2.0	3.0	12.0	30	360	0
light Parmesan (*Ragú Cheese Creations!*)	80	2.0	2.0	6.0	25	440	0
cheddar, double (*Ragú Cheese Creations!*)	110	4.0	2.0	10.0	25	420	0
cheddar and tomato, spicy (*Ragú Cheese Creations!*)	50	1.0	6.0	2.0	10	460	<1.0
four (*Ragú Cheese Creations!*)	120	2.0	2.0	11.0	30	300	0
garlic, roasted, Parmesan (*Ragú Cheese Creations!*)	120	2.0	3.0	11.0	25	420	0
Romano, cream tomato (*Ragú Cheese Creations!*)	60	2.0	7.0	2.5	10	290	1.0

Food and Measure	cal.	prot. (gms)	carbo. (gms)	fat (gms)	chol. (mgs)	sod. (mgs)	fiber (gms)
Cheese sauce mix, four (*Knorr* Pasta Sauces), 2 tbsp.	70	3.0	4.0	4.0	10	810	0
Cheese spread (see also "Cheese" and "Cheese product"), 2 tbsp., except as noted:							
(*Cheez Whiz*)	90	5.0	2.0	7.0	20	560	0
(*Cheez Whiz* Squeezable)	100	2.0	4.0	8.0	15	470	0
(*Cheez Whiz Light*)	80	6.0	6.0	3.0	15	540	0
(*Land O Lakes* Golden Velvet), 1 oz.	80	5.0	2.0	6.0	20	370	0
(*Squeez-A-Snak*)	90	5.0	<1.0	8.0	25	440	0
(*Velveeta*), 1 oz.	80	5.0	3.0	6.0	20	420	0
(*Velveeta Italiana*), 1 oz.	80	5.0	2.0	6.0	20	430	0
American:							
(*Easy Cheese*)	100	6.0	2.0	7.0	25	400	0
(*Harvest Moon*), ⅔ oz.	50	4.0	1.0	3.0	10	280	0
w/bacon (*Kraft*)	90	5.0	<1.0	8.0	25	570	0
blue cheese (*Kraft Roka*)	80	3.0	2.0	7.0	20	340	0
cheddar:							
(*Easy Cheese*)	100	5.0	3.0	7.0	25	410	0
medium (*Spreadery*)	80	5.0	3.0	4.5	15	290	0
plain or w/bacon or w/horseradish (*Heluva* Good Cold Pack)	90	5.0	3.0	7.0	20	210	0
sharp (*Spreadery*)	80	5.0	3.0	4.5	15	290	0
sharp, Vermont white (*Spreadery*)	80	5.0	3.0	4.5	15	290	0
garlic herb (*Alpine Lace* Reduced Fat)	60	4.0	2.0	4.0	10	190	0
w/jalapeños:							
(*Cheez Whiz*)	90	5.0	2.0	8.0	25	530	0
(*Kraft* Loaf), 1 oz.	80	5.0	2.0	6.0	20	470	0
hot (*Velveeta*), 1 oz.	80	5.0	2.0	6.0	20	520	0

Food and Measure	cal.	prot. (gms)	carbo. (gms)	fat (gms)	chol. (mgs)	sod. (mgs)	fiber (gms)
Cheese spread, w/jalapeños *(cont.)*							
mild (*Velveeta*), 1 oz.	80	5.0	3.0	6.0	20	440	0
Limburger (*Mohawk Valley*)	80	4.0	0	7.0	20	500	0
Neufchâtel:							
garden vegetable (*Spreadery*)	70	3.0	2.0	6.0	20	230	0
garlic herb (*Spreadery*)	80	3.0	1.0	7.0	20	180	0
ranch (*Spreadery*)	80	3.0	1.0	7.0	20	210	0
olive and pimiento (*Kraft*)	70	2.0	3.0	6.0	20	220	0
pimiento:							
(*Kraft*)	80	2.0	3.0	6.0	20	170	0
(*Spreadery*)	100	4.0	3.0	8.0	20	320	0
pineapple (*Kraft*)	70	2.0	4.0	5.0	15	120	0
port wine (*Heluva Good Cold Pack*) . . .	90	5.0	3.0	7.0	20	210	0
salsa:							
hot (*Cheez Whiz*)	90	5.0	2.0	7.0	25	540	0
mild (*Cheez Whiz*)	90	5.0	2.0	7.0	25	530	0
sharp (*Old English*)	90	5.0	<1.0	8.0	25	520	0
slices, 1 slice:							
(*Velveeta*), 3/4 oz.	60	4.0	2.0	4.5	15	300	0
(*Velveeta*), 4/5 oz.	70	4.0	2.0	4.5	15	310	0
(*Velveeta*), 1/2 oz.	100	6.0	3.0	7.0	25	480	0
sun-dried tomato-basil (*Alpine Lace* Reduced Fat)	70	4.0	2.0	5.0	15	300	0
Cheese steak pocket, see "Beef pocket"							
Cheese stick, frozen, breaded, w/sauce, 2 pcs., except as noted:							
Italian 4-cheese (*Rich-SeaPak* Dippers) . . .	140	6.0	10.0	8.0	10	350	0
jalapeño:							
cheddar (*Rich-SeaPak* Fiesta Dippers) . . . . :	140	4.0	15.0	7.0	10	280	<1.0

Food and Measure	cal.	prot. (gms)	carbo. (gms)	fat (gms)	chol. (mgs)	sod. (mgs)	fiber (gms)
cream cheese (*Rich-SeaPak* Fiesta Dippers)	130	3.0	15.0	7.0	10	250	<1.0
mozzarella (*Rich-SeaPak* Dippers) ...	190	12.0	15.0	10.0	10	420	<1.0
mozzarella, w/out sauce (*Banquet*), 6 pcs.	280	9.0	19.0	18.0	40	1060	1.0
pizza, approx. 3 pcs.: double cheese (*Rich-SeaPak* Dippers)	210	10.0	23.0	9.0	15	210	<1.0
pepperoni (*Rich-SeaPak* Dippers)	230	9.0	23.0	11.0	15	360	<1.0
Cheese turnover, frozen, cheddar w/jalapeño (*Cohen's Famous*), 4 pcs. ...	260	4.0	17.0	20.0	5	290	1.0
Cheeseburger, see "Beef sandwich"							
Cherimoya (see also "Custard apple"):							
(*Frieda's*), 5 oz.	130	2.0	34.0	.5	0	0	3.0
1 medium, 1.9 lbs.	515	7.1	131.3	2.2	0	n.a.	13.1
Cherry, fresh, ½ cup, except as noted:							
sour, red:							
w/pits	26	.5	6.3	.2	0	2	.6
pitted	39	.8	9.4	.2	0	3	.9
sweet:							
w/pits	52	.9	12.0	.7	0	1	1.7
10 medium, 2.6 oz.	49	.8	11.3	.7	0	<1	1.6
Cherry, candied, green or red (*Paradise/White Swan*), 1 pc.	15	0	4.0	0	0	0	0
w/pineapple (*Paradise/White Swan*), 2 tbsp., 1.3 oz.	110	0	29.0	0	0	25	1.0
Cherry, canned, ½ cup:							
(*Comstock/Wilderness* Dessert)	140	1.0	36.0	0	0	10	1.0

Food and Measure	cal.	prot. (gms)	carbo. (gms)	fat (gms)	chol. (mgs)	sod. (mgs)	fiber (gms)
Cherry, canned *(cont.)*							
sour, pitted:							
in water (*Comstock/ Wilderness* Tart Red)	50	1.0	11.0	0	0	10	1.0
in heavy syrup	116	.9	29.8	.1	0	9	1.0
sweet, w/pits, dark, in heavy syrup (*Oregon*)	100	<1.0	24.0	0	0	5	1.0
sweet, pitted:							
bing, in heavy syrup (*Oregon*)	110	1.0	26.0	0	0	10	1.0
dark, in heavy syrup (*Comstock/Wilderness*)	110	1.0	26.0	0	0	15	2.0
dark, in heavy syrup (*Del Monte*)	100	<1.0	24.0	0	0	10	<1.0
in heavy syrup	107	.8	27.4	.2	0	3	.9
Royal Anne, in heavy syrup (*Comstock/Wilderness*)	110	1.0	26.0	0	0	10	1.0
Royal Anne, in heavy syrup (*Oregon*)	110	1.0	26.0	0	0	10	1.0
Cherry, dried:							
(*L'Esprit*), 1/3 cup	160	2.0	36.0	0	0	0	2.0
bing, 1/4 cup, 1.4 oz.:							
(*Frieda's*)	120	2.0	26.0	0	0	5	3.0
(*Sonoma*)	140	1.0	34.0	0	0	0	2.0
sweet-tart (*Sonoma*), 1/4 cup, 1.4 oz.	140	1.0	33.0	0	0	0	2.0
tart (*Frieda's*), 1/3 cup, 1.4 oz.	150	2.0	33.0	0	0	0	2.0
w/liquid, 1 oz.	33	.1	8.3	.1	0	n.a.	<1.0
Cherry, frozen, sweetened, 4 oz.	101	1.3	25.4	.1	0	1	1.1
Cherry drink:							
(*Kool-Aid Bursts*), 6.75 fl. oz.	100	0	25.0	0	0	35	0

Food and Measure	cal.	prot. (gms)	carbo. (gms)	fat (gms)	chol. (mgs)	sod. (mgs)	fiber (gms)
(*Ocean Spray Black Cherry Blast*), 8 fl. oz.	140	— 0	33.0	0	0	35	0
(*Veryfine* Natural), 8 fl. oz.	0	0	0	0	0	5	0
Cherry drink mix*, 8 fl. oz.:							
(*Kool-Aid*)	100	0	25.0	0	0	10	0
(*Kool-Aid* Presweetened)	60	0	16.0	0	0	0	0
black (*Kool-Aid*)	100	0	25.0	0	0	20	0
Cherry dumpling, frozen (*Pepperidge Farm*), 3-oz. pc. ...	280	3.0	47.0	9.0	0	280	2.0
Cherry filling, see "Pastry filling" and "Pie filling"							
Cherry glacé, see "Cherry, candied"							
Cherry juice, 8 fl. oz.:							
(*After the Fall* Very)	100	0	26.0	0	0	20	0
(*Dole* Mountain)	150	0	38.0	0	0	30	0
(*Eden* Organic)	140	1.0	33.0	1.0	0	30	0
(*Juicy Juice*)	130	1.0	32.0	0	0	10	0
(*Veryfine* Juice-Up)	130	0	33.0	0	0	15	0
black (*R.W. Knudsen*)	180	2.0	43.0	0	0	40	0
Cherry juice blend, 8 fl. oz.:							
black, concentrate* (*R.W. Knudsen*) ...	130	0	23.0	0	0	15	0
cider (*R.W. Knudsen* Aseptic)	120	1.0	31.0	0	0	35	0
cider, concentrate* (*R.W. Knudsen*) ...	130	0	33.0	0	0	35	0
Cherry nectar (*Santa Cruz* Organic), 8 fl. oz.	110	0	26.0	0	0	20	0
Cherry pastry, see specific listings							

Food and Measure	cal.	prot. (gms)	carbo. (gms)	fat (gms)	chol. (mgs)	sod. (mgs)	fiber (gms)
Cherry syrup, mara-schino (*Trader Vic's*), 1 fl. oz.	90	0	23.0	0	0	15	0
Chervil, dried, 1 tsp.	1	.1	.3	<.1	0	<1	.1
Chestnut, Chinese, shelled, 1 oz.:							
dried	103	1.9	22.7	.5	0	2	<1.0
boiled or steamed	44	.8	9.6	.2	0	1	<1.0
roasted	68	1.3	14.9	.3	0	1	<1.0
Chestnut, European:							
raw:							
in shell, 1 lb.	714	8.1	152.8	7.6	0	9	27.2
shelled, w/peel, 1 cup, 13 kernels	308	3.5	66.0	3.3	0	4	11.7
dried, peeled, 1 oz.	105	1.4	22.3	1.1	0	11	<2.0
boiled, 1 oz.	37	.8	7.9	.4	0	8	<1.0
roasted, peeled:							
1 oz.	70	.9	15.0	.6	0	1	3.3
1 cup, 17 kernels	350	4.3	75.7	3.2	0	3	16.7
in jars (*Minerve*), 4 whole, 1.1 oz.	50	1.0	12.0	0	0	0	2.0
Chestnut, Japanese:							
dried, 1 oz.	102	1.5	23.1	.4	0	10	n.a.
boiled or steamed, 1 oz.	16	.2	3.6	.1	0	1	<1.0
roasted, 1 oz.	57	.8	12.8	.2	0	n.a.	<1.0
Chicken, fresh, 4 oz., except as noted:							
broiler-fryer, roasted:							
w/skin, ½ chicken, 10½ oz. (15.8 oz. w/bone)	715	81.6	0	40.7	263	244	0
w/skin	271	31.0	0	15.4	100	93	0
meat only	215	32.8	0	8.4	101	98	0
meat only, chopped or diced, 1 cup	266	40.5	0	10.4	125	120	0
skin only, 1 oz.	129	5.8	0	11.5	24	18	0
dark meat only	232	31.0	0	11.0	105	105	0
light meat only	196	35.1	0	5.1	96	87	0
breast, w/skin, ½ breast, 3½ oz. (8½ oz. w/bone)	193	29.2	0	7.6	83	69	0

Food and Measure	cal.	prot. (gms)	carbo. (gms)	fat (gms)	chol. (mgs)	sod. (mgs)	fiber (gms)
drumstick, w/skin, 1.8 oz. (2.9 oz. w/bone)	112	14.1	0	5.8	48	47	0
leg, w/skin (5.7 oz. w/bone)	265	29.6	0	15.4	105	99	0
thigh, w/skin, 2.2 oz. (2.9 oz. w/bone)	153	15.5	0	9.6	58	52	0
wing, w/skin, 1.2 oz. (2.3 oz. w/bone)	99	9.1	0	6.6	29	28	0
capon, roasted, w/skin:							
½ capon, 1.4 lbs. (2 lbs. w/bone)	1457	184.5	0	74.2	549	313	0
w/skin	260	32.8	0	13.2	98	56	0
Cornish hen, see "Cornish hen"							
ground, see "Chicken, ground"							
roaster, roasted:							
w/skin, ½ chicken, 1 lb. (1½ lbs. w/bone)	1071	115.0	0	64.3	365	349	0
meat w/skin	253	27.2	0	15.2	86	83	0
stewing, stewed:							
w/skin, ½ chicken, 9.2 oz. (13½ oz. w/bone)	744	70.2	0	49.2	205	190	0
meat w/skin	323	30.5	0	21.4	90	83	0
meat only	269	34.5	0	13.5	94	88	0
meat only, chopped or diced, 1 cup	332	42.6	0	16.6	117	109	0
Chicken, canned, chunk, 2 oz.:							
(*Hormel*)	70	12.0	0	3.0	35	200	0
breast:							
(*Hormel*)	60	12.0	0	1.5	25	200	0
(*Hormel* No Salt) . . .	60	12.0	0	1.5	30	20	0
in water (*Swanson* Premium)	60	11.0	<1.0	1.0	25	230	<1.0

Food and Measure	cal.	prot. (gms)	carbo. (gms)	fat (gms)	chol. (mgs)	sod. (mgs)	fiber (gms)
Chicken, freeze-dried, cooked, diced (*AlpineAire*), ½ oz.	60	13.0	0	.5	35	15	0
Chicken, frozen or re-frigerated, raw, ready-to-cook:							
breast, skinless, bone-less:							
(*Perdue*), 4 oz.	130	26.0	0	3.0	75	45	0
(*Perdue Fit 'n Easy/ Oven Stuffer*), 4 oz.	130	27.0	0	2.5	75	50	0
fillet, broth-marinated (*Tyson*), 4.7-oz. pc.	140	26.0	0	4.0	70	330	0
fillet, marinated (*Tyson*), 4.7-oz. pc.	140	26.0	0	3.5	60	410	0
half, broth-mari-nated (*Tyson*), 5.2-oz. pc.	230	29.0	0	12.0	100	440	0
tenderloin (*Perdue*), 4 oz.	110	25.0	0	1.0	65	15	0
tenderloin, broth-marinated (*Tyson*), 4 pcs., 4.6 oz.	110	25.0	0	1.0	55	330	0
tenders (*Perdue*), 4 oz.	120	27.0	0	1.0	75	55	0
thin-sliced (*Perdue*), 2.8 oz.	80	18.0	0	1.5	50	35	0
thin-sliced (*Perdue Fit 'n Easy/Oven Stuffer*), 3 oz.	90	19.0	0	1.5	50	35	0
breast, boneless, sea-soned:							
barbecue (*Perdue*), 4 oz.	130	24.0	8.0	1.0	79	600	0
barbecue (*Perdue Individually Fozen*), 5.7 oz.	190	34.0	7.0	3.0	100	440	<1.0

Food and Measure	cal.	prot. (gms)	carbo. (gms)	fat (gms)	chol. (mgs)	sod. (mgs)	fiber (gms)
Italian (*Perdue*), 4 oz.	110	22.0	4.0	1.0	60	740	0
Italian (*Perdue Individually Frozen*), 5.7 oz.	170	34.0	2.0	3.0	100	490	<1.0
lemon pepper (*Perdue*), 4 oz.	110	23.0	2.0	1.0	60	700	0
lemon pepper (*Perdue Individually Frozen*), 5.7 oz.	170	34.0	2.0	3.0	100	590	<1.0
Oriental (*Perdue*), 4 oz.	120	23.0	5.0	1.0	60	720	0
teriyaki (*Perdue Individually Frozen*), 5.7 oz.	180	34.0	4.0	3.0	100	580	<1.0
drums, broth-marinated (*Tyson*), 2 pcs., 4 oz.	140	17.0	0	7.0	90	290	0
stuffed, 5.9-oz. pc.:							
w/broccoli and cheese (*Tyson*)	320	20.0	23.0	16.0	50	870	3.0
Cordon Bleu (*Tyson*)	350	25.0	24.0	17.0	55	740	3.0
Kiev (*Tyson*)	460	20.0	24.0	32.0	115	980	2.0
w/wild rice and mushrooms (*Tyson*)	300	23.0	25.0	12.00	50	860	1.0
thigh, 1 pc.:							
boneless, roasted (*Perdue Oven Stuffer*), 3½ oz.	180	25.0	0	9.0	125	40	0
broth-marinated (*Tyson*), 4.9 oz.	380	17.0	1.0	34.0	110	350	0
fajita (*Perdue*), 3.2 oz.	100	15.0	2.0	3.0	65	500	0
honey mustard (*Perdue*), 3.2 oz.	110	15.0	5.0	3.5	65	470	0
wing:							
(*Tyson*), 5 pcs., 4.3 oz.	250	23.0	0	18.0	145	85	0
broth-marinated (*Tyson*), 4 pcs., 4.2 oz.	240	20.0	0	18.0	95	340	0

Food and Measure	cal.	prot. (gms)	carbo. (gms)	fat (gms)	chol. (mgs)	sod. (mgs)	fiber (gms)
Chicken, frozen or re-frigerated, cooked (see also "Chicken entree, frozen"), 3 oz., except as noted:							
whole, roasted:							
dark (*Perdue*)	210	17.0	0	16.0	110	55	0
dark (*Perdue* Cut-Up)	210	17.0	0	15.0	110	55	0
white (*Perdue*)	170	21.0	0	3.0	85	45	0
white (*Perdue* Cut-Up)	160	20.0	0	2.5	85	40	0
half, barbecue:							
dark (*Perdue*)	160	17.0	0	10.0	110	380	0
white (*Perdue*)	120	17.0	0	3.5	80	380	0
half, roasted:							
dark (*Perdue*)	170	17.0	0	11.0	110	320	0
white (*Perdue*)	140	19.0	0	7.0	80	320	0
breast, split, roasted:							
bone-in (*Perdue*), 5 oz.	190	34.0	0	6.0	115	350	0
bone-in (*Perdue* Value Pack), 6.8 oz.	370	48.0	0	20.0	180	100	0
boneless, skinless (*Perdue Fit 'n Easy*), 3½ oz. . . .	150	30.0	0	3.0	85	35	0
skinless, bone-in (*Perdue*), 5.8 oz.	240	45.0	0	6.0	150	75	0
breast, crispy baked, 3½-oz. pc.:							
(*Butterball Chicken Requests* Origi-nal)	180	16.0	16.0	6.0	45	500	2.0
Italian herb (*Butter-ball Chicken Re-quests*)	190	17.0	16.0	6.0	55	610	1.0
lemon pepper (*But-terball Chicken Requests*)	190	16.0	16.0	6.0	50	420	2.0

Food and Measure	cal.	prot. (gms)	carbo. (gms)	fat (gms)	chol. (mgs)	sod. (mgs)	fiber (gms)
Parmesan (*Butterball Chicken Requests*)	200	17.0	16.0	7.0	55	650	1.0
Southwestern (*Butterball Chicken Requests*)	170	17.0	13.0	6.0	35	590	2.0
breast, oven-roasted (*Tyson*), 2 oz.	80	8.0	1.0	4.5	20	490	0
breast, seasoned:							
barbecue (*Perdue*)	110	22.0	5.0	.5	60	420	0
barbecue (*Perdue Individually Frozen*), 4.3-oz. pc.	160	31.0	4.0	2.5	90	320	0
w/barbecue sauce (*Perdue*), ½ cup	200	19.0	19.0	5.0	105	670	0
honey roasted (*Perdue Short Cuts*), ½ cup	100	18.0	4.0	1.0	40	490	<1.0
Italian (*Perdue*)	100	20.0	2.0	.5	55	520	0
Italian (*Perdue Individually Frozen*), 4.3-oz pc.	150	31.0	1.0	2.5	90	370	0
Italian (*Perdue Short Cuts*), ½ cup	90	18.0	1.0	2.0	45	450	<1.0
lemon pepper (*Perdue*)	90	19.0	2.0	.5	55	520	0
lemon pepper (*Perdue Individually Frozen*), 4.3-oz. pc.	150	31.0	1.0	2.5	90	300	0
lemon pepper (*Perdue Short Cuts*), ½ cup	90	19.0	2.0	1.5	50	530	<1.0
mesquite (*Perdue Short Cuts*), ½ cup	90	18.0	2.0	1.5	45	430	<1.0
Oriental (*Perdue*)	100	20.0	3.0	1.0	55	550	0
roasted (*Perdue Short Cuts* Original), ½ cup	90	19.0	2.0	1.5	45	430	<1.0

Food and Measure	cal.	prot. (gms)	carbo. (gms)	fat (gms)	chol. (mgs)	sod. (mgs)	fiber (gms)
Chicken, frozen or refrigerated, cooked *(cont.)*							
breast, slow-roasted (*Shady Brook Farms*), 2 oz.	60	12.0	n.a.	.5	30	400	0
breast fillet:							
breaded (*Tyson*), 2 pcs., 2.9 oz. . . .	180	12.0	15.0	8.0	25	440	1.0
Southern fried (*Tyson*), 2 pcs., 3½ oz.	210	15.0	14.0	11.0	30	480	1.0
breast meat (*Tyson*)	90	20.0	0	1.0	45	240	0
breast strips:							
(*Tyson*)	90	20.0	0	1.0	45	240	0
Italian (*Louis Rich*)	100	19.0	2.0	1.5	60	730	0
seasoned (*Tyson*)	140	20.0	1.0	6.0	55	420	0
Southwestern (*Tyson*)	110	18.0	2.0	3.0	40	400	0
breast tenderloins:							
(*Perdue*)	100	23.0	0	1.0	55	25.0	0
breaded (*Perdue Original*)	170	13.0	13.0	7.0	25	360	<1.0
breaded (*Perdue Individually Frozen*)	200	15.0	13.0	10.0	30	510	<1.0
breaded (*Perdue Kick 'n Chicken*)	170	12.0	12.0	8.0	25	670	<1.0
breast tenders:							
(*Banquet*), 3 pcs.	240	12.0	15.0	15.0	40	480	<1.0
(*Perdue Done It!*)	160	18.0	7.0	7.0	65	320	2.0
baked (*Banquet Fat Free*), 3 pcs.	120	13.0	16.0	0	30	480	2.0
baked (*Butterball Chicken Requests*), 3 pcs.	170	14.0	15.0	6.0	35	410	2.0
w/barbecue sauce (*Banquet*), 3 pcs.	340	13.0	36.0	16.0	60	800	3.0
breaded (*Tyson*), 5 pcs.	220	14.0	8.0	15.0	35	290	1.0
breaded (*Tyson* Tenderloins), 2 pcs.	180	15.0	11.0	9.0	30	300	2.0
breaded, honey batter (*Tyson*), 5 pcs.	200	13.0	12.0	11.0	35	440	1.0

Food and Measure	cal.	prot. (gms)	carbo. (gms)	fat (gms)	chol. (mgs)	sod. (mgs)	fiber (gms)
breaded, patties (*Tyson*), 3 pcs.	100	13.0	11.0	0	20	540	1.0
Southern (*Banquet*), 3 pcs.	260	12.0	16.0	16.0	15	460	1.0
chunks, breaded:							
(*Tyson*), 6 pcs.	220	13.0	11.0	14.0	40	480	0
Southern (*Banquet*), 5 pcs.	270	12.0	16.0	18.0	35	570	2.0
Southern (*Tyson*), 6 pcs.	260	11.0	11.0	19.0	40	540	1.0
cutlets, breaded:							
(*Perdue*), 3½ oz.	240	12.0	14.0	15.0	35	550	<1.0
(*Perdue Done It!*), 3½ oz.	230	10.0	18.0	13.0	40	450	2.0
drumsticks:							
barbecue (*Perdue*)	110	18.0	0	4.0	100	360	0
barbecue, hot (*Tyson*), 2 pcs., 3½ oz.	160	22.0	3.0	7.0	100	620	1.0
roasted (*Perdue*), 2 pcs., 2½ oz.	100	17.0	0	4.0	95	350	0
roasted (*Perdue* Value Pack), 2.2 oz.	110	14.0	0	6.0	80	65	0
roasted (*Perdue* Oven Stuffer), 3.6 oz.	190	22.0	0	11.0	120	100	0
roasted, skinless (*Perdue*), 2 pcs., 3½ oz.	150	25.0	0	6.0	125	85	0
fried, bone-in:							
(*Banquet* Original)	280	14.0	15.0	18.0	65	620	1.0
(*Banquet* Original Jumbo Pack)	270	14.0	13.0	18.0	65	620	1.0
breasts (*Banquet* Original), 5½-oz. pc.	410	23.0	18.0	26.0	85	600	4.0
country (*Banquet*)	270	14.0	13.0	18.0	65	620	1.0
drums and thighs (*Banquet*)	260	15.0	10.0	18.0	65	540	2.0

Food and Measure	cal.	prot. (gms)	carbo. (gms)	fat (gms)	chol. (mgs)	sod. (mgs)	fiber (gms)
Chicken, frozen or refrigerated, cooked, fried, bone-in *(cont.)*							
honey barbecue, skinless (*Banquet*)	230	18.0	9.0	13.0	55	480	2.0
hot and spicy (*Banquet*)	260	14.0	13.0	18.0	65	590	1.0
lemon pepper, skinless (*Banquet*) . . .	210	18.0	7.0	13.0	55	560	2.0
skinless (*Banquet*)	210	18.0	7.0	13.0	55	480	2.0
Southern (*Banquet*)	280	14.0	15.0	18.0	65	700	1.0
wings, hot and spicy (*Banquet*), 4 pcs.	260	18.0	7.0	18.0	85	400	<1.0
grilled, lemon pepper fillet (*Tyson*), 1 pc., 2.7 oz.	100	14.0	3.0	3.5	40	370	0
leg:							
whole, roasted (*Perdue*), 5½-oz. leg	370	35.0	0	26.0	215	105	0
quarters (*Perdue* Value Pack)	220	17.0	0	5.0	105	55	0
nuggets, see "Chicken entree, frozen"							
patties, breaded, 1 pc., except as noted:							
(*Banquet* Fat Free)	100	9.0	15.0	0	20	400	1.0
(*Banquet* Original)	190	7.0	10.0	14.0	30	440	1.0
(*Perdue Individually Frozen*)	220	10.0	11.0	15.0	35	590	<1.0
(*Tyson*)	190	11.0	9.0	12.0	25	320	1.0
(*Tyson Thick'n Crispy*)	200	10.0	10.0	14.0	40	320	1.0
breast (*Tyson*)	80	10.0	9.0	0	15	430	1.0
cheddar (*Tyson Chick'n Quick Chick'n Cheddar*)	220	11.0	12.0	14.0	40	270	0
nugget shape (*Tyson*), 6 pcs., 3.8 oz.	250	14.0	15.0	15.0	45	300	2.0
Southern (*Banquet*)	170	10.0	10.0	10.0	20	430	1.0
Southern, breast (*Tyson*)	180	11.0	8.0	12.0	30	360	0

Food and Measure	cal.	prot. (gms)	carbo. (gms)	fat (gms)	chol. (mgs)	sod. (mgs)	fiber (gms)
patties, mesquite (*Tyson*), 2.8-oz. pc.	110	13.0	1.0	6.0	40	370	0
shredded, w/barbecue sauce (*Lloyd's*), ¼ cup	70	6.0	8.0	2.5	20	390	0
thigh, 1 pc.:							
barbecue (*Perdue*)	180	17.0	0	12.0	115	390	0
boneless, roasted (*Perdue*), 3.3 oz.	170	23.0	0	9.0	115	55	0
boneless, skinless, roasted (*Perdue Fit 'n Easy/Oven Stuffer*), 3½ oz.	180	25.0	0	9.0	125	40	0
fajita (*Perdue*), 2.4 oz.	120	15.0	1.0	6.0	55	380	0
honey mustard (*Perdue*), 2.4 oz.	130	15.0	4.0	7.0	55	360	0
roasted (*Perdue*) . . .	170	16.0	0	12.0	105	360	0
roasted (*Perdue Value Pack*), 3.2 oz.	240	17.0	0	19.0	115	65	0
skinless, roasted (*Perdue*), 2½ oz.	160	18.0	0	10.0	100	55	0
wings:							
(*Tyson* Wings of Fire), 3 pcs., 3.4 oz.	220	21.0	1.0	15.0	110	560	0
(*Tyson Tabasco*), 3 pcs., 2.7 oz. . . .	170	17.0	1.0	10.0	100	330	1.0
barbecue (*Perdue Done It!*)	200	18.0	4.0	12.0	35	760	0
barbecue (*Tyson*), 3 pcs., 3.2 oz. . . .	200	19.0	2.0	13.0	110	330	0
hot and spicy (*Perdue*)	190	16.0	2.0	13.0	110	610	<1.0
hot and spicy (*Perdue Done It!*)	200	19.0	18.0	13.0	40	450	2.0
hot and spicy (*Perdue Individually Frozen*)	180	16.0	1.0	12.0	95	430	<1.0

Food and Measure	cal.	prot. (gms)	carbo. (gms)	fat (gms)	chol. (mgs)	sod. (mgs)	fiber (gms)
Chicken, frozen or refrigerated, cooked, wings *(cont.)*							
roasted (*Perdue* Value Pack), 3.2 oz.	210	19.0	0	15.0	115	75	0
teriyaki (*Tyson*), 4 pcs., 3.4 oz. . . .	190	21.0	2.0	12.0	120	210	2.0
wingettes, roasted:							
(*Perdue*), 3 pcs. . . .	200	19.0	0	14.0	120	65	0
(*Perdue Oven Stuffer*), 3 pcs., 3.4 oz.	220	21.0	0	15.0	120	80	0
Chicken, ground:							
raw, 4 oz.:							
(*Perdue*)	190	19.0	0	13.0	150	65	0
(*Perdue* Burgers)	180	19.0	0	11.0	125	65	0
(*Wampler*)	220	22.0	0	14.0	90	85	0
cooked, 3 oz.:							
(*Perdue*)	180	19.0	0	11.0	135	45	0
(*Perdue* Burger) . . .	170	18.0	0	11.0	115	50	0
"Chicken," vegetarian:							
canned:							
diced (*Worthington* Chik), ¼ cup	40	7.0	1.0	0	0	270	1.0
fried (*Worthington* FriChik), 2 pcs.	120	10.0	1.0	8.0	0	430	1.0
fried (*Worthington* FriChik Lowfat), 2 pcs.	80	10.0	2.0	3.0	0	430	1.0
fried, w/gravy (*Loma Linda* Chik'n), 2 pcs.	160	12.0	4.0	10.0	0	440	2.0
sliced (*Worthington* Chik), 3 slices . . .	70	14.0	2.0	.5	0	430	2.0
frozen:							
(*Worthington Chic-Ketts*), 2 slices, ³/₈"	120	13.0	2.0	7.0	0	390	2.0
(*Worthington Chik-Stiks*), 1 pc.	110	9.0	3.0	7.0	0	360	2.0

Food and Measure	cal.	prot. (gms)	carbo. (gms)	fat (gms)	chol. (mgs)	sod. (mgs)	fiber (gms)
nuggets (*Loma Linda*), 5 pcs.	240	12.0	13.0	16.0	0	710	5.0
nuggets (*Morningstar Farms*), 4 pcs.	160	13.0	17.0	4.0	0	670	5.0
patty (*Morningstar Farms* Chik), 1 pc.	150	8.0	15.0	6.0	0	600	2.0
patty (*Worthington CrispyChik*), 1 pc.	150	8.0	5.0	9.0	0	600	2.0
slice or roll (*Morningstar Farms*), 2 slices	80	9.0	1.0	4.5	0	370	<1.0
mix (*Loma Linda* Supreme), 1/3cup	90	15.0	6.0	1.0	0	720	4.0
refrigerated, nuggets (*Morningstar Farms*), 4 pcs.	160	13.0	17.0	4.0	0	670	5.0
Chicken Dijon seasoning mix (*Knorr* Dijonne), 1 tbsp.	30	0	5.0	1.0	0	430	0
Chicken dinner, frozen, 1 pkg.:							
boneless (*Swanson Hungry Man*), 17¼ oz.	640	29.0	82.0	22.0	55	1650	8.0
breaded, country (*Healthy Choice*), 10¼ oz.	350	16.0	51.0	9.0	45	480	5.0
broccoli Alfredo (*Healthy Choice*), 11½ oz.	300	25.0	38.0	6.0	40	530	4.0
cacciatore (*Healthy Choice*), 12½ oz.	270	22.0	36.0	4.0	35	550	5.0
Cantonese (*Healthy Choice*), 10¾ oz.	280	22.0	34.0	6.0	50	480	2.0
Dijon (*Healthy Choice*), 11 oz.	270	23.0	33.0	5.0	40	470	6.0
Francesca (*Healthy Choice*), 12½ oz.	330	23.0	46.0	6.0	30	600	5.0

Food and Measure	cal.	prot. (gms)	carbo. (gms)	fat (gms)	chol. (mgs)	sod. (mgs)	fiber (gms)
Chicken dinner, frozen *(cont.)*							
fried:							
(*Banquet Extra Helping*), 18 oz.	910	34.0	70.0	55.0	160	2600	5.0
(*Swanson*), 11½ oz.	600	24.0	58.0	31.0	70	1360	5.0
(*Swanson Hungry Man* Classic), 16½ oz.	790	33.0	75.0	40.0	80	1940	6.0
boneless white meat (*Swanson*), 11 oz.	430	23.0	49.0	16.0	40	1010	5.0
country, w/gravy (*Marie Callender's*), 16 oz.	620	24.0	63.0	30.0	75	2300	6.0
white meat (*Swanson Hungry Man*), 16¾ oz.	660	34.0	73.0	26.0	60	1740	5.0
ginger, Hunan (*Healthy Choice*), 12.6 oz.	350	24.0	59.0	2.5	25	430	5.0
grilled:							
mushroom sauce (*Marie Callender's*), 14 oz.	480	33.0	54.0	15.0	65	1030	7.0
Southwestern (*Healthy Choice*), 10.2 oz.	260	21.0	30.0	6.0	40	450	4.0
herb, country (*Healthy Choice*), 12.15 oz.	320	17.0	49.0	6.0	45	540	4.0
mesquite, barbecue (*Healthy Choice*), 10½ oz.	310	18.0	48.0	5.0	55	480	6.0
parmigiana:							
(*Healthy Choice*), 11½ oz.	330	19.0	46.0	8.0	40	490	3.0
(*Marie Callender's*), 16 oz.	620	31.0	63.0	27.0	50	730	9.0
(*Swanson*), 11¼ oz.	370	13.0	40.0	17.0	25	1010	4.0
picante (*Healthy Choice*), 10¾ oz.	260	210.	30.0	6.0	45	550	4.0

Food and Measure	cal.	prot. (gms)	carbo. (gms)	fat (gms)	chol. (mgs)	sod. (mgs)	fiber (gms)
roasted (*Healthy Choice*), 11 oz.	230	20.0	25.0	5.0	45	480	6.0
sesame, Shanghai (*Healthy Choice*), 12 oz.	300	24.0	40.0	5.0	40	550	6.0
sweet and sour:							
(*Healthy Choice*), 11 oz.	360	20.0	53.0	7.0	45	360	5.0
(*Marie Callender's*), 14 oz.	530	25.0	86.0	9.0	35	700	1.0
teriyaki (*Healthy Choice*), 11 oz.	270	17.0	37.0	6.0	45	600	3.0
Chicken entree, canned or packaged, 1 cup, except as noted:							
chow mein:							
(*Chun King* Bi-Pack)	110	7.5	12.0	4.0	0	1070	3.0
(*La Choy* Bi-Pack)	100	8.0	10.0	4.0	15	1160	2.0
(*La Choy* Entree) ...	80	8.0	6.0	3.5	20	1190	3.0
and dumplings (*Dinty Moore* Microwave Cup)........	200	15.0	21.0	6.0	35	890	1.0
fajita (*Nalley* Superba)	230	13.0	13.0	6.0	15	810	13.0
w/mushrooms (*Hunt's*)	200	10.0	32.0	4.0	25	910	4.0
and noodles (*Dinty Moore American Classics*), 1 bowl	270	22.0	28.0	8.0	90	1310	2.0
noodles and, see "Noodle entree, canned or packaged"							
w/potatoes (*Dinty Moore American Classics*), 1 bowl	240	20.0	25.0	4.0	35	990	2.0
stew:							
(*Dinty Moore* Canned)	220	12.0	16.0	11.0	40	980	2.0
(*Dinty Moore* Microwave Cup)	180	10.0	18.0	8.0	30	920	2.0

Food and Measure	cal.	prot. (gms)	carbo. (gms)	fat (gms)	chol. (mgs)	sod. (mgs)	fiber (gms)
Chicken entree, canned or packaged *(cont.)*							
sweet and sour:							
(*Chun King* Bi-Pack)	160	8.0	29.0	2.5	20	650	2.0
(*La Choy* Bi-Pack)	160	8.0	29.0	2.0	10	730	4.5
teriyaki (*La Choy* Bi-Pack)	115	8.0	15.0	3.5	20	1360	3.0
Chicken entree, dried, 1 serving:							
(*AlpineAire* Kung Fu)	360	17.0	67.0	2.0	25	830	3.0
(*AlpineAire* Sierra) ...	250	22.0	34.0	3.0	25	550	2.0
(*AlpineAire* Summer)	310	24.0	34.0	8.0	50	630	1.0
à la king w/noodles (*Mountain House*)	290	19.0	31.0	10.0	70	1070	1.0
almond (*AlpineAire*)	240	20.0	28.0	5.0	20	450	4.0
brown rice, w/vegetables (*AlpineAire*)	320	20.0	54.0	2.0	30	960	6.0
gumbo (*AlpineAire*)	280	18.0	46.0	2.5	35	1150	3.0
noodles and (*Mountain House*)	200	11.0	33.0	3.0	40	940	3.0
peach, sweet, and pecan (*AlpineAire*) ...	380	18.0	54.0	10.0	35	590	3.0
Polynesian w/rice (*Mountain House*)	200	9.0	34.0	4.0	25	770	1.0
primavera (*AlpineAire*)	250	18.0	41.0	1.5	25	680	4.0
rice and (*Mountain House*)	300	8.0	44.0	10.0	15	1150	1.0
rotelle (*AlpineAire*) ...	330	23.0	40.0	8.0	60	870	1.0
stew (*Mountain House*)	220	11.0	24.0	9.0	30	1080	3.0
stew, creamy (*AlpineAire*)	300	20.0	39.0	7.0	45	860	4.0
sweet and sour w/noodles (*AlpineAire*)	330	20.0	58.0	2.0	35	610	3.0
teriyaki w/rice (*Mountain House*)	210	10.0	37.0	2.0	20	770	2.0

Food and Measure	cal.	prot. (gms)	carbo. (gms)	fat (gms)	chol. (mgs)	sod. (mgs)	fiber (gms)
Chicken entree, frozen (see also "Chicken, frozen or refrigerated, cooked"), 1 pkg., except as noted:							
à la king:							
(*Freezer Queen* Cook-in-Pouch), 4 oz.	70	8.0	7.0	1.5	15	390	2.0
(*Stouffer's*), 9½ oz.	350	17.0	41.0	13.0	40	800	2.0
à l'orange (*Lean Cuisine Cafe Classics*), 9 oz.	260	22.0	40.0	1.0	40	320	2.0
Alfredo (*Stouffer's Skillet Sensations*), ½ of 25-oz. pkg.	490	23.0	63.0	16.0	30	1240	9.0
baked (*Lean Cuisine American Favorites*), 8⅝ oz.	230	18.0	31.0	4.0	35	520	5.0
barbecue:							
w/potato, vegetables (*Tyson*), 14.8 oz.	560	19.0	73.0	21.0	30	1190	9.0
w/sauce (*Lean Cuisine Hearty Portions*), 13 oz.	380	24.0	54.0	8.0	50	790	6.0
smokey (*Wampler*), 1 cup or ⅑ pkg.	430	42.0	31.0	15.0	140	1020	1.0
Tabasco sauce (*Tyson*), 9 oz.	260	13.0	37.0	7.0	25	610	5.0
basil (*Weight Watchers Main Street Bistro*), 9½ oz.	280	19.0	35.0	7.0	25	790	2.0
w/basil cream sauce (*Lean Cuisine Cafe Classics*), 8½ oz.	270	16.0	35.0	7.0	35	580	3.0
biryani (*Curry Classics*), 10 oz.	460	2.0	58.0	13.0	100	820	4.0
and biscuits (*Freezer Queen* Deluxe Family), 1 cup	210	14.0	29.0	4.5	40	710	4.0

Food and Measure	cal.	prot. (gms)	carbo. (gms)	fat (gms)	chol. (mgs)	sod. (mgs)	fiber (gms)
Chicken entree, frozen (cont.)							
blackened, w/rice, corn (*Tyson*), 9 oz.	260	17.0	36.0	5.0	30	480	4.0
breast:							
baked (*Stouffer's* Homestyle), 8⅞ oz.	260	22.0	18.0	11.0	65	680	3.0
in barbecue sauce (*Stouffer's* Homestyle), 10 oz.	510	17.0	56.0	24.0	80	1270	0
w/con queso burrito (*Healthy Choice*), 10.55 oz.	350	14.0	60.0	6.0	35	590	6.0
w/mushroom gravy (*Stouffer's* Homestyle), 10 oz.	360	23.0	32.0	15.0	60	880	2.0
in wine sauce (*Lean Cuisine Cafe Classics*), 8 oz.	210	15.0	23.0	6.0	35	560	2.0
and broccoli:							
(*Healthy Choice Hearty Handfuls*), 6.1 oz.	320	17.0	51.0	5.0	20	580	5.0
and cheese, carrots, pasta (*Tyson*), 9 oz.	270	20.0	19.0	12.0	40	690	3.0
w/cheese and rice (*Banquet* Family), 1 cup	280	14.0	25.0	14.0	45	980	2.0
cacciatore (*Wampler*), 1 cup or ⅑ pkg. . . .	280	30	10.0	9.0	90	600	2.0
carbonara:							
(*Lean Cuisine Cafe Classics*), 9 oz.	280	18.0	33.0	8.0	30	580	2.0
(*Weight Watchers Main Street Bistro*), 9½ oz.	300	21.0	36.0	6.0	40	780	2.0
cheese, three (*Birds Eye Chicken Voila*), 1¾ cups	240	16.0	26.0	9.0	25	630	9.0
chow mein:							
(*Smart Ones*), 9 oz.	230	15.0	34.0	4.5	35	790	3.0

Food and Measure	cal.	prot. (gms)	carbo. (gms)	fat (gms)	chol. (mgs)	sod. (mgs)	fiber (gms)
w/egg rolls (*Banquet Meal*), 9 oz.	210	9.0	280	7.0	30	850	3.0
w/rice (*Lean Cuisine*), 9 oz.	220	12.0	33.0	5.0	35	560	3.0
w/rice (*Stouffer's*), 10⅝ oz.	220	13.0	33.0	4.5	30	1420	0
Cordon Bleu (*Marie Callender's*), 13 oz.	590	33.0	58.0	25.0	55	1920	7.0
creamed (*Stouffer's*), 6½ oz.	260	15.0	8.0	19.0	80	680	0
croquettes, gravy and (*Freezer Queen* Family), 1 patty w/gravy	160	8.0	16.0	8.0	10	690	2.0
divan, w/carrots, pasta (*Tyson*), 10 oz.	370	20.0	38.0	15.0	50	530	2.0
and dumplings: (*Marie Callender's*), 1 cup	250	13.0	22.0	12.0	80	1030	3.0
(*Marie Callender's* Family), 1 cup ...	320	18.0	26.0	16.0	80	1190	3.0
(*Stouffer's* Homestyle), 11 oz.	280	19.0	33.0	8.0	55	1000	0
country style (*Banquet* Family), 1 cup	290	12.0	30.0	14.0	40	1270	2.0
w/gravy (*Banquet*), 10 oz.	270	13.0	35.0	9.0	40	780	3.0
enchilada, see "Enchilada"							
fajita:							
(*Healthy Choice Fiesta*), 7 oz.	260	21.0	36.0	4.0	30	410	4.0
(*Tyson*), 3½ pcs., 13.2 oz.	460	28.0	61.0	11.0	45	1220	6.0
(*Wampler*), 1 cup or ⅑ pkg.	210	23.0	13.0	7.0	70	1360	2.0
(*Weight Watchers Main Street Bistro* Supreme), 9¼ oz.	280	19.0	33.0	7.0	30	790	2.0

Food and Measure	cal.	prot. (gms)	carbo. (gms)	fat (gms)	chol. (mgs)	sod. (mgs)	fiber (gms)
Chicken entree, frozen *(cont.)*							
fettuccine:							
(*The Budget Gourmet*), 8½ oz. ...	340	12.0	40.0	14.0	50	640	2.0
(*Lean Cuisine*), 9¼ oz.	300	24.0	38.0	6.0	50	590	3.0
(*Stouffer's* Homestyle), 10½ oz.	350	28.0	28.0	14.0	50	1040	2.0
(*Stouffer's* Hearty Portions), 16¾ oz.	640	39.0	67.0	24.0	40	1610	4.0
(*Weight Watchers Main Street Bistro*), 10 oz.	300	21.0	39.0	8.0	70	630	4.0
Alfredo (*Banquet*), 10¼ oz.	420	15.0	37.0	24.0	70	1000	4.0
Alfredo (*Healthy Choice*), 8½ oz.	260	22.0	35.0	4.5	40	410	3.0
fiesta:							
(*Lean Cuisine Cafe Classics*), 8½ oz.	270	19.0	36.0	5.0	30	590	4.0
(*Smart Ones*), 8½ oz.	210	13.0	35.0	2.0	25	570	5.0
fingers, w/barbecue sauce, 9 oz.:							
(*Banquet*)	340	13.0	36.0	16.0	60	800	3.0
(*Freezer Queen*) ...	310	16.0	32.0	13.0	40	900	5.0
Florentine (*Lean Cuisine Hearty Portions*), 13¼ oz. ...	440	35.0	56.0	8.0	35	850	7.0
Française, w/red potato, green beans (*Tyson*), 9 oz.	260	19.0	23.0	10.0	45	790	6.0
French recipe (*The Budget Gourmet Low Fat*), 8½ oz.	180	8.0	20.0	7.0	15	750	2.0
fried:							
(*Banquet Original*), 9 oz.	470	21.0	35.0	27.0	90	1500	2.0
(*Kid Cuisine* High Flying), 10.1 oz.	440	18.0	48.0	20.0	70	940	5.0

Food and Measure	cal.	prot. (gms)	carbo. (gms)	fat (gms)	chol. (mgs)	sod. (mgs)	fiber (gms)
breast (*Stouffer's Homestyle*), 8⅞ oz.	400	23.0	38.0	17.0	55	950	2.0
breast (*Stouffer's Hearty Portions*), 15 oz.	500	29.0	60.0	16.0	55	1220	6.0
country w/gravy, potato (*Marie Callender's* Family), 1 pc. w/½ cup potato	520	20.0	51.0	26.0	70	2000	4.0
w/gravy, w/mashed potato (*Tyson*), 10.9 oz.	360	16.0	39.0	15.0	30	840	4.0
Southern (*Banquet*), 8¾ oz.	560	26.0	40.0	33.0	100	1540	3.0
white meat (*Banquet*), 8¾ oz. ...	480	18.0	40.0	28.0	100	1100	3.0
garlic:							
(*Birds Eye Chicken Voila*), 2 cups ...	260	14.0	27.0	11.0	25	540	1.0
(*Healthy Choice Hearty Handfuls*), 6.1 oz.	330	20.0	53.0	5.0	25	600	6.0
golden baked (*Weight Watchers Main Street Bistro*), 10 oz.	280	19.0	40.0	6.0	25	650	3.0
Milano (*Healthy Choice*), 9½ oz.	240	18.0	34.0	4.0	35	510	3.0
glazed:							
(*Lean Cuisine Cafe Classics*), 8½ oz.	240	22.0	25.0	6.0	55	480	0
country (*Healthy Choice*), 8½ oz.	230	17.0	30.0	4.0	45	480	3.0
w/rice (*Stouffer's*), ⅕ of 59-oz. pkg.	290	21.0	39.0	6.0	45	810	2.0
grilled:							
(*Banquet*), 9.9 oz.	330	16.0	37.0	13.0	50	1210	3.0
(*Lean Cuisine Cafe Classics*), 8 oz.	260	18.0	28.0	8.0	35	580	3.0

Food and Measure	cal.	prot. (gms)	carbo. (gms)	fat (gms)	chol. (mgs)	sod. (mgs)	fiber (gms)
Chicken entree, frozen, grilled *(cont.)*							
breast, and rice pilaf (*Marie Callender's*), 11¾ oz.	360	20.0	38.0	14.0	40	1070	6.0
w/corn O'Brian, beans (*Tyson*), 9 oz.	230	19.0	30.0	4.0	30	590	7.0
fire, and vegetables (*Weight Watchers Main Street Bistro*), 10 oz.	280	18.0	40.0	5.0	40	780	2.0
Italian, w/pasta, vegetables (*Tyson*), 9 oz.	190	21.0	19.0	3.5	30	440	3.0
w/mashed potato (*Healthy Choice*), 8 oz.	170	18.0	18.0	3.5	40	600	3.0
and penne pasta (*Lean Cuisine Hearty Portions*), 14 oz.	380	30.0	50.0	7.0	40	850	6.0
salsa (*Lean Cuisine Cafe Classics*), 8 oz.	270	15.0	36.0	7.0	45	570	4.0
Sonoma (*Healthy Choice*), 9 oz.	230	18.0	30.0	4.0	45	530	3.0
herb, and roast potatoes (*Lean Cuisine Skillet Sensations*), ½ of 24-oz. pkg.	270	18.0	39.0	5.0	40	790	5.0
herb-roasted: (*Lean Cuisine Cafe Classics*), 8 oz.	200	15.0	24.0	5.0	25	510	3.0
w/potato (*Marie Callender's*), 14 oz.	670	43.0	32.0	31.0	205	2100	7.0
homestyle (*Stouffer's Skillet Sensations*), ½ of 25-oz. pkg.	390	22.0	47.0	13.0	50	1040	7.0
honey mustard: (*Healthy Choice*), 9½ oz.	270	21.0	38.0	4.0	40	520	2.0

Food and Measure	cal.	prot. (gms)	carbo. (gms)	fat (gms)	chol. (mgs)	sod. (mgs)	fiber (gms)
(*Lean Cuisine Cafe Classics*), 8 oz.	260	15.0	40.0	4.0	35	550	3.0
(*Smart Ones*), 8½ oz.	210	11.0	38.0	3.5	30	620	2.0
Dijon, w/pasta, peas (*Tyson*), 11.4 oz.	340	20.0	49.0	7.0	25	900	6.0
honey-roasted (*Lean Cuisine American Favorites*), 8½ oz.	270	13.0	42.0	6.0	25	590	4.0
imperial:							
(*Healthy Choice*), 9 oz.	230	17.0	31.0	4.0	50	470	3.0
w/rice (*Freezer Queen*), 8½ oz.	220	12.0	39.0	1.5	25	710	3.0
Kiev, w/rice pilaf, broccoli, and carrots (*Tyson*), 9 oz.	440	18.0	36.0	25.0	85	900	2.0
lemongrass basil, w/rice (*Thai Chef*), 11 oz.	390	22.0	55.0	10.0	40	105	4.0
mandarin:							
(*The Budget Gourmet* Low Fat), 8½ oz.	240	8.0	35.0	6.0	20	730	2.0
(*Healthy Choice*), 10 oz.	280	20.0	44.0	2.5	35	520	4.0
(*Lean Cuisine*), 9 oz.	250	15.0	38.0	4.0	25	590	3.0
Marsala:							
(*Marie Callender's*), 14 oz.	450	33.0	42.0	17.0	70	1260	6.0
w/vegetables (*Healthy Choice*), 11½ oz.	240	20.0	32.0	4.0	30	440	3.0
medallions, w/cheese sauce (*Lean Cuisine American Favorites*), 9 oz.	260	17.0	27.0	9.0	25	520	3.0
Mediterranean (*Lean Cuisine Cafe Classics*), 10½ oz.	260	17.0	38.0	4.0	25	590	2.0

Food and Measure	cal.	prot. (gms)	carbo. (gms)	fat (gms)	chol. (mgs)	sod. (mgs)	fiber (gms)
Chicken entree, frozen *(cont.)*							
mesquite, w/corn, peas, au gratin potato (*Tyson*), 9 oz.	320	18.0	44.0	8.0	25	780	4.0
Mirabella (*Smart Ones*), 9.2 oz.	180	11.0	30.0	2.0	20	480	4.0
and mushroom (*Healthy Choice Hearty Handfuls*), 6.1 oz.	310	17.0	49.0	5.0	20	590	4.0
w/mushroom sauce, rice pilaf, carrots (*Tyson*), 9 oz.	220	15.0	27.0	6.0	30	510	2.0
and noodles:							
(*The Budget Gourmet*), 8½ oz. ...	390	14.0	31.0	23.0	100	740	2.0
(*Marie Callender's*), 13 oz.	520	21.0	42.0	30.0	65	1320	5.0
escalloped (*Stouffer's*), 10 oz.	460	18.0	31.0	29.0	100	1310	3.0
escalloped (*Stouffer's 40 oz.*), 1 cup ...	370	15.0	25.0	23.0	45	1130	2.0
nuggets:							
(*Banquet* Original), 6 pcs.	270	14.0	12.0	19.0	35	540	1.0
(*Freezer Queen* Family), 6 pcs.	260	12.0	17.0	16.0	25	840	2.0
(*Kid Cuisine* Cosmic), 9.1 oz.	460	18.0	50.0	21.0	35	1070	5.0
(*Perdue*), 5 pcs. ...	240	11.0	14.0	15.0	35	530	<1.0
(*Perdue Done It!*), 5 pcs.	200	9.0	15.0	12.0	35	390	2.0
(*Perdue Individually Frozen*), 5 pcs.	250	11.0	15.0	16.0	40	720	1.0
(*Tyson*), 4 pcs.	240	12.0	16.0	14.0	40	330	2.0
(*Tyson*), 3-oz. pc. ...	220	13.0	11.0	14.0	35	320	2.0
w/apple compote, potato puffs (*Freezer Queen*), 6 oz.	320	11.0	34.0	16.0	20	910	3.0

Food and Measure	cal.	prot. (gms)	carbo. (gms)	fat (gms)	chol. (mgs)	sod. (mgs)	fiber (gms)
w/cheese (*Perdue*), 5 pcs.	270	11.0	13.0	18.0	40	640	<1.0
w/cheese (*Perdue Done It!*), 5 pcs.	220	11.0	11.0	15.0	95	550	1.0
Southern, w/barbecue sauce (*Banquet* Micro), 6 pcs. w/sauce	340	16.0	22.0	20.0	45	840	2.0
w/sweet and sour sauce (*Banquet* Micro), 6 pcs. w/sauce	320	16.0	25.0	18.0	45	670	2.0
orange-glazed (*The Budget Gourmet Low Fat*), 8½ oz.	280	11.0	48.0	5.0	30	720	1.0
Oriental:							
(*Lean Cuisine Skillet Sensations*), ½ of 24-oz. pkg.	280	17.0	46.0	3.0	15	790	6.0
w/egg rolls (*Banquet*), 9 oz.	260	10.0	36.0	9.0	40	790	3.0
glazed (*Lean Cuisine Hearty Portions*), 14 oz.	350	27.0	54.0	2.5	35	840	8.0
and vegetables (*The Budget Gourmet Low Fat*), 8½ oz.	260	9.0	40.0	6.0	15	590	3.0
Parmesan (*Lean Cuisine Cafe Classics*), 10 oz.	260	19.0	31.0	7.0	30	590	4.0
parmigiana:							
(*Banquet*), 9½ oz.	320	10.0	29.0	18.0	50	900	3.0
(*Banquet* Family), 1 patty w/gravy	240	11.0	18.0	13.0	20	690	2.0
(*Stouffer's* Homestyle), 12 oz.	460	24.0	54.0	16.0	45	1060	5.0
pasta:							
fiesta (*Marie Callender's*), 12½ oz.	640	27.0	44.0	40.0	80	860	4.0
primavera (*Banquet*), 9½ oz. . . .	320	11.0	40.0	12.0	25	840	6.0

Food and Measure	cal.	prot. (gms)	carbo. (gms)	fat (gms)	chol. (mgs)	sod. (mgs)	fiber (gms)
Chicken entree, frozen (cont.)							
patties, breaded							
(*Freezer Queen*),							
7½ oz.	290	14.0	29.0	14.0	20	750	7.0
in peanut sauce:							
(*Lean Cuisine Cafe*							
Classics), 9 oz.	290	23.0	35.0	6.0	30	590	4.0
satay (*Thai Chef*),							
11 oz.	400	20.0	50.0	14.0	35	740	3.0
penne, rosemary (*Tyson* Kit), 12½ oz.	330	25.0	45.0	5.0	45	860	5.0
pesto (*Birds Eye Chicken Voila*), 2¼ cups	250	16.0	25.0	9.0	25	720	1.0
piccata:							
(*Lean Cuisine Cafe*							
Classics), 9 oz.	270	13.0	41.0	6.0	25	530	2.0
(*Tyson*), 9 oz.	190	17.0	18.0	6.0	35	500	5.0
lemon herb (*Smart Ones*), 9 oz.	210	14.0	31.0	2.0	50	550	3.0
pie/pot pie:							
(*Banquet*), 7 oz.	380	10.0	36.0	22.0	40	950	1.0
(*Banquet* Family),							
1 cup	480	14.0	39.0	29.0	35	1010	6.0
(*Lean Cuisine*),							
9½ oz.	290	18.0	35.0	9.0	30	570	5.0
(*Marie Callender's*),							
9½ oz.	600	14.0	53.0	37.0	15	1070	4.0
(*Marie Callender's*),							
½ of 16½-oz. pie	520	13.0	45.0	32.0	15	1070	3.0
(*Pepperidge Farm*),							
1 cup, ½ pkg. . . .	450	12.0	40.0	26.0	25	1070	0
(*Stouffer's*), 10 oz.	490	19.0	38.0	29.0	35	1320	4.0
(*Stouffer's*), ½ of							
16-oz. pie	430	17.0	35.0	25.0	40	1150	5.0
(*Stouffer's Hearty*							
Portions), 16 oz.	590	15.0	49.0	37.0	40	1240	4.0
(*Swanson*), 7 oz.	410	10.0	43.0	22.0	25	780	2.0
(*Swanson Hungry*							
Man), 14 oz.	620	20.0	62.0	32.0	45	1450	5.0
au gratin (*Marie Callender's*), 9½ oz.	690	19.0	50.0	46.0	30	1300	4.0
au gratin (*Marie Cal-*							

Food and Measure	cal.	prot. (gms)	carbo. (gms)	fat (gms)	chol. (mgs)	sod. (mgs)	fiber (gms)
lender's), ¹/₂ of 16¹/₂-oz. pie	710	18.0	56.0	46.0	30	1190	3.0
and broccoli (Banquet), 7 oz.	330	10.0	32.0	18.0	35	810	2.0
and broccoli (Marie Callender's), 9¹/₂ oz.	670	16.0	54.0	43.0	25	1000	4.0
and broccoli (Marie Callender's), ¹/₂ of 16¹/₂-oz. pie	710	17.0	51.0	49.0	25	1060	4.0
primavera: (Lean Cuisine Skillet Sensations), ¹/₂ of 24-oz. pkg.	320	20.0	50.0	4.5	30	790	4.0
(Tyson), 11.4 oz.	350	25.0	48.0	6.0	30	610	5.0
rice, cheesy, w/chicken and broccoli (Marie Callender's), 12 oz. . . .	390	24.0	44.0	13.0	55	1220	6.0
rice, fried (Tyson Kit), 14 oz., 2¹/₂ cups . . .	440	27.0	69.0	6.0	30	1810	5.0
roasted: w/garlic sauce, pasta, vegetables (Tyson), 9 oz. . . .	210	17.0	20.0	7.0	25	460	3.0
w/mushrooms (Lean Cuisine Hearty Portions), 12¹/₂ oz.	340	27.0	44.0	6.0	35	850	4.0
oven (Weight Watchers Main Street Bistro), 9 oz.	300	18.0	38.0	7.0	30	790	2.0
sandwich, see "Chicken sandwich"							
sesame (Healthy Choice), 9³/₄ oz. . . .	240	16.0	38.0	3.0	30	600	3.0
sliced, gravy and (Freezer Queen Cook-in-Pouch), 4 oz.	60	6.0	4.0	2.5	15	620	1.0

Food and Measure	cal.	prot. (gms)	carbo. (gms)	fat (gms)	chol. (mgs)	sod. (mgs)	fiber (gms)
Chicken entree, frozen *(cont.)*							
stir-fry (*Tyson* Kit),							
14 oz., 2¾ cups ...	430	24.0	73.0	4.5	45	1700	5.0
sweet and sour:							
(*Wampler*), 1 cup, ⅑							
pkg.	250	20.0	35.0	4.0	55	510	1.0
w/rice (*Freezer*							
Queen), 8½ oz.	280	15.0	51.0	2.0	25	710	2.0
tenderloins, in gravy							
w/potatoes							
(*Stouffer's*), ⅕ of							
61-oz. pkg.	330	25.0	25.0	14.0	60	1070	3.0
teriyaki:							
(*Birds Eye Chicken*							
Voila), 2 cups ...	230	15.0	26.0	6.0	15	610	2.0
(*Stouffer's Skillet*							
Sensations), ½ of							
25-oz. pkg.	340	20.0	59.0	3.0	30	1350	3.0
tikka (*Curry Classics*							
Makhanwala),							
10 oz.	480	31.0	15.0	33.0	160	850	6.0
and vegetables:							
(*Lean Cuisine Cafe*							
Classics),							
10½ oz.	270	20.0	33.0	6.0	25	590	4.0
grilled (*Stouffer's*							
Skillet Sensa-							
tions), ½ of 25-oz.							
pkg.	440	27.0	62.0	9.0	30	1330	6.0
w/linguini (*Freezer*							
Queen Family),							
1 cup	250	16.0	30.0	8.0	20	540	4.0
w/noodles (*Freezer*							
Queen), 8 oz. ...	170	12.0	27.0	2.0	15	530	4.0
wraps:							
blackened (*Tyson*							
Kit), ½ pkg., 1½							
wraps	550	30.0	76.0	14.0	40	1470	5.0
mandarin (*Tyson*							
Kit), ½ pkg., 1½							
wraps	630	30.0	92.0	15.0	50	1840	5.0

Food and Measure	cal.	prot. (gms)	carbo. (gms)	fat (gms)	chol. (mgs)	sod. (mgs)	fiber (gms)
Chicken entree, re-frigerated, ½ of 12-oz. pkg.:							
à la king, w/noodles (*Perdue*)	160	2.0	15.0	5.0	25	330	1.0
Alfredo, w/fettuccine (*Perdue*)	410	2.0	19.0	29.0	100	780	3.0
cacciatore, w/pasta (*Perdue*)	150	11.0	18.0	4.5	15	680	2.0
jambalaya, w/rice (*Perdue*)	180	10.0	14.0	0	25	850	2.0
Chicken entree mix, 1 cup*:							
fettuccine Alfredo (*Chicken Helper*) . . .	300	27.0	28.0	9.0	65	870	0
stir-fried (*Skillet Chicken Helper*)	270	18.0	30.0	9.0	105	760	1.0
and stuffing (*Chicken Helper*)	290	25.0	28.0	9.0	60	830	0
Chicken fat:							
1 oz.	178	1.1	0	19.3	16	9	0
rendered (*Empire* Kosher), 1 tbsp.	120	0	<1.0	13.0	10	0	0
Chicken frankfurter, see "Frankfurter"							
Chicken giblets, sim-mered:							
4 oz.	178	29.3	1.1	5.4	446	66	0
chopped, 1 cup	228	37.5	1.4	6.9	570	85	0
Chicken gravy, ¼ cup:							
canned or in jars:							
(*Franco-American*)	40	0	3.0	3.0	<5	240	0
(*Franco-American* Fat Free)	15	<1.0	3.0	0	<5	320	0
(*Franco-American* Slow Roasted) . . .	25	1.0	3.0	1.0	<5	260	0
(*Franco-American* Slow Roasted Fat Free)	20	1.0	4.0	0	<5	220	0
(*Heinz* Home Style Classic)	25	1.0	3.0	1.0	0	360	0

Food and Measure	cal.	prot. (gms)	carbo. (gms)	fat (gms)	chol. (mgs)	sod. (mgs)	fiber (gms)
Chicken gravy, canned or in jars *(cont.)*							
giblet (*Franco-American*)	30	1.0	3.0	2.0	10	310	0
Chicken gravy mix,							
¼ cup*:							
roasted (*Knorr*)	30	2.0	3.0	1.0	5	310	0
style (*Pillsbury*)	20	<1.0	4.0	0	0	260	0
vegetarian (*Loma Linda Gravy Quik*)	20	1.0	3.0	0	0	410	0
Chicken lunch meat,							
breast, 2 oz., except as noted:							
(*Wampler* Gourmet)	80	10.0	2.0	1.5	30	450	0
(*Wampler* Premium)	90	8.0	2.0	5.0	30	540	0
barbecue (*Black Bear*)	70	11.0	1.0	1.5	30	450	0
browned:							
(*Healthy Choice*) . . .	60	12.0	1.0	1.0	25	360	0
oil (*Wampler*)	60	11.0	1.0	1.0	30	370	0
honey:							
(*Tyson* Fat Free), 2 slices, 1½ oz.	35	7.0	2.0	0	15	450	0
glazed (*Oscar Mayer Deli-Thin*), 4 slices, 1.8 oz. . . .	60	10.0	2.0	.5	25	730	0
mesquite:							
(*Healthy Choice*) . . .	60	12.0	0	1.0	25	360	0
(*Tyson* Fat Free), 2 slices, 1½ oz.	35	7.0	1.0	0	15	440	0
oven-roasted:							
(*Boar's Head*)	50	11.0	<1.0	1.0	30	420	0
(*Healthy Choice*), 1-oz. slice	25	5.0	2.0	0	10	240	0
(*Healthy Choice*) 10 oz., 1-oz. slice	35	5.0	2.0	1.0	10	240	0
(*Healthy Choice* Deli-Thin), 6 slices, 1.8 oz.	60	11.0	3.0	0	20	470	0
(*Oscar Mayer Free*), 4 slices, 1.8 oz.	45	10.0	1.0	0	25	650	0
(*Tyson* Fat Free), 2 slices, 1½ oz.	35	7.0	1.0	0	15	460	0

Food and Measure	cal.	prot. (gms)	carbo. (gms)	fat (gms)	chol. (mgs)	sod. (mgs)	fiber (gms)
peppered (*Tyson* Fat Free), 2 slices, 1½ oz.	35	7.0	1.0	0	15	480	0
rotisserie seasoned (*Healthy Choice* Hearty Deli), 3 slices, 2 oz.	60	11.0	2.0	.5	30	480	0
skinless (*Healthy Choice*)	45	10.0	0	0	25	420	0
smoked:							
(*Healthy Choice*), 1-oz. slice	30	5.0	2.0	1.0	15	240	9
(*Healthy Choice* Deli-Thin), 6 slices, 1.9 oz.	60	10.0	3.0	1.5	25	470	0
hickory (*Boar's Head*)	60	11.0	<1.0	1.0	30	440	0
hickory (*Tyson* Fat Free), 2 slices, 1½ oz.	35	7.0	1.0	0	15	450	0
honey-roasted (*Healthy Choice* Deli-Thin Savory Selections), 6 slices, 1.9 oz.	70	10.0	4.0	1.5	25	470	0
white meat:							
(*Tyson*), 2 slices, 1.3 oz.	60	7.0	0	4.0	15	300	0
rolled (*Tyson*)	90	10.0	0	6.0	25	440	0
Chicken patty, see "Chicken entree, frozen"							
Chicken pie, see "Chicken entree, frozen"							
Chicken pocket, frozen, 4½-oz. pc.:							
broccoli (*Lean Pockets* Supreme)	270	12.0	37.0	7.0	30	510	2.0
broccoli and cheddar (*Croissant Pockets*)	290	13.0	38.0	9.0	40	660	2.0

Food and Measure	cal.	prot. (gms)	carbo. (gms)	fat (gms)	chol. (mgs)	sod. (mgs)	fiber (gms)
Chicken pocket *(cont.)*						
and cheddar w/broccoli (*Hot Pockets*)	300	13.0	40.0	10.0	40	510	2.0
Parmesan (*Lean Pockets*)	280	14.0	41.0	7.0	25	490	3.0
Chicken salad, ⅓ cup:						
(*Wampler*)	200	9.0	9.0	14.0	30	420	1.0
(*Wampler* Low Fat) ...	90	8.0	9.0	1.5	20	440	0
Chicken sandwich, frozen, 1 pc., except as noted:						
(*Mrs. Paterson's Aussie Pie*)	460	12.0	45.0	25.0	90	770	2.0
(*Mrs. Paterson's Aussie Pie* Low Fat) ...	380	13.0	44.0	17.0	35	800	1.0
(*White Castle*), 2 pcs.	250	17.0	24.0	9.0	20	490	5.0
breaded (*Hormel Quick Meal*)	340	15.0	40.0	13.0	35	520	1.0
breast (*Tyson* Microwave)	320	14.0	33.0	15.0	30	630	2.0
grilled:						
(*Hormel Quick Meal*)	310	19.0	36.0	10.0	55	580	1.0
(*Tyson* Microwave)	210	13.0	25.0	6.0	25	460	2.0
Chicken sauce, cooking (see also specific listings), ½ cup, except as noted:						
cacciatore (*Chicken Tonight*)	70	2.0	11.0	1.5	0	480	2.0
Dijon:						
country (*Lawry's Chicken Saute*), 2 tbsp.	40	<1.0	7.0	1.0	0	360	0
white wine (*Jacques Pépin's Kitchen Chicken & Pork*)	70	3.0	5.0	2.5	0	940	0
French, country (*Chicken Tonight*)	120	<1.0	6.0	10.0	15	860	1.0

Food and Measure	cal.	prot. (gms)	carbo. (gms)	fat (gms)	chol. (mgs)	sod. (mgs)	fiber (gms)
honey mustard, light (*Chicken Tonight*)	60	1.0	13.0	.5	0	420	3.0
lemon herb (*Lawry's Chicken Saute*), 2 tbsp.	25	0	4.0	1.0	0	400	0
mushroom, creamy (*Chicken Tonight*)	80	<1.0	5.0	6.0	10	750	1.0
sweet and sour (*Chicken Tonight*)	120	<1.0	29.0	0	0	340	1.0
wing, see "Buffalo wing sauce"							
Chicken sausage, see "Sausage"							
Chicken seasoning and coating mix, 1/8 pkg.:							
(*Shake'n Bake* Original)	40	1.0	7.0	1.0	0	230	0
barbecue (*Shake'n Bake*)	45	1.0	9.0	1.0	0	410	0
extra crispy (*Oven Fry*)	60	2.0	10.0	1.0	0	420	0
homestyle flour (*Oven Fry*)	40	1.0	7.0	1.0	0	470	0
hot and spicy (*Shake'n Bake*)	40	1.0	7.0	1.0	0	190	0
Chicken spread (*Underwood*), 1/4 cup	120	9.0	2.0	8.0	40	390	0
Chick-fil-A, 1 serving:							
chicken soup, hearty breast of, 1 cup	110	16.0	10.0	1.0	45	760	1.0
chicken dishes:							
chargrilled chicken garden salad	170	26.0	10.0	3.0	25	650	5.0
chicken salad plate	290	21.0	40.0	5.0	35	570	6.0
Chick-fil-A Chicken Strips, 4 pcs. . . .	230	29.0	10.0	8.0	20	380	0
Chick-fil-A Nuggets, 8-pack	290	28.0	12.0	14.0	60	770	0
Chick-n-Strips salad	290	32.0	21.0	9.0	20	430	5.0
Chick-fil-A sandwich:							
regular	290	24.0	29.0	9.0	50	870	1.0
deluxe	300	25.0	31.0	9.0	50	870	2.0

Food and Measure	cal.	prot. (gms)	carbo. (gms)	fat (gms)	chol. (mgs)	sod. (mgs)	fiber (gms)
Chick-fil-A, *Chick-fil-A* sandwich *(cont.)*							
chicken only, no bun/pickles	160	21.0	1.0	8.0	45	690	0
Chick-fil-A chicken salad sandwich, on whole wheat	320	25.0	42.0	5.0	10	810	1.0
Chick-fil-A Chargrilled Chicken Sandwich:							
regular	280	27.0	36.0	3.0	40	640	1.0
deluxe	290	28.0	38.0	3.0	40	640	2.0
club, w/out dressing	390	33.0	38.0	12.0	70	980	2.0
chicken only, no bun/pickles	130	27.0	0	3.0	30	630	0
side items, small:							
carrot-raisin salad	150	5.0	28.0	2.0	6	650	2.0
Chick-fil-A Waffle Potato Fries, salted	290	1.0	49.0	10.0	5	960	0
Chick-fil-A Waffle Potato Fries, un-salted	290	1.0	49.0	10.0	5	80	0
cole slaw	130	6.0	11.0	6.0	15	430	1.0
tossed salad	70	5.0	13.0	0	0	0	1.0
desserts:							
brownie, fudge nut	350	10.0	41.0	16.0	30	650	0
cheese cake, slice	270	13.0	7.0	21.0	10	510	0
w/blueberry	290	14.0	9.0	23.0	10	550	0
w/strawberry	290	14.0	8.0	23.0	10	580	0
Icedream, small cone	140	11.0	16.0	4.0	40	240	0
Icedream, small cup	350	16.0	50.0	10.0	70	390	0
lemon pie, slice	320	7.0	40.0	16.0	135	280	1.0
Chickpeas, see "Garbanzo beans"							
Chicory, witloof:							
(*Frieda's* Belgium Endive), 2 cups, 3 oz.	15	1.0	3.0	0	0	20	3.0
5–7″ head, 2.1 oz. ...	9	.5	2.1	.1	0	1	1.6
½ cup	8	.4	1.8	<.1	0	1	1.4
Chicory greens:							
trimmed, 1 oz.	7	.5	1.3	.1	0	13	1.1
chopped, ½ cup	21	1.5	4.2	.3	0	41	3.6

Food and Measure	cal.	prot. (gms)	carbo. (gms)	fat (gms)	chol. (mgs)	sod. (mgs)	fiber (gms)
Chicory root:							
1 medium, 2.6 oz. ...	44	.8	10.5	.1	0	30	n.a.
1″ pcs., 1/2 cup	33	.6	7.9	.1	0	23	n.a.
Chili, canned or pack- **aged,** 1 cup, except as noted:							
w/beans:							
(*El Rio*)	240	19.0	34.0	10.0	35	1050	14.0
(*Gebhardt*)	320	15.0	32.0	15.0	30	675	14.5
(*Hormel* Micro- wave cup)	220	15.0	27.0	6.0	30	1050	6.0
(*Just Rite*)	380	18.0	31.0	26.0	35	50	13.0
(*Nalley* Con Carne), 71/2 oz.	260	18.0	28.0	8.0	20	810	10.0
(*Nalley* Real Hearty)	310	20.0	27.0	14.0	30	990	12.0
(*Old El Paso*)......	240	17.0	19.0	11.0	30	770	6.0
(*Open Range*)	280	17.0	25.0	16.0	25	1290	10.0
(*Wolf's*)	265	19.0	23.0	12.0	25	830	7.0
(*Wolf's* Chunky) ...	310	19.0	31.0	15.0	30	910	7.0
(*Wolf's* Micro)	275	17.0	23.0	15.0	25	965	6.0
black bean (*El Rio*)	220	17.0	19.0	10.0	40	1090	5.0
cheddar cheese (*Nalley*)	320	23.0	28.0	12.0	35	1250	8.0
cheddar cheese (*Nalley*), 71/2 oz. .	260	18.0	22.0	11.0	25	850	9.0
chunky (*Hormel*) ...	270	18.0	34.0	7.0	35	1240	7.0
hot (*Nalley*), 71/2 oz.	240	16.0	26.0	8.0	15	800	9.0
hot (*Nalley* Jalapeño Hot)	280	20.0	30.0	8.0	25	1010	12.0
lean (*Wolf's*)	185	19.0	19.0	5.0	20	910	11.0
regular or hot (*Hor- mel*)	270	16.0	34.0	7.0	30	1220	7.0
thick (*Nalley*)	290	21.0	32.0	9.0	30	1100	11.0
3-bean (*Hormel* Health Selections)	170	9.0	28.0	2.0	10	410	6.0
w/out beans:							
(*Gebhardt*), 1/2 cup	230	9.5	10.5	17.0	30	690	2.5
(*Nalley* Big Chunk)	280	25.0	13.0	14.0	50	1040	3.0
(*Open Range*)	350	17.5	19.0	25.5	50	1215	6.0
(*Wolf's*)	310	19.0	22.0	18.0	35	940	6.0
(*Wolf's* Chunky) ...	385	23.0	21.0	24.0	50	940	11.0

Food and Measure	cal.	prot. (gms)	carbo. (gms)	fat (gms)	chol. (mgs)	sod. (mgs)	fiber (gms)
Chili, canned or packaged, w/out beans *(cont.)*							
(*Wolf's* Chunky Steak Cut)	320	22.0	17.0	19.0	45	1120	2.0
(*Wolf's* Micro)	320	21.0	15.0	21.0	35	980	4.0
lean (*Wolf's*)	200	21.0	15.0	8.0	30	1090	6.0
onion (*Nalley* Walla Walla)	300	23.0	20.0	15.0	30	1130	4.0
regular or hot (*Hormel*)	210	16.0	17.0	9.0	40	970	3.0
regular or hot (*Hormel* Micro cup)	190	14.0	15.0	8.0	30	800	2.0
w/franks, see "Beans and franks"							
w/macaroni (*Hormel* Micro cup)	200	11.0	17.0	9.0	25	980	2.0
turkey:							
w/beans (*Hormel*)	210	17.0	26.0	3.0	45	1200	5.0
w/beans (*Hormel Health Selections*)	190	17.0	25.0	2.5	40	540	6.0
w/out beans (*Hormel*)	190	24.0	17.0	3.0	75	1250	3.0
w/out beans (*Wolf's*)	155	18.0	17.0	3.0	35	1450	8.0
vegetarian:							
(*Arrowhead Mills* Panhandle)	200	10.0	34.0	2.5	0	960	12.0
(*Hormel*)	200	12.0	38.0	1.0	0	780	7.0
(*Natural Touch*)	170	18.0	21.0	1.0	0	870	11.0
(*Wolf's* Chunky) . . .	130	7.5	27.0	5.0	0	1010	7.0
(*Worthington*)	290	19.0	21.0	15.0	0	1130	9.0
(*Worthington* Lowfat)	170	18.0	21.0	1.0	0	870	11.0
black bean, mild (*Arrowhead Mills*)	190	10.0	32.0	2.5	0	970	8.0
black bean, spicy (*Arrowhead Mills*)	200	10.0	34.0	3.0	0	950	8.0
black bean or 3-bean, mild or spicy (*Health Valley*), ½ cup	80	7.0	15.0	0	0	160	7.0

Food and Measure	cal.	prot. (gms)	carbo. (gms)	fat (gms)	chol. (mgs)	sod. (mgs)	fiber (gms)
burrito flavor (*Health Valley*), ½ cup	80	7.0	15.0	0	0	180	7.0
fajita or enchilada flavor (*Health Valley*), ½ cup	80	7.0	15.0	0	0	160	7.0
lentil (*Health Valley*), ½ cup	80	7.0	14.0	0	0	100	6.0
lentil (*Health Valley No Salt*), ½ cup	80	7.0	14.0	0	0	50	6.0
mild, medium, or hot (*Muir Glen*)	150	9.0	30.0	1.0	0	580	8.0
mild or spicy (*Health Valley*), ½ cup ...	80	7.0	15.0	0	0	100	7.0
mild or spicy (*Health Valley No Salt*), ½ cup	80	7.0	15.0	0	0	35	7.0
Chili, frozen, see "Chili dinner" and "Chili entree, frozen"							
Chili, mix, all varieties (*Health Valley* Chili in a Cup), ¾ cup ...	120	10.0	21.0	1.0	0	290	6.0
Chili beans (see also "Chili starter" and "Mexican beans"), canned, ½ cup:							
(*Eden* Organic)	130	9.0	21.0	0	0	250	7.0
(*Gebhardt*)	135	7.0	31.0	1.0	0	0630	7.0
all varieties (*Brooks*)	130	6.0	23.0	.5	0	530	9.0
hot (*Bush's Best*)	120	6.0	20.0	1.0	0	480	6.0
Mexican style (*Van Camp's*)	110	7.0	21.0	2.0	0	430	8.0
spicy:							
(*Eden* Organic Pintos)	125	6.0	24.0	0	0	195	7.0
(*Green Giant/Joan of Arc*)	110	6.0	20.0	1.0	0	490	5.0
zesty sauce (*Campbell's*)	130	6.0	21.0	3.0	5	490	6.0

Food and Measure	cal.	prot. (gms)	carbo. (gms)	fat (gms)	chol. (mgs)	sod. (mgs)	fiber (gms)
Chili dinner, frozen, black bean, w/corn bread (*Amy's*), 10½ oz.	320	11.0	59.0	6.0	10	780	8.0
Chili dip (see also "Salsa"), chunky (*La Victoria*), 2 tbsp.	10	0	2.0	0	0	140	0
Chili dishes, mix, 1 pkg., except as noted:							
black bean, w/corn (*Fantastic Foods Chile Ole!* Cup)	250	13.0	47.0	2.0	0	480	14.0
mac, w/ziti (*Fantastic Foods Chile Ole!* Cup)	270	16.0	48.0	1.5	0	480	10.0
nacho, w/tortillas (*Fantastic Foods Chile Ole!* Cup)	260	13.0	50.0	3.0	5	560	11.0
vegetarian (*Fantastic Foods*), ⅛ cup	50	5.0	10.0	0	0	280	3.0
white bean, spicy (*Fantastic Foods Chile Ole!* Cup)	260	12.0	46.0	2.5	5	540	10.0
Chili entree, dried, 1 serving:							
(*AlpineAire* Mountain)	290	22.0	46.0	2.0	0	1060	8.0
(*AlpineAire* Texas) ...	240	20.0	34.0	2.5	0	860	6.0
w/beef, beans:							
(*AlpineAire* Black Bart)	320	29.0	39.0	4.5	65	1430	10.0
(*Mountain House*)	190	11.0	27.0	4.0	10	1090	7.0
Chili entree, frozen:							
w/beans (*Stouffer's*), 8¾ oz.	270	15.0	29.0	10.0	35	1130	8.0
3-bean, w/rice (*Lean Cuisine*), 10 oz. ...	250	10.0	38.0	6.0	5	590	9.0
and corn bread (*Marie Callender's*), 1 cup, 2 oz. corn bread ...	350	14.0	45.0	13.0	30	1380	5.0

Food and Measure	cal.	prot. (gms)	carbo. (gms)	fat (gms)	chol. (mgs)	sod. (mgs)	fiber (gms)
turkey, w/beans (*Wampler*), 1 cup or ⅑ pkg.	250	23.0	22.0	7.0	75	1840	4.0
Chili paste, roasted, red (*Thai Kitchen*), 1 tbsp.	55	1.0	4.0	4.0	0	80	0
Chili pepper, see "Pepper, chili"							
Chili powder:							
(*Gebhardt Eagle*), ¼ tsp.	0	0	0	0	0	0	0
1 tbsp.	24	.9	4.1	1.3	0	76	2.6
1 tsp.	8	.3	1.4	.4	0	26	.9
Chili sauce, tomato (see also "Pepper sauce"):							
(*Del Monte*), 1 tbsp.	20	0	5.0	0	0	480	0
(*Gebhardt* Hot Dog), ¼ cup	60	2.5	8.0	3.0	<5	275	2.0
(*Heinz*), 1 tbsp.	15	0	4.0	0	0	230	0
(*Hunt's*), 2 tbsp.	35	1.0	8.0	0	0	395	1.0
(*Just Rite* Hot Dog), 1 oz.	25	1.0	3.0	1.0	<5	120	1.0
(*Nance's*), 2 tbsp. . . .	25	0	5.0	0	0	150	0
(*Open Range* Hot Dog), ¼ cup	60	3.0	6.5	3.5	<5	255	2.5
(*Stubb's* Chili Fixin's), ¼ cup	50	2.0	9.0	1.0	0	730	3.0
(*Wolf's* Hot Dog), ¼ cup	45	2.0	7.0	1.5	<5	260	2.0
Chili seasoning mix:							
(*Gebhardt Chili Quik*), 2 tbsp.	45	1.0	8.0	<1.0	0	985	2.0
(*Old El Paso*), 1 tbsp.	15	<1.0	3.0	.5	0	570	<1.0
Chili starter (see also "Chili beans"), canned:							
(*Bush's Chili Magic* Traditional), ½ cup	110	5.0	19.0	1.0	0	890	5.0
(*Bush's Chili Magic* Traditional), 1 cup*	220	22.0	15.0	8.0	55	770	3.0

Food and Measure	cal.	prot. (gms)	carbo. (gms)	fat (gms)	chol. (mgs)	sod. (mgs)	fiber (gms)
Chili starter *(cont.)*							
Louisiana:							
(*Bush's Chili*							
Magic), ½ cup . . .	110	4.0	21.0	1.5	0	1070	5.0
(*Bush's Chili*							
Magic), 1 cup*	220	22.0	16.0	7.0	60	820	3.0
Mexican:							
(*Bush's Chili*							
Magic), ½ cup . . .	120	5.0	22.0	1.5	0	1030	4.0
(*Bush's Chili*							
Magic), 1 cup*	230	24.0	15.0	9.0	55	860	4.0
Texas:							
(*Bush's Chili*							
Magic), ½ cup . . .	120	5.0	20.0	2.0	0	1130	5.0
(*Bush's Chili*							
Magic), 1 cup*	230	22.0	15.0	9.0	55	880	4.0
Chimichanga, frozen, 4½-oz. pc.:							
beef (*Old El Paso*)	360	9.0	37.0	20.0	10	470	3.0
chicken (*Old El Paso*)	340	11.0	39.0	16.0	20	540	2.0
Chimichanga dinner, frozen, 16-oz. pkg.:							
beef (*Chi-Chi's*)	630	28.0	75.0	24.0	55	2050	10.0
chicken (*Chi-Chi's*) . . .	580	25.0	78.0	19.0	50	2100	15.0
Chitterlings, pork, simmered, 4 oz. . . .	344	11.6	0	32.6	162	44	0
Chives:							
fresh:							
1 oz.	9	.9	1.2	.2	0	1	.9
chopped, 1 tbsp.	1	.1	.1	<.1	0	<1	.1
freeze-dried:							
¼ cup	2	.2	.5	<.1	0	24	<1.0
1 tbsp.	1	<.1	.1	<.1	0	6	<1.0
Chocolate, see "Candy"							
Chocolate, baking, ½ oz., except as noted:							
(*Choco Bake*)	80	1.0	4.0	8.0	0	0	2.0
bar:							
(*Baker's German*)	60	1.0	8.0	3.5	0	0	<1.0

Food and Measure	cal.	prot. (gms)	carbo. (gms)	fat (gms)	chol. (mgs)	sod. (mgs)	fiber (gms)
(*Hershey's*)	90	2.0	4.0	7.0	0	0	2.0
bittersweet (*Ghirardelli*), 3 pcs., 1½ oz.	210	3.0	24.0	15.0	0	0	1.0
bittersweet (*Hershey's*)	70	<1.0	8.0	4.5	0	0	0
dark, sweet (*Ghirardelli*), 3 pcs., 1½ oz.	210	2.0	26.0	14.0	0	0	0
milk (*Ghirardelli*), 1 oz.	140	2.0	17.0	8.0	5	20	0
milk (*Ghirardelli*), 3 pcs., 1½ oz.	220	3.0	25.0	14.0	10	30	0
semisweet (*Baker's*), 1 oz.	130	2.0	17.0	9.0	0	0	2.0
semisweet (*Ghirardelli*), 3 pcs., 1½ oz.	210	2.0	25.0	14.0	5	0	0
semisweet (*Hershey's*)	70	<1.0	9.0	4.0	0	0	0
semisweet (*Nestlé*)	70	<1.0	9.0	4.0	0	0	<1.0
unsweetened (*Baker's*), 1 oz.	140	3.0	9.0	14.0	0	0	4.0
unsweetened (*Ghirardelli*), 3 pcs., 1½ oz.	210	5.0	12.0	23.0	0	0	1.0
unsweetened (*Nestlé*)	80	2.0	4.0	7.0	0	0	2.0
white (*Baker's*), 1 oz.	160	2.0	17.0	9.0	5	25	0
white (*Ghirardelli*), 3 pcs., 1½ oz.	240	2.0	25.0	15.0	5	40	0
white (*Nestlé*)	80	1.0	8.0	5.0	<5	15	0
bits, 1 tbsp.:							
milk (*M&M's*)	70	1.0	10.0	3.5	5	10	0
semisweet (*M&M's*)	70	1.0	9.0	3.5	0	0	1.0
chips or morsels:							
milk (*Baker's*)	70	1.0	9.0	4.0	0	0	10
milk (*Ghirardelli*), 2 tbsp.	70	0	10.0	4.0	0	10	0
milk (*Hershey's*) ...	80	1.0	9.0	4.5	<5	10	0

Food and Measure	cal.	prot. (gms)	carbo. (gms)	fat (gms)	chol. (mgs)	sod. (mgs)	fiber (gms)
Chocolate, baking, chips or morsels *(cont.)*							
milk (*Nestlé*)	70	<1.0	9.0	4.0	<5	0	0
mint (*Hershey's*) . . .	80	<1.0	10.0	4.0	0	0	0
mint (*Nestlé*)	70	<1.0	9.0	4.0	0	0	<1.0
peanut butter (*Hershey's*)	80	3.0	7.0	4.0	0	35	0
raspberry (*Hershey's*)	80	<1.0	10.0	4.0	0	0	0
semisweet (*Baker's*)	60	1.0	9.0	3.5	0	10	<1.0
semisweet (*Ghirardelli*), 2 tbsp.	70	0	10.0	4.0	0	0	0
semisweet (*Hershey's*)	80	<1.0	10.0	4.0	0	0	0
semisweet (*Hershey's Lowfat*)	60	<1.0	11.0	3.5	0	0	0
semisweet (*Nestlé/ Nestlé Mini/Mega*)	70	<1.0	9.0	4.0	0	0	<1.0
white (*Ghirardelli*), 2 tbsp.	80	1.0	10.0	4.0	0	15	0
white (*Hershey's*)	80	1.0	9.0	4.0	0	30	0
white (*Nestlé*)	80	<1.0	9.0	4.0	0	20	0
kisses (*Hershey's Mini*), 11 pcs.	80	1.0	9.0	4.5	<5	15	0
pieces, broken (*Ghirardelli*), 1.4 oz.	200	3.0	25.0	12.0	10	30	0
sprinkles, chocolate, milk (*Hershey's Chocolate Shoppe*), 2 tbsp.	140	1.0	21.0	6.0	<5	15	0
Chocolate dip, 2 tbsp.:							
(*Marzetti Fat Free*) . . .	100	1.0	25.0	0	0	150	0
(*Smucker's Fat Free*)	130	2.0	31.0	0	0	75	0
(*T. Marzetti's* Natural Fruit Dip 4 oz.)	140	2.0	22.0	5.0	0	150	1.0
(*T. Marzetti's* Natural Fruit Dip 15 oz.) . . .	120	1.0	21.0	4.0	0	50	0
Chocolate drink:							
(*Yoo-Hoo*), 9 fl. oz.	150	2.0	33.0	1.0	0	200	0

Food and Measure	cal.	prot. (gms)	carbo. (gms)	fat (gms)	chol. (mgs)	sod. (mgs)	fiber (gms)
(*Yoo-Hoo*), ½ of 15.5-fl. oz. can	130	2.0	29.0	1.0	0	180	0
Chocolate drink mix:							
(*Nestlé Quik*), 4 tbsp.	100	1.0	22.0	1.0	0	35	1.0
fudge shake (*Weight Watchers*), ¾ oz.	80	6.0	12.0	1.0	0	140	2.0
Chocolate milk, dairy, 1 cup:							
(*Hershey's Fat Free*)	150	9.0	29.0	0	<5	140	<1.0
(*Hershey's Reduced Fat*)	190	8.0	30.0	4.5	15	140	1.0
(*Hood* 1% Lowfat) ...	170	8.0	30.0	1.5	15	210	<1.0
(*Quik*)	230	7.0	33.0	8.0	30	100	1.0
Chocolate mousse, frozen (*Weight Watchers*), 2.7 oz.	190	6.0	31.0	5.0	5	150	3.0
Chocolate mousse mix, see "Mousse mix"							
Chocolate pastry (see also specific listings), frozen:							
dark (*Pepperidge Farm Clouds*), 2 pcs. ...	580	6.0	53.0	38.0	25	380	4.0
milk (*Pepperidge Farm Clouds*), 2 pcs. ...	580	6.0	54.0	38.0	55	400	3.0
Chocolate shake:							
(*Hershey's*), 7 fl. oz.	230	6.0	41.0	4.5	20	290	1.0
(*Milky Way*), 1 cup ...	220	7.0	44.0	3.0	10	135	2.0
Chocolate syrup, 2 tbsp.:							
(*Fox's U-Bet*)	120	1.0	29.0	0	0	35	0
(*Hershey's*)	100	1.0	24.0	0	0	25	0
dark (*Hershey's Special Dark*)	110	<1.0	27.0	0	0	35	0
malt (*Hershey's*)	100	<1.0	25.0	0	0	55	0
Chocolate topping, 2 tbsp.:							
(*Hershey's Heath* Fat Free)	100	0	24.0	0	0	130	0
(*Kraft*)	110	2.0	26.0	0	0	30	1.0

Food and Measure	cal.	prot. (gms)	carbo. (gms)	fat (gms)	chol. (mgs)	sod. (mgs)	fiber (gms)
Chocolate topping (cont.)							
caramel (*Hershey's* Fat							
Free)	100	<1.0	25.0	0	0	95	0
dark (*Dove*)	140	<1.0	22.0	5.0	0	80	5.0
double (*Hershey's* Fat							
Free)	100	<1.0	24.0	0	0	20	1.0
fudge:							
(*Smucker's*)	130	0	28.0	1.5	0	60	1.0
(*Smucker's* Micro)	130	0	28.0	1.5	0	60	1.0
dark chocolate (*Mrs.							
Richardson's*) ...	140	1.0	20.0	6.0	0	75	1.0
hot (*Kraft*)	140	1.0	24.0	4.0	0	100	<1.0
hot (*Mrs. Richard-							
son's*)	140	1.0	20.0	6.0	0	75	<1.0
hot (*Mrs. Richard-							
son's* Fat Free) ...	110	1.0	25.0	0	0	60	<1.0
hot (*Smucker's*) ...	140	2.0	24.0	4.0	0	60	1.0
hot (*Smucker's*							
Light)	90	2.0	23.0	0	0	95	2.0
hot (*Smucker's*							
Micro)	130	2.0	24.0	2.5	0	50	<1.0
hot (*Smucker's*							
Micro Fat Free)	110	2.0	26.0	0	0	70	<1.0
hot (*Smucker's* Spe-							
cial Recipe)	140	2.0	22.0	4.0	0	70	<1.0
milk (*Dove*)	130	2.0	21.0	4.0	0	75	4.0
mint (*Hershey's* Fat							
Free)	110	<1.0	26.0	0	0	25	0
nut (*Smucker's Magic							
Shell*)	220	1.0	16.0	16.0	0	25	0
Chorizo, see "Sau-							
sage"							
Chow chow pickle:							
(*Crosse & Blackwell*),							
1 tbsp.	10	0	1.0	0	0	105	<1.0
relish, 1/2 cup:							
(*Stubb's* Original)	70	2.0	13.0	1.0	0	610	2.0
spicy (*Stubb's*)	70	2.0	13.0	1.0	0	600	2.0
Chrysanthemum gar-							
land, 1/2 cup:							
raw, 1″ pcs.	2	.2	.5	<.1	0	7	.4

Food and Measure	cal.	prot. (gms)	carbo. (gms)	fat (gms)	chol. (mgs)	sod. (mgs)	fiber (gms)
boiled, drained, 1" pcs.	10	.8	2.2	.1	0	27	1.2
Church's Chicken:							
chicken, 1 pc.:							
breast, 2.8 oz.	200	19.0	4.3	12.4	65	510	0
leg, 2 oz.	140	12.7	2.4	9.1	45	160	0
Tenderstrip, 1.1 oz.	80	6.0	4.5	4.0	15	140	.5
thigh, 2.8 oz.	230	16.2	5.3	16.2	80	520	0
wing, 3.1 oz.	250	18.5	7.7	16.1	60	540	0
sides:							
biscuit, 2.1 oz.	250	2.2	25.6	16.4	<5	640	1.0
cole slaw, 3 oz. . . .	92	4.2	8.4	5.5	0	230	2.0
corn on cob, 5.7 oz.	139	4.4	23.5	3.2	0	15	9.0
french fries, 2.7 oz.	210	3.3	28.5	10.5	0	60	2.0
okra, 2.8 oz.	210	2.7	19.1	16.1	0	520	4.0
potatoes and gravy, 3.7 oz.	90	1.2	14.0	3.3	0	520	1.0
rice, Cajun, 3.1 oz.	130	1.3	15.6	7.0	5	260	<1.0
Churro, cinnamon (*Tio Pepe's*), 1-oz. pc. . .	110	1.0	14.0	5.0	15	100	2.0
Chutney:							
(*Crosse & Blackwell* Major Grey's), 1 tbsp.	60	0	14.0	0	0	170	0
(*Trader Vic's* Calcutta), 2 tbsp.	44	.5	11.0	0	0	270	0
apple curry (*Crosse & Blackwell*), 1 tbsp.	25	0	7.0	0	0	20	0
cranberry (*Crosse & Blackwell*), 1 tbsp.	40	0	10.0	0	0	0	0
mango:							
(*Bombay Brand* Major Grey's), 2 tbsp.	110	0	25.0	0	0	210	0
hot (*Crosse & Blackwell*), 1 tbsp. . . .	60	0	14.0	0	0	170	0
mango-ginger (*Bombay Brand*), 2 tbsp.	90	0	23.0	0	0	25	1.0
tomato, dried (*Sonoma*), 1 tbsp.	35	0	9.0	0	0	0	0

Food and Measure	cal.	prot. (gms)	carbo. (gms)	fat (gms)	chol. (mgs)	sod. (mgs)	fiber (gms)
Cilantro, see "Coriander"							
Cinnamon:							
ground, 1 tsp.	6	.1	2.1	.1	0	1	1.4
Cisco, meat only, raw,							
4 oz.	112	21.5	0	2.2	n.a.	62	0
Citron, candied, diced							
(*Paradise/White*							
Swan), 2 tbsp.	80	0	19.0	0	0	15	1.0
Citrus drink blends,							
8 fl. oz., except as							
noted:							
(*Sunny Delight* Calcium Enriched)	140	0	34.0	0	0	70	0
(*Sunny Delight* California Style)	130	0	33.0	0	0	130	0
(*Sunny Delight* Florida Style)	120	0	30.0	0	0	190	
(*Tropicana*)	140	0	36.0	0	0	15	0
(*Tropicana Twister*), 10 fl. oz.	180	0	45.0	0	0	15	0
(*V8 Splash*)	120	0	29.0	0	0	40	0
(*Whipper Snapple* Power Smoothie), 10 fl. oz.	150	0	39.0	0	0	60	0
Citrus fruit salad, see "Fruit, mixed" and specific listings							
Citrus juice blends, 8 fl. oz.:							
(*R.W. Knudsen* Morning Blend)	120	1.0	31.0	0	0	15	0
(*R.W. Knudsen* Natural Breakfast Juice) . . .	110	1.0	27.0	0	0	35	0
(*R.W. Knudsen* Vita Juice)	120	2.0	29.0	0	0	35	0
punch (*R.W. Knudsen*)	120	1.0	29.0	0	0	30	0
Clam, meat only:							
raw:							
4 oz.	84	14.5	2.9	1.1	39	64	0

Food and Measure	cal.	prot. (gms)	carbo. (gms)	fat (gms)	chol. (mgs)	sod. (mgs)	fiber (gms)
9 large or 20 small, 6.3 oz.	133	23.0	4.6	1.8	60	100	0
boiled, poached or steamed, 4 oz.	168	29.0	5.8	2.2	76	127	0
Clam, canned, ¼ cup or 2 oz., except as noted:							
chopped:							
ocean (*Chincoteague*)	30	6.0	1.0	0	10	290	0
sea, Eastern (*Chincoteague*)	25	6.0	0	0	15	260	0
minced (*Progresso*)	25	4.0	2.0	0	10	250	0
smoked, baby (*Reese*), ⅓ cup	120	9.0	3.0	9.0	30	130	0
Clam, fried, frozen:							
(*Gorton's*), 3 oz.	250	8.0	20.0	15.0	10	310	n.a.
(*Mrs. Paul's*), 4½-oz. pkg.	370	14.0	39.0	18.0	30	840	2.0
(*Van de Kamp's*), 5-oz. pkg.	410	16.0	44.0	20.0	35	930	2.0
crisps (*Acadian Gourmet*), 22 pcs., 3.1 oz.	310	9.0	27.0	18.0	10	1130	2.0
Clam, stuffed, 2 pcs., except as noted:							
(*Matlaw's* Large)	180	8.0	21.0	8.0	0	730	3.0
(*Morning Catch*), 1 pc.	130	6.0	15.0	6.0	0	530	2.0
casino (*Matlaw's*)	60	3.0	7.0	3.0	0	260	1.0
oreganata (*Matlaw's*)	90	3.0	7.0	6.0	0	180	1.0
Clam chowder, see "Soup"							
Clam dip, 2 tbsp.:							
(*Heluva* Good New England)	50	1.0	2.0	4.5	20	130	0
(*Kraft*)	60	1.0	3.0	4.0	0	250	0
(*Kraft* Premium)	45	1.0	2.0	4.0	10	210	0
(*Nalley*)	100	1.0	3.0	10.0	10	260	0
Chesapeake (*Breakstone's*)	50	1.0	2.0	4.0	30	190	0

Food and Measure	cal.	prot. (gms)	carbo. (gms)	fat (gms)	chol. (mgs)	sod. (mgs)	fiber (gms)
Clam juice, 8 fl. oz.:							
ocean (*Chincoteague*)	10	2.0	1.0	0	0	1490	0
sea (*Chincoteague*)	15	1.0	0	0	0	590	0
Clam sauce, canned, ½ cup:							
red (*Progresso*)	60	4.0	8.0	1.0	10	350	1.0
white:							
(*Chincoteague*)	120	4.0	9.0	8.0	10	490	0
(*Contadina*)	130	6.0	4.0	10.0	10	700	0
(*Progresso*)	140	7.0	5.0	10.0	15	510	0
(*Progresso* Authentic)	150	9.0	5.0	10.0	20	710	0
(*Rienzi*)	130	3.0	7.0	10.0	<5	510	1.0
creamy (*Progresso*)	110	5.0	8.0	6.0	10	440	0
Cloves, ground:							
1 tbsp.	21	.4	4.0	1.3	0	16	<1.0
1 tsp.	7	.1	1.3	.4	0	5	.2
Cobbler, frozen:							
apple:							
(*Marie Callender's*), ¼ of 17-oz. pkg.	350	2.0	45.0	18.0	0	170	2.0
(*Mrs. Smith's*), pkg., 4 oz.	240	2.0	39.0	9.0	0	370	3.0
cinnamon (*Pet-Ritz*), ⅙ pkg., 4.3 oz.	280	2.0	40.0	12.0	0	380	0
crumb (*Pet-Ritz*), ⅙ pkg., 4.3 oz.	280	2.0	49.0	9.0	5	270	0
berry (*Marie Callender's*), ¼ of 17-oz. pkg.	390	3.0	41.0	19.0	<5	170	1.0
blackberry:							
(*Mrs. Smith's*), pkg., 4 oz.	250	3.0	39.0	9.0	0	220	4.0
(*Pet-Ritz*), ⅙ pkg., 4.3 oz.	260	2.0	37.0	12.0	0	230	1.0
crumb (*Pet-Ritz*), ⅙ pkg., 4.3 oz.	260	3.0	45.0	8.0	5	170	1.0
blueberry (*Marie Callender's*), ¼ of 17-oz. pkg.	340	3.0	42.0	18.0	0	220	2.0

Food and Measure	cal.	prot. (gms)	carbo. (gms)	fat (gms)	chol. (mgs)	sod. (mgs)	fiber (gms)
cherry:							
(*Marie Callender's*),							
¼ of 17-oz. pkg.	390	3.0	50.0	19.0	<5	100	0
(*Mrs. Smith's*),							
⅛ pkg., 4 oz. . . .	250	3.0	39.0	9.0	0	280	3.0
(*Pet-Ritz*), ⅙ pkg.,							
4.3 oz.	300	2.0	48.0	11.0	0	300	1.0
crumb (*Pet-Ritz*),							
⅙ pkg., 4.3 oz.	280	2.0	54.0	6.0	5	330	0
peach:							
(*Marie Callender's*),							
¼ of 17-oz. pkg.	370	3.0	47.0	18.0	0	170	0
(*Mrs. Smith's*),							
⅛ pkg., 4 oz. . . .	240	3.0	38.0	9.0	0	250	3.0
(*Pet-Ritz*), ⅙ pkg.,							
4.3 oz.	240	1.0	37.0	10.0	0	220	1.0
crumb (*Pet-Ritz*),							
⅙ pkg., 4.3 oz.	230	2.0	38.0	7.0	5	170	1.0
strawberry (*Pet-Ritz*),							
⅙ pkg., 4.3 oz.	260	2.0	40.0	10.0	0	330	1.0
Cocktail sauce, see							
"Seafood sauce"							
Cocoa, baking:							
(*Ghirardelli*), 1 tbsp.	35	2.0	5.0	3.0	0	0	3.0
(*Hershey's*), 1 tbsp.	20	1.0	3.0	.5	0	0	1.0
(*Nestlé*), 1 tbsp.	15	1.0	3.0	.5	0	0	1.0
(*Watkins*), 1 tsp.	20	1.0	3.0	.5	0	0	1.0
European style (*Hershey's*), 1 tbsp. . . .	20	1.0	3.0	.5	0	0	1.0
sweetened							
(*Ghirardelli*),							
2½ tbsp.	80	1.0	19.0	1.5	0	30	0
Cocoa mix, hot, 1 pkt.,							
except as noted:							
(*Swiss Miss* Cocoa							
and Cream)	150	2.0	25.0	5.0	5	160	<1.0
(*Swiss Miss* Diet)	20	2.0	4.0	0	0	145	<1.0
(*Swiss Miss* Fat Free)	50	4.0	9.0	0	0	185	1.0
(*Swiss Miss* Lite)	80	2.0	17.0	<1.0	0	180	2.0
(*Swiss Miss* No Sugar)	50	0	10.0	1.0	0	165	1.0
(*Weight Watchers*) . . .	70	6.0	10.0	0	0	160	1.0

Food and Measure	cal.	prot. (gms)	carbo. (gms)	fat (gms)	chol. (mgs)	sod. (mgs)	fiber (gms)
Cocoa mix (cont.)							
chocolate:							
(*Swiss Miss* Rich)	110	2.0	23.0	2.0	<5	150	1.0
(*Swiss Miss Sensa-*							
tion)	150	2.0	27.0	4.0	0	170	1.5
almond (*Hershey's*)	150	3.0	27.0	3.0	0	150	1.0
amaretto (*Her-*							
shey's)	150	3.0	27.0	3.0	0	135	1.0
creme, French (*Car-*							
nation)	90	2.0	17.0	1.0	0	85	<1.0
double (*Ghirardelli*)	90	1.0	21.0	1.5	0	35	1.0
Dutch (*Hershey's*)	160	1.0	27.0	5.0	0	180	1.0
hazelnut							
(*Ghirardelli*)	90	1.0	21.0	1.5	0	35	1.0
milk (*Swiss Miss*)	115	1.5	22.0	2.5	<5	115	1.5
milk, w/mini marsh-							
mallows (*Swiss*							
Miss)	115	1.0	22.0	2.0	0	140	1.5
mint (*Hershey's*) ...	150	3.0	27.0	3.0	0	140	1.0
mocha (*Ghirardelli*)	90	1.0	21.0	2.0	0	35	1.0
raspberry (*Her-*							
shey's)	150	3.0	27.0	3.0	0	135	1.0
toffee, English							
(*Swiss Miss*)	140	2.0	28.0	2.5	<5	225	3.0
white (*Swiss Miss*)	110	3.0	21.0	1.5	0	130	0
Irish creme:							
(*Hershey's*)	150	3.0	27.0	3.0	0	140	1.0
(*Watkins*), 1 oz.,							
3 tbsp.	110	2.0	25.0	1.5	0	170	0
w/marshmallows:							
(*Swiss Miss* Marsh-							
mallow Lovers)	140	2.0	27.0	3.0	<5	150	1.0
(*Swiss Miss* Marsh-							
mallow Lovers Fat							
Free)	65	3.0	12.5	0	0	155	n.a.
(*Swiss Miss* No							
Sugar)	55	2.5	10.0	1.0	0	145	1.0
Swiss mocha (*Her-*							
shey's)	140	2.0	29.0	2.0	0	110	<1.0
vanilla, French:							
(*Hershey's*)	140	2.0	28.0	2.5	0	150	0

Food and Measure	cal.	prot. (gms)	carbo. (gms)	fat (gms)	chol. (mgs)	sod. (mgs)	fiber (gms)
(*Swiss Miss*)	110	2.0	21.0	1.0	0	150	1.0
(*Swiss Miss* Fat Free)	50	4.0	8.0	0	0	140	1.0
(*Watkins*), 1 oz., 3 tbsp.	110	1.0	23.0	1.5	0	120	1.0
Cocoa-coffee mix							
(*Trader Vic's* Kafe-La-Te), 2 rounded tsp., ½ oz.	50	0	13.0	0	0	30	0
Coconut:							
fresh, shelled:							
1 oz.	100	.9	4.3	9.5	0	6	2.6
shredded or grated, 1 cup not packed	283	2.7	12.2	26.8	0	16	7.2
canned, flake, sweetened, ⅓ cup	114	.9	10.5	8.1	0	5	1.2
dried, toasted, 1 oz.	168	1.5	12.6	13.4	0	11	n.a.
package, flake, 2 tbsp., except as noted:							
(*Baker's* Premium Shred)	60	1.0	6.0	4.0	0	35	1.0
(*Baker's* Angel Flake Bag)	70	1.0	7.0	4.5	0	45	1.0
(*Baker's* Angel Flake Can)	70	1.0	7.0	5.0	0	0	1.0
(*Mounds*)	70	<1.0	8.0	4.5	0	45	1.0
sweetened, ⅓ cup	117	.8	11.8	7.9	0	63	1.1
Coconut cream, canned:							
(*Goya* Coco Cream of Coconut), 2 tbsp.	140	0	22.0	5.0	0	15	0
1 tbsp.	36	.5	1.6	3.4	0	10	.4
Coconut milk, canned:							
(*Goya*), 1 tbsp.	50	1.0	1.0	5.0	0	5	0
(*Taste of Thai*), ⅓ cup	140	1.0	3.0	15.0	0	20	0
(*Taste of Thai* Lite), ⅓ cup	45	1.0	3.0	4.0	0	20	0
(*Thai Kitchen*), 2 oz.	90	1.0	1.0	9.0	0	10	0
(*Thai Kitchen* Lite), 2 oz.	53	.5	1.0	5.0	0	6	0

Food and Measure	cal.	prot. (gms)	carbo. (gms)	fat (gms)	chol. (mgs)	sod. (mgs)	fiber (gms)
Coconut milk, canned *(cont.)*							
(*Tropical Pepper Co.*),							
¼ cup	90	<1.0	1.0	9.0	0	10	0
(*Tropical Pepper Co.*							
Lite), ¼ cup	53	<1.0	1.0	5.0	0	10	0
Coconut nectar (*R.W.*							
Knudsen), 8 fl. oz.	140	1.0	26.0	5.0	0	55	0
Cod, meat only:							
Atlantic:							
raw, 4 oz.	93	20.2	0	.8	49	62	0
baked, broiled, or							
microwaved,							
4 oz.	119	25.9	0	1.0	62	88	0
Pacific:							
raw, 4 oz.	93	20.3	0	.7	42	81	0
baked, broiled, or							
microwaved,							
4 oz.	119	26.0	0	.9	53	103	0
Cod, canned, Atlantic,							
w/liquid, 4 oz.	119	25.8	0	1.0	62	247	0
Cod, dried, Atlantic,							
salted, 1 oz.	81	17.6	0	.7	42	1968	0
Cod, frozen, fillets							
(*Frionor*), 4 oz.	90	20.0	0	1.0	50	60	0
Cod entree, frozen:							
au gratin (*Oven Pop-*							
pers), 5-oz. pc.	220	24.0	5.0	11.0	75	450	1.0
fillets, 1 pc.:							
(*Frionor Bunch O*							
Crunch)	270	13.0	23.0	15.0	35	560	0
(*Mrs. Paul's*)	250	14.0	24.0	11.0	40	510	2.0
(*Van de Kamp's*) . . .	220	14.0	19.0	10.0	35	410	0
stuffed w/broccoli,							
cheese (*Oven Pop-*							
pers), 5-oz. pc. . . .	150	20.0	4.0	6.0	55	330	1.0
Cod liver oil, see "Oil"							
Coffee:							
brewed, 6 fl. oz.	4	.1	.8	0	0	4	0
instant, regular,							
1 rounded tsp.* . . .	4	.2	.7	tr.	0	1	0

Food and Measure	cal.	prot. (gms)	carbo. (gms)	fat (gms)	chol. (mgs)	sod. (mgs)	fiber (gms)
Coffee, flavored, see "Cappuccino"							
Coffee, flavored, mix, 8 fl. oz.*, except as noted:							
all varieties (*Taster's Choice*), 1 tsp.	5	0	1.0	0	0	0	0
Belgian hazelnut (*General Foods International*)	70	<1.0	12.0	2.0	0	65	0
cafe Amaretto (*General Foods International*)	60	<1.0	8.0	3.0	0	105	0
cafe Français (*General Foods International*)	60	<1.0	7.0	3.5	0	25	0
cafe Vienna:							
(*General Foods International*)	70	<1.0	11.0	2.5	0	110	0
(*General Foods International* Low Cal)	30	<1.0	3.0	1.5	0	75	0
cappuccino:							
cinnamon (*Maxwell House*)	90	2.0	16.0	1.5	0	70	0
coffee (*Maxwell House*)	90	1.0	18.0	1.0	0	65	0
Italian (*General Foods International*)	50	<1.0	10.0	1.5	0	50	0
mocha/mocha decaf (*Maxwell House*)	100	2.0	17.0	2.5	0	70	0
orange (*General Foods International*)	70	<1.0	11.0	2.0	0	100	0
orange (*General Foods International* Low Cal)	30	<1.0	3.0	1.5	0	75	0
vanilla/vanilla decaf (*Maxwell House*)	90	1.0	19.0	1.0	0	65	0
French vanilla:							
(*General Foods International*)	60	<1.0	10.0	2.5	0	55	0

Food and Measure	cal.	prot. (gms)	carbo. (gms)	fat (gms)	chol. (mgs)	sod. (mgs)	fiber (gms)
Coffee, flavored, mix, French vanilla *(cont.)*							
(*General Foods International* Low Cal)	35	<1.0	4.0	2.0	0	55	0
Kahlúa Cafe (*General Foods International*)	60	<1.0	10.0	2.0	0	55	0
Suisse mocha:							
(*General Foods International*)	60	<1.0	8.0	2.5	0	50	0
(*General Foods International* Low Cal)	30	<1.0	4.0	2.0	0	30	0
decaf (*General Foods International*)	60	<1.0	8.0	3.0	0	40	0
decaf (*General Foods International* Low Cal)	30	<1.0	4.0	1.5	0	35	0
Viennese chocolate (*General Foods International*)	60	<1.0	10.0	2.0	0	30	0
Coffee, iced, see "Cappuccino"							
Coffee creamer, see "Creamer, nondairy"							
Coffee substitute, cereal grain, 1 tsp., except as noted:							
(*Natural Touch Kaffree Roma*)	10	0	2.0	0	0	0	0
(*Natural Touch Roma Cappuccino*), 3 tbsp.	50	1.0	5.0	3.0	0	15	0
(*Postum*)	10	0	3.0	0	0	0	0
powder	9	.1	1.9	.1	0	2	0
Cold cuts, see "Lunch meat" and specific listings							
Cole slaw dressing, see "Salad dressing"							

Food and Measure	cal.	prot. (gms)	carbo. (gms)	fat (gms)	chol. (mgs)	sod. (mgs)	fiber (gms)
Collard greens, fresh:							
raw, 1 oz.	9	.4	2.0	.1	0	6	1.0
raw, chopped, ½ cup	6	.3	1.3	<.1	0	4	.7
boiled, drained,							
chopped, ½ cup . . .	17	.9	3.9	.1	0	10	1.3
Collard greens,							
canned, ½ cup:							
(*Allens/Sunshine*)	30	1.0	5.0	.5	0	20	3.0
(*Stubb's*)	30	1.0	5.0	.5	0	20	3.0
chopped (*Bush's Best*)	30	2.0	4.0	0	0	410	2.0
seasoned (*Sylvia's*)	45	1.0	8.0	1.0	0	475	3.0
Collard greens, fro-							
zen, chopped:							
(*Birds Eye Southern*),							
1 cup	30	2.0	2.0	0	0	20	2.0
(*McKenzie's*), 1 cup	30	2.0	2.0	0	0	20	2.0
boiled, drained, ½ cup	31	2.5	6.1	.4	0	42	n.a.
Cookie (see also							
"Cake, snack" and							
specific listings):							
almond:							
(*Anna'a*), 7 pcs.,							
1 oz.	141	2.0	19.0	7.0	0	360	1.0
(*Frieda's*), 2 pcs.,							
1 oz.	170	2.0	19.0	10.0	0	75	0
(*Stella D'oro Break-*							
fast Treats), .8-oz.							
pc.	100	1.0	16.0	3.0	10	80	<1.0
(*Stella D'oro* Chi-							
nese Dessert),							
1.2-oz. pc.	170	2.0	21.0	2.0	5	90	<1.0
butter (*Jules*							
Destrooper),							
11 pcs., 1.1 oz.	127	2.0	24.0	3.0	6	182	0
crescents (*Arch-*							
way), 2 pcs.,							
.8 oz.	100	1.0	17.0	3.5	5	75	1.0
toast (*Stella D'oro*							
Mandel), 2 pcs.,							
1 oz.	110	2.0	21.0	2.5	30	85	1.0

Food and Measure	cal.	prot. (gms)	carbo. (gms)	fat (gms)	chol. (mgs)	sod. (mgs)	fiber (gms)
Cookie *(cont.)*							
animal:							
(*Sunshine All American*), 14 pcs., 1.1 oz.	140	2.0	24.0	4.0	0	125	<1.0
chocolate chip (*Barbara's Snackimals*), 8 pcs., 1.1 oz.	120	2.0	18.0	5.0	0	85	1.0
chocolate chip (*Keebler*), 7 pcs., 1 oz.	130	2.0	22.0	4.5	0	120	0
iced (*Keebler*), 6 pcs., 1.1 oz.	150	2.0	24.0	5.0	0	110	0
oatmeal (*Barbara's Snackimals* Wheat Free), 8 pcs., 1.1 oz.	120	2.0	19.0	5.0	0	75	2.0
sprinkled (*Keebler*), 6 pcs., 1.1 oz.	150	2.0	24.0	4.5	0	105	0
vanilla (*Barbara's*), 8 pcs., 1 oz.	130	2.0	20.0	5.0	0	105	1.0
vanilla (*Barbara's Snackimals*), 8 pcs., 1.1 oz. ...	120	2.0	19.0	4.5	0	55	1.0
anisette:							
(*Stella D'oro* Jumbo Toast), 1.1-oz. pc.	100	2.0	23.0	.5	15	65	<1.0
(*Stella D'oro* Sponge), 2 pcs., 1 oz.	90	2.0	19.0	1.0	40	80	<1.0
(*Stella D'oro* Toast), 3 pcs., 1.2 oz. ...	130	2.0	27.0	1.0	35	150	<1.0
apple cinnamon:							
(*Newton Cobblers*), ³/₄-oz. pc.	70	1.0	17.0	0	0	40	<1.0
filled (*Barbara's* Fat Free Whole Wheat), ²/₃-oz. pc.	60	1.0	14.0	0	0	20	2.0
apple-filled (*Fig Newton* Fat Free), 2 pcs., 1 oz.	90	1.0	21.0	0	0	60	<1.0

Food and Measure	cal.	prot. (gms)	carbo. (gms)	fat (gms)	chol. (mgs)	sod. (mgs)	fiber (gms)
apple raisin:							
(*Archway* Gourmet),							
.9-oz. pc.	110	1.0	17.0	4.0	5	120	<1.0
(*Health Valley*							
Jumbo), 1 pc. ...	80	2.0	19.0	0	0	35	3.0
bar (*Weight Watch-*							
ers), ¾ oz.	70	1.0	14.0	2.0	0	60	2.0
apple spice (*Health*							
Valley), 3 pcs.	100	2.0	24.0	0	0	50	3.0
apricot:							
(*Health Valley* De-							
light), 3 pcs.	100	2.0	24.0	0	0	50	3.0
filled (*Archway*),							
.9-oz. pc.	100	1.0	16.0	3.5	5	80	0
apricot raspberry cup							
(*Pepperidge Farm*							
Fruitful), 3 pcs.,							
1.1 oz.	140	2.0	22.0	6.0	5	110	<1.0
arrowroot, see							
"Cracker"							
(*Bahlsen* Afrika),							
8 pcs., 1.1 oz.	170	2.0	17.0	10.0	5	20	2.0
(*Bahlsen* Nuss Des-							
sert), 3 pcs., 1.1 oz.	180	2.0	17.0	11.0	10	60	0
biscotti:							
all varieties (*Health*							
Valley), 2 pcs. ...	120	3.0	23.0	3.0	0	50	3.0
almond (*Pepperidge*							
Farm Caruso),							
.7-oz. pc.	90	2.0	12.0	3.5	5	65	<1.0
almond (*Perugina*),							
1 pc.	120	2.0	17.0	5.0	25	45	1.0
anise (*Pepperidge*							
Farm La Scala),							
.7-oz. pc.	90	2.0	14.0	3.0	5	75	0
chocolate chunk							
(*Stella D'oro*),							
.8-oz. pc.	90	2.0	16.0	2.5	10	60	0
chocolate dipped							
(*Pepperidge Farm*							
Figaro), .8-oz. pc.	110	2.0	14.0	4.0	10	70	1.0

Food and Measure	cal.	prot. (gms)	carbo. (gms)	fat (gms)	chol. (mgs)	sod. (mgs)	fiber (gms)
Cookie, biscotti *(cont.)*							
cranberry pistachio (*Pepperidge Farm Tosca*), .7-oz. pc.	90	2.0	13.0	3.0	5	65	<1.0
French vanilla (*Stella D'oro*), .8-oz. pc.	90	2.0	16.0	2.5	10	65	0
hazelnut (*Stella D'oro*), .8-oz. pc.	100	2.0	15.0	3.5	10	60	0
biscottini cashews (*Stella D'oro*), .7-oz. pc.	110	1.0	13.0	6.0	5	50	<1.0
blueberry-filled:							
(*Archway*), .8-oz. pc.	100	1.0	16.0	3.5	<5	85	0
(*Barbara's*), .7-oz. pc.	60	1.0	14.0	1.0	0	25	1.0
butter (see also "shortbread," below):							
(*Bahlsen* Leaves), 7 pcs., 1 oz.	140	2.0	19.0	7.0	15	50	<1.0
(*Bahlsen* Leibniz), 6 pcs., 1.1 oz. . . .	130	2.0	23.0	3.5	10	125	1.0
(*Keebler*), 5 pcs., 1.1 oz.	150	2.0	22.0	6.0	0	170	<1.0
(*Keebler Cookie Stix*), 4 pcs., 1 oz.	130	2.0	19.0	5.0	10	130	<1.0
(*Peek Freans* Petit Beurre), 6 pcs., 1.4 oz.	180	2.5	31.0	5.0	<5	165	1.0
(*Pepperidge Farm* Chessman), 3 pcs., .9 oz.	120	2.0	18.0	3.0	20	80	<1.0
(*Pepperidge Farm* Médaillon au Beurre), 4 pcs., 1.2 oz.	150	2.0	25.0	5.0	15	105	<1.0
(*Sunshine All American*), 5 pcs., 1.1 oz.	140	2.0	21.0	6.0	<5	135	<1.0

Food and Measure	cal.	prot. (gms)	carbo. (gms)	fat (gms)	chol. (mgs)	sod. (mgs)	fiber (gms)
chocolate topped (*Carr's*), 2 pcs., 1 oz.	150	2.0	19.0	7.0	0	40	2.0
sandwich, w/fudge (*E. L. Fudge*), 2 pcs., .9 oz.	120	1.0	17.0	6.0	<5	70	<1.0
waffles (*Jules Destrooper* Paris), 3 pcs., 1.3 oz.	190	3.0	25.0	9.0	55	140	0
butternut (*Archway* Gourmet), .9-oz. pc.	120	1.0	16.0	6.0	<5	115	0
caramel (*SnackWell's* Delights), .6-oz. pc.	70	1.0	13.0	2.0	0	50	0
caramel apple (*Barbara's Mini*), 6 pcs., 1.1 oz.	110	2.0	24.0	0	0	125	1.0
caramel pecan (*Pepperidge Farm*), .9-oz. pc.	130	2.0	16.0	7.0	20	55	<1.0
carrot cake (*Archway*), 1-oz. pc.	120	1.0	18.0	5.0	<5	180	<1.0
cashew nougat (*Archway*), 3 pcs., 1.1 oz.	170	2.0	16.0	11.0	0	95	0
cherry cobbler (*Pepperidge Farm*), .6-oz. pc.	70	<1.0	11.0	2.5	<5	45	0
cherry-filled (*Archway*), .8-oz. pc. . . .	100	1.0	16.0	3.5	5	80	0
chocolate:							
(*Bahlsen* Leibniz), 4 pcs., 1 oz.	140	2.0	18.0	7.0	5	60	1.0
(*Goldfish*), 19 pcs., 1.1 oz.	140	2.0	22.0	5.0	10	85	2.0
(*Stella D'oro* Breakfast Treat), .8-oz. pc.	100	2.0	15.0	3.5	10	70	<1.0
(*Stella D'oro* Castelets), 2 pcs., 1 oz.	130	2.0	19.0	6.0	<5	65	<1.0

Food and Measure	cal.	prot. (gms)	carbo. (gms)	fat (gms)	chol. (mgs)	sod. (mgs)	fiber (gms)
Cookie, chocolate *(cont.)*							
brownie nut (*Pepperidge Farm*), 3 pcs., 1.1 oz. . . .	160	2.0	18.0	9.0	15	115	2.0
dark (*Bahlsen* Star), 3 pcs., 1.1 oz. . . .	170	2.0	16.0	12.0	0	10	1.0
dark (*Peek Freans* Digestive), 3 pcs., 1.4 oz.	205	2.0	27.0	10.0	0	125	1.0
dark (*Pepperidge Farm* Espirits Noir), .6-oz. pc.	90	1.0	10	5.0	10	50	0
double (*Barbara's* Mini), 6 pcs., 1.1 oz.	100	2.0	23.0	0	0	135	1.0
double Dutch (*Barbara's* Crisp), .6-oz. pc.	80	1.0	10.0	4.0	5	60	1.0
milk (*Bahlsen* Star), 3 pcs., 1.1 oz. . . .	180	2.0	16.0	12.0	5	25	1.0
orange (*Pepperidge Farm* a l'Orange), 2 pcs., 1.1 oz. . . .	150	2.0	23.0	6.0	<5	20	0
topped, w/nuts (*Pepperidge Farm* Geneva), 3 pcs., 1.1 oz.	160	2.0	19.0	9.0	0	95	1.0
wafer (*Keebler* Reduced Fat), 8 pcs., 1.1 oz.	130	1.0	25.0	3.5	0	170	0
wafer (*Nabisco* Famous), 5 pcs., 1.2 oz.	140	2.0	24.0	4.0	<5	230	1.0
white, w/macadamias (*Entenmann's*), .7-oz. pc.	100	1.0	12.0	6.0	10	65	<1.0
chocolate chip/chunk: (*Archway*), 1-oz. pc.	130	1.0	19.0	6.0	5	150	0

Food and Measure	cal.	prot. (gms)	carbo. (gms)	fat (gms)	chol. (mgs)	sod. (mgs)	fiber (gms)
(*Archway* Drop), .8-oz. pc.	100	1.0	15.0	3.5	15	75	0
(*Archway* Gourmet Supreme), .9-oz. pc.	120	1.0	17.0	5.0	<5	120	0
(*Archway* Ice Box), .8-oz. pc.	120	1.0	15.0	6.0	10	60	0
Archway 2 Big), .9-oz. pc.	120	1.0	17.0	5.0	<5	105	0
(*Barbara's* Crisp), .6-oz. pc.	80	1.0	10.0	4.0	5	60	1.0
(*Chip-A-Roos*), 5 pcs., 1.1 oz. ...	160	1.0	21.0	8.0	0	140	<1.0
(*Chips Ahoy!*), 3 pcs., 1.1 oz. ...	160	2.0	21.0	8.0	0	105	1.0
(*Chips Ahoy!* Chewy), 3 pcs., 1.3 oz.	170	2.0	23.0	8.0	0	125	<1.0
(*Chips Ahoy!* Chunky), .6-oz. pc.	80	1.0	10.0	4.0	5	35	0
(*Chips Ahoy!* Munch Size), 6 pcs., 1.1 oz.	160	2.0	21.0	8.0	0	150	1.0
(*Entenmann's*), .7-oz. pc.	100	1.0	13.0	5.0	10	60	<1.0
(*Entenmann's* Chocolatey), .7-oz. pc.	199	1.0	13.0	5.0	10	60	<1.0
(*Entenmann's* Original), 3 pcs., 1.1 oz.	150	1.0	20.0	7.0	10	90	<1.0
(*Entenmann's* Light), 2 pcs., 1.1 oz	120	1.0	21.0	3.5	0	80	<1.0
(*Goldfish*), 19 pcs., 1.1 oz.	150	2.0	21.0	7.0	20	50	1.0
(*Grandma's* Big), 1.4-oz. pc.	190	2.0	25.0	9.0	0	135	1.0
Grandma's Rich N'Chewy), 1 pkg.	270	2.0	39.0	12.0	10	130	1.0

Food and Measure	cal.	prot. (gms)	carbo. (gms)	fat (gms)	chol. (mgs)	sod. (mgs)	fiber (gms)
Cookie, chocolate chip/chunk *(cont.)*							
(*Keebler Chips Deluxe*), 1/2-oz. pc.	80	1.0	9.0	4.5	0	60	0
(*Keebler Chips Deluxe* Chocolate Lovers'), .6-oz. pc.	90	1.0	11.0	5.0	5	80	0
(*Keebler Chips Deluxe* Reduced Fat), .6-oz. pc.	70	<1.0	11.0	3.0	0	70	0
(*Keebler Cookie Stix*), 4 pcs., 1 oz.	130	2.0	19.0	5.0	5	100	<1
(*Keebler Soft Batch* Homestyle), .9-oz. pc.	130	1.0	17.0	7.0	0	80	1.0
(*Pepperidge Farm* Old Fashioned), 3 pcs., 1 oz.	140	2.0	18.0	7.0	10	65	<1.0
(*Pepperidge Farm Chesapeake*), .9-oz. pc.	140	2.0	15.0	8.0	10	100	<1.0
(*Pepperidge Farm Nantucket*), .9-oz. pc.	130	1.0	16.0	7.0	10	75	<1.0
(*SnackWell's* Bite Size), 13 pcs., 1 oz.	130	2.0	22.0	4.0	0	160	<1.0
(*Weight Watchers*), 1.1 oz.	140	2.0	22.0	5.0	0	90	1.0
all varieties (*Health Valley Healthy Chips*), 3 pcs. . . .	100	3.0	24.0	0	0	40	4.0
chocolate, walnut, soft (*Pepperidge Farm*), .9-oz. pc.	130	2.0	16.0	6.0	5	45	1.0
coconut (*Keebler Chip Deluxe*), 1/2-oz. pc.	80	1.0	10.0	5.0	0	50	<1.0

Food and Measure	cal.	prot. (gms)	carbo. (gms)	fat (gms)	chol. (mgs)	sod. (mgs)	fiber (gms)
double (*Entenmann's*), .7-oz. pc.	100	1.0	14.0	5.0	10	65	<1.0
double (*Keebler Soft Batch*), .9-oz. pc.	130	1.0	17.0	7.0	0	90	1.0
double (*SnackWell's*), 13 pcs., 1.1 oz.	130	2.0	22.0	4.0	0	190	1.0
w/fudge (*Grandma's Big*), 1.4-oz. pc.	170	1.0	26.0	7.0	<5	160	1.0
w/macadamias (*Pepperidge Farm Sausalito*), .9-oz. pc.	140	2.0	16.0	7.0	10	110	<1.0
w/macadamias, soft (*Pepperidge Farm*), .9-oz. pc.	130	1.0	16.0	6.0	10	55	1.0
milk (*Pepperidge Farm Montauk*), .9-oz. pc.	130	1.0	17.0	7.0	10	90	0
w/peanut butter cups (*Keebler Chips Deluxe*), .6-oz. pc.	80	1.0	9.0	4.5	0	45	0
rainbow (*Keebler Chips Deluxe*), 1/2-oz. pc.	80	1.0	10.0	4.0	0	45	1
soft (*Keebler Soft Batch*), .6-oz. pc.	80	<1.0	10.0	3.5	0	70	<1.0
soft (*Pepperidge Farm* Chunk), .9-oz. pc.	130	1.0	16.0	6.0	10	35	2.0
soft, chewy (*Keebler Chips Deluxe*), .6-oz. pc.	80	1.0	11.0	3.5	5	60	0
w/toffee (*Archway Gourmet*), 1-oz. pc.	130	1.0	18.0	6.0	5	125	<1.0
w/toffee (*Pepperidge Farm Charleston*), .9-oz. pc.	60	1.0	16.0	7.0	20	110	<1.0

Food and Measure	cal.	prot. (gms)	carbo. (gms)	fat (gms)	chol. (mgs)	sod. (mgs)	fiber (gms)
Cookie, chocolate chip/chunk *(cont.)*							
w/walnuts (*Pepperidge Farm Beacon Hill*), .9-oz. pc.	130	2.0	16.0	7.0	5	100	<1.0
white, w/macadamias (*Pepperidge Farm Tahoe*), .9-oz. pc.	130	2.0	16.0	7.0	15	110	<1.0
chocolate fudge:							
(*Grandma's* Cookie Bits), 9 pcs.	150	2.0	21.0	7.0	0	125	<1.0
(*Keebler Classic Collection*), .6-oz. pc.	80	1.0	12.0	3.5	0	75	0
(*Stella D'oro* Swiss), 2 pcs., .9 oz.	130	1.0	17.0	6.0	15	65	<1.0
(*Stella D'oro* Swiss Super), 2 pcs., 1 oz.	130	1.0	16.0	7.0	15	65	0
center (*Health Valley*), 2 pcs.	70	2.0	17.0	0	0	25	3.0
mint (*Fudge Shoppe* Grasshoppers), 4 pcs., 1.1 oz.	150	1.0	20.0	7.0	0	70	<1.0
nutty (*Grandma's* Big), 1.4-oz. pc.	180	3.0	25.0	8.0	<5	150	1.0
S'mores (*Fudge Shoppe*), 3 pcs., 1.2 oz.	160	1.0	22.0	8.0	0	95	<1.0
sticks (*Fudge Shoppe*), 3 pcs., 1 oz.	150	1.0	20.0	8.0	0	55	<1.0
striped (*Fudge Favorites*), 3 pcs., 1.1 oz.	160	2.0	21.0	8.0	0	150	<1.0
striped (*Fudge Shoppe*), 3 pcs., 1.1 oz.	160	1.0	20.0	8.0	0	140	<1.0
chocolate sandwich:							
(*Hydrox*), 3 pcs., 1.1 oz.	150	2.0	21.0	7.0	0	125	1.0

Food and Measure	cal.	prot. (gms)	carbo. (gms)	fat (gms)	chol. (mgs)	sod. (mgs)	fiber (gms)
(*Oreo*), 3 pcs., 1.2 oz.	160	1.0	23.0	7.0	0	220	1.0
(*Oreo Double Stuf*), 2 pcs., 1 oz.	140	1.0	19.0	7.0	0	150	<1.0
(*Pepperidge Farm Bordeaux*), 4 pcs., 1 oz.	130	2.0	20.0	5.0	10	95	<1.0
(*Pepperidge Farm Brussels*), 3 pcs., 1.1 oz.	150	2.0	20.0	7.0	5	65	1.0
(*Pepperidge Farm Lido*), .6-oz. pc.	90	<1.0	11.0	4.5	5	45	0
(*Pepperidge Farm Milano*), 3 pcs., 1.2 oz.	180	2.0	21.0	10.0	10	80	<1.0
(*SnackWell's*), 2 pcs., .9 oz.	110	1.0	20.0	3.0	0	210	<1.0
(*Weight Watchers*), 1.1 oz.	140	2.0	23.0	3.5	0	160	1.0
chocolate (*Pepperidge Farm Milano*), 3 pcs., 1.2 oz.	180	2.0	21.0	10.0	<5	85	1.0
dark, w/vanilla (*E. L. Fudge*), 2 pcs., .9 oz.	120	1.0	17.0	6.0	0	90	<1.0
double chocolate (*Pepperidge Farm Milano*), 2 pcs., 1 oz.	150	2.0	17.0	8.0	10	70	<1.0
fudge (*E. L. Fudge*), 2 pcs., .9 oz.	120	2.0	17.0	6.0	0	70	<1.0
fudge (*Grandma's*), 1 pkg.	240	3.0	41.0	7.0	0	270	1.0
hazelnut (*Pepperidge Farm Milano*), 2 pcs., .9 oz.	130	2.0	15.0	7.0	5	65	1.0
milk (*Pepperidge Farm Bordeaux*), 3 pcs., 1.1 oz.	160	2.0	19.0	9.0	0	95	0

Food and Measure	cal.	prot. (gms)	carbo. (gms)	fat (gms)	chol. (mgs)	sod. (mgs)	fiber (gms)
Cookie, chocolate sandwich *(cont.)*							
milk (*Pepperidge Farm Milano*), 3 pcs., 1.3 oz. ...	180	2.0	21.0	10.0	10	80	<1.0
mint (*Pepperidge Farm Brussels*), 3 pcs., 1.3 oz. ...	190	2.0	22.0	10.0	0	100	1.0
mint (*Pepperidge Farm Milano*), 2 pcs., .9 oz.	140	1.0	16.0	8.0	<5	70	<1.0
orange (*Pepperidge Farm Milano*), 2 pcs., .9 oz.	140	1.0	16.0	8.0	5	70	<1.0
white fudge covered (*Oreo*), ¾-oz. pc.	110	1.0	13.0	6.0	0	70	0
cinnamon:							
apple (*Archway*), .9-oz. pc.	110	1.0	17.0	3.5	0	130	0
honey (*Archway* Fat Free Hearts), 3 pcs., 1.1 oz. ...	110	1.0	25.0	0	0	125	0
raisin (*Stella D'oro*), 1-oz. pc.	110	1.0	19.0	3.5	20	55	1.0
cocoa:							
Dutch (*Archway*), .8-oz. pc.	100	1.0	16.0	3.0	<5	85	<1.0
mocha (*Barbara's* Mini), 6 pcs., 1.1 oz.	100	2.0	23.0	0	0	125	1.0
coconut:							
almond (*Barbara's Nature's Choice* Dipped), 1.1-oz. bar	120	2.0	20.0	4.5	0	10	1.0
chocolate coated (*Larzaroni*), 5 pcs., 1.1 oz. ...	158	3.0	17.0	9.0	17	36	.8
cream sandwich (*Piccadeli*), 3 pcs., 1 oz.	140	2.0	21.0	6.0	0	75	<1.0

Food and Measure	cal.	prot. (gms)	carbo. (gms)	fat (gms)	chol. (mgs)	sod. (mgs)	fiber (gms)
macaroon (*Archway*), .8-oz. pc.	100	<1.0	12.0	6.0	0	40	<1.0
cranberry:							
(*Fig Newton* Fat Free), 2 pcs., 1 oz.	100	1.0	22.0	0	0	95	<1.0
(*Golden Fruit* Biscuits), .7-oz. pc.	80	1.0	14.0	2.0	0	55	<1.0
creme sandwich (*SnackWell's*), 2 pcs., .9 oz.	110	1.0	20.0	3.0	0	130	0
currant, black (*Peek Freans* Fruit Creme), 3 pcs., 1.4 oz.	190	2.0	28.0	7.0	0	0	<1.0
Danish (*Keebler* Wedding), 4 pcs., 1 oz.	120	1.0	20.0	5.0	0	120	<1.0
date (*Health Valley* Delight), 3 pcs.	100	2.0	24.0	0	0	50	3.0
devil's food:							
(*Archway* Fat Free), .7-oz. pc.	70	<1.0	16.0	0	0	80	<1.0
(*SnackWell's* Fat Free), .6-oz. pc.	50	1.0	13.0	0	0	25	0
(*SnackWell's* Golden), .6-oz. pc.	50	1.0	11.0	.5	0	25	0
egg biscuit (see also "kichel," below):							
(*Stella D'oro* Jumbo), 2 pcs., .8 oz.	90	2.0	18.0	1.0	30	60	<1.0
(*Stella D'oro* Very Low Sodium), 3 pcs., 1.1 oz. . . .	120	4.0	20.0	3.0	40	15	1.0
vanilla (*Stella D'oro* Roman), 1.2-oz. pc.	140	2.0	21.0	5.0	20	125	<1.0
espresso bean (*Barbara's Nature's Choice* Dipped), 1.1-oz. bar	120	2.0	22.0	3.0	0	10	1.0

Food and Measure	cal.	prot. (gms)	carbo. (gms)	fat (gms)	chol. (mgs)	sod. (mgs)	fiber (gms)
Cookie *(cont.)*							
fig-filled/fig bar:							
(*Barbara's* Fat/ Wheat Free), ⅔-oz. pc.	60	<1.0	15.0	0	0	20	1.0
(*Barbara's* Traditional), ⅔-oz. pc.	60	1.0	14.0	1.0	0	25	1.0
(*Barbara's* Whole Wheat), ⅔-oz. pc.	60	<1.0	16.0	0	0	20	2.0
(*Fig Newton*), 2 pcs., 1.1 oz. ...	110	1.0	22.0	2.5	0	125	1.0
(*Fig Newton* Fat Free), 2 pcs., 1 oz. ....:	90	1.0	20.0	0	0	110	1.0
(*Weight Watchers*), .7 oz.	70	1.0	16.0	0	0	50	0
fortune, 4 pcs.:							
(*Frieda's*), 1 oz. ...	120	2.0	23.0	1.0	5	65	1.0
(*La Choy*), 1.1 oz.	115	1.5	27.0	0	0.	10	<1.0
fruit:							
(*Stella D'oro* Holiday Slices), 2 pcs., 1.2 oz.	130	0	20.0	5.0	<5	90	1.0
bar (*Archway* Fat Free), .9-oz. pc.	80	<1.0	19.0	0	0	90	0
cake (*Archway*), 3 pcs., 1.1 oz. ...	140	2.0	20.0	6.0	0	150	1.0
filled (*Bahlsen* Deloba), 4 pcs., 1 oz.	120	2.0	19.0	5.0	0	80	1.0
and honey bar (*Archway*), .9-oz. pc.	100	1.0	18.0	3.5	5	105	0
tropical (*Health Valley*), 3 pcs.	100	2.0	24.0	0	0	50	3.0
ginger (*Pepperidge Farm* Gingerman), 4 pcs., 1 oz.	120	2.0	21.0	3.5	10	95	<1.0
ginger lemon creme (*Carr's*), 2 pcs., 1 oz.	140	1.0	19.0	7.0	<5	105	<1.0

Food and Measure	cal.	prot. (gms)	carbo. (gms)	fat (gms)	chol. (mgs)	sod. (mgs)	fiber (gms)
ginger snaps:							
(*Archway*), 5 pcs., 1.1 oz.	150	1.0	23.0	5.0	0	120	0
(*Archway* Reduced Fat), 5 pcs., 1.1 oz.	140	1.0	25.0	3.5	0	140	0
(*Nabisco*), 4 pcs., 1 oz.	120	1.0	22.0	2.5	0	230	<1.0
(*Sunshine*), 5 pcs., 1.2 oz.	150	2.0	24.0	6.0	0	120	0
iced (*Archway*), 5 pcs., 1.3 oz.	170	1.0	26.0	7.0	0	130	0
gingerbread, iced (*Archway*), 3 pcs., 1.1 oz.	140	1.0	22.0	5.0	5	120	0
golden bar (*Stella D'oro*), 1-oz. pc.	110	2.0	17.0	3.5	20	65	0
graham cracker:							
(*Cinnamon Crisps Graham Selects*), 8 pcs., 1.1 oz.	140	2.0	22.0	5.0	0	170	1.0
(*Cinnamon Crisps Graham Selects Reduced Fat*), 8 pcs., 1 oz.	110	2.0	24.0	1.5	0	190	<1.0
(*Goldfish*), 19 pcs., 1.1 oz.	150	2.0	20.0	7.0	15	150	2.0
(*Graham Selects*), 8 pcs., 1 oz.	130	2.0	23.0	3.0	0	135	<1.0
(*Honey Graham Selects*), 8 pcs., 1.1 oz.	150	2.0	21.0	6.0	0	140	1.0
(*Honey Graham Selects* Low Fat), 9 pcs., 1.1 oz.	120	2.0	25.0	1.5	0	210	1.0
(*Honey Maid*), 8 pcs., 1 oz.	120	2.0	22.0	3.0	0	180	1.0
(*Honey Maid* Low Fat), 8 pcs., 1 oz.	110	2.0	23.0	1.5	0	200	<1.0

Food and Measure	cal.	prot. (gms)	carbo. (gms)	fat (gms)	chol. (mgs)	sod. (mgs)	fiber (gms)
Cookie, graham cracker *(cont.)*							
(*Honey Snackin' Grahams* Bite Size), 23 pcs., 1.1 oz.	130	3.0	23.0	3.0	0	180	<1.0
(*Nabisco*), 4 pcs., 1 oz.	120	2.0	33.0	3.0	0	180	1.0
amaranth (*Health Valley*), 8 pcs.	100	4.0	23.0	0	0	30	3.0
amaranth (*Health Valley* Original), 6 pcs.	120	3.0	22.0	3.0	0	80	3.0
cinnamon (*Honey Maid*), 8 pcs., 1 oz.	120	2.0	23.0	2.5	0	180	<1.0
cinnamon (*Honey Maid* Low Fat), 8 pcs., 1 oz.	110	2.0	23.0	1.5	0	170	<1.0
cinnamon (*Snackin' Grahams* Bite Size), 21 pcs., 1 oz.	130	2.0	23.0	3.0	0	210	1.0
cinnamon (*Sweet Crispers* Snacks), 18 pcs., 1.1 oz.	130	2.0	26.0	2.5	0	180	<1.0
honey (*Sweet Crispers* Snacks), 18 pcs., 1.1 oz.	130	2.0	26.0	2.5	0	200	1.0
honey (*Teddy Grahams* Snacks), 24 pcs., 1.1 oz.	140	2.0	23.0	4.0	0	170	<1.0
oat bran (*Health Valley*), 8 pcs.	100	4.0	23.0	0	0	30	3.0
oatmeal crunch (*Honey Maid*), 8 pcs., 1 oz.	120	2.0	22.0	2.5	0	140	1.0
graham cracker, chocolate:							
(*Fudge Favorites*), 3 pcs., 1 oz.	140	2.0	18.0	7.0	0	125	<1.0

Food and Measure	cal.	prot. (gms)	carbo. (gms)	fat (gms)	chol. (mgs)	sod. (mgs)	fiber (gms)
(*Fudge Shoppe Deluxe*), 3 pcs., .9 oz.	140	1.0	19.0	7.0	0	105	<1.0
(*Fudge Shoppe Deluxe* Reduced Fat), 3 pcs., .9 oz.	120	1.0	19.0	5.0	0	130	0
(*Graham Selects*), 8 pcs., 1.1 oz.	130	2.0	23.0	4.0	0	115	0
(*Honey Maid*), 8 pcs., 1 oz.	120	2.0	22.0	3.0	0	170	1.0
(*Sweet Crispers* Snacks), 18 pcs., 1.1 oz.	130	2.0	25.0	2.5	0	190	1.0
(*Teddy Grahams* Snacks), 24 pcs., 1.1 oz.	140	2.0	22.0	4.5	0	150	1.0
(*Teddy Grahams Dizzy Grizzly*), 8 pcs., 1.1 oz.	150	1.0	24.0	5.0	0	110	<1.0
graham cracker, vanilla frosted (*Teddy Grahams Dizzy Grizzly*), 8 pcs., 1.1 oz.	150	1.0	24.0	6.0	0	105	<1.0
granola (*Archway* Fat Free), 2 pcs., 1.1 oz.	100	2.0	22.0	0	0	100	1.0
hazelnut:							
(*Bahlsen* Kipfrel), 4 pcs., 1 oz.	150	2.0	16.0	9.0	5	10	0
(*Pepperidge Farm*), 3 pcs., 1.1 oz. ...	160	2.0	21.0	8.0	0	135	<1.0
hermits (*Archway* Cookie Jar), .9-oz. pc.	90	1.0	16.0	2.5	<5	150	<1.0
holiday, 1.1 oz.:							
(*Archway* Bells & Stars), 3 pcs.	150	1.0	19.0	7.0	5	105	1.0
(*Archway* Party Treats), 3 pcs.	140	2.0	20.0	7.0	15	105	0
(*Archway* Wedding Cake), 3 pcs. ...	160	1.0	20.0	8.0	0	45	0

Food and Measure	cal.	prot. (gms)	carbo. (gms)	fat (gms)	chol. (mgs)	sod. (mgs)	fiber (gms)
Cookie, holiday *(cont.)*							
(*Stella D'oro* Rings & Stars), 3 pcs.	140	1.0	26.0	3.0	0	35	<1.0
(*Stella D'oro* Trinkets), 4 pcs.	160	2.0	20.0	8.0	10	125	<1.0
kichel:							
(*Manischewitz*), 4 pcs., .5 oz.	70	2.0	8.0	4.0	105	45	1.0
(*Stella D'oro* Low Sodium), 21 pcs., 1 oz.	150	4.0	13.0	9.0	80	25	<1.0
lemon:							
(*Archway* Drop), .8-oz. pc.	90	1.0	15.0	3.5	10	95	0
(*Archway* Frosty), .9-oz. pc.	110	1.0	17.0	4.5	0	95	0
(*Archway* Frosty 2 Big), .9-oz. pc.	110	1.0	19.0	5.0	0	100	0
(*Sunshine All American*), 5 pcs., 1.1 oz.	140	1.0	21.0	60	0	100	<1.0
w/hazelnuts (*Larzaroni*), 5 pcs., 1 oz.	140	2.0	16.0	8.0	5	30	2.0
nuggets (*Archway* Fat Free), 4 pcs., 1.1 oz.	110	1.0	27.0	0	0	115	0
nut crunch (*Pepperidge Farm*), 3 pcs., 1.1 oz. . . .	170	2.0	18.0	9.0	15	60	2.0
snaps (*Archway*), 5 pcs., 1.1 oz. . . .	140	1.0	25.0	3.5	0	140	0
thins (*Peek Freans*), 3 pcs., 1.4 oz. . . .	195	2.0	28.0	8.0	n.a.	110	n.a.
yogurt (*Barbara's Nature's Choice* Dipped), 1.1-oz. bar	120	2.0	22.0	3.5	0	10	1.0
macaroon, see "coconut," above							

Food and Measure	cal.	prot. (gms)	carbo. (gms)	fat (gms)	chol. (mgs)	sod. (mgs)	fiber (gms)
marshmallow, choco-late coated:							
(*Mallomars*), 2 pcs., .9 oz.	120	1.0	17.0	5.0	0	35	<1.0
original or cappuc-cino (*Peek Freans* Dream Puffs), 2 pcs., .9 oz.	110	<1.0	18.0	4.0	0	50	0
mint creme (*SnackWell's*), 2 pcs., .9 oz.	110	1.0	19.0	3.5	0	70	<1.0
molasses:							
(*Archway* 2 Big), .9-oz. pc.	110	1.0	19.0	3.0	5	135	0
(*Archway/Archway* Old Fashioned), .9-oz. pc.	100	1.0	18.0	3.0	10	140	0
(*Grandma's* Big), 1.4-oz. pc.	160	2.0	22.0	4.0	<5	230	<1.0
crisps (*Pepperidge Farm*), 5 pcs., 1.1 oz.	150	2.0	20.0	6.0	0	140	<1.0
dark (*Archway*), 1-oz. pc.	120	1.0	20.0	3.5	0	160	0
iced (*Archway*), 1-oz. pc.	120	1.0	20.0	3.5	0	130	0
soft (*Archway* Drop), .8-oz. pc.	90	<1.0	15.0	3.0	<5	140	0
mud pie (*Archway*), .9-oz. pc.	110	1.0	15.0	5.0	5	100	<1.0
nutty nougat (*Arch-way*), 3 pcs., 1.1 oz.	170	1.0	16.0	12.0	0	95	1.0
oatmeal:							
(*Archway*), .9-oz. pc.	110	2.0	17.0	3.5	<5	85	<1.0
(*Archway* Ruth's), .9-oz. pc.	110	2.0	17.0	4.0	<5	115	<1.0
(*Archway* Ruth's Golden), 1-oz. pc.	120	2.0	18.0	5.0	<5	110	<1.0
(*Archway* 2 Big), .9-oz. pc.	100	2.0	19.0	4.0	<5	90	<1.0

Food and Measure	cal.	prot. (gms)	carbo. (gms)	fat (gms)	chol. (mgs)	sod. (mgs)	fiber (gms)
Cookie, oatmeal *(cont.)*							
(*Barbara's* Crisp Old Fashioned), .6-oz. pc.	70	1.0	11.0	3.0	5	65	1.0
(*Keebler Classic Collection*), 2 pcs., 1.1 oz.	150	2.0	18.0	8.0	2	150	<1.0
(*Nabisco* Family Favorites), .6-oz. pc.	80	1.0	12.0	3.0	0	65	0
(*Pepperidge Farm* Irish), 3 pcs., 1 oz.	130	2.0	19.0	6.0	<5	70	2.0
(*Sunshine* Country), ½-oz. pc.	80	1.0	9.0	4.5	0	60	0
apple-filled (*Archway*), .9-oz. pc.	100	1.0	16.0	3.0	<5	105	<1.0
butterscotch (*Pepperidge Farm*), 3 pcs., 1.2 oz. . . .	170	2.0	22.0	9.0	10	110	1.0
crunch (*Archway* Gourmet), .9-oz. pc.	120	1.0	16.0	6.0	<5	120	<1.0
date-filled (*Archway*), .9-oz. pc.	100	1.0	17.0	3.0	<5	100	<1.0
iced (*Archway*), 1-oz. pc.	120	1.0	19.0	5.0	<5	95	<1.0
iced (*Nabisco* Family Favorites), .6-oz. pc.	80	1.0	12.0	3.0	0	55	0
pecan (*Archway* Gourmet), 1-oz. pc.	140	2.0	16.0	7.0	5	105	<1.0
raspberry (*Archway* Fat Free), 1.1-oz. pc.	110	1.0	25.0	0	0	170	<1.0
oatmeal raisin:							
(*Archway*), .9-oz. pc.	110	1.0	17.0	3.5	<5	100	<1.0

Food and Measure	cal.	prot. (gms)	carbo. (gms)	fat (gms)	chol. (mgs)	sod. (mgs)	fiber (gms)
(*Archway* Fat Free), 1.1-oz. pc.	110	1.0	25.0	0	0	170	<1.0
(*Archway* 2 Big), .9-oz. pc.	110	1.0	18.0	3.5	0	95	<1.0
(*Barbara's* Mini), 6 pcs., 1.1 oz. ...	110	2.0	24.0	0	0	105	2.0
(*Entenmann's Light*), 2 pcs., 1.1 oz. ....,..	100	2.0	23.0	0	0	150	1.0
(*Grandma's* Big), 1.4-oz. pc.	160	1.0	26.0	6.0	5	250	1.0
(*Keebler Soft Batch*), .9-oz. pc.	130	1.0	20.0	4.5	0	150	<1.0
(*Pepperidge Farm*), 3 pcs., 1.2 oz. ...	160	2.0	23.0	6.0	10	150	1.0
(*Pepperidge Farm* Santa Fe), .9-oz. pc.	120	2.0	18.0	4.5	<5	110	<1.0
(*Weight Watchers*), 1.1 oz.	120	2.0	22.0	2.0	0	90	1.0
soft (*Pepperidge Farm*), .9-oz. pc.	110	1.0	17.0	4.0	15	60	1.0
orange (*Archway Frosty*), .9-oz. pc.	110	1.0	17.0	4.5	0	95	0
peach tart (*Pepperidge Farm*), 2 pcs., 1.1 oz.	120	1.0	23.0	3.0	0	115	<1.0
peach-apricot (*Newton Cobblers*), ¾-oz. pc.	70	1.0	17.0	0	0	55	0
peanut:							
(*Archway* Jumble), .8-oz. pc.	110	2.0	13.0	6.0	<5	75	<1.0
roasted (*Barbara's Nature's Choice* Dipped), 1.1-oz. bar	130	3.0	20.0	4.5	0	50	1.0
peanut butter:							
(*Archway*), ¾-oz. pc.	100	2.0	12.0	5.0	10	85	<1.0

Food and Measure	cal.	prot. (gms)	carbo. (gms)	fat (gms)	chol. (mgs)	sod. (mgs)	fiber (gms)
Cookie, peanut butter *(cont.)*							
(*Archway* Ol'Fashion), .9-oz. pc. . . . .:. . .	120	2.0	15.0	6.0	10	120	<1.0
(*Grandma's* Big), 1.4-oz. pc.	190	2.0	22.0	9.0	<5	200	1.0
(*Grandma's* Cookie Bits), 9 pcs.	150	2.0	21.0	7.0	0	140	1.0
(*Keebler Classic Collection*), 2 pcs., 1.1 oz.	150	2.0	18.0	9.0	2	150	<1.0
(*Keebler Cookie Stix*), 4 pcs., 1 oz.	130	2.0	18.0	6.0	0	120	<1.0
chip (*SnackWell's* Bite Size), 13 pcs., 1 oz.	120	3.0	20.0	4.0	0	210	<1.0
w/chocolate chip (*Grandma's* Big), 1.4-oz. pc.	190	4.0	23.0	9.0	<5	170	1.0
peanut butter sandwich:							
(*Grandma's*), 5 pcs.	210	3.0	28.0	10.0	0	200	1.0
(*Nutter Butter*), 2 pcs., 1 oz.	130	2.0	19.0	6.0	<5	110	<1.0
chocolate (*Nutter Butter*), 2 pcs., 1 oz.	130	2.0	18.0	5.0	0	130	<1.0
pecan:							
(*Archway* Ice Box), .8-oz. pc.	120	1.0	15.0	6.0	5	75	0
malted nougat (*Archway*), 3 pcs., 1.1 oz.	160	2.0	17.0	10.0	0	60	2.0
pfeffernuss:							
(*Archway*), 2 pcs., 1 oz.	100	1.0	23.0	1.0	5	90	1.0
(*Stella D'oro*), 3 pcs., 1 oz.	120	1.0	21.0	3.0	15	55	0
pound cake (*Archway* Aunt Bea's), .9-oz. pc.	100	1.0	15.0	4.0	15	85	0

Food and Measure	cal.	prot. (gms)	carbo. (gms)	fat (gms)	chol. (mgs)	sod. (mgs)	fiber (gms)
praline, chocolate coated (*Bahlsen* Pralinette), 4 pcs., 1 oz.	150	2.0	15.0	9.0	0	25	1.0
pumpkin spice (*Archway*), 3 pcs., 1.1 oz.	120	1.0	19.0	4.0	<5	190	1.0
raisin:							
(*Golden Fruit* Biscuits), .7-oz. pc.	80	1.0	15.0	1.5	0	50	<1.0
(*Health Valley* Jumbo), 1 pc. . . .	80	2.0	19.0	0	0	35	3.0
raspberry:							
(*Health Valley* Jumbo), 1 pc. . . .	80	2.0	19.0	0	0	35	3.0
(*Pepperidge Farm* Linzer), .8-oz. pc.	100	1.0	15.0	4.0	5	65	<1.0
center (*Health Valley*), 1 pc.	70	2.0	18.0	0	0	20	2.0
filled (*Archway*), .9-oz. pc.	100	1.0	16.0	3.5	5	85	0
filled (*Barbara's* Fat/ Wheat Free), 2/3-oz. pc.	60	1.0	15.0	0	0	25	1.0
filled (*Fig Newton* Fat Free), 2 pcs., 1 oz.	100	1.0	23.0	0	0	115	<1.0
filled (*Weight Watchers*), .7 oz.	70	1.0	16.0	0	0	45	0
hazelnut (*Pepperidge Farm Chantilly*), .6-oz. pc.	80	<1.0	12.0	3.0	5	50	<1.0
nuggets (*Archway* Fat Free), 4 pcs., 1.1 oz.	120	1.0	27.0	0	0	125	0
tart (*Pepperidge Farm Fruitful*), 2 pcs., 1.1 oz. . . .	120	1.0	23.0	3.0	0	115	<1.0
vanilla, tart (*Pepperidge Farm Wholesome Choice*), 2 pcs., 1.1 oz. . . .	120	1.0	23.0	3.0	0	115	<1.0

Food and Measure	cal.	prot. (gms)	carbo. (gms)	fat (gms)	chol. (mgs)	sod. (mgs)	fiber (gms)
Cookie *(cont.)*							
rocky road (*Archway Gourmet*), 1-oz. pc.	130	2.0	18.0	6.0	10	70	<1.0
sesame (*Stella D'oro Regina*), 3 pcs., 1.1 oz.	150	2.0	210	6.0	10	85	1.0
shortbread:							
(*Barbara's* Crisp Traditional), .6-oz. pc.	80	1.0	10.0	4.0	10	40	1.0
(*Lorna Doone*), 4 pcs., 1 oz.	140	2.0	19.0	7.0	5	130	<1.0
(*Pecan Sandies*), .6-oz. pc.	80	<1.0	9.0	5.0	<5	75	<1.0
(*Pecan Sandies* Reduced Fat), .6-oz. pc.	70	<1.0	11.0	3.0	0	55	0
(*Peek Freans Butter*), 4 pcs., 1.4 oz.	205	5.5	23.0	10.0	0	105	1.0
(*Pepperidge Farm*), 2 pcs., .9 oz.	140	2.0	16.0	7.0	10	105	<1.0
(*Simply Sandies*), .6-oz. pc.	80	1.0	9.0	4.5	10	70	0
(*Sugar Kake*), 4 pcs., 1 oz.	140	1.0	19.0	6.0	0	110	0
almond (*Almond Sandies*), .6-oz. pc.	80	1.0	9.0	5.0	5	50	0
pecan (*Pepperidge Farm*), 2 pcs., .9 oz.	140	1.0	14.0	9.0	<5	85	1.0
shortcake (*Peek Freans*), 3 pcs., 1.4 oz.	205	2.0	27.0	10.0	0	100	<1.0
(*Social Tea*), 6 pcs., 1 oz.	120	2.0	22.0	3.5	5	115	<1.0
(*Stella D'oro Angel Wings*), 2 pcs., .9 oz.	140	2.0	13.0	9.0	<5	80	<1.0

Food and Measure	cal.	prot. (gms)	carbo. (gms)	fat (gms)	chol. (mgs)	sod. (mgs)	fiber (gms)
(*Stella D'oro Angelica Goodies*), .8-oz. pc.	100	2.0	15.0	4.0	15	45	0
(*Stella D'oro Anginetti*), 4 pcs., 1.1 oz.	140	2.0	23.0	4.0	40	10	<1.0
(*Stella D'oro Como Delight*), 1.1-oz. pc.	140	2.0	18.0	7.0	40	60	<1.0
(*Stella D'oro Hostess With the Mostest*), 3 pcs., 1 oz.	130	1.0	19.0	5.5	5	60	<1.0
(*Stella D'oro Lady Stella Assortment*), 3 pcs., 1 oz.	130	1.0	19.0	5.0	5	65	<1.0
(*Stella D'oro Margherite*), 2 pcs., 1.1 oz.	140	2.0	22.0	5.0	15	90	<1.0
(*Stella D'oro Royal Nuggets*), 100 pcs., 1.1 oz.	140	11.0	9.0	6.0	60	150	<1.0
strawberry-filled:							
(*Archway*), .9-oz. pc.	100	1.0	16.0	3.5	5	85	0
(*Fig Newton Fat Free*), 2 pcs., 1 oz.	100	1.0	23.0	0	0	115	<1.0
cup (*Pepperidge Farm Fruitful*), 3 pcs., 1.1 oz.	140	2.0	22.0	5.0	10	105	<1.0
sugar:							
(*Archway*), .8-oz. pc.	100	1.0	16.0	3.0	5	160	0
(*Archway Fat Free*), .7-oz. pc.	70	<1.0	17.0	0	0	80	0
(*Keebler Classic Collection*), 2 pcs., 1 oz.	140	2.0	18.0	7.0	2	150	0
(*Pepperidge Farm*), 3 pcs., 1.1 oz.	140	2.0	20.0	6.0	15	90	<1.0
soft (*Archway Drop*), .8-oz. pc.	90	1.0	15.0	3.0	15	80	0

Food and Measure	cal.	prot. (gms)	carbo. (gms)	fat (gms)	chol. (mgs)	sod. (mgs)	fiber (gms)
Cookie *(cont.)*							
sugar wafer:							
(*Keebler*), 3 pcs.,							
1 oz.	150	1.0	19.0	9.0	0	20	0
(*Sunshine*), 3 pcs.,							
.9 oz.	130	1.0	18.0	6.0	0	20	<1.0
creme filled (*Bis-*							
cos), 9 pcs., 1 oz.	140	<1.0	21.0	6.0	0	40	0
peanut butter (*Sun-*							
shine), 4 pcs.,							
1.1 oz.	170	3.0	19.0	9.0	0	75	1.0
vanilla:							
(*Goldfish*), 19 pcs.,							
1.1 oz.	150	2.0	21.0	7.0	20	50	1.0
(*Grandma's Cookie*							
Bits), 9 pcs.	150	2.0	22.0	7.0	<5	85	1.0
(*Keebler Classic Col-*							
lection), .6-oz.							
pc.	80	1.0	12.0	3.5	0	65	0
wafer (*Keebler*),							
8 pcs., 1.1 oz. . . .	150	1.0	20.0	7.0	0	120	<1.0
wafer (*Keebler Re-*							
duced Fat),							
8 pcs., 1.1 oz. . . .	130	2.0	25.0	3.5	0	140	<1.0
wafer (*Nilla*), 8 pcs.,							
1.1 oz.	140	1.0	24.0	5.0	<5	100	0
wafer (*Nilla Reduced*							
Fat), 8 pcs., 1 oz.	120	1.0	24.0	2.0	0	105	0
wafer, chocolate							
(*Nilla Reduced*							
Fat), 8 pcs., 1 oz.	110	2.0	23.0	2.0	0	120	<1.0
vanilla sandwich:							
(*Cameo*), 2 pcs.,							
1 oz.	130	1.0	21.0	5.0	0	105	0
(*Grandma's*), 1 pkg.	210	2.0	30.0	10.0	2	125	<1.0
(*Vienna Fingers*),							
2 pcs., 1 oz.	140	2.0	21.0	6.0	0	105	<1.0
(*Vienna Fingers Low*							
Fat), 2 pcs., 1 oz.	130	1.0	22.0	4.5	0	105	<1.0
(*Weight Watchers*),							
1.1 oz.	140	1.0	25.0	3.0	0	80	1.0

Food and Measure	cal.	prot. (gms)	carbo. (gms)	fat (gms)	chol. (mgs)	sod. (mgs)	fiber (gms)
waffle:							
(*Bahlsen Hannover*), 5 pcs., 1 oz.	160	1.0	16.0	10.0	0	35	0
(*Bahlsen Waffeletten*), 5 pcs., 1 oz.	160	1.0	18.0	9.0	5	40	1.0
walnut:							
black (*Archway Ice Box*), .8-oz. pc.	120	1.0	15.0	6.0	10	75	0
nutty (*Archway*), 3 pcs., 1 oz.	120	1.0	18.0	6.0	<5	125	<1.0
windmill (*Archway Old Fashioned*), .7-oz. pc.	90	1.0	14.0	3.5	0	90	<1.0
Cookie, refrigerated, 1 oz., except as noted:							
(*Pillsbury M&M's*) . . .	130	1.0	18.0	6.0	<5	75	<1.0
(*Pillsbury M&M's* One Step Pan), 1/8 pan	130	1.0	19.0	6.0	<5	85	<1.0
chocolate, double (*Pillsbury*)	130	1.0	17.0	6.0	<5	90	<1.0
chocolate chip:							
(*Nestlé/Nestlé* Big Batch), 2 tbsp.	140	1.0	20.0	6.0	10	110	1.0
(*Nestlé* Reduced Fat), 2 tbsp.	130	2.0	21.0	4.5	10	100	1.0
(*Pillsbury*)	130	1.0	17.0	6.0	<5	85	<1.0
(*Pillsbury* One Step Pan), 1/8 pan	130	1.0	19.0	6.0	<5	100	<1.0
(*Pillsbury* Reduced Fat) . . :	110	1.0	19.0	3.0	<5	85	<1.0
oatmeal (*Pillsbury*)	120	1.0	16.0	6.0	<5	95	<1.0
peanut butter (*Nestlé*), 2 tbsp.	160	2.0	19.0	8.0	10	120	1.0
w/walnuts (*Pillsbury*)	140	1.0	17.0	7.0	<5	90	<1.0
chocolate chunk:							
(*Pillsbury*)	130	1.0	17.0	6.0	<5	90	<1.0
white (*Pillsbury*) . . .	130	1.0	17.0	6.0	<5	100	0
holiday shapes (*Pillsbury*)	130	1.0	16.0	7.0	<5	100	0

Food and Measure	cal.	prot. (gms)	carbo. (gms)	fat (gms)	chol. (mgs)	sod. (mgs)	fiber (gms)
Cookie, refrigerated *(cont.)*							
oatmeal (*Nestlé Scotchies*), 2 tbsp.	140	1.0	20.0	6.0	10	110	3.0
peanut butter:							
(*Pillsbury*)	120	2.0	15.0	6.0	<5	130	<1.0
(*Pillsbury Reese's*)	130	3.0	15.0	6.0	<5	105	<1.0
sugar:							
(*Nestlé*), ½″ slice	120	1.0	18.0	5.0	<5	130	1.0
(*Pillsbury*)	130	1.0	19.0	5.0	<5	125	0
Cookie crumbs, graham (*Honey Maid*), 2½ tbsp.	70	1.0	12.0	1.5	0	100	0
Cookie mix*, 2 pcs., except as noted:							
chocolate chip:							
(*Arrowhead Mills*), 1 pc.	80	1.0	16.0	1.5	0	110	0
(*Betty Crocker*)	160	2.0	21.0	8.0	10	105	0
(*Duncan Hines*)	170	2.0	22.0	8.0	10	100	0
wheat free (*Arrowhead Mills*), 1 pc.	80	1.0	16.0	1.5	0	105	<1.0
chocolate chunk, double (*Betty Crocker*)	150	2.0	21.0	6.0	10	105	0
cookie bar, see "Cake, snack, mix"							
espresso chip (*Arrowhead Mills*), 1 pc.	80	1.0	16.0	1.5	0	50	0
fudge, candy splash (*Duncan Hines*)	140	1.0	21.0	7.0	10	120	0
oatmeal chocolate chip (*Betty Crocker*)	160	2.0	21.0	7.0	10	125	0
oatmeal raisin (*Arrowhead Mills*), 1 pc.	70	1.0	16.0	0	0	110	1.0
peanut butter:							
(*Betty Crocker*)	160	3.0	20.0	8.0	10	135	0
(*Duncan Hines*)	140	2.0	16.0	8.0	10	120	0
sugar:							
(*Betty Crocker*)	170	2.0	22.0	8.0	10	130	0
(*Duncan Hines*)	150	1.0	21.0	7.0	20	90	0

Food and Measure	cal.	prot. (gms)	carbo. (gms)	fat (gms)	chol. (mgs)	sod. (mgs)	fiber (gms)
Cookie pie crust, see "Pie crust"							
Cooking sauce, see specific listings							
Coq au vin seasoning mix (*Knorr*), 1 tbsp.	30	<1.0	5.0	1.0	0	250	0
Coquito nut (*Frieda's*), 11 pcs., 1 oz.	110	21.0	5.0	10.0	0	5	3.0
Coriander:							
fresh, ¼ cup	1	.1	.1	<.1	0	1	.1
dried:							
leaf, 1 tsp.	2	.1	.3	<.1	0	1	.1
seed, 1 tsp.	5	.2	1.0	.3	0	1	.5
Corkscrew pasta, see "Pasta"							
Corkscrew pasta dishes:							
four-cheese sauce:							
(*DeBoles*), 2 oz. mix	220	8.0	37.0	2.5	5	640	2.0
(*Pasta Roni*), 1 cup*	410	13.0	49.0	18.0	10	1050	2.0
garlic sauce, creamy (*Pasta Roni*), 1 cup*	420	9.0	41.0	24.5	5	1010	2.0
w/herb-garlic sauce (*Annie's*), ⅔ cup mix	260	10.0	50.0	3.0	5	450	2.0
Corn, fresh, kernels, boiled, drained, ½ cup	89	2.7	20.6	1.1	0	14	2.3
Corn, canned (see also "Hominy"), ½ cup, except as noted:							
baby, whole (*Haddon House*)	30	1.0	3.0	1.5	0	30	4.0
kernel, golden:							
(*Del Monte*)	90	2.0	18.0	1.0	0	360	3.0
(*Del Monte* Supersweet)	60	2.0	11.0	1.0	0	360	3.0
(*Del Monte* Supersweet No Salt) ...	60	2.0	11.0	1.0	0	10	3.0

Food and Measure	cal.	prot. (gms)	carbo. (gms)	fat (gms)	chol. (mgs)	sod. (mgs)	fiber (gms)
Corn, canned, kernel, golden *(cont.)*							
(*Del Monte* Super-sweet Vac Pack)	70	2.0	13.0	1.0	0	270	3.0
(*Del Monte* Super-sweet Vac Pack No Salt)	70	2.0	13.0	1.0	0	10	3.0
(*Green Giant*)	80	2.0	18.0	.5	0	360	2.0
(*Green Giant* 50% Less Sodium) ...	80	2.0	17.0	.5	0	180	2.0
(*Green Giant Niblets*), 1/3 cup	70	2.0	15.0	0	0	230	2.0
(*Green Giant Niblets* Extra Sweet), 1/3 cup	50	2.0	10.0	0	0	200	2.0
(*Green Giant Niblets* Less Sodium), 1/3 cup	60	2.0	14.0	0	0	115	1.0
(*Green Giant Niblets* No Salt/Sugar), 1/3 cup	60	2.0	13.0	0	0	0	2.0
(*Seneca*)	90	2.0	20.0	.5	0	250	2.0
(*Seneca No Salt*) ...	80	2.0	16.0	.5	0	40	<1.0
kernel, golden and white (*Del Monte* Supersweet)	80	2.0	18.0	.5	0	360	2.0
kernel, white:							
(*Del Monte*)	60	2.0	11.0	1.0	0	360	3.0
(*Seneca* Super Sweet)	100	2.0	21.0	1.0	0	220	3.0
kernel, w/peppers:							
(*Del Monte* Fiesta)	50	2.0	12.0	1.0	0	310	2.0
(*Green Giant Mexicorn*), 1/2 cup ...	60	2.0	14.0	0	0	430	2.0
cream style, golden:							
(*Del Monte*)	90	2.0	20.0	.5	0	360	2.0
(*Del Monte* No Salt)	90	2.0	20.0	.5	0	10	2.0
(*Del Monte* Super-sweet)	60	1.0	14.0	.5	0	360	2.0
(*Del Monte* Super-sweet No Salt) ...	60	1.0	14.0	.5	0	10	2.0
(*Green Giant*)	100	2.0	7.0	.5	0	430	1.0

Food and Measure	cal.	prot. (gms)	carbo. (gms)	fat (gms)	chol. (mgs)	sod. (mgs)	fiber (gms)
(*Seneca*)	80	1.0	19.0	0	0	360	2.0
cream style, white (*Del Monte*)	100	2.0	21.0	1.0	0	360	2.0
Corn, dried:							
(*Frieda's* Posole), 1/3 cup	30	1.0	6.0	0	0	95	1.0
toasted, sweet (*John Cope's*), 1/4 cup	130	2.0	15.0	1.0	0	0	1.0
Corn, freeze-dried, 1/2 cup:							
(*AlpineAire*)	90	3.0	16.0	1.5	0	0	3.0
(*Mountain House*) . . .	80	13.0	17.0	1.0	0	0	2.0
Corn, frozen:							
on cob, 1 ear, except as noted:							
(*Birds Eye/Freshlike* 3 or 4 Ears)	140	5.0	34.0	1.5	0	20	2.0
(*Birds Eye* 6/12 Little)	80	3.0	18.0	1.0	0	10	1.0
(*Birds Eye* 8 Little), 2 ears	110	4.0	26.0	1.0	0	0	3.0
(*Freshlike* 6/8/12/24 Ears)	80	3.0	18.0	1.0	0	10	1.0
(*Green Giant* Extra Sweet)	120	4.0	22.0	2.0	0	0	3.0
(*Green Giant* Niblers)	70	2.0	14.0	.5	0	5	1.0
(*Green Giant* Niblets)	160	4.0	32.0	1.5	0	10	3.0
(*John Cope's*)	140	5.0	34.0	1.5	0	20	2.0
(*John Cope's* Mini)	80	3.0	18.0	1.0	0	10	1.0
(*Seneca*)	140	4.0	29.0	1.0	0	370	<1.0
kernel, baby:							
(*Birds Eye* Farm Fresh/Freshlike Blend), 2/3 cup . . .	60	2.0	11.0	.5	0	15	2.0
gold and white (*Birds Eye* Farm Fresh), 2/3 cup . . .	80	3.0	15.0	1.0	0	10	2.0
kernel, golden:							
(*Birds Eye* Sweet), 1/3 cup	70	3.0	17.0	.5	0	0	2.0

Food and Measure	cal.	prot. (gms)	carbo. (gms)	fat (gms)	chol. (mgs)	sod. (mgs)	fiber (gms)
Corn, frozen, kernel, golden *(cont.)*							
(*Birds Eye* Tender Deluxe), 1/3 cup	60	2.0	14.0	1.0	0	0	2.0
(*Cascadian Farm*), 3/4 cup	90	3.0	21.0	1.0	0	0	5.0
(*Freshlike*), 2/3 cup	80	3.0	19.0	1.0	0	10	1.0
(*Green Giant Niblets*), 2/3 cup	80	2.0	17.0	.5	0	5	2.0
(*Green Giant Niblets Extra Sweet*), 2/3 cup	70	2.0	13.0	1.0	0	0	2.0
(*Green Giant Niblets Harvest Fresh*), 2/3 cup	80	3.0	17.0	.5	0	60	3.0
(*John Cope's* Shoepeg), 2/3 cup	80	3.0	19.0	1.0	0	10	1.0
(*Seneca*), 2/3 cup . . .	90	3.0	20.0	.5	0	45	3.0
kernel, gold and white (*Freshlike*), 2/3 cup	80	3.0	15.0	1.0	0	10	1.0
kernel, white:							
(*Freshlike*), 2/3 cup	80	2.0	14.0	1.5	0	10	3.0
(*Green Giant* Select Extra Sweet), 2/3 cup	50	2.0	10.0	.5	0	0	3.0
(*Green Giant* Select Shoepeg), 3/4 cup	100	3.0	20.0	1.0	0	0	3.0
(*Green Giant* Harvest Fresh Shoepeg), 1/2 cup	70	2.0	14.0	.5	0	45	2.0
in butter sauce:							
(*Birds Eye Side Orders*), 1/2 cup	110	3.0	23.0	3.0	5	230	2.0
(*Cascadian Farm*), 1/2 cup	100	3.0	19.0	3.0	5	310	2.0
(*Green Giant Niblets*), 2/3 cup	130	3.0	23.0	3.0	<5	350	3.0
white (*Green Giant*), 3/4 cup	120	3.0	21.0	2.5	<5	320	3.0
cream style, 1/2 cup:							
(*Green Giant*)	110	2.0	23.0	1.0	0	330	2.0

Food and Measure	cal.	prot. (gms)	carbo. (gms)	fat (gms)	chol. (mgs)	sod. (mgs)	fiber (gms)
(*Seabrook*)	170	3.0	17	4.0	10	200	2.0
seasoned (*Green Giant* Southwestern), ¾ cup	90	3.0	18.0	1.0	0	130	1.0
Corn, whole-grain:							
1 oz.	103	2.7	21.1	1.3	0	10	n.a.
1 cup	605	15.6	123.3	7.9	0	58	n.a.
Corn bran, crude:							
1 oz.	64	2.4	24.3	.3	0	2	24.0
1 cup	170	6.4	65.1	.7	0	5	64.3
Corn bread, mix, ⅙ pan*, except as noted:							
(*Aunt Jemima* Easy), ⅛ pkg.	145	2.0	24.0	4.5	0	440	1.0
(*Ballard*), ¹⁄₁₈ loaf* ...	130	4.0	23.0	2.5	25	520	<1.0
buttermilk, ⅕ pan*:							
(*Martha White*)	140	3.0	24.0	4.0	<5	450	1.0
(*Martha White Cotton Pickin'*)	170	2.0	23.0	3.5	0	430	2.0
chili (*Martha White* Fiesta)	190	4.0	20.0	10.0	55	510	<1.0
honey, golden (*Martha White*)...........	170	3.0	21.0	8.0	45	400	0
Mexican:							
(*Gladiola*)	130	4.0	20.0	4.0	40	420	<1.0
(*Martha White*)	140	4.0	20.0	4.5	40	430	<1.0
white:							
(*Burrus Light Crust*)	140	4.0	21.0	4.0	40	380	1.0
(*Gladiola*)	140	4.0	20.0	4.5	35	420	<1.0
yellow:							
(*Burrus Light Crust*)	140	4.0	21.0	4.0	40	420	<1.0
(*Gladiola*)	140	4.0	20.0	4.5	35	420	0
(*Martha White*), ⅕ pan*	160	4.0	27.0	4.0	<5	480	<1.0
Corn bread, refrigerated, twists (*Pillsbury*), 1 pc.	140	3.0	18.0	6.0	0	330	0
Corn cake, see "Popcorn cake"							

Food and Measure	cal.	prot. (gms)	carbo. (gms)	fat (gms)	chol. (mgs)	sod. (mgs)	fiber (gms)
Corn chips, puffs, and similar snacks (see also "Snack chips and crisps"), 1 oz., except as noted:							
(*Baked Bugels*), 1.1 oz.	130	2.0	23.0	3.5	0	380	0
(*Baked Bugels*), 1.4-oz. pkg.	170	2.0	30.0	4.5	0	500	<1.0
(*Barbara's Thangs* Major Corn)	120	2.0	22.0	3.0	0	240	0
(*Bugels*), 1.1 oz.	160	1.0	18.0	9.0	0	310	<1.0
(*Bugels*), 1½-oz. pkg.	230	2.0	25.0	13.0	0	440	<1.0
(*Dipsy Doodles*)	160	1.0	16.0	10.0	0	180	1.0
(*Frito-Lay Funyons*)	140	2.0	18.0	7.0	0	270	<1.0
(*Frito-Lay Munchos*)	160	1.0	16.0	10.0	0	230	1.0
(*Fritos*)	160	2.0	15.0	10.0	0	170	1.0
(*Fritos* King Size)	160	2.0	16.0	10.0	0	150	1.0
(*Fritos* Scoops)	160	2.0	17.0	10.0	0	105	1.0
barbecue:							
(*Bugels* Smokin), 1.1 oz.	150	1.0	19.0	8.0	0	330	0
(*Frito-Lay Munchos*)	160	1.0	15.0	10.0	0	250	1.0
(*Fritos*)	150	2.0	16.0	9.0	0	290	1.0
(*Moore's*)	160	2.0	16.0	10.0	0	250	1.0
(*Wise*)...........	150	1.0	16.0	9.0	0	200	1.0
honey (*Fritos* Texas Grill)	150	2.0	16.0	9.0	0	200	1.0
mesquite (*Dipsy Doodles*)	160	1.0	16.0	10.0	0	250	1.0
caramel puffs (*Health Valley*), 2 cups	120	2.0	25.0	1.5	0	80	1.0
cheese:							
(*Barbara's* Puffs)	90	2.0	16.0	10.0	0	130	0
(*Barbara's* Puffs Bakes)	160	2.0	13.0	11.0	0	190	0
(*Chee•tos* Checkers)	160	2.0	15.0	10.0	<5	340	<1.0
(*Chee•tos* Crunchy)	160	2.0	15.0	10.0	0	290	<1.0
(*Chee•tos* Curls) ...	150	2.0	15.0	10.0	0	290	1.0
(*Chee•tos* Puffed Balls)	150	2.0	15.0	10.0	0	300	<1.0

Food and Measure	cal.	prot. (gms)	carbo. (gms)	fat (gms)	chol. (mgs)	sod. (mgs)	fiber (gms)
(*Chee•tos Puffs*) . . .	160	2.0	15.0	10.0	0	370	<1.0
(*Old Dutch* Baked)	170	2.0	16.0	12.0	0	270	0
(*Weight Watchers* Curls), ½ oz. . . .	70	1.0	10.0	2.5	0	85	0
chili (*Fritos*)	160	2.0	16.0	10.0	0	240	1.0
crunch (*Husman's*), 1½ cups, 1½ oz.	200	3.0	29.0	8.0	0	340	0
crunch (*Snyder*) . . .	130	2.0	19.0	6.0	0	230	0
hot (*Chee•tos* Flamin')	160	2.0	15.0	10.0	0	280	<1.0
jalapeño (*Barbara's* Puffs)	150	2.0	15.0	9.0	0	250	0
nacho (*Bugels*), 1.1 oz.	160	2.0	18.0	9.0	0	300	0
nacho (*Chee•tos*)	160	2.0	15.0	10.0	0	260	<1.0
nacho (*Doodle Twisters*)	160	2.0	14.0	11.0	0	250	1.0
nacho (*Old Dutch*), 1.1 oz.	150	2.0	19.0	7.0	0	150	1.0
pizza (*Doodle O's*)	150	1.0	15.0	10.0	0	160	0
pizza (*Wise Crunchers*)	160	1.0	16.0	10.0	0	230	0
cheese, cheddar:							
(*Baked Bugels*), 1.1 oz.	130	2.0	22.0	3.5	0	440	0
(*Dipsy Doodles*) . . .	150	2.0	16.0	9.0	0	190	0
(*Dipsy Doodles* Reduced Fat)	130	2.0	20.0	4.5	0	180	0
(*Doodle Heads*)	150	2.0	15.0	9.0	<5	270	0
(*Wise* Baked Puffed Balls)	140	2.0	15.0	9.0	0	320	0
(*Wise* Baked Puffs)	150	2.0	17.0	8.0	0	360	0
(*Wise* Puffed Doodles)	120	2.0	20.0	4.0	0	350	0
hot (*Sabrositas* Flamin')	150	2.0	16.0	9.0	0	180	1.0
lime and chili (*Sabrositas*)	150	2.0	17.0	9.0	0	240	1.0
ranch:							
(*Barbara's Thangs* Wild)	120	2.0	21.0	3.0	0	240	0

Food and Measure	cal.	prot. (gms)	carbo. (gms)	fat (gms)	chol. (mgs)	sod. (mgs)	fiber (gms)
Corn chips, puffs, and similar snacks, ranch *(cont.)*							
(*Bugels*), 1.1 oz.	160	2.0	18.0	9.0	0	310	<1.0
(*Fritos* Wild N'Mild)	160	2.0	15.0	10.0	0	160	1.0
salsa (*Barbara's*							
Thangs Sassy)	120	2.0	21.0	3.0	0	220	0
sour cream and onion							
(*Bugels*), 1.1 oz.	160	1.0	18.0	9.0	0	290	0
tortilla:							
(*Doritos* Toasted)	140	2.0	18.0	7.0	0	120	1.0
(*Moore's* Tostado							
Rounds)	150	2.0	18.0	8.0	0	140	1.0
(*Old Dutch*)	140	2.0	21.0	6.0	0	90	1.0
(*Old Dutch* Bite Size)	150	2.0	18.0	8.0	0	105	1.0
(*Old Dutch* Restau-							
rant)	140	2.0	20.0	7.0	0	95	2.0
(*Santitas* Chips) ...	140	2.0	19.0	6.0	0	75	1.0
(*Santitas* Strips) ...	140	2.0	19.0	6.0	0	60	1.0
(*Tostitos* Baked) ...	110	3.0	21.0	1.0	3	200	1.0
(*Tostitos* Baked Bite							
Size)	110	3.0	24.0	1.0	0	200	2.0
(*Tostitos* Baked Un-							
salted)	110	3.0	24.0	1.0	0	0	2.0
(*Tostitos* Bite Size)	140	2.0	17.0	8.0	0	110	1.0
(*Tostitos* Crispy							
Rounds)	150	2.0	17.0	8.0	0	85	1.0
(*Tostitos* Restau-							
rant)	140	2.0	19.0	6.0	0	110	1.0
(*Tostitos* Restaurant							
Unsalted)	140	2.0	18.0	8.0	0	10	1.0
(*Tostitos* Santa Fe							
Gold)	140	2.0	19.0	6.0	0	80	1.0
(*Tyson* Salted)	150	2.0	20.0	7.0	0	65	2.0
(*Wise/LaFamous*)	150	2.0	18.0	8.0	0	80	1.0
all varieties (*Valley*							
of Mexico)	140	3.0	19.0	6.0	0	150	<1.0
blue corn (*Bar-*							
bara's), 1.1 oz.	140	3.0	16.0	7.0	0	40	1.0
blue corn (*Barbara's*							
No Salt), 1.1 oz.	140	3.0	16.0	7.0	0	0	1.0
hot (*Doritos* Flamin')	140	2.0	17.0	7.0	0	210	1.0

Food and Measure	cal.	prot. (gms)	carbo. (gms)	fat (gms)	chol. (mgs)	sod. (mgs)	fiber (gms)
lime and chili (*Tostitos*)	150	2.0	17.0	7.0	0	180	1.0
pizza (*Doritos* Cravers)	140	2.0	18.0	7.0	0	170	1.0
ranch (*Doritos* Cooler)	140	2.0	18.0	7.0	0	170	1.0
ranch (*Doritos* 3D's Cooler)	140	2.0	18.0	6.0	<5	350	1.0
ranch (*Wise*)	150	2.0	19.0	8.0	0	200	1.0
salsa sour cream (*Tostitos* Baked)	120	2.0	21.0	3.0	0	190	1.0
taco (*Taco Bell* Supreme)	150	2.0	21.0	7.0	0	170	1.0
white corn (*Santitas*)	140	2.0	19.0	6.0	0	80	1.0
yellow corn (*Tyson*)	150	2.0	20.0	7.0	0	65	2.0
yellow corn (*Wise*)	150	2.0	18.0	8.0	0	60	1.0
tortilla, cheese and salsa (*Tostitos*)	140	2.0	18.0	7.0	0	180	1.0
tortilla, nacho cheese:							
(*Doritos* Cheesier)	140	2.0	17.0	7.0	0	200	1.0
(*Doritos* Spicy)	140	2.0	18.0	6.0	0	210	1.0
(*Doritos* 3D's Cheesier)	140	2.0	17.0	7.0	<5	360	1.0
(*Doritos Wow!*)	90	2.0	18.0	1.0	0	240	1.0
(*Tostitos*)	140	2.0	19.0	6.0	0	100	1.0
(*Wise* Bravo)	150	2.0	17.0	8.0	0	180	1.0
Corn dog, see "Frankfurter sandwich"							
Corn flake crumbs (*Kellogg's*), 2 tbsp.	40	1.0	9.0	0	0	105	0
Corn flour:							
whole-grain, 1 oz. . . .	102	2.0	21.8	1.1	0	1	3.8
whole-grain, 1 cup . . .	422	8.1	89.9	4.5	0	6	15.7
masa, 1 oz.	103	2.6	21.6	1.1	0	1	2.7
masa, 1 cup	416	10.7	87.0	4.3	0	6	10.9
Corn fritter mix, dry (*Casbah*), mix for 2 fritters	130	3.0	25.0	2.0	0	265	2.0

Food and Measure	cal.	prot. (gms)	carbo. (gms)	fat (gms)	chol. (mgs)	sod. (mgs)	fiber (gms)
Corn grits, dry, ¼ cup, except as noted:							
(*Albers*)	140	3.0	31.0	.5	0	0	1.0
(*Jim Dandy*)	170	4.0	38.0	1.0	0	0	1.0
(*Jim Dandy* Quick) . . .	160	4.0	35.0	1.0	0	0	<1.0
(*Jim Dandy* Quick Iron Fortified)	140	3.0	31.0	1.0	0	0	<1.0
(*Martha White* Original Instant), 1 oz.	100	2.0	22.0	0	0	320	2.0
(*Quaker* Instant), 1 pkt.	95	2.0	22.0	0	0	305	1.0
w/bacon:							
(*Martha White* Instant), 1 oz.	110	3.0	21.0	.5	0	300	2.0
bits (*Quaker* Instant), 1 pkt.	100	3.0	22.0	.5	0	340	1.0
bits and cheddar (*Quaker* Instant), 1 pkt.	100	3.0	20.0	1.5	0	430	1.0
butter flavor:							
(*Martha White* Instant), 1 oz.	100	2.0	21.0	.5	0	420	2.0
(*Quaker* Instant), 1 pkt.	100	2.0	20.0	1.0	0	325	1.0
cheese flavor:							
(*Martha White* Instant), 1 oz.	100	2.0	21.0	.5	0	400	1.0
American (*Quaker* Instant), 1 pkt.	100	3.0	21.0	1.0	0	425	1.0
w/sausage bits (*Quaker* Instant), 1 pkt.	100	3.0	20.0	1.0	0	430	1.0
w/ham bits (*Quaker* Instant), 1 pkt.	95	3.0	21.0	.5	0	490	1.0
white:							
(*Arrowhead Mills*)	140	3.0	30.0	0	0	0	1.0
(*Quaker* Quick Hominy)	130	3.0	29.0	.5	0	0	2.0
yellow:							
(*Arrowhead Mills*)	130	3.0	29.0	0	0	0	1.0
(*Martha White*)	150	3.0	35.0	0	0	0	1.0

Food and Measure	cal.	prot. (gms)	carbo. (gms)	fat (gms)	chol. (mgs)	sod. (mgs)	fiber (gms)
(*Quaker* Quick Hominy)	125	3.0	29.0	.5	0	0	2.0
Corn relish:							
(*Green Giant*), 1 tbsp.	20	0	2.0	0	0	40	0
(*Nance's*), 2 tbsp. ...	25	0	6.0	0	0	75	0
Corn soufflé, frozen (*Stouffer's* Side Dish), ½ cup	170	5.0	21.0	7.0	55	540	1.0
Cornichon, see "Pickle"							
Cornish hen:							
fresh or frozen, cooked, 3 oz.:							
dark (*Perdue*)	210	18.0	0	15.0	130	45	0
white (*Perdue*)	170	21.0	0	10.0	100	40	0
frozen, raw (*Tyson*), 4 oz.	180	18.0	0	12.0	130	65	0
oven-roasted, 3 oz.:							
dark (*Perdue*)	140	15.0	0	9.0	110	320	0
white (*Perdue*)	130	17.0	0	7.0	85	320	0
Cornmeal (see also "Corn flour" and "Polenta"), 3 tbsp., except as noted:							
(*Arrowhead Mills* Hi-Lysine), ¼ cup	120	3.0	25.0	1.0	0	0	3.0
(*Frieda's*), ¼ cup	110	2.0	23.0	1.0	0	10	2.0
(*Goya Fine*)	100	2.0	23.0	0	0	0	1.0
blue (*Arrowhead Mills*), ¼ cup	130	3.0	25.0	1.5	0	0	3.0
buttermilk, mix:							
(*Aunt Jemima* White Self-Rising)	80	2.0	18.0	.5	0	440	1.0
(*Gladiola/Martha* White Self-Rising)	110	3.0	22.0	1.0	0	440	1.0
masa harina:							
(*Quaker*), ¼ cup ...	110	3.0	24.0	1.5	0	0	2.5
(*Quaker* Preparada ParaTortillas), ⅓ cup	160	4.0	27.0	4.5	0	400	1.0

Food and Measure	cal.	prot. (gms)	carbo. (gms)	fat (gms)	chol. (mgs)	sod. (mgs)	fiber (gms)
Cornmeal (cont.)							
white:							
(*Albers*)	110	2.0	24.0	0	0	0	<1.0
(*Aunt Jemima* Self-Rising)	90	2.0	20.0	.5	0	360	1.0
(*Jim Dandy*)	120	2.0	25.0	1.0	0	0	2.0
(*Jim Dandy* Self-Rising)	110	2.0	24.0	1.0	0	470	2.0
(*Martha White/Hay Market*)	120	3.0	24.0	1.0	0	0	2.0
(*Martha White* Self-Rising)	110	3.0	23.0	1.0	0	470	2.0
white, mix:							
(*Aunt Jemima* Self-Rising)	85	2.0	18.0	.5	0	340	1.0
(*Gladiola/Hay Market/Honey Suckle/ Martha White/ Mother's Best/ Omega* Self-Rising)	110	2.0	22.0	1.0	0	450	2.0
whole ground:							
(*Cabin Home*)	110	2.0	24.0	1.0	0	0	2.0
(*Cabin Home* Self-Rising)	110	2.0	24.0	0	0	0	<1.0
yellow:							
(*Albers*)	110	2.0	24.0	0	0	0	<1.0
(*Arrowhead Mills*), 1/4 cup	120	3.0	27.0	1.0	0	0	3.0
(*Martha White*)	120	3.0	25.0	1.0	0	10	2.0
yellow, mix:							
(*Aunt Jemima* Self-Rising)	85	2.0	19.0	.5	0	320	1.0
(*Martha White* Self-Rising)	110	2.0	23.0	1.0	0	460	2.0
Cornstarch (*Argo/ Kingsford*), 1 tbsp.	30	0	7.0	0	0	0	0
Cottonseed kernels, roasted, 1 tbsp. . . .	51	3.3	2.2	3.6	0	3	.6
Cottonseed meal, partially defatted, 1 oz.	104	13.9	10.9	1.4	0	10	<1.0

Food and Measure	cal.	prot. (gms)	carbo. (gms)	fat (gms)	chol. (mgs)	sod. (mgs)	fiber (gms)
Country gravy mix							
(*Loma Linda Gravy Quik*), 1 tbsp.	25	<1.0	4.0	1.0	0	260	0
Couscous:							
dry, 1/4 cup, except as noted:							
(*Arrowhead Mills*)	170	6.0	35.0	0	0	0	2.0
(*Fantastic Foods*)	210	7.0	43.0	0	0	5	3.0
(*Near East*), 1/3 cup	220	8.0	45.0	1.0	0	5	2.0
whole wheat (*Fantastic Foods*)	210	8.0	45.0	1.0	0	0	7.0
cooked:							
1/2 cup	101	3.4	20.9	.1	0	4	1.3
dried (*AlpineAire*), 1 oz.	100	3.0	20.0	.5	0	0	1.0
Couscous dishes, mix, dry, 1/3 cup, except as noted:							
(*Marrakesh Express Lucky Seven*)	190	7.0	38.0	.5	0	300	1.0
black bean salsa (*Fantastic Foods* Cup), 2.4 oz.	240	11.0	46.0	1.5	0	450	8.0
broccoli (*Near East*), 2 oz.	195	7.0	42.0	1.0	0	460	3.0
cheddar, nacho (*Fantastic Foods* Cup), 1.9 oz.	200	8.0	36.0	3.0	0	590	6.0
corn, sweet (*Fantastic Foods* Cup), 1.8 oz.	180	7.0	36.0	1.0	0	510	6.0
cranberry (*Marrakesh Express Calypso*)	200	7.0	42.0	0	0	220	1.0
Creole vegetable (*Fantastic Foods* Cup), 2.1 oz.	220	10.0	41.0	1.5	0	590	6.0
garlic, w/red pepper (*Fantastic Foods Healthy Complements*)	200	7.0	41.0	2.0	0	440	2.0
garlic, roasted:							
(*Marrakesh Express*)	170	7.0	34.0	1.0	0	370	1.0

Food and Measure	cal.	prot. (gms)	carbo. (gms)	fat (gms)	chol. (mgs)	sod. (mgs)	fiber (gms)
Couscous dishes, garlic, roasted (cont.)							
and olive oil (*Casbah*), 1/4 cup	230	9.0	38.0	0	0	410	3.0
garlic and olive oil (*Near East*), 2 oz.	200	7.0	41.0	1.0	0	480	2.0
lemon spinach (*Casbah*), 1/4 cup	220	8.0	40.0	0	0	420	3.0
lentil curry (*Marrakesh Express*)	170	7.0	35.0	0	0	290	1.0
mango salsa (*Marrakesh Express*) . . .	190	6.0	40.0	0	0	270	1.0
mushroom, wild:							
(*Casbah Forest*), 1/4 cup	220	9.0	35.0	0	0	420	3.0
(*Marrakesh Express*)	190	8.0	38.0	0	0	310	1.0
nutted, w/currants and spice (*Casbah*), 1/4 cup	240	8.0	42.0	1.5	0	420	3.0
Parmesan (*Near East*), 2 oz.	200	8.0	40.0	1.5	<5	505	2.0
pilaf (*Casbah*), 3/4 cup	220	8.0	40.0	.5	0	480	.5
sesame ginger (*Marrakesh Express*) . . .	180	7.0	36.0	1.0	0	350	0
sun-dried tomato (*Marrakesh Express*)	190	8.0	36.0	1.0	0	230	1.0
Thai, royal (*Fantastic Foods Healthy Complements*)	200	8.0	41.0	1.0	0	480	2.0
tomato lentil (*Near East*), 2 oz.	190	8.0	42.0	.5	0	650	3.0
Cowpeas, 1/2 cup, except as noted:							
fresh:							
raw, trimmed	65	2.1	13.6	.3	0	3	3.6
boiled, drained	79	2.6	16.7	.3	0	3	4.1
fresh, leafy tips:							
raw, chopped	5	.7	.9	<.1	0	1	n.a.
boiled, drained, 4 oz.	25	5.3	3.2	.1	0	7	n.a.

Food and Measure	cal.	prot. (gms)	carbo. (gms)	fat (gms)	chol. (mgs)	sod. (mgs)	fiber (gms)
fresh, pods, w/seeds:							
raw, trimmed	21	1.6	4.5	.1	0	2	n.a.
boiled, drained	16	1.2	3.3	.1	0	1	n.a.
canned, see "Black-eyed peas"							
frozen, boiled, drained	112	7.2	20.2	.6	0	5	4.3
Cowpeas, catjang, see "Catjang"							
Crab, meat only, 4 oz.:							
Alaska king:							
raw	95	20.8	0	.7	47	948	0
boiled, poached, or steamed	110	21.9	0	1.7	60	1216	0
blue:							
raw	99	20.5	.1	1.2	89	332	0
boiled, poached, or steamed	116	22.9	0	2.0	113	316	0
Dungeness:							
raw	98	19.8	.8	1.1	67	335	0
boiled, poached, or steamed	125	25.3	1.1	1.4	86	429	0
queen:							
raw	102	21.0	0	1.4	62	611	0
boiled, poached, or steamed	130	26.9	0	1.7	81	784	0
Crab, canned:							
blue, 4 oz.	112	23.3	0	1.4	101	378	0
"Crab," imitation, frozen or refrigerated:							
chunk or flakes (*Louis Kemp Crab Delights*), ½ cup	90	10.0	12.0	0	10	410	2.0
flakes, ½ cup:							
(*Captain Jac Crab Tasties*)	100	6.0	15.0	1.5	5	430	0
(*Pacific Mate*)	100	7.0	15.0	1.0	5	600	0
(*Seafest*)	100	7.0	14.0	1.5	5	400	0
leg style, 3 legs, 3 oz.:							
(*Captain Jac Crab Tasties*)	90	6.0	14.0	1.5	5	430	0

Food and Measure	cal.	prot. (gms)	carbo. (gms)	fat (gms)	chol. (mgs)	sod. (mgs)	fiber (gms)
"Crab," imitation, leg style *(cont.)*							
(*Louis Kemp Crab*							
Delights)	90	10.0	12.0	0	10	410	2.0
(*Seafest*)	90	7.0	14.0	1.5	5	390	0
from surimi, 1 oz. . . .	29	3.4	3.0	.4	6	238	0
Crab apple, fresh:							
(*Frieda's*), 5 oz.	140	1.0	28.0	0	0	0	0
1 oz.	22	.1	5.7	.1	0	<1	n.a.
sliced, ½ cup	42	.2	11.0	.2	0	1	n.a.
Crab apple, canned,							
in heavy syrup							
(*Comstock/Wilder-*							
ness), .9-oz. pc. . . .	35	0	8.0	0	0	15	0
Crab cake, see "Crab							
entree, frozen"							
Crab dip mix, dry							
(*Watkins*), 1 tsp.	10	0	3.0	0	0	170	0
Crab entree, frozen,							
1 pc., except as							
noted:							
bites (*Matlaw's*),							
2 pcs.	60	2.0	8.0	2.0	0	80	1.0
cakes:							
(*Van de Kamp's*) . . .	170	6.0	17.0	9.0	15	460	<1.0
deviled (*Mrs. Paul's*)	170	8.0	20.0	7.0	20	440	1.0
deviled, mini (*Mrs.*							
Paul's), 6 pcs.	230	8.0	25.0	11.0	15	620	2.0
stuffed (*Five Star*)	230	8.0	11.0	17.0	90	769	<1.0
Cracker:							
almond (*Blue Diamond*							
Nut Thins), 16 pcs.,							
1.1 oz.	130	3.0	19.0	4.5	0	75	<1.0
arrowroot:							
(*Nabisco*), 1 pc.,							
.2 oz.	20	0	4.0	.5	0	15	0
(*Peek Freans*),							
5 pcs., 1.4 oz. . . .	180	3.0	31.0	5.0	0	215	1.0
(*Barbara's Rite* Lite							
Rounds), 5 pcs.,							
½ oz.	55	1.0	12.0	<1.0	0	150	0
butter/butter flavor:							
(*Goya*), ¼-oz. pc.	30	1.0	5.0	0	0	50	0

Food and Measure	cal.	prot. (gms)	carbo. (gms)	fat (gms)	chol. (mgs)	sod. (mgs)	fiber (gms)
(*Hi Ho*), 4 pcs., ½ oz.	70	1.0	8.0	4.0	0	130	<1.0
(*Hi Ho* Reduced Fat), 5 pcs., ½ oz.	70	1.0	10.0	2.5	0	140	<1.0
(*Keebler Club*), 4 pcs., ½ oz.	70	1.0	9.0	3.0	0	160	0
(*Keebler Club* Low Salt), 4 pcs., ½ oz.	70	1.0	9.0	3.0	0	80	0
(*Keebler Club* Reduced Fat), 5 pcs., .6 oz.	70	1.0	12.0	2.0	0	200	0
(*Pepperidge Farm* Thins), 4 pcs., ½ oz.	70	1.0	10.0	3.0	10	95	0
(*Ritz* Air Crisps), 24 pcs., 1 oz. ...	140	2.0	22.0	5.0	0	240	<1.0
(*Ritz* Low Sodium), 5 pcs., .6 oz.	80	1.0	10.0	4.0	0	35	0
(*Ritz* Original), 5 pcs., .6 oz.	80	1.0	10.0	4.0	0	135	0
(*Town House*), 5 pcs., .6 oz.	80	1.0	9.0	4.5	0	150	<1.0
(*Town House* Low Salt), 5 pcs., .6 oz.	80	1.0	10.0	4.5	0	75	<1.0
(*Town House* Reduced Fat), 6 pcs., ½ oz.	70	1.0	11.0	2.0	0	180	<1.0
crisp (*Toasteds*), 5 pcs., .6 oz.	80	1.0	10.0	3.5	0	150	0
cheddar cheese:							
(*Better Cheddars*), 22 pcs., 1.1 oz.	150	4.0	17.0	8.0	<5	290	<1.0
(*Better Cheddars* Low Sodium), 22 pcs., 1.1 oz.	150	3.0	18.0	7.0	<5	75	<1.0
(*Better Cheddars* Lowfat), 24 pcs., 1.1 oz.	140	4.0	19.0	6.0	<5	350	<1.0
(*Combos*), 1 oz. ...	150	3.0	16.0	8.0	5	300	0

Food and Measure	cal.	prot. (gms)	carbo. (gms)	fat (gms)	chol. (mgs)	sod. (mgs)	fiber (gms)
Cracker, cheddar cheese *(cont.)*							
(*Combos*), 1.7-oz. bag	250	5.0	28.0	13.0	5	510	1.0
(*Goldfish*), 55 pcs., 1.1 oz.	140	4.0	19.0	6.0	10	200	<1.0
(*Krispy*), 5 pcs., ½ oz.	60	2.0	10.0	2.0	0	180	<1.0
(*Munch'ems*), 30 pcs., 1 oz. ...	130	3.0	21.0	4.0	0	330	<1.0
white (*Cheez-It*), 26 pcs., 1.1 oz.	150	3.0	18.0	7.0	<5	280	<1.0
cheese:							
(*Barbara's Bites*), 26 pcs., 1.1 oz.	120	3.0	24.0	1.5	0	290	1.0
(*BIG Cheez-It*), 13 pcs., 1 oz. ...	150	4.0	16.0	8.0	0	230	<1.0
(*Cheese Nips*), 29 pcs., 1.1 oz.	150	3.0	18.0	6.0	0	310	<1.0
(*Cheese Nips* Reduced Fat), 31 pcs., 1.1 oz.	130	3.0	21.0	3.5	0	310	<1.0
(*Cheese Nips Air Crisps*), 32 pcs., 1.1 oz.	130	3.0	21.0	4.0	<5	300	<1.0
(*Cheez-It*), 27 pcs., 1.1 oz.	160	4.0	16.0	8.0	0	240	<1.0
(*Cheez-It* Low Sodium), 27 pcs., 1.1 oz.	160	4.0	16.0	8.0	0	70	<1.0
(*Cheez-It Lowfat*), 29 pcs., 1.1 oz.	140	4.0	20.0	4.5	0	280	<1.0
(*SnackWell's* Zesty), 38 pcs., 1.1 oz.	130	2.0	23.0	3.0	0	310	<1.0
(*Tid Bits*), 32 pcs., 1.1 oz.	160	2.0	16.0	9.0	0	360	<1.0
hot, spicy (*Cheez-It*), 26 pcs., 1.1 oz.	160	3.0	17.0	8.0	0	220	<1.0
nacho (*Cheez-It*), 28 pcs., 1.1 oz.	150	3.0	18.0	7.0	0	280	<1.0

Food and Measure	cal.	prot. (gms)	carbo. (gms)	fat (gms)	chol. (mgs)	sod. (mgs)	fiber (gms)
pizza (*Cheese Nips*), 29 pcs., 1.1 oz.	140	3.0	19.0	6.0	0	330	<1.0
and sesame (*Twigs*), 15 pcs., 1.1 oz.	150	4.0	17.0	7.0	0	300	<1.0
Swiss (*Nabisco*), 15 pcs., 1.1 oz.	140	2.0	18.0	7.0	0	350	<1.0
whole wheat (*Health Valley*), 5 pcs.	50	2.0	11.0	0	0	100	2.0
cheese sandwich: (*Handi-Snacks*), 1.1-oz. pkg.	130	4.0	10.0	8.0	15	340	0
(*Ritz Bits*), 14 pcs., 1.1 oz.	170	2.0	17.0	10.0	5	300	0
cheddar (*Frito-Lay*), 1.3-oz. pkg.	200	5.0	27.0	10.0	<5	530	1.0
cheddar (*Keebler Club*), 1.3-oz. pkg.	190	3.0	20.0	11.0	10	320	<1.0
cheddar (*Keebler Townhouse*), 1.3-oz. pkg.	200	3.0	19.0	13.0	10	300	<1.0
cheesy (*Chee•tos*), 1 pkg.	210	3.0	23.0	11.0	<5	340	1.0
w/bacon (*Chee•tos*), 1 pkg.	190	3.0	25.0	9.0	<5	410	1.0
nacho (*Doritos Cheesier*), 1 pkg.	240	4.0	25.0	14.0	<5	340	1.0
w/peanut butter (*Keebler*), 1.3-oz. pkg.	190	6.0	22.0	9.0	<5	420	<1.0
w/peanut butter (*Peter Pan* Cheese), 1 pkg.	210	5.0	23.0	11.0	0	280	1.0
spicy (*Doritos*), 1 pkg.	230	3.0	26.0	14.0	<5	450	1.0
(*Chicken In A Biskit*), 12 pcs., 1.1 oz. ...	160	2.0	17.0	9.0	0	270	<1.0
croissant (*Carr's*), 3 pcs., ½ oz.	70	1.0	10.0	3.0	<5	115	0

Food and Measure	cal.	prot. (gms)	carbo. (gms)	fat (gms)	chol. (mgs)	sod. (mgs)	fiber (gms)
Cracker *(cont.)*							
garlic, roasted: (*Health Valley Low Fat*), 6 pcs.	60	2.0	10.0	1.5	0	90	2.0
garlic herb (*Barbara's* Wafer Crisps), 3 pcs., ½ oz.	60	1.0	12.0	1.0	0	140	<1.0
(*Goldfish* Original), 55 pcs., 1.1 oz. . . .	140	3.0	19.0	6.0	0	230	<1.0
(*Goya*), 1 pc., .3 oz.	40	1.0	6.0	1.0	0	80	0
graham cracker, see "Cookie"							
hazelnut (*Blue Diamond* Nut Thins), 16 pcs., 1.1 oz. . . .	120	2.0	20.0	4.0	0	75	1.0
herb:							
garden (*Triscuit*), 6 pcs., 1 oz.	130	3.0	20.0	4.5	0	135	3.0
Italian (*Harvest Crisp*), 13 pcs., 1 oz.	130	3.0	22.0	3.5	0	320	1.0
whole wheat (*Health Valley*), 5 pcs. . . .	50	2.0	11.0	0	0	80	2.0
jalapeño, mild (*Health Valley*), 6 pcs.	60	2.0	10.0	1.5	0	90	2.0
matzo:							
(*Manischewitz* Everything!), 12 pcs., 1 oz. . . .	110	3.0	22.0	.5	0	150	1.0
(*Manischewitz* No Salt), 1-oz. pc.	110	3.0	24.0	0	0	0	0
garlic (*Manischewitz*), 12 pcs., 1 oz.	100	3.0	23.0	0	0	200	1.0
Passover (*Manischewitz* Tam Tam), 10 pcs., 1.1 oz.	140	3.0	22.0	4.0	10	100	<1.0
thins (*Manischewitz*), .8-oz. pc.	90	2.0	20.0	0	0	0	0

Food and Measure	cal.	prot. (gms)	carbo. (gms)	fat (gms)	chol. (mgs)	sod. (mgs)	fiber (gms)
multigrain:							
(*Harvest Crisp*),							
13 pcs., 1.1 oz.	130	3.0	23.0	3.5	0	270	1.0
(*Saltines*), 5 pcs.,							
½ oz.	60	1.0	10.0	1.5	0	150	<1.0
(*Munch'ems*), 35 pcs.,							
1.1 oz.	130	2.0	21.0	4.0	0	450	<1.0
nori maki (*Eden*),							
15 pcs., 1.1 oz. . . .	110	3.0	24.0	0	0	160	2.0
oat bran (*Health Valley*), 6 pcs.	120	3.0	22.0	3.0	0	80	3.0
onion:							
(*Toasteds*), 5 pcs.,							
.6 oz.	80	1.0	10.0	3.0	0	230	0
French (*Barbara's* Wafer Crisps),							
3 pcs., ½ oz.	60	1.0	12.0	1.0	0	140	<1.0
French (*SnackWell's*),							
38 pcs., 1.1 oz.	130	2.0	23.0	3.0	0	270	<1.0
French (*Triscuit* Thin Crisps), 14 pcs.,							
1.1 oz.	130	3.0	20.0	4.5	0	160	3.0
whole wheat (*Health Valley*), 5 pcs. . . .	50	2.0	11.0	0	0	80	2.0
Parmesan (*Goldfish*),							
60 pcs., 1.1 oz. . . .	140	4.0	19.0	5.0	0	300	1.0
peanut butter sandwich:							
(*Handi-Snacks*),							
1.1-oz. pkg.	130	5.0	12.0	12.0	0	150	1.0
(*Ritz Bits*), 14 pcs.,							
1.1 oz.	150	3.0	18.0	8.0	0	200	1.0
cheese, see "cheese sandwich," above							
toast (*Keebler*),							
1 pkg.	190	5.0	23.0	9.0	0	300	1.0
toast (*Keebler* Reduced Fat), 1 pkg.	170	4.0	23.0	7.0	0	450	<1.0
toast (*Peter Pan*),							
1 pkg.	210	5.0	23.0	11.0	0	280	<1.0

Food and Measure	cal.	prot. (gms)	carbo. (gms)	fat (gms)	chol. (mgs)	sod. (mgs)	fiber (gms)
Cracker *(cont.)*							
pecan (*Blue Diamond Nut Thins*), 16 pcs., 1.1 oz.	130	2.0	20.0	5.0	0	75	<1.0
pizza flavor:							
(*Goldfish*), 55 pcs., 1.1 oz.	140	3.0	19.0	6.0	0	160	1.0
all varieties (*Health Valley* Healthy Pizza), 6 pcs. . . .	50	2.0	11.0	0	0	140	2.0
potato:							
barbecue (*Air Crisps*), 22 pcs., 1 oz.	120	2.0	21.0	3.5	0	220	1.0
ranch (*Air Crisps*), 23 pcs., 1.1 oz.	140	2.0	21.0	4.5	0	290	1.0
pretzel (*Air Crisps*), 23 pcs., 1 oz.	110	2.0	23.0	0	0	550	<1.0
ranch, 1.1 oz.:							
(*Munch'ems*), 33 pcs.	130	3.0	21.0	4.0	0	310	<1.0
(*SnackWell's*), 38 pcs.	130	2.0	28.0	3.0	0	320	<1.0
(*Wheatables*), 25 pcs.	150	3.0	16.0	7.0	0	310	1.0
(*Wheatables* Reduced Fat), 29 pcs.	130	3.0	21.0	4.0	0	340	1.0
rice:							
bran (*Health Valley*), 6 pcs.	110	3.0	19.0	3.0	0	70	3.0
brown (*Eden*), 5 pcs., 1.1 oz. . . .	120	2.0	22.0	2.0	0	230	2.0
salsa (*Munch'ems* Southwest), 28 pcs., 1.1 oz.	130	2.0	23.0	4.0	0	260	1.0
saltines, 5 pcs., 1/2 oz.:							
(*Krispy*)	60	2.0	10.0	1.5	0	180	<1.0
(*Krispy* Fat Free) . . .	50	1.0	11.0	0	0	150	0
(*Krispy* Unsalted)	60	2.0	10.0	1.5	0	120	<1.0
(*Saltines*)	60	1.0	10.0	1.5	0	180	0

Food and Measure	cal.	prot. (gms)	carbo. (gms)	fat (gms)	chol. (mgs)	sod. (mgs)	fiber (gms)
(*Saltines* Fat Free)	60	2.0	12.0	0	0	180	0
(*Saltines* Unsalted)	60	1.0	10.0	1.5	0	105	0
(*Zesta*)	60	1.0	10.0	2.0	0	190	<1.0
(*Zesta* Fat Free)	50	1.0	11.0	0	0	150	0
(*Zesta* Low Salt) . . .	70	1.0	11.0	2.0	0	95	<1.0
(*Zesta* Unsalted) . . .	70	1.0	10.0	2.0	0	90	<1.0
sandwich (*Chee•tos* Golden Toast), 1 pkg.	240	4.0	25.0	14.0	5	440	1.0
sesame: (*Pepperidge Farm*), 3 pcs., ½ oz.	70	1.0	9.0	2.5	0	95	2.0
(*Toasteds*), 5 pcs., .6 oz.	80	1.0	10.0	3.5	0	160	<1.0
(*Toasteds Reduced Fat*), 5 pcs., ½ oz.	60	1.0	10.0	2.0	0	160	<1.0
toast (*Barbara's* Wafer Crisp), 3 pcs., ½ oz.	60	1.0	11.0	1.5	0	135	<1.0
(*Sociables*), 7 pcs., ½ oz.	80	1.0	9.0	4.0	0	150	0
soda/water: (*Crown Pilot*), .6-oz. pc.	70	2.0	13.0	1.5	0	85	0
(*Export*), 3 pcs., ½ oz.	60	1.0	10.0	2.0	0	80	<1.0
(*Royal Lunch*), .4-oz. pc.	60	<1.0	8.0	2.0	0	70	0
cracked pepper (*Carr's*), 5 pcs., .6 oz.	70	2.0	13.0	1.5	0	100	<1.0
cracked pepper (*SnackWell's*), 5 pcs., ½ oz.	60	1.0	10.0	1.5	0	115	0
poppy-sesame seeds (*Carr's*), 4 pcs., .6 oz.	80	2.0	9.0	5.0	<5	135	<1.0
roasted garlic and herbs (*Carr's*), 5 pcs., .6 oz.	70	2.0	13.0	1.5	0	140	<1.0

Food and Measure	cal.	prot. (gms)	carbo. (gms)	fat (gms)	chol. (mgs)	sod. (mgs)	fiber (gms)
Cracker *(cont.)*							
soup and oyster:							
(*Zesta*), 45 pcs.,							
½ oz.	70	1.0	9.0	3.0	0	220	0
sour cream–onion,							
1.1 oz.:							
(*Munch'ems*),							
28 pcs.	140	3.0	19.0	6.0	0	330	<1.0
(*Munch'ems* Re-							
duced Fat),							
33 pcs.	130	2.0	22.0	3.5	0	390	0
(*Ritz Air Crisps*),							
23 pcs.	140	2.0	22.0	5.0	0	310	<1.0
sun-dried tomato-basil							
(*Barbara's* Wafer							
Crisp), 3 pcs., ½ oz.	60	1.0	12.0	1.0	0	140	<1.0
(*Uneeda* Biscuit),							
2 pcs., ½ oz.	60	1.0	11.0	1.5	0	110	0
vegetable:							
(*Nabisco Thins*),							
14 pcs., 1.1 oz.	160	2.0	19.0	9.0	0	310	1.0
garden (*Harvest*							
Crisp), 15 pcs.,							
1.1 oz.	130	2.0	22.0	3.5	0	230	1.0
garden (*Wheat-*							
ables), 25 pcs.,							
1.1 oz.	140	3.0	18.0	7.0	0	310	3.0
whole wheat (*Health*							
Valley), 5 pcs. . . .	50	2.0	11.0	0	0	80	2.0
wheat:							
(*Pepperidge Farm*							
Hearty), 3 pcs.,							
.6 oz.	80	2.0	10.0	3.5	0	100	1.0
(*SnackWell's*),							
5 pcs., ½ oz.	70	1.0	11.0	1.5	0	160	<1.0
(*Toasteds*), 5 pcs.,							
.6 oz.	80	1.0	11.0	3.0	0	160	0
(*Toasteds* Reduced							
Fat), 5 pcs., ½ oz.	60	1.0	10.0	2.0	0	160	<1.0
(*Triscuit* Low So-							
dium), 7 pcs.,							
1.1 oz.	140	3.0	22.0	5.0	0	75	4.0

Food and Measure	cal.	prot. (gms)	carbo. (gms)	fat (gms)	chol. (mgs)	sod. (mgs)	fiber (gms)
(*Triscuit* Original), 7 pcs., 1.1 oz. . . .	140	3.0	21.0	5.0	0	170	4.0
(*Triscuit* Reduced Fat), 8 pcs., 1.2 oz.	130	3.0	24.0	3.0	0	180	4.0
(*Triscuit* Thin Crisps), 15 pcs., 1.1 oz.	130	3.0	21.0	5.0	0	170	3.0
(*Waverly*), 5 pcs., ½ oz.	70	1.0	10.0	3.5	0	135	0
(*Wheat Thins* Air Crisps), 24 pcs., 1.1 oz.	130	2.0	21.0	4.5	0	290	1.0
(*Wheat Thins* Big), 11 pcs., 1.1 oz.	140	3.0	20.0	6.0	0	260	1.0
(*Wheat Thins* Low Sodium), 16 pcs., 1.1 oz.	140	2.0	20.0	6.0	0	75	2.0
(*Wheat Thins* Multigrain), 17 pcs., 1.1 oz.	130	2.0	21.0	4.0	0	290	2.0
(*Wheat Thins* Original), 16 pcs., .8 oz	140	2.0	19.0	6.0	0	180	2.0
(*Wheat Thins* Reduced Fat), 18 pcs., 1 oz. . . .	120	2.0	21.0	4.0	0	220	2.0
(*Wheatables*), 26 pcs., 1.1 oz.	150	3.0	18.0	7.0	0	320	1.0
(*Wheatables* 50% Reduced Fat), 29 pcs., 1.1 oz.	130	3.0	21.0	3.5	0	320	1.0
(*Wheatables* Reduced Fat), 27 pcs., 1.1 oz.	130	3.0	21.0	4.0	0	330	<1.0
(*Wheatsworth*), 5 pcs., .6 oz.	80	2.0	10.0	3.5	0	170	1.0
all varieties (*Barbara's Wheatines*), ½-oz. sq.	50	<1.0	10.0	1.5	0	110	0

Food and Measure	cal.	prot. (gms)	carbo. (gms)	fat (gms)	chol. (mgs)	sod. (mgs)	fiber (gms)
Cracker, wheat *(cont.)*							
cracked (*Pepperidge Farm*), 2 pcs., ½ oz.	70	1.0	9.0	2.5	0	150	<1.0
wheat, whole:							
(*Health Valley*), 5 pcs.	50	2.0	11.0	0	0	80	2.0
(*Hi Ho*), 4 pcs., ½ oz.	70	1.0	8.0	3.5	0	125	<1.0
(*Krispy*), 5 pcs., ½ oz.	60	2.0	10.0	1.5	0	130	<1.0
zweiback (*Nabisco*), 1 pc., .3 oz.	35	1.0	6.0	1.0	0	10	0
Cracker crumbs and meal, ¼ cup, except as noted:							
crumbs:							
(*Ritz*), ⅓ cup	140	2.0	17.0	7.0	0	270	1.0
graham cracker (*Sunshine*), 3 tbsp.	80	2.0.	13.0	2.0	0	150	<1.0
saltine (*Premium* Fat Free)	100	3.0	23.0	0	0	0	1.0
meal:							
(*Nabisco*)	110	3.0	22.0	0	0	15	<1.0
matzo (*Manische-witz*)	130	3.0	27.0	.5	0	0	0
matzo (*Streit's*)	110	3.0	24.0	.5	0	0	1.0
Cranberry, fresh:							
(*Ocean Spray*), 2 oz.	25	0	6.0	0	0	0	0
whole, ½ cup	23	.2	6.0	.1	0	1	2.0
chopped, ½ cup	27	.2	7.0	.1	0	1	2.3
Cranberry, dried, ⅓ cup, 1.4 oz.:							
(*Craisins*)	130	0	33.0	0	0	0	2.0
(*Frieda's*)	120	0	28.0	0	0	0	3.0
(*L'Esprit*)	131	0	36.0	0	0	0	0
(*Sonoma*)	120	0	29.0	0	0	0	2.0
Cranberry beans:							
boiled, ½ cup	120	8.2	21.5	.4	0	1	3.0
canned, ½ cup	108	7.2	19.7	.4	0	431	n.a.

Food and Measure	cal.	prot. (gms)	carbo. (gms)	fat (gms)	chol. (mgs)	sod. (mgs)	fiber (gms)
Cranberry drink, see "Cranberry juice cocktail"							
Cranberry drink, mix* (*Crystal Light Cranberry Breeze*), 8 fl. oz.	5	0	0	0	0	0	0
Cranberry drink blend, 8 fl. oz., except as noted:							
apple:							
(*Cranapple*)	160	0	41.0	0	0	35	1.0
(*Tropicana Twister*)	140	0	34.0	0	0	30	0
reduced calorie (*Cranapple*)	50	0	13.0	0	0	35	0
apricot (*Cranicot*)	160	0	40.0	0	0	35	0
(*Cran•Blueberry*)	160	0	41.0	0	0	35	0
(*Cran•Cherry*)	160	0	39.0	0	0	35	0
(*Cran•Currant*)	140	0	33.0	0	0	35	0
(*Cran•Strawberry*) . . .	140	0	36.0	0	0	35	1.0
(*Cran•Tangerine*)	130	0	33.0	0	0	35	0
grape:							
(*Cran•Grape*)	170	0	41.0	0	0	35	0
(*Cran•Grape Lightstyle*)	40	0	9.0	0	0	75	0
guava nectar (*Santa Cruz* Organic)	110	0	24.0	0	0	25	0
hibiscus: (*R.W. Knudsen*)	120	0	30.0	0	0	35	0
lemon (*Santa Cruz* Organic)	120	0	29.0	0	0	35	0
mango:							
(*Cran•Mango*)	130	0	33.0	0	0	35	0
(*Cran•Mango Lightstyle*)	40	0	10.0	0	0	75	0
nectar (*Santa Cruz* Organic)	110	0	27.0	0	0	25	0
punch (*Tropicana Twister*), 10 fl. oz.	170	0	43.0	0	0	20	0
raspberry:							
(*Cran•Raspberry*)	140	0	36.0	0	0	35	0

Food and Measure	cal.	prot. (gms)	carbo. (gms)	fat (gms)	chol. (mgs)	sod. (mgs)	fiber (gms)
Cranberry drink blend, raspberry *(cont.)*							
(*Cran•Raspberry* Reduced Calorie)	50	0	13.0	0	0	35	0
(*Cran•Raspberry* Lightstyle)	40	0	10.0	0	0	35	0
(*R.W. Knudsen*) . . .	140	0	36.0	0	0	35	0
(*Snapple* Diet)	10	0	2.0	0	0	10	0
(*Veryfine*)	160	0	41.0	0	0	10	0
strawberry (*Tropicana Twister*)	120	0	31.0	0	0	5	0
strawberry (*Tropicana Twister* Light)	35	0	8.0	0	0	70	0
Cranberry juice, 8 fl. oz., except as noted:							
(*After the Fall* Cape Cod)	100	0	24.0	0	0	20	0
(*After the Fall* Nantucket)	60	1.0	15.0	0	0	25	0
(*Apple & Eve*)	120	1.0	30.0	0	0	20	0
(*R.W. Knudsen* Just Cranberry)	60	0	14.0	0	0	25	0
(*R.W. Knudsen* Yankee)	120	0	30.0	0	0	25	0
(*Season's Best* Cocktail)	140	0	34.0	0	0	35	0
(*Snapple* Royale), 10 fl. oz.	150	0	37.0	0	0	25	0
(*Wellfleet Farms*)	130	0	33.0	0	0	35	0
concentrate* (*R.W. Knudsen*)	70	0	13.0	0	0	15	0
Cranberry juice blend, 8 fl. oz., except as noted:							
(*Apple & Eve* Ruby Red)	120	1.0	30.0	0	0	10	.5
(*Season's Best* Medley)	120	<1.0	29.0	0	0	25	0
apple:							
(*Dole*)	120	0	30.0	0	0	35	0

Food and Measure	cal.	prot. (gms)	carbo. (gms)	fat (gms)	chol. (mgs)	sod. (mgs)	fiber (gms)
(*Snapple*), 12 fl. oz.	200	0	51.0	0	0	20	0
(*Wellfleet Farms Granny Smith*) ...	130	0	33.0	0	0	35	0
grape (*Apple & Eve*), 10 fl. oz.	175	1.0	42.0	0	0	31	0
grapefruit (*After the Fall Ruby of the Cape*)	110	1.0	29.0	0	0	10	0
kiwi (*After the Fall Ruby of the Cape*)	100	1.0	26.0	0	0	18	0
lime, key (*Wellfleet Farms*)	140	0	35.0	0	0	35	0
mango (*After the Fall Ruby of the Cape*)	110	1.0	26.0	0	0	15	0
orange (*After the Fall Ruby of the Cape*)	110	1.0	28.0	0	0	15	0
peach (*Wellfleet Farms Georgia*)	140	0	35.0	0	0	35	0
raspberry (*After the Fall*)	100	1.0	23.0	0	0	20	0
strawberry (*After the Fall Ruby of the Cape*)	100	1.0	26.0	0	0	15	0
Cranberry juice cock- tail, 8 fl. oz., except as noted:							
(*Ocean Spray*)	140	0	34.0	0	0	35	0
(*Ocean Spray Reduced Calorie*)	50	0	13.0	0	0	35	0
(*Ocean Spray Light- style*)	40	0	10.0	0	0	75	0
(*Veryfine*)	160	0	39.0	0	0	10	0
(*Veryfine*), 10 fl. oz.	200	0	49.0	0	0	10	0
Cranberry nectar (*R.W. Knudsen*), 8 fl. oz.	150	1.0	38.0	0	0	45	0
Cranberry sauce, canned, ¼ cup:							
whole (*Ocean Spray*)	110	0	28.0	0	0	35	1.0
jellied (*Ocean Spray*)	110	0	27.0	0	0	35	1.0

Food and Measure	cal.	prot. (gms)	carbo. (gms)	fat (gms)	chol. (mgs)	sod. (mgs)	fiber (gms)
Cranberry sauce blend, 1/4 cup:							
w/orange (*Cran•Fruit*)	120	0	29.0	0	0	35	1.0
w/raspberry or strawberry (*Cran•Fruit*)	120	0	29.0	0	0	35	2.0
Cranberry-orange relish, in jars (*New England*), 1/4 cup	120	0	31.0	0	0	0	0
Crayfish, mixed species, meat only:							
farmed:							
raw, 4 oz.	82	16.9	0	1.1	122	70	0
boiled or steamed, 4 oz.	99	19.9	0	1.5	155	110	0
wild:							
raw, 4 oz.	87	18.1	0	1.1	130	66	0
raw, 8 medium, 1 oz.	22	4.5	0	.3	32	16	0
boiled or steamed, 4 oz.	100	19.0	0	1.4	151	107	0
Cream (see also "Crème fraîche"):							
all-purpose (*Hood*), 1 tbsp.	45	0	<1.0	4.5	20	5	0
half-and-half:							
(*Hood*), 2 tbsp.	40	1.0	1.0	3.5	15	20	0
1 cup	315	7.2	10.4	27.8	89	98	0
1 tbsp.	20	.4	.6	1.7	6	6	0
light, coffee or table:							
(*Hood*), 1 tbsp.	30	0	<1.0	3.0	10	10	0
1 cup	469	6.5	8.8	46.3	159	95	0
1 tbsp.	29	.4	.6	2.9	10	6	0
medium (25% fat):							
1 cup	583	5.9	8.3	59.8	209	88	0
1 tbsp.	37	.4	.5	3.8	13	6	0
sour, see "Cream, sour"							
whipped topping, see "Cream topping"							

Food and Measure	cal.	prot. (gms)	carbo. (gms)	fat (gms)	chol. (mgs)	sod. (mgs)	fiber (gms)
whipping[1], light:							
1 cup	699	5.2	7.1	73.9	265	82	0
1 tbsp.	44	.3	.4	4.6	17	5	0
whipping[1], heavy:							
(*Hood*), 1 tbsp.	50	0	0	5.0	20	0	0
1 cup	821	4.9	6.6	88.1	326	89	0
1 tbsp.	52	.3	.4	5.6	21	6	0
Cream, sour, 2 tbsp., except as noted:							
(*Breakstone's*)	60	1.0	1.0	5.0	25	15	0
(*Friendship*)	60	1.0	1.0	5.0	20	15	0
(*Heluva* Good)	60	1.0	2.0	5.0	20	15	0
(*Hood*)	60	1.0	2.0	5.0	20	20	0
(*Knudsen Hampshire*)	60	1.0	1.0	6.0	25	15	0
(*Land O Lakes*)	60	1.0	2.0	6.0	15	15	0
(*Sealtest*)	60	<1.0	1.0	5.0	20	15	0
1 cup	493	7.3	9.8	48.2	102	123	0
half-and-half (*Break-stone's*)	45	1.0	2.0	3.5	15	20	0
light:							
(*Friendship*)	40	1.0	3.0	1.5	10	25	0
(*Heluva* Good)	40	1.0	3.0	2.5	10	20	0
(*Hood*)	35	1.0	3.0	1.5	5	20	0
(*Knudsen Light*) ...	40	2.0	2.0	2.5	10	20	0
(*Land O Lakes*)	35	1.0	4.0	2.0	10	30	0
(*Sealtest Light*)	40	2.0	2.0	2.5	10	20	0
nonfat:							
(*Breakstone's Free*)	35	2.0	6.0	0	<5	25	0
(*Friendship*)	25	2.0	4.0	0	0	20	0
(*Heluva* Good)	20	1.0	3.0	0	0	45	0
(*Hood*)	25	1.0	4.0	0	0	25	0
(*Knudsen Free*)	35	2.0	6.0	0	0	25	0
(*Land O Lakes*)	30	1.0	5.0	0	<5	40	0
(*Sealtest Free*)	35	2.0	6.0	0	<5	25	0
Cream, sour, fla-vored, 2 tbsp.:							
roasted garlic (*Friend-ship*)	60	1.0	2.0	5.0	20	130	0
salsa (*Friendship*)	60	1.0	2.0	4.0	20	130	0

[1] *Unwhipped; volume approximately doubled when whipped.*

Food and Measure	cal.	prot. (gms)	carbo. (gms)	fat (gms)	chol. (mgs)	sod. (mgs)	fiber (gms)
Cream, sour, powder							
(*AlpineAire*), 2 oz.	310	13.0	20.0	20.0	80	200	0
Cream cheese dip,							
fruit, 2 tbsp.:							
(*Marzetti* Fruit Dip) . . .	70	1.0	10.0	3.0	10	85	0
brown sugar cinna-							
mon (*Marzetti* Fruit							
Dip)	70	0	10.0	4.0	15	95	0
Cream of tartar							
(*Tone's*), 1 tsp.	2	0	.6	0	0	n.a.	0
Cream topping,							
2 tbsp.:							
(*Cool Whip* Extra							
Creamy)	30	0	2.0	2.0	10	5	0
(*Cool Whip* Lite)	20	0	2.0	1.0	0	0	0
(*Cool Whip* Nondairy)	25	0	0	1.5	0	0	0
(*Hood*)	20	0	1.0	1.5	5	0	0
(*Hood* Light)	15	0	1.0	.5	<5	0	0
(*Kraft* Real)	20	0	1.0	1.5	5	0	0
(*Kraft* Whipped)	20	0	1.0	1.5	0	0	0
(*La Creme* Lite)	15	0	2.0	1.0	0	10	0
(*Pet Whip*)	30	0	2.0	2.0	0	0	0
(*Reddi-wip* Extra							
Creamy)	30	0	<1.0	3.0	10	0	0
(*Reddi-wip* Original)	20	0	<1.0	2.0	5	0	0
mix*:							
(*D-Zerta*)	10	0	1.0	1.0	0	10	0
(*Dream Whip*)	20	0	2.0	1.0	0	10	0
Creamer, nondairy:							
fluid, 1 tbsp.:							
(*Coffee-mate*)	20	0	2.0	1.0	0	0	0
(*Coffee-mate* Fat							
Free)	10	0	1.0	0	0	0	0
(*Coffee-mate* Lite)	10	0	1.0	.5	0	5	0
(*Hood*)	20	0	2.0	1.5	0	0	0
powder, 1 tsp.							
(*Coffee-mate*)	10	0	1.0	.5	0	0	0
(*Coffee-mate* Fat							
Free)	10	0	2.0	0	0	0	0
(*N-Rich*)	10	0	1.0	0	0	0	0

Food and Measure	cal.	prot. (gms)	carbo. (gms)	fat (gms)	chol. (mgs)	sod. (mgs)	fiber (gms)
Creamer, nondairy, flavored:							
fluid, all varieties (*Coffee-mate*), 1 tbsp.	40	0	5.0	2.0	0	5	0
powder, 1⅓ tbsp.:							
all varieties (*Coffee-mate*)	60	0	9.0	3.0	0	15	0
all varieties (*Coffee-mate* Lite)	10	0	2.0	0	0	0	0
Crème fraîche (*Santè*), 2 tbsp. ...	100	<1.0	<1.0	11.0	40	10	0
Cress, garden, ½ cup:							
raw	8	.7	1.4	.2	0	4	.3
boiled, drained	16	1.3	2.6	.4	0	5	.5
Cress, water, see "Watercress"							
Croaker, meat only, raw, Atlantic, 4 oz.	119	20.2	0	3.6	69	63	0
Croissant, 1 pc.:							
butter:							
(*Awrey's*), 1½ oz.	140	3.0	13.0	9.0	25	230	0
(*Awrey's*), 2 oz. ...	190	4.0	17.0	12.0	35	310	<1.0
(*Awrey's* Tip-to-Tip), 3 oz.	290	6.0	26.0	18.0	55	470	<1.0
(*Pepperidge Farm* Petite)	130	3.0	13.0	8.0	20	180	<1.0
dill and onion (*Awrey's*), 2½ oz.	210	5.0	24.0	10.0	0	180	1.0
margarine:							
(*Awrey's* Sandwich), 1.8 oz.	180	3.0	17.0	11.0	0	170	<1.0
(*Awrey's* Sandwich), 2½ oz.	250	5.0	23.0	15.0	0	230	<1.0
(*Awrey's* Tip-to-Tip), ¾ oz.	140	2.0	14.0	8.0	0	140	0
wheat (*Awrey's* Sandwich), 2½ oz.	250	5.0	22.0	15.0	0	220	1.0
pesto Parmesan (*Awrey's*), 2½ oz.	210	5.0	23.0	11.0	5	270	<1.0

Food and Measure	cal.	prot. (gms)	carbo. (gms)	fat (gms)	chol. (mgs)	sod. (mgs)	fiber (gms)
Croissant, frozen:							
French style (*Sara Lee*), 1 pc.	170	4.0	20.0	8.0	<5	200	1.0
French style, petite (*Sara Lee*), 2 pcs.	230	6.0	26.0	11.0	<5	260	1.0
Crookneck squash:							
fresh, sliced, 1/2 cup:							
raw, ends trimmed	12	.6	2.6	.2	0	1	.7
boiled, drained	18	.8	3.9	.3	0	1	1.3
canned, cut, drained, no salt, 1/2 cup	14	.7	3.2	.1	0	5	1.1
frozen, boiled, sliced, 1/2 cup	24	1.2	5.3	.2	0	6	1.2
Croutons (see also "Salad toppers"):							
Caesar:							
(*Brownberry*), 2 tbsp.	30	1.0	4.0	1.5	0	80	<1.0
(*Brownberry* Fat Free), 1/4 cup	30	1.0	5.0	0	0	85	<1.0
(*Chatham Village*), 2 tbsp.	35	1.0	4.0	1.5	0	50	0
(*Pepperidge Farm*), 6 pcs., 1/4 oz.	35	1.0	4.0	1.5	0	90	0
cheddar and Romano (*Pepperidge Farm*), 9 pcs., 1/4 oz.	30	1.0	4.0	1.0	0	95	0
cracked pepper and Parmesan (*Pepperidge Farm*), 6 pcs., 1/4 oz.	35	1.0	4.0	1.5	0	90	0
garden herb (*Brownberry* Fat Free), 1/4 cup	30	1.0	5.0	0	0	95	<1.0
garlic butter or garden herb (*Chatham Village*), 2 tbsp.	35	1.0	4.0	1.5	0	55	0
garlic herb (*Arnold* Home Style), 1/4 cup	30	1.0	5.0	1.0	0	80	<1.0

Food and Measure	cal.	prot. (gms)	carbo. (gms)	fat (gms)	chol. (mgs)	sod. (mgs)	fiber (gms)
Italian, zesty:							
(*Arnold Home Style*), 1/4 cup	30	1.0	5.0	1.0	0	60	<1.0
(*Pepperidge Farm*), 9 pcs., 1/4 oz.	35	1.0	4.0	1.5	<5	65	0
olive oil–garlic (*Pepperidge Farm*), 6 pcs., 1/4 oz.	30	1.0	5.0	1.0	0	80	0
onion and garlic:							
(*Brownberry*), 2 tbsp.	30	1.0	5.0	1.0	0	75	<1.0
(*Pepperidge Farm*), 9 pcs., 1/4 oz.	30	1.0	5.0	1.0	0	80	0
ranch:							
(*Brownberry*), 2 tbsp.	30	1.0	5.0	1.0	0	90	<1.0
(*Pepperidge Farm*), 9 pcs., 1/4 oz.	35	1.0	4.0	1.5	<5	65	0
seasoned:							
(*Arnold* Classic), 2 tbsp.	30	1.0	5.0	1.0	0	75	<1.0
(*Pepperidge Farm*), 9 pcs., 1/4 oz.	35	1.0	4.0	1.5	0	85	0
sourdough cheese (*Pepperidge Farm*), 6 pcs., 1/4 oz.	30	1.0	4.0	1.0	0	80	0
sun-dried tomato (*Chatham Village* Fat Free), 2 tbsp.	30	1.0	5.0	0	0	90	0
Cruller, see "Donut"							
Cucumber, w/peel:							
1 medium, 81/4″ long	38	2.1	8.3	.4	0	6	2.4
sliced, 1/2 cup	7	.4	1.4	.1	0	1	.4
Cucumber, Japanese or hothouse (*Frieda's*), 2/3 cup, 3 oz.	10	1.0	2.0	0	0	0	1.0
Cucumber, pickled, see "Pickle"							

Food and Measure	cal.	prot. (gms)	carbo. (gms)	fat (gms)	chol. (mgs)	sod. (mgs)	fiber (gms)
Cucumber dip, creamy (*Kraft Premium*), 2 tbsp.	50	<1.0	2.0	4.0	10	160	0
Cucumber-dill dip mix, dry (*Watkins*), 1 tsp.	10	0	2.0	0	0	210	0
Cucuzza squash (*Frieda's*), ¾ cup, 3 oz.	10	1.0	3.0	0	0	0	0
Cumin seed, ground: 1 tsp.	8	.4	.9	.5	0	4	.2
Cupcake, see "Cake, snack"							
Currant, ½ cup, except as noted:							
fresh, black, Europe	36	.8	8.6	.2	0	1	3.0
fresh, red or white ...	31	.8	7.7	.1	0	1	2.4
dried, zante:							
½ cup	204	2.9	53.3	.2	0	6	4.9
(*Sun•Maid*), ¼ cup	130	1.0	31.0	0	0	10	2.0
Curry oil, see "Oil"							
Curry paste:							
(*Patak's*), 2 tbsp.	170	2.0	4.0	16.0	5	900	0
red (*Thai Kitchen*), 1 tbsp.	10	0	2.0	0	0	140	0
Curry powder:							
1 tbsp.	20	.8	3.7	.9	0	3	1.0
1 tsp.	6	.3	1.2	.3	0	1	.3
Curry sauce, cooking:							
(*Kylin Thai*), ¼ cup ...	25	1.0	5.0	.5	0	600	<1.0
(*Thai Kitchen Thai Tonight* Bangkok), ½ cup	60	0	4.0	4.0	0	600	0
hot, ½ cup:							
Madras (*Patak's*)	300	4.0	17.0	25.0	5	1330	5.0
vindaloo (*Patak's*)	320	4.0	16.0	27.0	<5	1540	5.0
Jalfrezzi (*Patak's*), ½ cup	160	3.0	15.0	10.0	0	430	4.0
Masala, ¼ cup:							
(*Shahi* Cream)	50	1.0	5.0	4.0	0	550	1.0
(*Shahi* Curry)	50	1.0	4.0	4.0	0	680	1.0

Food and Measure	cal.	prot. (gms)	carbo. (gms)	fat (gms)	chol. (mgs)	sod. (mgs)	fiber (gms)
spinach (*Shahi*) ...	40	1.0	3.0	2.5	0	550	1.0
tikka (*Patak's*)	240	4.0	14.0	18.0	10	1390	3.0
red or green (*Thai Kitchen Thai Tonight*), ½ cup	60	0	4.0	4.0	0	600	0
Rogan Josh (*Patak's*), ½ cup	190	3.0	12.0	15.0	<5	1270	4.0
Curry sauce, Thai, green (*Ka•Me*), 1 tbsp.	10	0	2.0	0	0	440	0
Curry sauce, w/vegetables, see "Vegetable entree, packaged"							
Cusk, meat only:							
raw, 4 oz.	99	21.6	0	.8	47	36	0
baked, broiled, or microwaved, 4 oz. ...	127	27.6	0	1.0	60	45	0
Custard, see "Pudding"							
Custard apple, trimmed, 1 oz.	29	.5	7.1	.2	0	1	1.0
Custard marrow, see "Chayote"							
Cuttlefish, meat only:							
raw, 4 oz.	90	18.4	.9	.8	127	422	0
boiled or steamed, 4 oz.	179	36.8	1.9	1.6	254	844	0
Cuttlefish, canned, in ink (*Goya*), ¼ cup	120	8.0	2.0	9.0	15	350	0

D

Food and Measure	cal.	prot. (gms)	carbo. (gms)	fat (gms)	chol. (mgs)	sod. (mgs)	fiber (gms)
Daikon, see "Radish, Oriental"							
Daiquiri mixer:							
Hawaiian (*Trader Vic's*), 4 fl. oz.	170	0	42.0	0	0	20	0
Dairy Queen/Brazier, 1 serving:							
burgers:							
DQ Homestyle:							
cheeseburger ...	340	20.0	29.0	17.0	55	850	2.0
cheeseburger, double	540	35.0	30.0	31.0	115	1130	2.0
cheeseburger, double, w/bacon......	610	41.0	31.0	36.0	130	1380	2.0
hamburger ....:	290	17.0	29.0	12.0	45	630	2.0
DQ Ultimate burger	670	40.0	29.0	43.0	135	1210	2.0
sandwiches:							
chicken, grilled	310	24.0	30.0	10.0	50	1040	3.0
chicken breast fillet	430	24.0	37.0	20.0	55	760	2.0
chili 'n' cheese dog	330	14.0	22.0	21.0	45	1090	2.0
hot dog	240	9.0	19.0	14.0	25	730	1.0
chicken strip basket	1000	35.0	102.0	50.0	55	2260	5.0
side dishes:							
fries, medium	350	4.0	42.0	18.0	0	630	3.0
fries, large	440	5.0	53.0	23.0	0	790	4.0
onion rings	320	5.0	39.0	16.0	0	180	3.0
desserts and shakes:							
banana split	510	8.0	96.0	12.0	30	180	3.0
Blizzard, small:							
chocolate chip cookie dough	660	12.0	99.0	24.0	55	440	1.0

Food and Measure	cal.	prot. (gms)	carbo. (gms)	fat (gms)	chol. (mgs)	sod. (mgs)	fiber (gms)
chocolate sandwich cookie . . .	520	10.0	79.0	18.0	40	380	1.0
Blizzard, medium:							
chocolate chip cookie dough	950	17.0	143.0	36.0	75	660	1.0
chocolate sandwich cookie . . .	640	12.0	97.0	23.0	45	500	1.0
Breeze yogurt:							
Heath, small	470	11.0	85.0	10.0	10	380	1.0
Heath, medium	710	15.0	123.0	18.0	20	580	1.0
strawberry, small	320	10.0	68.0	.5	5	190	1.0
strawberry, medium	460	13.0	99.0	1.0	10	270	1.0
Buster Bar	450	10.0	41.0	28.0	15	280	2.0
Chocolate Dilly	210	3.0	21.0	13.0	10	75	0
cone, chocolate:							
DQ soft serve,							
½ cup	150	4.0	22.0	5.0	15	75	0
small	240	6.0	37.0	8.0	20	115	0
medium	340	8.0	53.0	11.0	30	160	0
cone, dipped:							
small	340	6.0	42.0	17.0	20	130	1.0
medium	480	8.0	59.0	24.0	30	190	1.0
cone, vanilla:							
DQ soft serve,							
½ cup	140	3.0	22.0	4.5	15	70	0
small	230	6.0	38.0	7.0	20	115	0
medium	330	8.0	53.0	9.0	30	160	0
large	410	10.0	65.0	12.0	40	200	0
DQ frozen, ⅛ of 8″ cake	340	7.0	53.0	12.0	25	250	1.0
DQ fudge bar	50	4.0	13.0	0	0	70	0
DQ sandwich	150	3.0	24.0	5.0	5	115	1.0
DQ Treatzza Pizza:							
Heath, ⅛ pizza . . .	180	3.0	28.0	7.0	5	160	1.0
M&M's, ⅛ pizza	190	3.0	29.0	7.0	5	160	1.0
DQ vanilla orange bar	60	2.0	17.0	0	0	40	0
Fudge Cake Supreme	890	11.0	124.0	38.0	65	960	3.0

Food and Measure	cal.	prot. (gms)	carbo. (gms)	fat (gms)	chol. (mgs)	sod. (mgs)	fiber (gms)
Dairy Queen/Brazier, desserts and shakes *(cont.)*							
lemon *DQ Freez'r,*							
½ cup	80	0	20.0	0	0	10	0
malt, chocolate:							
small	650	15.0	111.0	16.0	55	370	0
medium	880	19.0	153.0	22.0	70	500	0
Misty slush:							
small	220	0	56.0	0	0	20	0
medium	290	0	74.0	0	0	30	0
Peanut Buster par-							
fait	730	16.0	99.0	31.0	35	400	2.0
shake, chocolate:							
small	560	13.0	94.0	15.0	50	310	0
medium	770	17.0	130.0	20.0	70	420	0
Starkiss	80	0	21.0	0	0	10	0
strawberry short-							
cake	430	7.0	70.0	14.0	60	360	1.0
sundae, chocolate:							
small	280	5.0	49.0	7.0	20	140	0
medium	400	8.0	71.0	10.0	30	210	0
yogurt, frozen:							
cone, medium . . .	260	9.0	56.0	1.0	5	160	0
cup, medium	230	8.0	48.0	.5	5	150	0
DQ nonfat, ½ cup	100	3.0	21.0	0	<5	70	0
strawberry sun-							
dae, medium . .	280	8.0	61.0	.5	5	160	1.0
Dandelion greens:							
raw:							
(*Frieda's*), 2 cups,							
3 oz.	40	2.0	8.0	.5	0	65	3.0
½ cup chopped,							
1 oz.	13	.8	2.6	.2	0	22	1.0
boiled, drained,							
chopped, ½ cup . . .	17	1.0	3.3	.3	0	23	1.5
Danish, 1 pc., except							
as noted:							
all varieties:							
(*Awrey's*)	300	3.0	32.0	17.0	10	210	<1.0
(*Awrey's* Petite) . . .	130	1.0	14.0	8.0	5	85	0
apple (*Awrey's*							
Grande)	450	4.0	51.0	26.0	15	270	1.0

Food and Measure	cal.	prot. (gms)	carbo. (gms)	fat (gms)	chol. (mgs)	sod. (mgs)	fiber (gms)
cheese (*Awrey's* Grande)	480	4.0	51.0	26.0	15	270	1.0
cherry cheese (*Awrey's* Marquise)	350	4.0	38.0	21.0	20	250	<1.0
cinnamon:							
(*Awrey's* Marquise)	470	5.0	60.0	24.0	15	310	<1.0
roll (*Awrey's* Home-style)	270	4.0	46.0	8.0	10	240	1.0
swirl (*Awrey's* Grande)	420	6.0	57.0	21.0	10	410	2.0
lemon cheese (*Awrey's* Marquise)	350	4.0	38.0	21.0	20	250	<1.0
raspberry cheese swirl (*Awrey's* Grande)	400	6.0	51.0	19.0	20	400	1.0
rolls (*Dolly Madison* Rollers), 3 pcs. ...	290	3.0	46.0	10.0	0	130	1.0
strawberry (*Awrey's* Grande)	480	5.0	49.0	30.0	20	360	<1.0
Danish, frozen, 1 pc.:							
apple or raspberry (*Pepperidge Farm*)	210	4.0	29.0	9.0	15	190	2.0
cheese (*Pepperidge Farm*)	230	6.0	25.0	11.0	55	230	1.0
cinnamon roll (*Pepperidge Farm*)	250	4.0	33.0	12.0	15	220	2.0
Danish cake, see "Cake"							
Dasheen, see "Taro"							
Date, dried, pitted:							
(*Calavo* California), 5-6 pcs., 1.4 oz. ...	120	1.0	31.0	0	0	0	3.0
(*Pavich* California), 5-6 pcs., 1.4 oz. ...	120	1.0	31.0	0	0	0	3.0
(*Sonoma*), 5 pcs., 1.4 oz.	110	1.0	30.0	0	0	15	5.0
10 pcs., 2.9 oz.	228	1.6	61.0	.4	0	2	6.2
Date filling, see "Pastry filling"							
Date loaf, see "Bread mix, sweet"							

Food and Measure	cal.	prot. (gms)	carbo. (gms)	fat (gms)	chol. (mgs)	sod. (mgs)	fiber (gms)
Delicata squash							
(*Frieda's*), ¾ cup,							
3 oz.	30	1.0	7.0	0	0	0	1.0
Demi-glace sauce							
mix (*Knorr*),							
1 tbsp.	30	<1.0	4.0	1.0	0	380	0
Denny's, general							
menu, 1 serving:							
breakfast dishes:							
All American Slam	1028	48.0	24.0	87.0	724	1924	2.0
Big Texas Chicken							
Fajita Skillet	1184	59.0	43.0	88.0	679	2406	5.0
Canadian Scramble							
skillet	842	50.0	34.0	62.0	642	2183	3.0
chicken fried steak							
and eggs	723	28.0	31.0	56.0	452	1505	8.0
eggs Benedict	860	35.0	55.0	56.0	525	1943	3.0
Farmer's Omelette	912	34.0	38.0	69.0	633	1816	3.0
French Slam	1029	44.0	58.0	71.0	777	1428	2.0
French toast, plain	510	19.0	51.0	25.0	317	413	2.0
Grand Slam original	795	34.0	65.0	50.0	460	2237	2.0
ham 'n cheddar om-							
elette	743	36.0	24.0	55.0	657	1518	2.0
hotcakes, plain	491	12.0	95.0	7.0	0	1818	3.0
Meat Lover's Skillet	1344	59.0	34.0	108.0	673	3063	3.0
Moons Over My							
Hammy	807	44.0	46.0	48.0	430	2247	2.0
pork chop and eggs	555	33.0	21.0	36.0	469	968	2.0
porterhouse steak							
and eggs	1223	70.0	21.0	95.0	570	1360	2.0
Sausage Supreme							
Skillet	1170	40.0	36.0	96.0	620	2371	4.0
Scram Slam	974	42.0	30.0	80.0	694	1750	4.0
sirloin steak and							
eggs	808	37.0	21.0	64.0	476	952	2.0
Slim Slam, no syrup	495	34.0	98.0	12.0	34	1746	1.0
Southern Slam	1065	37.0	47.0	84.0	484	2449	0
Super/Play It Again							
Slam	1192	51.0	98.0	75.0	690	3555	3.0
T-bone steak and							
eggs	1045	56.0	21.0	82.0	530	1191	2.0

Food and Measure	cal.	prot. (gms)	carbo. (gms)	fat (gms)	chol. (mgs)	sod. (mgs)	fiber (gms)
Ultimate Omelette	780	31.0	29.0	62.0	639	1360	4.0
veggie-cheese omelette	714	28.0	29.0	53.0	644	955	4.0
waffle, plain	304	7.0	23.0	21.0	146	200	0
breakfast items:							
bacon, 4 slices	162	12.0	1.0	18.0	36	640	0
bacon, Canadian ...	110	17.0	1.0	5.0	43	1039	0
bagel, dry	235	9.0	46.0	1.0	0	495	0
biscuit, plain	375	5.0	40.0	22.0	0	750	0
biscuit and sausage gravy	570	11.0	45.0	38.0	24	1475	0
egg, 1	134	6.0	1.0	12.0	205	61	0
Egg Beaters	71	5.0	1.0	5.0	1.0	138	0
English muffin, dry	125	5.0	24.0	1.0	0	198	1.0
grits, 4 oz.	80	2.0	18.0	0	0	520	0
hash browns	218	2.0	20.0	14.0	0	424	2.0
covered	318	9.0	21.0	23.0	30	604	2.0
covered, smothered	359	9.0	26.0	26.0	30	790	2.0
oatmeal, 4 oz.	100	5.0	18.0	2.0	0	175	3.0
sausage links, 4 ...	354	16.0	0	32.0	64	944	0
sausage patties, 2	506	18.0	2.0	47.0	76	760	0
syrup, 1.5 oz.:							
blueberry.......	102	0	26.0	0	0	15	0
maple	143	0	36.0	0	0	26	0
maple, sugar-free	23	0	9.0	0	0	71	0
strawberry......	91	0	23.0	0	0	36	0
toast, 1 slice, dry	92	3.0	17.0	1.0	0	166	1.0
topping, 3 oz.:							
blueberry.......	106	0	26.0	0	0	15	0
cherry	86	0	21.0	0	0	5	0
strawberry......	115	1.0	26.0	1.0	0	12	1.0
whipped cream	23	0	2.0	2.0	7	3	0
sandwiches:							
BLT	634	18.0	37.0	46.0	54	1116	2.0
burger:							
bacon cheddar	935	53.0	43.0	63.0	164	1732	3.0
Big Texas BBQ ...	929	53.0	53.0	58.0	163	2271	3.0
classic	673	37.0	42.0	40.0	106	1142	3.0
classic w/cheese	836	47.0	43.0	53.0	137	1595	3.0
garden.........	665	18.0	75.0	33.0	36	1051	8.0

Food and Measure	cal.	prot. (gms)	carbo. (gms)	fat (gms)	chol. (mgs)	sod. (mgs)	fiber (gms)
Denny's, sandwiches, burger (cont.)							
garden, patty only	172	8.0	25.0	4.0	20	424	5.0
Charleston Chicken	632	35.0	53.0	32.0	81	1967	4.0
chicken, grilled	509	34.0	52.0	19.0	83	1809	3.0
chicken melt	520	26.0	43.0	29.0	39	1096	2.0
Classic Combos:							
turkey, multigrain	476	23.0	39.0	26.0	57	1107	5.0
ham/Swiss, rye	533	23.0	40.0	31.0	36	1638	5.0
club	718	32.0	62.0	38.0	75	1666	3.0
Delidinger	852	56.0	62.0	45.0	80	3142	3.0
deluxe grilled							
cheese	482	18.0	44.0	26.0	1	1135	2.0
fisherman's choice	905	29.0	74.0	56.0	69	1704	4.0
patty melt	695	38.0	39.0	44.0	114	1007	2.0
The Super Bird	620	35.0	48.0	32.0	60	1880	2.0
soup, 8 oz.:							
broccoli, cream of	193	4.0	15.0	12.0	0	818	2.0
cheese	293	6.0	13.0	23.0	19	895	4.0
chicken noodle	60	2.0	8.0	2.0	10	640	0
clam chowder	214	5.0	22.0	11.0	5	903	1.0
potato, cream of . . .	222	4.0	23.0	12.0	0	761	2.0
split pea	146	8.0	18.0	6.0	5	819	2.0
vegetable beef	79	6.0	11.0	1.0	5	820	2.0
appetizers, w/out con-							
diments, except as							
noted:							
Buffalo wings, 12	856	92.0	1.0	54.0	500	5552	1.0
chicken quesadilla	827	50.0	43.0	55.0	181	1982	2.0
chicken strips, 5 . . .	720	47.0	56.0	33.0	95	1666	0
chicken strips, Buf-							
falo, 5	734	48.0	43.0	42.0	96	1673	0
mozzarella sticks, 8,							
w/sauce	756	37.0	56.0	43.0	48	5423	7.0
onion ring basket,							
13	824	11.0	83.0	50.0	14	2173	1.0
Sampler	1405	47.0	124.0	80.0	75	5305	4.0
dinner entrees, meat/							
fish:							
chicken, Charleston,							
w/gravy	327	25.0	16.0	18.0	65	993	1.0
chicken, grilled	130	24.0	0	4.0	67	560	0

Food and Measure	cal.	prot. (gms)	carbo. (gms)	fat (gms)	chol. (mgs)	sod. (mgs)	fiber (gms)
chicken strip,							
w/honey mustard	635	47.0	55.0	25.0	95	1510	0
chopped steak,							
grilled, w/gravy	400	30.0	12.0	26.0	91	447	2.0
cod, battered,							
w/tartar sauce ...	732	30.0	48.0	47.0	105	1335	3.0
pork chop	386	39.0	0	24.0	121	844	0
porterhouse steak	708	56.0	0	54.0	161	713	0
pot roast	260	39.0	5.0	11.0	140	1085	0
salmon, Alaskan,							
grilled	296	43.0	1.0	14.0	102	257	0
shrimp, fried	558	19.0	49.0	32.0	135	1114	3.0
sirloin steak	271	22.0	0	21.0	62	273	0
steak, chicken-fried,							
w/gravy	265	15.0	14.0	17.0	27	668	1.0
steak and shrimp	645	36.0	31.0	42.0	150	1143	2.0
T-bone steak	530	42.0	0	40.0	121	534	0
turkey, roast,							
w/stuffing, gravy	701	47.0	63.0	27.0	100	2346	0
sides:							
applesauce	60	0	13.0	0	0	13	1.0
broccoli, butter							
sauce	50	3.0	7.0	2.0	5	280	3.0
carrots, honey glaze	80	1.0	12.0	3.0	0	220	3.0
corn, butter sauce	120	3.0	19.0	4.0	5	260	5.0
corn bread stuffing,							
plain	182	4.0	20.0	9.0	0	405	0
cottage cheese	72	9.0	2.0	3.0	10	281	0
fries, no salt	323	5.0	44.0	14.0	0	130	0
fries, seasoned	261	5.0	35.0	12.0	0	556	0
gravy, brown	13	0	2.0	0	0	184	0
gravy, chicken	14	0	2.0	.5	2	139	0
gravy, country	17	0	2.0	1.0	0	93	0
green beans							
w/bacon	60	1.0	6.0	4.0	5	390	3.0
green peas, butter							
sauce	100	5.0	14.0	2.0	5	360	4.0
hashed browns	218	2.0	20.0	14.0	0	424	2.0
mushrooms, grilled	14	2.0	2.0	0	0	0	1.0
onion rings	381	5.0	38.0	23.0	6	1003	1.0

Food and Measure	cal.	prot. (gms)	carbo. (gms)	fat (gms)	chol. (mgs)	sod. (mgs)	fiber (gms)
Denny's, sides *(cont.)*							
potato, plain:							
baked	186	4.0	43.0	0	0	14	4.0
mashed	105	3.0	21.0	1.0	0	378	2.0
rice pilaf	112	2.0	21.0	2.0	0	328	0
roll, dinner	132	4.0	26.0	2.0	0	265	1.0
toast, herb	200	4.0	21.0	11.0	0	372	1.0
tomato, 3 slices ...	13	1.0	3.0	0	0	6	1.0
salads:							
chicken:							
Buffalo	615	39.0	36.0	37.0	88	1258	3.0
fried	506	38.0	30.0	31.0	94	1174	3.0
garden delite	277	30.0	30.0	5.0	67	785	6.0
grilled, Caesar ...	655	37.0	23.0	47.0	86	1728	4.0
Oriental	568	33.0	49.0	26.0	67	1656	7.0
side, Caesar	338	8.0	20.0	25.0	7	725	3.0
side, garden	113	3.0	16.0	4.0	0	147	3.0
dressings/condiments, 1 oz., except as noted:							
BBQ sauce, 1.5 oz.	47	0	11.0	1.0	0	595	0
blue cheese	124	4.0	4.0	12.0	18	405	0
Caesar	142	1.0	1.0	15.0	2	340	0
French	106	0	3.0	10.0	7	274	0
French, reduced cal	76	0	8.0	5.0	0	265	0
honey mustard	38	0	9.0	0	0	121	0
horseradish sauce, 1.5 oz.	170	1.0	3.0	20.0	43	227	0
Italian, creamy	106	0	4.0	10.0	0	306	0
Italian, reduced cal	23	0	3.0	1.0	0	515	0
mayonnaise, 2 tbsp.	200	0	1.0	22.0	16	159	0
Oriental peanut	106	1.0	6.0	8.0	0	399	0
ranch	101	1.0	1.0	11.0	8	215	0
sour cream, 1.5 oz.	91	1.0	2.0	9.0	19	23	0
Thousand Island ...	104	0	2.0	10.0	21	208	0
desserts:							
banana royale	548	6.0	80.0	25.0	64	184	6.0
banana split sundae	894	15.0	121.0	43.0	78	177	6.0

Food and Measure	cal.	prot. (gms)	carbo. (gms)	fat (gms)	chol. (mgs)	sod. (mgs)	fiber (gms)
chocolate cake	370	4.0	53.0	17.0	29	374	2.0
hot fudge cake sundae	687	9.0	83.0	38.0	62	486	3.0
ice cream/*Coke* float	280	3.0	47.0	10.0	39	109	0
pie, *Mother Butler*, ⅙ pie:							
apple	430	3.0	59.0	20.0	<5	390	1.0
apple, Dutch	440	3.0	65.0	19.0	0	290	1.0
apple, w/*Equal* ...	370	3.0	43.0	20.0	<5	360	2.0
cheesecake	470	8.0	48.0	27.0	90	280	0
cheesecake topping:							
blueberry	106	0	26.0	0	0	15	0
cherry	86	0	21.0	0	0	5	0
strawberry	115	1.0	26.0	1.0	0	12	1.0
cherry	540	5.0	83.0	21.0	<5	430	2.0
chocolate peanut butter	653	12.0	64.0	39.0	27.0	319	3.0
chocolate pecan	790	6.0	107.0	37.0	70	460	3.0
French silk	650	6.0	60.0	43.0	165	220	2.0
Key lime	600	10.0	79.0	27.0	35	300	0
lemon meringue	460	5.0	71.0	17.0	95	310	1.0
pecan	600	5.0	81.0	28.0	50	430	2.0
pumpkin	233	5.0	38.0	7.0	36	213	2.0
shake/malt:							
chocolate	579	12.0	77.0	27.0	108	278	0
vanilla	581	11.0	77.0	27.0	108	236	0
sherbet, rainbow ...	120	1.0	25.0	1.5	5	30	0
sundae:							
double scoop ...	375	6.0	29.0	27.0	74	86	0
single scoop	188	3.0	14.0	14.0	37	43	0
yogurt, chocolate/ chocolate chip ...	110	4.0	19.0	2.0	5	60	1.0
Dessert, see specific listings							
Dessert filling, see "Pastry filling" and "Pie filling"							
Dhal, see "Lentil dishes, canned"							

Food and Measure	cal.	prot. (gms)	carbo. (gms)	fat (gms)	chol. (mgs)	sod. (mgs)	fiber (gms)
Dill dip, 2 tbsp.:							
(*Bernstein's* Zesty) . . .	120	0	2.0	12.0	20	160	0
(*Heluva* Good)	60	1.0	2.0	5.0	20	150	0
(*T. Marzetti's* Veggie Dip)	140	1.0	2.0	14.0	25	190	0
(*T. Marzetti's* Veggie Dip Fat Free)	30	1.0	6.0	0	0	410	0
w/hummus (*Heluva* Good)	50	1.0	3.0	4.0	15	180	0
Dill dip mix, garden (*Knorr*), ½ tsp. . . .	5	0	0	0	0	110	0
Dill seed, 1 tsp.	6	.3	1.2	.3	0	<1	.4
Dill weed:							
fresh:							
5 sprigs	<1	<1.0	.1	<.1	0	1	n.a.
½ cup loose-packed	2	.2	.3	.1	0	3	n.a.
dried, 1 tsp.	3	.2	.6	<.1	0	2	.1
Dip, see "Salad dress-ings" and specific listings							
Dock, boiled, drained, 4 oz.	23	2.1	3.3	.7	0	3	<1.0
Dolmas mix, see "Rice dishes, mix"							
Dolphinfish, meat only:							
raw, 4 oz.	97	21.0	0	.8	83	99	0
baked, broiled, or mi-crowaved, 4 oz. . . .	124	26.9	0	1.0	107	128	0
Domino's Pizza:							
cheese pizza, medium, 12″, 2 of 8 slices, except as noted:							
deep dish	477	18.4	55.3	21.6	19	1085	3.3
hand-tossed	347	14.5	49.6	10.7	15	723	2.8
thin crust, ¼ pie . . .	271	11.8	30.8	11.8	15	809	1.8
"Add a Topping":							
anchovies	23	3.1	0	1.0	9	395	0
bacon	82	4.3	.1	7.0	12	226	0
beef, precooked	55	2.7	0	4.9	10	154	0
cheddar	57	3.5	.2	4.7	15	88	0

Food and Measure	cal.	prot. (gms)	carbo. (gms)	fat (gms)	chol. (mgs)	sod. (mgs)	fiber (gms)
cheese, extra	48	3.2	.6	3.8	7	150	.2
ham...........	17	2.4	.1	.7	7	162	0
Italian sausage	55	2.4	1.6	4.3	11	171	.1
mushroom, canned.......	4	.3	.9	.1	0	75	.4
mushroom, fresh	4	.3	.7	.1	0	1	.2
olives, green	12	.2	.1	1.3	0	255	.1
olives, ripe......	14	.1	.6	1.2	0	71	.5
onion..........	4	.1	.8	0	0	0	.1
pepper, banana	4	.1	.9	0	0	91	0
pepper, green ...	3	.1	.6	0	0	0	.1
pepperoni	75	3.2	.2	6.7	15	238	.1
pineapple	10	.1	2.5	0	0	1	.1
cheese pizza, large, 14", 2 of 12 slices, except as noted:							
deep dish	456	17.6	54.4	19.7	18	1029	3.2
hand-tossed	317	13.3	44.9	9.9	13	669	2.5
thin crust, ⅙ pie ...	253	11.1	28.7	11.0	13	757	1.6
"Add a Topping":							
anchovies	23	3.1	0	1.0	9	395	0
bacon	75	4.0	.1	6.4	11	207	0
beef, precooked	44	2.1	0	3.9	8	123	0
cheddar	48	2.9	.1	3.9	12	73	0
cheese, extra	44	3.0	.6	3.5	7	140	.2
ham...........	17	2.3	.3	.7	7	156	0
Italian sausage	44	1.9	1.2	3.5	9	137	.1
mushroom, canned......	3	.2	.6	0	0	50	.3
mushroom, fresh	3	.2	.5	0	0	0	.1
olives, green	11	.1	.1	1.2	0	227	.1
olives, ripe......	12	.1	.5	1.1	0	63	.5
onion..........	3	.1	.7	0	0	0	0
pepper, banana	3	.1	.5	0	0	81	0
pepper, green ...	2	.1	.5	0	0	0	.1
pepperoni	66	2.9	.2	6.0	14	212	.1
pineapple	8	.1	2.0	0	0	1	.1
cheese pizza, 6" deep dish, 1 pie	595	22.7	68.0	27.5	23	1300	3.9
"Add a Topping":							
anchovies	45	6.2	0	2.1	18	790	0

Food and Measure	cal.	prot. (gms)	carbo. (gms)	fat (gms)	chol. (mgs)	sod. (mgs)	fiber (gms)
Domino's Pizza, cheese pizza, 6″ deep dish, 1 pie *(cont.)*							
bacon	82	4.3	.1	7.0	12	226	0
beef, precooked	44	2.1	0	3.9	8	123	0
cheddar	86	5.3	.2	7.0	22	132	0
cheese, extra	57	3.9	.8	4.5	9	180	.2
ham	17 ·	2.3	.3	.7	7	156	0
Italian sausage	44	1.9	1.2	3.5	9	137	.1
mushroom, canned	2	.2	.4	0	0	36	.2
mushroom, fresh	2	.2	.4	0	0	0	.1
olives, green	10	.1	.1	1.1	0	204	.1
olives, ripe	11	.1	.5	1.0	0	57	.4
onion	3	.1	.6	0	0	0	0
pepper, banana	3	.1	.5	0	0	73	0
pepper, green . . .	2	.1	.6	0	0	0	.1
pepperoni	49	2.3	.2	4.5	10	159	0
pineapple	5	0	1.2	0	0	1	.1
Buffalo wings, 1 pc.:							
barbecue	50	5.5	1.6	2.4	26	175	.2
hot	45	5.5	.5	2.4	26	354	.2
salad, no dressing:							
small	22	1.3	4.2	.3	0	14	1.8
large	39	2.2	7.3	.5	0	26	3.2
Marzetti dressings, 1½ oz.:							
blue cheese	220	2.0	2.0	24.0	40	440	0
Caesar, creamy	200	1.0	2.0	22.0	10	470	0
honey French	210	0	14.0	18.0	0	780	0
Italian, house	220	0	1.0	24.0	0	440	0
Italian, light	20	0	2.0	1.0	0	780	0
ranch	260	0	1.0	29.0	5	380	0
ranch, fat free	40	0	10.0	0	0	560	1.0
Thousand Island . . .	200	0	5.0	20.0	0	320	0
breadstick, 1 pc.	78	1.7	10.7	3.3	0	158	.3
cheesy bread, 1 pc.	103	3.2	10.3	5.4	5	187	.3
Donut, 1 pc., except as noted:							
(*Dolly Madison* Old Fashioned)	280	4.0	28.0	16.0	20	360	0

Food and Measure	cal.	prot. (gms)	carbo. (gms)	fat (gms)	chol. (mgs)	sod. (mgs)	fiber (gms)
plain:							
(*Awrey's*), 1½ oz.	170	2.0	19.0	10.0	15	220	0
(*Awrey's*), 2 oz. ...	240	3.0	21,0	16.0	15	290	<1.0
(*Dolly Madison*) ...	140	2.0	15.0	7.0	10	190	0
(*Entenmann's* Dippers)	160	1.0	19.0	9.0	10	130	<1.0
(*Entenmann's* Popettes), 4 pcs.	270	3.0	29.0	16.0	20	260	<1.0
(*Hostess*)	140	2.0	15.0	7.0	10	190	0
blueberry:							
(*Hostess*)	210	2.0	21.0	13.0	10	220	0
filled, powdered (*Krispy Kreme*)	200	4.0	26.0	9.0	5	160	2.0
glazed (*Krispy Kreme*)	300	2.0	37.0	15.0	5	200	1.0
cake:							
(*Krispy Kreme* Traditional)	200	3.0	22.0	11.0	15	280	<1.0
chocolate-iced (*Entenmann's*)	280	3.0	27.0	19.0	10	220	1.0
chocolate-iced (*Krispy Kreme*)	230	3.0	28.0	12.0	15	280	<1.0
chocolate-iced, mini (*Entenmann's*)	150	1.0	12.0	11.0	5	100	<1.0
crumb-topped (*Entenmann's*)	260	3.0	34.0	13.0	15	230	<1.0
milk chocolate–iced (*Entenmann's*)	320	3.0	36.0	19.0	15	180	1.0
powdered (*Krispy Kreme*)	220	3.0	26.0	11.0	15	250	0
chocolate (*Dolly Madison* Gems), 4 pcs., 2 oz.	260	3.0	28.0	15.0	10	230	1.0
chocolate-iced/ frosted:							
(*Awrey's*), 1¾ oz.	200	2.0	23.0	11.0	15	240	<1.0
(*Awrey's*), 2½ oz.	300	3.0	31.0	18.0	20	340	<1.0
(*Awrey's* Ring), 3 oz.	350	5.0	33.0	21.0	0	370	1.0
(*Dolly Madison*) ...	140	1.0	15.0	8.0	5	130	1.0
(*Hostess*)	180	2.0	19.0	11.0	5	170	0

Food and Measure	cal.	prot. (gms)	carbo. (gms)	fat (gms)	chol. (mgs)	sod. (mgs)	fiber (gms)
Donut, chocolate-iced/frosted *(cont.)*							
(*Hostess Donettes*), 3 pcs., 1½ oz.	200	2.0	21.0	12.0	10	170	0
(*Krispy Kreme*)	260	3.0	30.0	14.0	<5	105	1.0
(*Tastykake* Rich) ...	270	3.0	30.0	16.0	5	180	2.0
chocolate (*Awrey's*), 1¾ oz.	190	2.0	25.0	10.0	5	150	<1.0
chocolate (*Awrey's*), 2½ oz.	280	3.0	34.0	16.0	5	200	1.0
creme-filled (*Krispy Kreme*)	270	4.0	32.0	14.0	<5	150	2.0
custard (*Awrey's* Bismark)	350	5.0	36.0	20.0	0	370	1.0
custard (*Krispy Kreme*)	250	4.0	38.0	9.0	5	150	3.0
sour cream (*Awrey's*)	430	4.0	52.0	23.0	0	360	<1.0
w/sprinkles (*Krispy Kreme*)	220	2.0	31.0	10.0	<5	95	<1.0
cinnamon apple–filled (*Krispy Kreme*)	210	4.0	29.0	9.0	<5	150	3.0
coconut top (*Awrey's*)	210	2.0	25.0	12.0	10	190	0
creme-filled, glazed (*Krispy Kreme*)	270	4.0	32.0	14.0	<5	150	2.0
cruller:							
(*Dolly Madison* English)	250	2.0	31.0	14.0	30	190	1.0
(*Entenmann's*)	220	2.0	26.0	13.0	15	190	<1.0
chocolate-iced (*Krispy Kreme*)	240	2.0	26.0	14.0	10	160	<1.0
glazed (*Krispy Kreme*)	220	2.0	22.0	14.0	10	150	0
crumb (*Hostess Donettes*), 3 pcs., 1½ oz.	170	2.0	23.0	8.0	10	190	0
crunch:							
(*Awrey's*), 2½ oz.	280	3.0	35.0	15.0	15	320	<1.0
(*Dolly Madison* Gems), 3 pcs., 2 oz.	220	3.0	31.0	10.0	10	250	0

Food and Measure	cal.	prot. (gms)	carbo. (gms)	fat (gms)	chol. (mgs)	sod. (mgs)	fiber (gms)
top (*Awrey's*), 1¾ oz.	160	2.0	19.0	8.0	10	190	0
devil's food:							
(*Entenmann's*)	310	3.0	34.0	19.0	15	170	2.0
glazed (*Krispy Kreme*)	240	2.0	29.0	13.0	10	180	3.0
honey-glazed (*Awrey's*)	310	4.0	43.0	14.0	15	530	2.0
glazed:							
(*Dolly Madison Whirl*)	210	2.0	31.0	11.0	25	150	0
(*Dolly Madison Yeast*)	190	2.0	23.0	9.0	10	130	0
(*Entenmann's Popems*), 4 pcs.	210	2.0	29.0	10.0	15	190	<1.0
(*Hostess* Old Fashioned)	260	2.0	33.0	13.0	25	220	1.0
(*Krispy Kreme* Original)	170	2.0	17.0	10.0	<5	95	<1.0
honey (*Awrey's* Ring)	310	5.0	30.0	19.0	0	330	1.0
glazed (*Awrey's*) . . .	420	4.0	52.0	23.0	0	340	0
stick (*Awrey's* Twin)	330	4.0	32.0	21.0	20	390	<1.0
honey, wheat (*Tastykake*)	230	2.0	33.0	10.0	5	180	1.0
jelly, powdered sugar (*Awrey's* Bismark)	320	18.0	35.0	18.0	0	310	1.0
lemon-filled (*Krispy Kreme*)	210	4.0	28.0	10.0	5	150	<1.0
maple-iced (*Krispy Kreme*)	200	3.0	28.0	9.0	0	100	2.0
orange-glazed (*Tastykake*)	220	2.0	33.0	9.0	5	200	1.0
powdered sugar:							
(*Awrey's*), 1½ oz.	170	2.0	19.0	10.0	15	220	0
(*Awrey's*), 2¼ oz.	390	5.0	44.0	22.0	25	470	1.0
(*Dolly Madison*) . . .	120	1.0	14.0	6.0	10	140	0
(*Dolly Madison* Gems), 4 pcs., 2 oz.	230	3.0	30.0	11.0	15	260	0
(*Hostess*)	150	2.0	19.0	8.0	10	180	0

Food and Measure	cal.	prot. (gms)	carbo. (gms)	fat (gms)	chol. (mgs)	sod. (mgs)	fiber (gms)
Donut, powdered sugar (cont.)							
(*Hostess Donettes*),							
3 pcs., 1½ oz. . . .	180	2.0	23.0	9.0	10	190	0
raspberry-filled:							
(*Hostess O's*)	230	3.0	34.0	10.0	5	230	1.0
(*Krispy Kreme*)	210	4.0	27.0	10.0	<5	160	3.0
sour cream (*Awrey's*)	370	4.0	41.0	22.0	0	340	0
sprinkle top (*Awrey's*)	160	2.0	19.0	8.0	10	190	0
stick:							
(*Dolly Madison* Dunkin'Stix)	170	1.0	20.0	9.0	15	130	0
cinnamon (*Dolly Madison* Stix) . . .	170	1.0	21.0	9.0	15	140	0
vanilla-iced:							
(*Awrey's* Bismark)	320	4.0	35.0	18.0	0	320	1.0
(*Awrey's* Long John)	380	5.0	44.0	20.0	0	350	1.0
white-iced (*Awrey's*)	200	2.0	24.0	10.0	15	240	0
Donut mix, dry (*Manischewitz Passover Gold*), ¾ cup	270	3.0	36.0	12.0	0	105	2.0
Dressing, see "Salad dressing" and specific listings							
Drum, freshwater, meat only:							
raw, 4 oz.	135	19.9	0	5.6	73	85	0
baked, broiled, or microwaved, 4 oz. . . .	173	25.5	0	7.2	93	109	0
Duck, domesticated, roasted:							
meat w/skin, 4 oz. . . .	382	21.5	0	32.1	95	67	0
meat only, 4 oz.	228	26.6	0	12.7	101	74	0
Duck, wild, raw:							
meat w/skin, 4 oz. . . .	239	19.8	0	17.2	91	64	0
breast meat, 4 oz. . . .	139	22.5	0	4.8	n.a.	65	0
Duck sauce, see "Sweet and sour sauce"							
Duck sausage, see "Sausage"							

Food and Measure	cal.	prot. (gms)	carbo. (gms)	fat (gms)	chol. (mgs)	sod. (mgs)	fiber (gms)
Dumpling entree, Oriental, frozen (*Lean Cuisine*), 9 oz.	300	10.0	51.0	6.0	20	520	2.0
Dumpling squash, see "Sweet dumpling squash"							
Dutch loaf, see "Lunch meat"							

E

Food and Measure	cal.	prot. (gms)	carbo. (gms)	fat (gms)	chol. (mgs)	sod. (mgs)	fiber (gms)
Eclair, chocolate, 1 pc.:							
(*Entenmann's*)	260	3.0	24.0	9.0	80	210	<1.0
frozen:							
(*Rich's*)	190	2.0	24.0	9.0	40	115	0
(*Weight Watchers*)	150	2.0	25.0	4.0	30	170	1.0
triple (*Weight Watchers*)	160	3.0	25.0	5.0	30	190	1.0
Eel, meat only:							
raw, 4 oz.	209	20.9	0	3.2	143	58	0
baked, broiled, or microwaved, 4 oz. . . .	268	26.8	0	17.0	183	74	0
Egg, chicken:							
raw, 1 large egg:							
whole	75	6.3	.6	5.0	213	63	0
white only	17	3.5	.3	0	0	55	0
yolk only[1]	59	2.8	.3	5.1	213	7	0
cooked:							
hard-boiled, chopped, 1 cup	210	17.1	1.5	14.4	578	169	0
poached, 1 large . . .	74	6.2	.6	5.0	212	140	0
dried, 1 oz.:							
whole	168	13.0	1.4	11.9	544	148	0
whole, stabilized . . .	174	13.7	.7	12.5	572	155	0
white, stabilized, flakes	100	21.8	1.2	<.1	0	328	0
yolk	195	8.7	.1	17.4	830	26	0
Egg, duck, 1 egg	130	9.0	1.0	9.6	619	102	0
Egg, goose, 1 egg . . .	267	20.0	1.9	19.1	n.a.	n.a.	0
Egg, quail, 1 egg	14	1.2	<.1	1.0	76	n.a.	0

[1] *Includes a small portion of white.*

Food and Measure	cal.	prot. (gms)	carbo. (gms)	fat (gms)	chol. (mgs)	sod. (mgs)	fiber (gms)
Egg, substitute,							
¼ cup:							
(*Egg Beaters*)	30	6.0	1.0	0	0	125	0
(*Healthy Choice*)	30	5.0	1.0	<1.0	0	90	0
(*Morningstar Farms*							
Better'n Eggs)	20	5.0	0	0	0	90	0
(*Morningstar Scram-*							
blers)	35	6.0	2.0	0	0	95	0
Egg, turkey, 1 egg . . .	135	10.8	.9	9.4	737	n.a.	0
Egg breakfast, dried,							
1 serving:							
w/bacon:							
(*Mountain House*)	150	11.0	5.0	9.0	345	460	0
precooked (*Moun-*							
tain House)	120	10.0	5.0	7.0	190	550	0
omelet:							
cheese (*Mountain*							
House)	180	13.0	7.0	11.0	335	530	0
ranch, w/beef (*Al-*							
pineAire)	400	36.0	3.0	27.0	1100	420	0
scrambled:							
(*AlpineAire*)	170	11.0	2.0	13.0	345	180	0
(*AlpineAire* Bandito)	240	15.0	17.0	12.0	430	500	2.0
scrambling/omelet mix							
(*AlpineAire*)	330	27.0	3.0	23.0	980	300	0
Egg breakfast, frozen,							
1 pkg.:							
omelet:							
cheese, three							
(*Papetti Foods*							
Chef's)	230	14.0	5.0	16.0	150	660	0
ham (*Papetti Foods*							
Chef's)	180	14.0	5.0	12.0	140	600	0
ham and cheese							
(*Weight Watch-*							
ers)	220	13.0	30.0	5.0	30	440	2.0
sausage and cheese							
(*Papetti Foods*							
Chef's)	240	15.0	4.0	18.0	145	590	0
Western (*Papetti*							
Foods Chef's) . . .	150	11.0	6.0	9.0	130	440	0

Food and Measure	cal.	prot. (gms)	carbo. (gms)	fat (gms)	chol. (mgs)	sod. (mgs)	fiber (gms)
Egg breakfast, frozen *(cont.)*							
scrambled:							
w/bacon, home fries *(Swanson Great Starts)*	290	11.0	17.0	19.0	240	700	1.0
w/sausage, hash browns *(Swanson Great Starts)*	360	12.0	21.0	26.0	280	800	3.0
Egg breakfast sandwich, see "Breakfast sandwich"							
Egg pocket, see "Breakfast sandwich"							
Egg roll, frozen:							
(Matlaw's), 2 rolls . . .	45	1.0	8.0	1.0	0	120	1.0
chicken:							
(Chun King Restaurant Style), 3-oz. roll	190	6.0	22.0	9.0	20	550	2.0
mini *(Chun King)*, 6 rolls	210	6.0	25.0	9.0	15	650	2.0
pork and shrimp, mini *(Chun King)*, 6 rolls	210	6.0	27.0	9.0	15	540	2.0
shrimp:							
(Chun King Restaurant Style), 3-oz. roll	180	5.0	25.0	7.0	15	490	2.0
mini *(Chun King)*, 6 rolls	190	5.0	28.0	6.0	10	730	2.0
vegetarian *(Worthington)*, 1 roll	180	6.0	20.0	8.0	0	380	2.0
Egg roll entree, frozen, vegetable *(Lean Cuisine)*, 9 oz.	340	7.0	64.0	6.0	0	590	3.0
Egg roll wrapper:							
(Frieda's), 2 pcs.	130	5.0	28.0	.5	0	250	1.0
(Nasoya), 1½ oz.	117	4.5	23.7	.5	14	290	1.0
Eggnog, dairy, ½ cup:							
(Crowley)	190	4.0	23.0	9.0	65	130	0
(Crowley Light)	120	4.0	22.0	2.0	n.a.	95	0

Food and Measure	cal.	prot. (gms)	carbo. (gms)	fat (gms)	chol. (mgs)	sod. (mgs)	fiber (gms)
(*Crowley* Nonfat)	130	5.0	25.0	0	20	75	0
(*Hood* Fat Free)	110	8.0	19.0	.4	<5	210	0
(*Hood* Golden)	180	4.0	22.0	8.0	65	100	0
(*Hood* Light)	140	4.0	22.0	4.0	45	100	0
vanilla (*Hood*)	180	4.0	22.0	8.0	65	100	0
Eggplant, fresh:							
raw, 1″ pcs., ½ cup	11	.4	2.5	.1	0	1	1.0
raw, Japanese, w/peel, (*Frieda's*), ⅔ cup, 3 oz.	20	1.0	5.0	0	0	0	2.0
boiled, drained, 1″ cubes, ½ cup ...	13	.4	3.2	.1	0	2	1.2
Eggplant appetizer:							
(*Cedar's* Baba Ghannouj), 2 tbsp.	50	2.0	5.0	2.0	0	80	3.0
(*Progresso* Caponata), 2 tbsp.	25	0	2.0	2.0	0	130	2.0
(*Sabra* Babaganoush), 1 oz.	77	.3	1.5	7.7	8	110	.9
roasted, hummus (*Vita*), 2 tbsp.	31	1.0	3.0	1.5	0	73	1.0
salad, grilled, chopped (*Sabra*), 1 oz.	61	.1	.7	6.4	0	138	.9
Spanish (*Sabra*), 1 oz.	70	.4	2.3	6.7	0	78	.4
w/tomato (*Sabra* Matbucha Salad), 1 oz.	18	.3	1.6	1.1	0	116	.5
Eggplant appetizer mix, dry (*Casbah* Baba Ganoush), 2 oz.	150	8.0	25.0	1.5	0	280	2.0
Eggplant cutlet, frozen, breaded (*The Eggplant People*), 3 oz.	100	2.0	14.0	9.0	0	160	2.0
Eggplant entree, frozen, Parmesan (*Cedar Lane*), 5-oz. pkg.	160	7.0	16.0	8.0	15	390	3.0

Food and Measure	cal.	prot. (gms)	carbo. (gms)	fat (gms)	chol. (mgs)	sod. (mgs)	fiber (gms)
Eggplant pickle relish							
(*Patak's* Brinjal),							
1 tbsp.	60	0	10.0	2.0	0	180	<1.0
Elderberry, ½ cup . . .	53	.5	13.3	.4	0	n.a.	5.1
Empanadillas, frozen,							
2 pcs.:							
cheese (*Goya*)	350	10.0	44.0	15.0	20	659	2.0
pizza (*Goya*)	370	11.0	56.0	12.0	15	930	4.0
Enchilada, canned							
(*Gebhardt*), 2 pcs.	250	5.0	22.0	16.5	20	590	4.0
Enchilada dinner, fro-							
zen, 1 pkg.:							
(*Chi-Chi's* Baja),							
16 oz.	590	27.0	75.0	20.0	50	1920	15.0
beef:							
(*Banquet Extra Help-*							
ing), 15.65 oz.	610	20.0	73.0	26.0	30	2320	7.0
(*Patio*), 12 oz.	370	12.0	52.0	12.0	25	1700	9.0
(*Patio* Chili 'n							
Beans), 15½ oz.	540	12.0	73.0	22.0	50	2690	12.0
beef and cheese (*Patio*							
Chili 'n Beans),							
15½ oz.	610	20.0	80.0	24.0	60	2400	12.0
black bean (*Amy's*),							
10 oz.	250	7.0	41.0	8.0	0	680	5.0
cheese:							
(*Amy's*), 9 oz.	330	15.0	38.0	14.0	30	680	6.0
(*Patio*), 12 oz.	370	11.0	54.0	12.0	25	1570	7.0
chicken:							
(*Chi-Chi's* Su-							
preme), 16 oz.	600	26.0	80.0	20.0	70	2310	11.0
(*Healthy Choice*							
Suprema),							
11.3 oz.	300	13.0	46.0	7.0	40	560	4.0
(*Patio*), 12 oz.	400	13.0	60.0	12.0	35	1470	8.0
Enchilada entree, fro-							
zen, 1 pkg., except							
as noted:							
beef:							
(*Banquet* Meal),							
11 oz.	370	10.0	54.0	12.0	20	1330	8.0

Food and Measure	cal.	prot. (gms)	carbo. (gms)	fat (gms)	chol. (mgs)	sod. (mgs)	fiber (gms)
(*Patio* Family),							
2 pcs. w/sauce	210	5.0	29.0	8.0	20	940	5.0
and tamale (*Banquet*), 11 oz.	400	10.0	56.0	15.0	30	1530	9.0
black bean vegetable:							
(*Amy's*), 4¾ oz. ...	130	4.0	20.0	4.0	0	390	2.0
(*Amy's* Family),							
4.38 oz.	120	4.0	18.0	4.0	0	360	2.0
cheese:							
(*Amy's*), 4¾ oz. ...	210	10.0	13.0	12.0	35	440	2.0
(*Amy's* Family),							
5 oz.	240	11.0	13.0	13.0	35	490	2.0
(*Banquet*), 11 oz.	360	12.0	56.0	10.0	20	1500	8.0
(*Patio* Family),							
2 pcs. w/sauce	210	6.0	30.0	7.0	20	880	2.0
chicken:							
(*Banquet*), 11 oz.	350	12.0	54.0	10.0	25	1580	9.0
(*Stouffer's*), ¹⁄₁₂ of							
58-oz. pkg.	220	8.0	22.0	11.0	30	570	2.0
Suiza (*Healthy*							
Choice), 10 oz.	280	14.0	43.0	6.0	25	440	5.0
Suiza (*Smart Ones*),							
9 oz.	270	15.0	33.0	9.0	50	660	2.0
Suiza, w/rice (*Lean*							
Cuisine), 9 oz.	280	11.0	48.0	5.0	25	520	3.0
combo (*Banquet*							
Meal), 11 oz.	360	10.0	55.0	11.0	20	1390	9.0
Enchilada sauce,							
¼ cup:							
(*Chi-Chi's*)	30	0	3.0	2.0	0	210	0
(*Gebhardt*)	35	1.0	4.0	2.0	<5	265	1.0
(*La Victoria*)	20	0	3.0	1.0	0	400	0
(*Rosarita*)	20	<1.0	3.0	1.0	0	400	0
green chili (*Old El*							
Paso)	30	<1.0	3.0	1.5	0	330	0
hot, medium, or mild							
(*Old El Paso*)	30	0	4.0	1.5	0	190	0
Enchilada sauce mix							
(*Old El Paso*), 2 tsp.	10	0	2.0	0	0	540	<1.0
Endive, chopped,							
½ cup	4	.3	.8	.1	0	6	.8

Food and Measure	cal.	prot. (gms)	carbo. (gms)	fat (gms)	chol. (mgs)	sod. (mgs)	fiber (gms)
Endive, Belgian, see "Chicory, witloof"							
Entree mix, frozen, see "Vegetable entree mix" and specific listings							
Eppaw, ½ cup	75	2.3	15.8	.9	0	6	n.a.
Escarole, see "Endive"							

F

Food and Measure	cal.	prot. (gms)	carbo. (gms)	fat (gms)	chol. (mgs)	sod. (mgs)	fiber (gms)
Fajita dinner mix:							
(*Chi-Chi's* Kit), seasoning, 2 shells ...	300	6.0	54.0	7.0	0	1280	2.0
(*Old El Paso* Kit), 2 pcs.*	300	15.0	34.0	12.0	25	810	1.0
Fajita entree, see specific listings							
Fajita pocket, frozen, 4½-oz. pc.:							
beef (*Hot Pockets*) ...	340	14.0	39.0	14.0	40	680	5.0
chicken (*Lean Pockets*)	270	11.0	41.0	7.0	30	580	5.0
Fajita sauce (*World Harbors* Guadalupe Mountain), 2 tbsp.	45	0	10	0	0	290	0
Fajita seasoning (*El Rio*), 1 tbsp.	5	0	0	0	0	60	0
Fajita seasoning mix:							
(*Lawry's* Chicken), 1 tsp.	10	0	2.0	0	0	320	0
(*Old El Paso*), 1½ tsp.	10	0	2.0	0	0	200	0
Falafel mix, dry:							
(*Casbah*), 1½ oz.	160	6.0	20.0	3.0	0	530	2.0
(*Fantastic Foods*), ½ cup	250	15.0	42.0	4.0	0	610	11.0
(*Near East*), ¼ cup ...	100	10.0	18.0	1.0	0	560	5.0
Farfalle dishes, mix, dry, w/Alfredo sauce (*Al Dente*), 1 cup ...	230	8.0	44.0	1.5	5	310	2.0
Farina, whole-grain (see also "Cereal"):							
dry, 1 oz.	105	3.0	22.1	.1	0	1	.8

Food and Measure	cal.	prot. (gms)	carbo. (gms)	fat (gms)	chol. (mgs)	sod. (mgs)	fiber (gms)
Farina, whole-grain *(cont.)*							
cooked, 1 cup.......	116	3.4	24.6	.2	0	1	3.3
Farro, see "Spelt"							
Fat, see specific listings							
Fava beans, see "Broad beans"							
Feijoa, raw:							
(*Frieda's*), 5 oz.	70	2.0	15.0	1.0	0	0	0
w/skin, 1 medium, 2.3 oz.	25	.6	5.3	.4	0	2	0
pureed, ½ cup	60	1.5	12.9	1.0	0	4	0
Fennel, bulb, raw:							
(*Frieda's*), ¾ cup, 3 oz.	25	1.0	6.0	0	0	45	0
8.3-oz. bulb	72	2.9	17.1	.5	0	122	n.a.
sliced, ½ cup	27	1.1	6.3	.2	0	45	0
Fennel seed, 1 tsp.	7	.3	1.1	.3	0	2	<1.0
Fenugreek seed, 1 tsp.	12	.9	2.2	.2	0	2	<1.0
Fettuccine:							
dry, see "Pasta" refrigerated:							
refrigerated:							
(*Contadina*), 1¼ cups	240	10.0	45.0	2.5	90	20	2.0
(*Di Giorno*), 2½ oz.	190	7.0	39.0	1.5	0	125	2.0
spinach (*Contadina*), 1¼ cups	260	12.0	43.0	4.0	100	110	3.0
spinach (*Di Giorno*), 2½ oz.	190	7.0	38.0	1.5	0	140	2.0
Fettuccine dishes, mix, dry, except as noted:							
(*AlpineAire* Leonardo da Fettuccine), 2¾ oz.	320	16.0	41.0	10.0	30	710	1.0
Alfredo:							
(*DeBoles*), 2.4 oz.	270	11.0	44.0	3.0	10	730	2.0
(*Knorr*), ¾ cup	280	11.0	43.0	7.0	70	960	2.0
(*Knorr* Cup), 1 cont.	230	7.0	41.0	4.0	10	980	1.0

Food and Measure	cal.	prot. (gms)	carbo. (gms)	fat (gms)	chol. (mgs)	sod. (mgs)	fiber (gms)
(*Pasta Roni*), 1 cup*	240	13.0	48.0	26.0	10	1110	2.0
(*Pasta Roni* Reduced Fat), 1 cup*	310	11.0	50.0	8.0	10	1080	2.0
w/basil sauce, creamy (*Knorr* Cup), 1 cont.	220	6.0	40.0	4.0	10	850	2.0
curly, cheddar-broccoli sauce (*Annie's*), ²/₃ cup	260	10.0	48.0	3.0	5	450	2.0
tomato-basil sauce (*DeBoles*), 2 oz. . . .	240	7.0	41.0	.5	0	460	2.0
Fettuccine entree, frozen, 1 pkg., except as noted:							
Alfredo:							
(*Banquet*), 9½ oz.	350	11.0	40.0	16.0	25	850	4.0
(*Banquet* Family), 1 cup	350	7.0	37.0	19.0	50	700	2.0
(*Freezer Queen*), 9 oz.	360	13.0	42.0	15.0	45	840	3.0
(*Healthy Choice*), 8 oz.	250	11.0	39.0	5.0	15	480	3.0
(*Lean Cuisine*), 9 oz.	300	12.0	47.0	7.0	15	550	2.0
(*Marie Callender's* Supreme), 1 cup, ½ of 13-oz. pkg.	450	15.0	35.0	27.0	80	680	4.0
(*Michelina's*), 9½ oz.	400	15.0	48.0	16.0	40	690	2.0
(*Smart Ones*), 9¼ oz.	270	14.0	39.0	6.0	15	650	3.0
(*Stouffer's*), 10 oz.	460	16.0	47.0	23.0	70	910	3.0
four-cheese (*The Budget Gourmet Value Classics*), 8 oz.	320	13.0	40.0	12.0	60	640	5.0
w/garlic bread (*Marie Callender's*), 14 oz.	800	23.0	71.0	47.0	95	1270	5.0
w/broccoli and chicken (*Marie Callender's*), ½ of 13 oz. pkg. . . .	410	16.0	32.0	24.0	45	550	4.0

Food and Measure	cal.	prot. (gms)	carbo. (gms)	fat (gms)	chol. (mgs)	sod. (mgs)	fiber (gms)
Fettuccine entree, frozen *(cont.)*							
and meatballs, in wine sauce (*The Budget Gourmet* Low Fat), 8½ oz.	270	15.0	40.0	7.0	25	560	3.0
w/mushrooms and herbs (*The Budget Gourmet*), 8 oz. ...	320	10.0	40.0	13.0	65	600	2.0
primavera:							
(*Lean Cuisine*), 10 oz.	270	13.0	38.0	7.0	15	580	4.0
(*Stouffer's*), 10 oz.	370	14.0	45.0	15.0	40	950	4.0
herb sauce (*The Budget Gourmet* Low Fat), 8½ oz.	260	12.0	36.0	6.0	20	590	3.0
w/tortellini (*Marie Callender's*), 1 cup, 7 oz.	430	11.0	35.0	27.0	35	670	4.0
Fig, fresh:							
large, 2.3 oz.	47	.5	12.3	.2	0	1	2.1
medium, 1.8 oz.	37	.4	9.6	.2	0	1	1.7
Fig, canned, ½ cup:							
in syrup	114	.5	29.7	.1	0	2	2.8
Kadota, in heavy syrup (*Oregon*)	130	<1.0	30.0	1.0	0	5	3.0
Fig, dried:							
10 figs, 6.6 oz.	477	5.7	122.2	2.2	0	20	17.4
California, 4 figs, 2 oz.	143	2.4	38.8	.7	0	6	9.5
Calimyrna (*Sun•Maid*), 3 pcs., 1.5 oz.	120	1.0	28.0	0	0	0	5.0
Calimyrna or Mission (*Sonoma* Organic), 3 pcs., 1.4 oz.	110	1.0	26.0	0	0	0	5.0
Filbert:							
dried:							
1 oz.	179	3.7	4.4	17.8	0	1	1.7
chopped, 1 cup	727	15.0	17.6	72.0	0	3	7.0
blanched, 1 oz. ...	191	3.6	4.5	19.1	0	1	<2.0
dry-roasted:							
1 oz.	188	2.8	5.1	18.8	0	1	<2.0

Food and Measure	cal.	prot. (gms)	carbo. (gms)	fat (gms)	chol. (mgs)	sod. (mgs)	fiber (gms)
salted, 1 oz.	188	2.8	5.1	18.8	0	221	<2.0
oil-roasted:							
1 oz.	187	4.1	5.4	18.1	0	1	1.8
salted, 1 oz.	187	4.1	5.4	18.1	0	223	1.8
Fillo pastry, frozen:							
(*Apollo*), 1/8 pkg.	180	5.0	35.0	0	0	300	1.0
mini shells (*Athens Foods*), 2 pcs.	45	1.0	5.0	2.0	0	20	0
Fish, see specific listings							
"Fish," vegetarian:							
frozen (*Worthington*), 2 pcs.	180	16.0	8.0	10.0	0	750	4.0
mix (*Loma Linda* Ocean Platter), 1/3 cup	90	14.0	8.0	1.0	0	450	4.0
Fish dinner, frozen, battered, 'n chips (*Swanson*), 10-oz. pkg.	490	19.0	59.0	20.0	45	1030	5.0
Fish entree, frozen (see also specific fish listings):							
baked (*Lean Cuisine American Favorites*), 9 oz.	270	17.0	36.0	6.0	45	540	3.0
bites, battered (*Gorton's* Tenders), 3½ pcs., 4 oz.	250	11.0	20.0	14.0	30	530	0
w/cheese, salsa (*Oven Poppers*), 4½-oz. pc.	130	16.0	3.0	6.0	70	150	1.0
fillet:							
in butter sauce (*Mrs. Paul's*), 1 pc.	120	16.0	4.0	5.0	25	450	0
w/macaroni and cheese (*Stouffer's* Homestyle), 9 oz.	430	24.0	39.0	21.0	70	930	2.0

Food and Measure	cal.	prot. (gms)	carbo. (gms)	fat (gms)	chol. (mgs)	sod. (mgs)	fiber (gms)
Fish entree *(cont.)*							
fillet, baked, 1 pc.:							
au gratin (*Gorton's* Homestyle)	130	14.0	7.0	5.0	50	400	0
garlic-herb (*Mrs. Paul's/Van de Kamp's* Crunchy)	150	8.0	17.0	5.0	20	540	0
lemon pepper (*Mrs. Paul's/Van de Kamp's* Crunchy)	140	8.0	17.0	5.0	20	410	0
fillet, battered:							
(*Mrs. Paul's*), 1 pc.	170	6.0	13.0	11.0	15	470	1.0
(*Van de Kamp's*), 1 pc.	180	8.0	12.0	11.0	20	340	0
crispy (*Gorton's*), 2 pcs.	240	11.0	19.0	13.0	40	540	0
lemon pepper (*Gorton's*), 2 pcs. ...	270	9.0	18.0	18.0	35	610	0
fillet, breaded:							
(*Mrs. Paul's*), 2 pcs.	240	13.0	20.0	12.0	25	390	1.0
(*Mrs. Paul's/Van de Kamp's* Crisp & Healthy), 2 pcs.	150	12.0	20.0	2.5	30	380	0
(*Van de Kamp's*), 2 pcs.	280	11.0	17.0	19.0	35	270	0
cornmeal (*Mrs. Paul's/Van de Kamp's* Country), 1 pc.	180	7.0	15.0	11.0	20	580	0
crunchy (*Gorton's*), 2 pcs.	250	10.0	21.0	14.0	35	480	0
w/fries (*Van de Kamp's* Fish 'n Fries), 6.6 oz. ...	380	13.0	41.0	18.0	25	370	2.0
garlic and herb (*Gorton's*), 2 pcs.	220	10.0	21.0	11.0	30	670	0
Parmesan (*Gorton's*), 2 pcs. ...	260	10.0	20.0	15.0	30	650	0
southern-fried (*Gorton's*), 2 pcs. ...	230	10.0	16.0	14.0	30	660	0

Food and Measure	cal.	prot. (gms)	carbo. (gms)	fat (gms)	chol. (mgs)	sod. (mgs)	fiber (gms)
fillet, grilled, 1 pc.:							
garlic butter (*Gorton's*)	120	16.0	1.0	6.0	60	300	0
garlic butter or Italian herb (*Mrs. Paul's/Van de Kamp's*)	130	18.0	0	6.0	60	230	0
lemon pepper (*Mrs. Paul's/Van de Kamp's*)	130	18.0	0	6.0	60	250	0
herb baked (*Healthy Choice*), 10.9 oz.	340	16.0	54.0	7.0	35	480	5.0
lemon pepper (*Healthy Choice*), 10.7 oz.	320	14.0	50.0	7.0	30	480	5.0
nuggets:							
(*Frionor Bunch O Crunch*), 6 pcs., 3 oz.	210	10.0	17.0	11.0	25	430	0
battered (*Van de Kamp's*), 8 pcs.	280	11.0	20.0	18.0	25	600	0
portions:							
battered (*Mrs. Paul's*), 1 pc. . . .	160	6.0	13.0	9.0	20	400	0
battered (*Van de Kamp's*), 1 pc.	180	6.0	13.0	11.0	20	350	0
breaded (*Mrs. Paul's*), 2 pcs.	190	9.0	16.0	10.0	15	280	1.0
w/shrimp, crab, vegetables (*Oven Poppers*), 4½-oz. pc.	200	13.0	13.0	11.0	85	380	0
w/spinach, cheese (*Oven Poppers*), 4½-oz. pc.	160	15.0	8.0	8.0	70	310	0
sticks:							
(*Banquet*), 6.6 oz.	290	11.0	33.0	13.0	30	820	4.0
(*Frionor Bunch O Crunch*), 5 pcs.	230	10.0	19.0	13.0	30	640	0
(*Kid Cuisine Funtastic*), 8¼ oz.	410	9.0	57.0	16.0	20	550	4.0
sticks, battered (*Gorton's*), 5 pcs.	290	10.0	20.0	19.0	25	530	0

Food and Measure	cal.	prot. (gms)	carbo. (gms)	fat (gms)	chol. (mgs)	sod. (mgs)	fiber (gms)
Fish entree, sticks, battered *(cont.)*							
(*Mrs. Paul's*),							
6 pcs.	270	8.0	21.0	17.0	30	810	1.0
(*Van de Kamp's*),							
6 pcs.	260	11.0	18.0	16.0	30	540	0
sticks, breaded, 6 pcs.,							
except as noted:							
(*Gorton's*)	250	12.0	21.0	13.0	30	340	0
(*Mrs. Paul's*)	210	11.0	21.0	10.0	20	540	2.0
(*Mrs. Paul's* Value							
Pack)..........	220	9.0	20.0	11.0	20	420	1.0
(*Mrs. Paul's/Van de*							
Kamp's Crisp &							
Healthy)	180	13.0	26.0	3.0	25	440	0
(*Van de Kamp's*) ...	290	13.0	23.0	17.0	35	390	0
(*Van de Kamp's*							
Snack/Value							
Pack)..........	260	11.0	21.0	14.0	25	350	0
mini (*Gorton's*),							
13 pcs.	230	11.0	18.0	13.0	25	430	0
mini (*Van de*							
Kamp's), 13 pcs.	250	11.0	19.0	14.0	30	330	0
Fish roll, frozen, 2 oz.:							
(*Season* Rolle Classic							
Original)	75	7.0	5.0	3.0	30	380	1.0
almond (*Season* Rolle)	90	7.0	6.0	4.0	50	360	1.0
lemon dill (*Season*							
Rolle)	90	7.0	6.0	4.0	40	340	1.0
salmon (*Season* Rolle)	90	8.0	6.0	4.0	45	340	1.0
Fish sandwich, fillet,							
frozen (*Hormel*							
Quick Meal), 1 pc.	420	15.0	49.0	18.0	40	960	1.0
Fish seasoning, see							
specific listings							
Fish seasoning and							
coating mix (*Shake*							
'n Bake), 1/4 pkt.	70	1.0	14.0	1.5	0	420	1.0
Flan, see "Pudding"							
and "Pudding and							
pie filling mix"							

Food and Measure	cal.	prot. (gms)	carbo. (gms)	fat (gms)	chol. (mgs)	sod. (mgs)	fiber (gms)
Flatfish, meat only:							
raw, 4 oz.	104	21.4	0	1.4	54	92	0
baked, broiled, or microwaved, 4 oz. ...	133	27.4	0	1.7	77	119	0
Flavor enhancer, ¼ tsp. dry, except as noted:							
(*Ac'cent*), ⅛ tsp.	0	0	0	0	0	80	0
(*Sa-so'n Ac'cent*)	0	0	0	0	0	150	0
(*Sa-so'n Ac'cent* con Ajo Cebolla)	0	0	0	0	0	140	0
(*Sa-so'n Ac'cent* con Azafran)	0	0	0	0	0	125	0
(*Sa-so'n Ac'cent* Culantro)	0	0	0	0	0	170	0
liquid (*Watkins* Meat Magic), 1 tsp.	10	0	2.0	0	0	180	0
Flax powder (*Arrowhead Mills* Nutri Flax), 2 tbsp.	70	6.0	6.0	2.0	0	10	6.0
Flax seeds (*Arrowhead Mills*), 3 tbsp.	140	5.0	11.0	10.0	0	0	6.0
Flounder:							
fresh, see "Flatfish"							
frozen (*Van de Kamp's*), 4-oz. fillet	110	22.0	0	2.0	45	105	0
Flounder entree, frozen:							
au gratin (*Oven Poppers*), 5-oz. pc. ...	220	24.0	5.0	11.0	75	450	1.0
breaded, fillet, 1 pc.:							
(*Mrs. Paul's*), 2.8 oz.	170	8.0	16.0	8.0	25	370	1.0
(*Van de Kamp's*), 4 oz.	230	15.0	19.0	11.0	40	400	0
primavera (*Frionor*), 1 pc., 9 oz.	270	32.0	0	13.0	100	930	0
stuffed, 5-oz. pc.:							
w/broccoli and cheese (*Oven Poppers*)	150	20.0	4.0	6.0	55	330	1.0

Food and Measure	cal.	prot. (gms)	carbo. (gms)	fat (gms)	chol. (mgs)	sod. (mgs)	fiber (gms)
Flounder entree, stuffed *(cont.)*							
w/crab (*Oven Poppers*)	250	17.0	15.0	13.0	70	400	1.0
w/garlic, shrimp, almonds (*Oven Poppers*)	250	19.0	15.0	13.0	80	430	2.0
Flour, see "Wheat flour" and specific listings							
Frankfurter (see also "Knockwurst"), 1 link, except as noted:							
(*Ball Park Franks*)	180	6.0	2.0	16.0	40	660	0
(*Ball Park Franks* Fat Free)	45	6.0	4.0	0	10	450	0
(*Ball Park Lite Franks*)	100	6.0	3.0	7.0	25	640	0
(*Boar's Head* Natural Casing/Skinless) . . .	150	7.0	0	14.0	25	460	0
(*Healthy Choice* Low Fat), 1.4 oz.	60	5.0	5.0	2.0	10	320	0
(*Healthy Choice* Low Fat/Bunsize), 1.8 oz.	70	6.0	6.0	2.5	15	400	0
(*Hormel Light & Lean* Fat Free)	45	5.0	5.0	0	15	580	0
(*Oscar Mayer* Fat Free Wieners)	40	6.0	3.0	0	15	490	0
(*Oscar Mayer* Little Wieners), 6 links . . .	180	6.0	2.0	17.0	35	570	0
(*Oscar Mayer* Wieners)	140	5.0	1.0	13.0	35	440	0
(*Oscar Mayer* Bun-Length Wieners) . . .	190	6.0	2.0	17.0	40	570	0
(*Oscar Mayer Free* Hot Dogs)	40	7.0	2.0	0	15	490	0
beef:							
(*Alan King's "Perfect"*)	120	6.0	0	10.0	25	310	0
(*Ball Park Franks*)	180	6.0	2.0	16.0	35	670	0

Food and Measure	cal.	prot. (gms)	carbo. (gms)	fat (gms)	chol. (mgs)	sod. (mgs)	fiber (gms)
(*Ball Park Franks* Fat Free)	45	6.0	5.0	0	10	470	0
(*Ball Park Lite Franks*)	100	6.0	3.0	7.0	25	620	0
(*Boar's Head* Lite)	90	7.0	0	6.0	25	270	0
(*Boar's Head* Natural Casing)	160	7.0	1.0	14.0	30	440	0
(*Boar's Head* Skinless)	120	6.0	0	11.0	20	350	0
(*Healthy Choice*) ...	80	6.0	7.0	2.5	15	400	0
(*Hebrew National*)	150	6.0	1.0	14.0	30	370	0
(*Hebrew National* 99% Fat Free) ...	45	6.0	3.0	1.5	15	400	0
Hebrew National Reduced Fat)	120	8.0	1.0	10.0	25	350	0
(*Hormel Light & Lean* Fat Free) ...	45	6.0	5.0	0	10	590	0
(*Hormel Wranglers*)	170	7.0	1.0	15.0	40	560	0
(*Oscar Mayer*)	140	5.0	1.0	13.0	30	460	0
(*Oscar Mayer Big & Juicy* Deli Style)	230	9.0	1.0	22.0	50	680	0
(*Oscar Mayer Big & Juicy* Original) ...	240	9.0	1.0	22.0	45	700	0
(*Oscar Mayer Free*)	35	7.0	2.0	0	20	480	0
(*Oscar Mayer Light*)	110	6.0	2.0	8.0	30	620	0
cocktail (*Cohen's Famous*), 7 pcs.	320	8.0	13.0	26.0	30	500	1.0
cocktail (*Hebrew National*), 4 pcs., 2 oz.	180	7.0	0	16.0	40	450	0
dinner (*Hebrew National* 1/4 Pound)	350	14.0	1.0	34.0	75	890	0
cheese:							
(*Hormel Wranglers*)	170	7.0	1.0	15.0	40	630	0
(*Oscar Mayer* Cheese Dogs) ...	150	5.0	1.0	13.0	40	490	0
chicken, 2-oz. link:							
(*Empire* Kosher) ...	100	8.0	1.0	7.0	70	465	0
(*Wampler*)	120	7.0	0	11.0	50	480	1.0

Food and Measure	cal.	prot. (gms)	carbo. (gms)	fat (gms)	chol. (mgs)	sod. (mgs)	fiber (gms)
Frankfurter *(cont.)*							
hot and spicy:							
(*Oscar Mayer* Little							
Wieners), 6 links	170	7.0	1.0	16.0	40	580	0
(*Oscar Mayer Big &*							
Juicy Wieners)	220	10.0	1.0	20.0	45	750	0
smoked:							
(*Hormel Wranglers*)	170	7.0	1.0	15.0	40	560	0
(*Oscar Mayer Big &*							
Juicy Smokie) . . .	220	10.0	1.0	19.0	50	770	0
turkey:							
(*Ball Park Franks* Fat							
Free)	40	6.0	4.0	0	13	530	0
(*Empire* Kosher) . . .	90	9.0	<1.0	6.0	35	410	0
(*Wampler*), 1.6 oz.	90	6.0	0	8.0	35	430	2.0
and beef (*Oscar*							
Mayer Hot Dogs)	40	7.0	2.0	0	15	460	0
"Frankfurter," vege-							
tarian, 1 link, except							
as noted:							
canned:							
(*Loma Linda* Big)	110	10.0	2.0	7.0	0	240	2.0
(*Loma Linda* Big							
Lowfat)	80	11.0	3.0	3.0	0	220	2.0
(*Loma Linda* Little							
Links), 2 links . . .	90	8.0	2.0	6.0	0	230	2.0
(*Loma Linda*							
Linketts)	70	7.0	1.0	4.5	0	160	1.0
(*Worthington Super*							
Links)	110	7.0	2.0	8.0	0	350	1.0
(*Worthington Veja*							
Links)	50	5.0	1.0	3.0	0	190	0
(*Worthington Veja*							
Links Lowfat) . . .	40	5.0	1.0	1.5	0	190	0
frozen:							
(*Morningstar Farms*							
Original)	80	11.0	6.0	.5	0	580	1.0
(*Natural Touch* Vege							
Frank)	100	10.0	2.0	6.0	0	470	2.0
(*VegiDogs*)	45	9.0	1.0	0	0	170	0

Food and Measure	cal.	prot. (gms)	carbo. (gms)	fat (gms)	chol. (mgs)	sod. (mgs)	fiber (gms)
(*Worthington Leanies*)	100	7.0	2.0	7.0	0	430	1.0
corn (*Loma Linda*)	150	7.0	22.0	4.0	0	500	3.0
corn (*Morningstar Farms*)	150	7.0	22.0	4.0	0	500	3.0
Frankfurter sandwich, frozen, 1 pc., except as noted:							
(*Ball Park Fun Franks*), 4 oz.	350	12.0	29.0	21.0	45	900	3.0
beef (*Ball Park Fun Franks*), 4 oz.	340	12.0	29.0	20.0	40	800	3.0
corn dog:							
(*Ball Park*)	220	5.0	21.0	13.0	20	840	1.0
(*Hormel Quick Meal*)	220	6.0	25.0	11.0	45	520	1.0
(*Kid Cuisine* Circus Show Entree), 8.8-oz. pkg.	450	8.0	70.0	15.0	30	750	5.0
beef (*Ball Park*)	220	5.0	21.0	12.0	20	820	1.0
mini (*Hormel Quick Meal*), 10 pcs.	490	6.0	47.0	29.0	90	1130	1.0
Franks and beans, see "Beans and franks"							
French toast, frozen, 2 pcs.:							
(*Aunt Jemima* Homestyle)	240	10.0	35.0	7.0	95	310	2.0
cinnamon (*Aunt Jemima*)	240	10.0	35.0	7.0	90	330	2.0
French toast breakfast, frozen, 1 pkg.:							
sticks, w/syrup (*Swanson Great Starts*)	320	7.0	25.0	50.0	25	260	2.0
w/sausage:							
(*Swanson Great Starts*)	410	12.0	36.0	24.0	95	490	3.0
cinnamon swirl (*Swanson Great Starts*)	440	14.0	35.0	28.0	150	580	2.0
Frog's legs, meat only, raw, 4 oz. ...	83	18.6	0	.3	n.a.	n.a.	0

Food and Measure	cal.	prot. (gms)	carbo. (gms)	fat (gms)	chol. (mgs)	sod. (mgs)	fiber (gms)
Frosting, ready-to-spread, 2 tbsp.:							
banana creme (*Pillsbury Creamy Supreme*)	150	0	23.0	6.0	0	70	0
butter cream:							
(*Creamy Deluxe*) . . .	150	0	25.0	6.0	0	70	0
(*Duncan Hines*)	140	0	22.0	5.0	0	60	0
chocolate (*Duncan Hines*)	130	0	20.0	5.0	0	95	0
butterscotch (*Duncan Hines*)	140	0	22.0	5.0	0	60	0
caramel (*Duncan Hines*)	140	0	22.0	5.0	0	60	0
caramel pecan (*Pillsbury Creamy Supreme*)	150	0	19.0	8.0	0	65	0
cherry (*Creamy Deluxe*)	140	0	24.0	5.0	0	40	0
cherry, wild, vanilla (*Duncan Hines*)	140	0	22.0	5.0	0	60	0
chocolate:							
(*Creamy Deluxe*) . . .	130	0	22.0	5.0	0	95	0
(*Duncan Hines*)	130	0	20.0	5.0	0	95	0
(*Pillsbury Creamy Supreme*)	140	0	21.0	6.0	0	80	0
(*Sweet Rewards*)	120	<1.0	24.0	2.5	0	55	0
(*Whipped Deluxe*)	100	<1.0	14.0	5.0	0	45	0
dark (*Creamy Deluxe*)	140	1.0	22.0	6.0	0	50	1.0
dark (*Pillsbury Creamy Supreme*)	130	0	20.0	6.0	0	45	0
fudge (*Pillsbury Creamy Supreme*)	140	0	21.0	6.0	0	75	0
fudge (*SnackWell's*)	120	0	22.0	3.0	0	65	0
milk (*Creamy Deluxe*)	150	0	24.0	6.0	0	70	0
milk (*Pillsbury Creamy Supreme*)	140	0	21.0	6.0	0	60	<1.0
milk (*SnackWell's*)	120	0	22.0	3.0	0	80	<1.0

Food and Measure	cal.	prot. (gms)	carbo. (gms)	fat (gms)	chol. (mgs)	sod. (mgs)	fiber (gms)
milk (*Sweet Re-wards*)	120	0	24.0	2.5	0	60	0
milk (*Whipped Deluxe*)	100	0	14.0	4.5	0	50	0
milk, swirl, w/fudge glaze (*Pillsbury Creamy Supreme*)	140	0	22.0	6.0	0	60	<1.0
milk or dark (*Duncan Hines*)	130	0	20.0	5.0	0	95	0
mocha (*Duncan Hines*)	130	0	20.0	5.0	0	95	0
mocha (*Pillsbury Creamy Supreme*)	140	0	22.0	6.0	0	55	0
w/stars (*Creamy Deluxe*)	140	0	22.0	5.0	0	105	0
coconut pecan:							
(*Creamy Deluxe*)	140	1.0	17.0	8.0	0	50	0
(*Pillsbury Creamy Supreme*)	160	0	17.0	10.0	0	60	<1.0
cream cheese:							
(*Creamy Deluxe*)	140	1.0	24.0	5.0	0	65	0
(*Duncan Hines*)	140	0	22.0	5.0	0	60	0
(*Pillsbury Creamy Supreme*)	150	0	240	6.0	0	70	0
(*Whipped Deluxe*)	100	0	15.0	4.5	0	45	0
creamy candy (*Pillsbury Creamy Supreme*)	150	0	22.0	7.0	0	95	0
fudge, hot (*Pillsbury Creamy Supreme*)	140	0	21.0	6.0	0	55	0
Funfetti:							
(*Pillsbury Creamy Supreme* Halloween)	140	0	22.0	6.0	0	80	0
chocolate (*Pillsbury Creamy Supreme*)	140	0	22.0	6.0	0	80	0
pink vanilla (*Pillsbury Creamy Supreme*)	150	0	24.0	6.0	0	70	0
vanilla (*Pillsbury Creamy Supreme*)	150	0	25.0	6.0	0	75	0

Food and Measure	cal.	prot. (gms)	carbo. (gms)	fat (gms)	chol. (mgs)	sod. (mgs)	fiber (gms)
Frosting (cont.)							
lemon:							
(Creamy Deluxe) . . .	140	0	24.0	5.0	0	65	0
(Whipped Deluxe)	100	0	15.0	4.5	0	25	0
cream (Duncan							
Hines)	140	0	22.0	5.0	0	60	0
cream (Pillsbury							
Creamy Supreme)	150	0	24.0	6.0	0	75	0
Oreo (Pillsbury							
Creamy Supreme)	150	0	23.0	6.0	0	75	0
rainbow chip (Creamy							
Deluxe)	140	0	23.0	6.0	0	25	0
raspberries or straw-							
berries and cream							
(Duncan Hines)	140	0	22.0	5.0	0	60	0
sour cream:							
chocolate (Creamy							
Deluxe)	150	<1.0	23.0	6.0	0	105	0
white (Creamy							
Deluxe)	150	0	25.0	6.0	0	45	0
strawberry:							
cream cheese							
(Creamy Deluxe)	150	0	26.0	6.0	0	70	0
creme (Pillsbury							
Creamy Supreme)	150	0	24.0	6.0	0	75	0
vanilla:							
(Creamy Deluxe)	140	0	24.0	5.0	0	35	0
(Duncan Hines)	140	0	22.0	5.0	0	60	0
(Pillsbury Creamy							
Supreme)	150	0	21.0	6.0	0	70	0
(Sweet Rewards)	120	0	26.0	2.0	0	65	0
(Whipped Deluxe)	100	0	15.0	4.5	0	25	0
French (Creamy							
Deluxe)	140	0	24.0	5.0	0	20	0
French (Pillsbury							
Creamy Supreme)	160	0	26.0	6.0	0	75	0
w/stars (Creamy							
Deluxe)	140	0	25.0	5.0	0	65	0
swirl, w/fudge glaze							
(Pillsbury Creamy							
Supreme)	150	0	25.0	6.0	0	75	0

Food and Measure	cal.	prot. (gms)	carbo. (gms)	fat (gms)	chol. (mgs)	sod. (mgs)	fiber (gms)
white, fluffy (*Whipped Deluxe*)	100	0	15.0	4.5	0	25	0
white chocolate (*Creamy Deluxe*) . . .	140	0	24.0	5.0	0	70	0
Frosting mix*:							
coconut pecan (*Betty Crocker*), 2 tbsp.	160	<1.0	21.0	8.0	0	55	<1.0
white, fluffy (*Betty Crocker*), 6 tbsp.	100	<1.0	24.0	0	0	60	0
Frozen desserts, see "Ice cream"							
Fructose (*Estee*), 1 tsp.	16	0	4.0	0	0	0	0
Fruit, see specific listings							
Fruit, candied, see specific listings							
Fruit, mixed, candied:							
(*Paradise/Queen Anne* Fruit Cake Mix), 2 tbsp.	100	0	25.0	0	0	20	1.0
(*Paradise* Old English/ *White Swan*), 1 tbsp.	70	0	18.0	0	0	15	1.0
(*White Swan* Deluxe), 2 tbsp.	100	0	25.0	0	0	20	1.0
Fruit, mixed, canned or chilled (see also "Fruit cocktail"), ½ cup, except as noted:							
(*Del Monte* Very Cherry)	90	<1.0	22.0	0	0	10	<1.0
in juice:							
(*Del Monte* Fruit Naturals Chunky)	60	0	15.0	0	0	10	1.0
(*Del Monte* Fruit Naturals cup), 4 oz.	50	0	13.0	0	0	10	<1.0
(*Libby's* Chunky Lite)	60	0	14.0	0	0	5	1.0

Food and Measure	cal.	prot. (gms)	carbo. (gms)	fat (gms)	chol. (mgs)	sod. (mgs)	fiber (gms)
Fruit, mixed, canned or chilled, in juice *(cont.)*							
(*Sunfresh* Mixed Fruit Chilled), 4 oz.	70	1.0	17.0	0	0	25	1.0
citrus (*Sunfresh* Chilled), 4 oz. . . .	70	1.0	16.0	0	0	20	1.0
citrus (*Sunfresh* Chilled), 6 oz. . . .	110	1.0	25.0	0	0	30	1.0
tropical (*Sunfresh* Chilled), 4 oz. . . .	70	1.0	17.0	0	0	10	.0
tropical (*Sunfresh* Chilled), 6 oz. . . .	110	1.0	26.0	0	0	15	0
in extra-light syrup:							
(*Del Monte* Lite Chunky)	60	0	15.0	0	0	10	1.0
(*Del Monte* Lite cup), 4 oz.	50	0	13.0	0	0	10	<1.0
(*Sunfresh* Fruit Salad Chilled) . . .	70	1.0	22.0	0	0	5	2.0
(*Sunfresh* Mixed Fruit Chilled)	90	1.0	20.0	0	0	25	2.0
Ambrosia (*Sunfresh* Chilled)	70	0	16.0	0	0	25	1.0
citrus (*Sunfresh* Chilled)	80	0	20.0	0	0	20	0
tropical (*Sunfresh* Chilled)	80	1.0	20.0	0	0	10	0
in light syrup:							
(*Del Monte* Cut-Ups)	80	0	20.0	0	0	10	<1.0
(*Del Monte* Fruit Express), 6-oz. cup	110	1.0	29.0	0	0	10	2.0
California (*Del Monte* Orchard Select)	80	<1.0	19.0	0	0	10	<1.0
cherry flavor (*Del Monte*)	90	<1.0	22.0	0	0	10	<1.0
citrus salad (*Sunfresh* Can)	50	0	12.0	0	0	0	1.0
tropical (*Del Monte*)	80	0	21.0	0	0	10	1.0

Food and Measure	cal.	prot. (gms)	carbo. (gms)	fat (gms)	chol. (mgs)	sod. (mgs)	fiber (gms)
tropical (*Del Monte* Fruit Express), 6-oz. cup	130	1.0	30.0	0	0	20	2.0
tropical (*Sunfresh* Can)	120	0	28.0	1.0	0	0	1.0
in heavy syrup:							
(*Del Monte* Chunky)	100	0	24.0	0	0	10	1.0
(*Del Monte* Cup), 4 oz.	80	0	20.0	0	0	10	<1.0
tropical salad	110	.5	28.6	.1	0	3	1.7
in cherry-flavor syrup (*Del Monte* Fruit Rageous), 4-oz. cup	90	<1.0	22.0	0	0	10	<1.0
in pineapple–passion fruit juices (*Del Monte* Tropical) . . .	60	0	16.0	0	0	15	1.0
in wildberry flavor juice (*Del Monte* Cut-Ups)	80	0	20.0	0	0	10	<1.0
Fruit, mixed, dried:							
(*Sonoma* Organic), 7 pcs., 1.4 oz.	120	1.0	30.0	0	0	0	3.0
(*Sun•Maid*), 1/4 cup	110	1.0	26.0	0	0	55	3.0
diced:							
(*Sonoma* Organic), 1/3 cup, 1.4 oz.	120	1.0	31.0	0	0	0	3.0
(*Sun•Maid* Bits), 1/4 cup	120	1.0	28.0	0	0	55	2.0
and nuts, see "Trail mix"							
Fruit, mixed, frozen:							
(*Birds Eye*), 1/2 cup	90	<1.0	23.0	0	0	0	n.a.
Fruit bar, frozen (see also "Yogurt bar"), 1 pc.:							
(*Starburst* Single)	80	0	20.0	0	0	0	0
(*Starburst* 12-Pack)	50	0	12.0	0	0	0	0
(*Starburst* No Sugar)	20	0	6.0	0	0	0	0
(*Welch's* Variety Pack)	45	0	11.0	0	0	0	0
(*Welch's* Variety Pack No Sugar)	25	0	6.0	0	0	0	0

Food and Measure	cal.	prot. (gms)	carbo. (gms)	fat (gms)	chol. (mgs)	sod. (mgs)	fiber (gms)
Fruit bar, frozen *(cont.)*							
all flavors:							
(*Mr. Freeze*)	50	0	14.0	0	0	20	0
(*Mr. Freeze* Sugar							
Free)	20	0	5.0	0	0	45	0
banana, and cream:							
(*Frozfruit*)	150	1.0	20.0	8.0	30	20	<1.0
chocolate coated							
(*Frozfruit*)	210	1.0	21.0	14.0	20	15	1.0
cherry (*Frozfruit*)	70	1.0	17.0	0	0	60	<1.0
coconut, and cream:							
(*Dole* Fruit 'n Juice)	210	3.0	33.0	7.0	10	50	0
(*Edy's/Dreyer's*) . . .	130	3.0	20.0	5.0	5	40	0
(*Frozfruit*)	200	2.0	18.0	14.0	35	25	2.0
chocolate coated							
(*Frozfruit*)	240	2.0	19.0	18.0	25	20	2.0
grape:							
(*Dole* Fruit Juice)	45	0	11.0	0	0	5	0
(*Dole* Fruit Juice No							
Sugar)	25	0	6.0	0	0	5	0
(*Welch's*)	80	0	19.0	0	0	0	0
lemon:							
(*Frozfruit*)	90	0	21.0	0	0	75	0
and strawberry							
(*Real Fruit*)	80	0	21.0	0	0	5	0
lemonade:							
(*Dole* Fruit 'n Juice),							
4 oz.	120	1.0	28.0	0	0	55	0
lemon (*Minute*							
Maid)	90	0	23.0	0	0	15	0
lime:							
(*Dole* Fruit 'n Juice),							
4 oz.	110	0	28.0	0	0	55	0
(*Edy's/Dreyer's*) . . .	80	0	20.0	0	0	0	0
(*Frozfruit*)	90	0	22.0	0	0	80	0
mango (*Frozfruit*)	100	0	25.0	0	0	5	1.0
peach passion (*Dole*							
Fruit 'n Juice),							
2.5 oz.	70	0	17.0	0	0	5	0
piña colada, and							
cream (*Frozfruit*) . . .	180	2.0	22.0	10.0	30	20	1.0

Food and Measure	cal.	prot. (gms)	carbo. (gms)	fat (gms)	chol. (mgs)	sod. (mgs)	fiber (gms)
pineapple (*Frozfruit*)	60	0	16.0	0	0	0	0
pine-coconut (*Dole* Fruit 'n Juice), 4 oz.	150	1.0	27.0	4.0	0	5	0
pine-orange-banana:							
(*Dole* Fruit 'n Juice), 2.5 oz.	70	0	16.0	0	0	5	0
(*Dole* Fruit 'n Juice), 4 oz.	110	0	26.0	0	0	5	0
raspberry:							
(*Dole* Fruit Juice)	45	0	11.0	0	0	5	0
(*Dole* Fruit Juice No Sugar)	25	0	6.0	0	0	5	0
(*Dole* Fruit 'n Juice), 2.5 oz.	70	0	16.0	0	0	5	0
raspberry kiwi (*Edy's/ Dreyer's*)	80	0	21.0	0	0	0	0
strawberry:							
(*Dole* Fruit Juice)	45	0	11.0	0	0	5	0
(*Dole* Fruit Juice No Sugar)	25	0	6.0	0	0	5	0
(*Dole* Fruit 'n Juice), 2.5 oz.	70	0	17.0	0	0	5	0
(*Dole* Fruit 'n Juice), 4 oz.	110	0	26.0	0	0	5	0
(*Edy's/Dreyer's*) . . .	80	0	21.0	0	0	0	0
(*Frozfruit*)	90	0	22.0	0	0	0	<1.0
strawberry, and cream:							
(*Frozfruit*)	150	1.0	22.0	7.0	25	20	<1.0
chocolate coated (*Frozfruit*)	200	1.0	21.0	13.0	15	15	1.0
tropical:							
(*Frozfruit*)	110	0	26.0	0	0	0	<1.0
(*Welch's*)	45	0	11.0	0	0	0	0
Fruit cocktail, canned, 1/2 cup:							
in juice:							
(*Del Monte* Fruit Naturals)	60	0	15.0	0	0	10	1.0
(*Libby's* Lite)	60	0	15.0	0	0	10	1.0

Food and Measure	cal.	prot. (gms)	carbo. (gms)	fat (gms)	chol. (mgs)	sod. (mgs)	fiber (gms)
Fruit cocktail *(cont.)*							
in extra-light syrup							
(*Del Monte* Lite) . . .	60	0	15.0	0	0	10	1.0
in light syrup	72	.5	18.8	.1	0	7	1.4
in heavy syrup (*Del*							
Monte)	100	0	24.0	0	0	10	1.0
Fruit dip, see "Apple							
dip," "Cream cheese							
dip," and "Choco-							
late dip"							
Fruit dip mix (see also							
"Apple dip"), dry,							
1 tsp.:							
caramel (*Watkins*) . . .	5	0	2.0	0	0	10	0
mandarin orange							
(*Watkins*)	10	0	2.0	0	0	15	0
tropical fruit (*Watkins*)	10	0	3.0	0	0	0	0
Fruit drink blends (see							
also specific list-							
ings), 8 fl. oz., ex-							
cept as noted:							
(*Capri Sun Mountain*							
Cooler), 6.75 fl. oz.	100	0	26.0	0	0	20	0
(*Capri Sun Pacific*							
Cooler), 6.75 fl. oz.	110	0	29.0	0	0	20	0
(*Capri Sun Surfer*							
Cooler), 6.75 fl. oz.	100	0	27.0	0	0	20	0
(*Dole* Fruit Fiesta)	140	0	34.0	0	0	20	0
(*Dole* Tropical Breeze)	120	0	30.0	0	0	20	0
(*Fruitopia Fruit Inte-*							
gration)	111	0	29.0	0	0	58	0
(*Fruitopia Tropical*							
Temptation)	107	0	29.0	0	0	58	0
(*Season's Best* Med-							
ley)	130	<1.0	32.0	0	0	25	0
(*Snapple* Bali Blast/Sa-							
moan Splash)	110	0	28.0	0	0	10	0
berry (*Capri Sun Yo*							
Yogi Berry),							
6.75 fl. oz.	100	0	30.0	0	0	20	0

Food and Measure	cal.	prot. (gms)	carbo. (gms)	fat (gms)	chol. (mgs)	sod. (mgs)	fiber (gms)
berry, red (*Capri Sun*),							
6.75 fl. oz.	100	0	28.0	0	0	20	0
cherry, wild (*Capri Sun*), 6.75 fl. oz.	110	0	30.0	0	0	20	0
citrus, see "Citrus drink blends"							
grape (*Capri Sun*),							
6.75 fl. oz.	110	0	28.0	0	0	20	0
orange (*Capri Sun*),							
6.75 fl. oz.	100	0	26.0	0	0	20	0
punch:							
(*Arizona*)	90	0	25.0	0	0	20	0
(*Capri Sun*),							
6.75 fl. oz.	100	0	26.0	0	0	20	0
(*Capri Sun Maui Punch*),							
6.75 fl. oz.	110	0	28.0	0	0	20	0
(*Capri Sun Safari Punch*),							
6.75 fl. oz.	100	0	25.0	0	0	20	0
(*Dole*), 10 fl. oz. ...	160	0	39.0	0	0	25	0
(*R.W. Knudsen* Rain Forest/Tropical)	120	0	29.0	0	0	20	0
(*Snapple*)	110	0	29.0	0	0	10	0
(*Tropicana*)	130	0	32.0	0	0	15	0
(*Tropicana Twister*)	140	0	35.0	0	0	30	0
(*Veryfine*)	130	0	33.0	0	0	20	0
(*Veryfine*), 10 fl. oz.	170	0	42.0	0	0	25	0
Veryfine), 11.5 fl. oz.	200	0	49.0	0	0	30	0
(*Veryfine* Chiller Freeze)	110	0	28.0	0	0	20	0
(*Veryfine* Chiller Freeze), 11.5 fl. oz.	160	0	40.0	0	0	25	0
(*Veryfine* Chiller Freeze 20 oz.) ...	130	0	33.0	0	0	20	0
strawberry (*Capri Sun Strawberry Cooler*),							
6.75 fl. oz.	100	0	26.0	0	0	20	0

Food and Measure	cal.	prot. (gms)	carbo. (gms)	fat (gms)	chol. (mgs)	sod. (mgs)	fiber (gms)
Fruit drink blends *(cont.)*							
tropical:							
(*Kool-Aid Bursts*),							
6.75 fl. oz.	100	0	24.0	0	0	30	0
(*Tropicana Twister*)	140	0	35.0	0	0	30	0
(*V8 Splash*)	110	0	28.0	0	0	35	0
(*Veryfine* Chiller Freeze)	120	0	30.0	0	0	10	0
(*Veryfine* Chiller Freeze),							
11.5 fl. oz.	170	0	43.0	0	0	15	0
nectar (*Kern's*),							
11.5 fl. oz.	210	3.0	48.0	0	0	10	0
Fruit drink mix*, tropical punch, 8 fl. oz.:							
(*Kool-Aid*)	100	0	25.0	0	0	20	0
(*Kool-Aid* Presweetened)	60	0	16.0	0	0	0	0
Fruit glacé, see "Fruit, mixed, candied" and specific listings							
Fruit glaze, see "Glaze"							
Fruit juice blends (see also specific fruit listings), 8 fl. oz., except as noted:							
(*Dole*)	160	0	38.0	0	0	30	0
(*Minute Maid*)	119	0	32.0	0	0	5	0
(*Snapple* Vitamin Supreme), 10 fl. oz.	150	0	38.0	0	0	25	0
punch:							
(*After the Fall Maui Grove*)	90	1.0	23.0	0	0	15	0
(*Apple & Eve*),							
8.45 fl. oz.	120	1.0	30.0	0	0	30	0
(*Hood*)	130	0	32.0	0	0	7	0
(*Juicy Juice*)	130	1.0	32.0	0	0	10	0
(*Minute Maid*)	112	0	30.0	0	0	22	0
(*Ocean Spray*)	130	0	32.0	0	0	35	0
(*Veryfine* Juice-Up)	130	0	33.0	0	0	20	0

Food and Measure	cal.	prot. (gms)	carbo. (gms)	fat (gms)	chol. (mgs)	sod. (mgs)	fiber (gms)
citrus, see "Citrus juice blends"							
Concord (*Minute Maid*)	127	0	32.0	0	0	26	0
tropical (*R.W. Knudsen* Aseptic)	120	1.0	29.0	0	0	20	0
tropical, frozen* (*R.W. Knudsen*)	120	0	29.0	0	0	20	0
tropical (*Juicy Juice*)	130	1.0	31.0	0	0	10	0
Fruit and nut mix, see "Trail mix"							
Fruit pectin (*Sure•Jell*), ¼ tsp.	5	0	1.0	0	0	0	0
Fruit protector (*Ever-Fresh*), ¼ tsp.	5	0	1.0	0	0	0	0
Fruit salsa, see "Salsa"							
Fruit snack (see also specific fruit listings), all varieties:							
(*Fruit by the Foot*), ¾-oz. roll	80	0	17.0	1.5	0	50	0
(*Fruit Gushers*), .9-oz. pouch	90	0	20.0	1.0	0	40	0
(*Fruit Roll-Ups*), ½-oz. roll	50	0	12.0	.5	0	55	0
(*Fruit String Thing*), ¾-oz. pouch	80	0	17.0	1.0	0	45	0
Fruit spread (see also "Jam and preserves"), 1 tbsp.:							
all flavors (*Kraft* Reduced Calorie)	20	0	5.0	0	0	20	0
apricot, blackberry, red raspberry, or strawberry (*Kraft*)	50	0	13.0	0	0	10	0
peach, pineapple, or orange marmalade (*Kraft*)	50	0	14.0	0	0	10	0

Food and Measure	cal.	prot. (gms)	carbo. (gms)	fat (gms)	chol. (mgs)	sod. (mgs)	fiber (gms)
Fruit syrup, see specific listings							
Fruit-nut mix, see "Trail mix"							
Fudge topping, see "Chocolate topping"							
Fusilli dishes, mix, dry:							
black beans, Mediterranean (*Bean Cuisine* Pasta & Rice), 1.5 oz	150	7.0	30.0	1.0	0	10	4.0
w/garlic herb sauce (*Al Dente*), ¾ cup	230	8.0	45.0	1.5	0	390	2.0
w/pesto sauce, creamy (*Knorr*), ⅔ cup	250	9.0	46.0	3.5	<5	860	3.0

G

Food and Measure	cal.	prot. (gms)	carbo. (gms)	fat (gms)	chol. (mgs)	sod. (mgs)	fiber (gms)
Gai choy, see "Cabbage, mustard"							
Gai lan, see "Kale, Chinese"							
Garbanzo beans, dried:							
(*Arrowhead Mills*), ¼ cup	170	10.0	29.0	2.0	0	10	6.0
(*Frieda's*), ⅓ cup, 3 oz.	150	7.0	23.0	3.0	0	230	n.a.
boiled, ½ cup	134	7.3	22.5	2.1	0	6	2.9
Garbanzo beans, canned, ½ cup:							
(*Allens/East Texas Fair*)	120	5.0	19.0	2.5	0	330	8.0
(*Bush's Best* Chick Peas)	130	6.0	22.0	2.0	0	500	9.0
(*Eden* Organic)	120	7.0	19.0	1.5	0	10	5.0
(*Goya* Chick Peas)	100	6.0	20.0	2.0	0	360	7.0
(*Green Giant/Joan of Arc*)	110	6.0	18.0	1.5	0	380	5.0
(*Old El Paso*)	100	6.0	16.0	1.5	0	340	4.0
(*Progresso*)	110	6.0	18.0	1.5	0	380	5.0
(*Progresso* Chick peas)	120	5.0	20.0	2.5	0	280	5.0
(*Seneca*)	110	6.0	19.0	1.5	0	330	5.0
w/liquid	143	5.9	27.1	1.4	0	359	5.3
Garbanzo flour (*Arrowhead Mills*), ¼ cup	90	5.0	15.0	1.0	0	0	3.0
Garlic:							
(*Frieda's* Elephant), 1 tbsp.	5	0	1.0	0	0	0	0

Food and Measure	cal.	prot. (gms)	carbo. (gms)	fat (gms)	chol. (mgs)	sod. (mgs)	fiber (gms)
Garlic *(cont.)*							
trimmed, 1 oz.	42	1.8	9.4	.1	0	5	.6
clove, .1 oz.	4	.2	1.0	<.1	0	1	.1
chopped, in oil *(Christopher Ranch)*,							
1 tsp.	10	0	1.0	1.0	0	0	0
granulated/minced:							
1 tsp.	13	.7	2.9	0	0	1	0
pickled *(Christopher Ranch)*, 3 pcs.	5	0	0	0	0	80	0
roasted *(Christopher Ranch)*, 2-3 cloves	10	0	2.0	0	0	5	0
Garlic, crushed, 1 tsp.:							
(Christopher Ranch)	10	0	1.0	0	0	0	0
(McCormick)	10	0	4.0	0	0	0	0
Garlic basting sauce *(Tabasco)*, 1 tbsp.	20	0	4.0	0	0	250	0
Garlic dip *(Nalley)*,							
2 tbsp.	130	1.0	2.0	13.0	10	190	0
Garlic oil, see "Oil"							
Garlic pepper, 1 tsp.	8	.3	1.8	0	0	360	.3
Garlic pickle relish *(Patak's)*, 1 tbsp.	45	<1.0	4.0	3.0	0	430	<1.0
Garlic powder:							
(Lawry's), ¼ tsp.	0	0	1.0	0	0	0	0
1 tsp.	10	.5	2.3	0	0	1	0
Garlic salt:							
(Lawry's), ¼ tsp.	0	0	0	0	0	240	0
1 tsp.	3	.1	.5	0	0	2233	0
Garlic spread:							
(Lawry's Concentrate), 2 tsp.	50	0	1.0	6.0	0	80	0
(Lawry's Ready-to-Spread), 1 tbsp. . . .	100	0	2.0	10.0	0	190	0
and herb *(McCormick)*, ½ tbsp.	45	0	1.0	4.5	0	125	0
Garlic-dill dip mix, dry *(Watkins)*,							
1 tsp.	10	0	2.0	0	0	100	0

Food and Measure	cal.	prot. (gms)	carbo. (gms)	fat (gms)	chol. (mgs)	sod. (mgs)	fiber (gms)
Gefilte fish, drained, 1 pc.:							
in jelled broth (*Manischewitz*)	80	7.0	3.0	3.0	15	540	<1.0
sweet (*Manischewitz*)	90	5.0	4.0	2.0	15	340	<1.0
whitefish and pike (*Manischewitz*)	50	7.0	3.0	1.5	35	300	<1.0
Gelatin, unflavored (*Knox*), 1 pkt.	25	6.0	0	0	0	10	0
Gelatin dessert:							
all flavors:							
(*Hunt's Snack Pack Juicy Gels*), 3½ oz.	100	0	25.0	0	0	40	0
(*Jell-O*), ½ cup	80	1.0	18.0	0	0	45	0
(*Jell-O* Sugar Free), ½ cup	10	1.0	0	0	0	50	0
grapefruit, lemon-lime, or strawberry, w/fruit (*Sunfresh FruitJelite*), 4 oz.	90	0	22.0	0	0	30	1.0
orange, w/fruit (*Sunfresh FruitJelite*), 4 oz.	90	0	22.0	0	0	45	0
Gelatin dessert mix*:							
all flavors, ½ cup, except as noted:							
(*Jell-O* Sugar Free)	10	1.0	0	0	0	—[1]	0
except black raspberry (*Jell-O*)	80	2.0	19.0	0	0	—[2]	0
black raspberry (*Jell-O*)	80	2.0	20.0	0	0	35	0
strawberry:							
(*D-Zerta*)	10	2.0	0	0	0	5	0
(*Jell-O 1-2-3*), ⅔ cup	130	2.0	26.0	1.5	0	45	0
Gelatin drink mix, orange (*Knox*), 1 pkt.	40	6.0	4.0	(0)	0	15	0

[1] *Sodium values vary between 50 and 70 mgs according to flavor.*
[2] *Sodium values vary between 35 and 75 mgs according to flavor.*

Food and Measure	cal.	prot. (gms)	carbo. (gms)	fat (gms)	chol. (mgs)	sod. (mgs)	fiber (gms)
Gemelli dishes, mix, French beans, country (*Bean Cuisine* Pasta & Beans), 1.5 oz.	150	7.0	30.0	1.0	0	10	4.0
Giardiniera, see "Vegetables, mixed, pickled"							
Gil choy (*Frieda's*), 1 tbsp.	0	0	0	0	0	0	0
Ginger, trimmed root:							
(*Frieda's*), 1 tbsp. . . .	0	0	1.0	0	0	0	0
1 oz.	20	.5	4.3	.2	0	4	.6
sliced:							
¼ cup	17	.4	3.6	.2	0	3	.5
(*Ka•Me*), 20 pcs., ½ oz.	0	0	0	0	0	70	0
Ginger, candied or crystallized:							
(*Christopher Ranch*), 1 tsp.	15	0	3.0	0	0	0	0
(*Frieda's*), 9 pcs., 1 oz.	100	0	26.0	0	0	10	0
(*Paradise/White Swan*), 3 pcs., 1½″ diam., 1 oz.	100	0	26.0	0	0	10	1.0
(*Sonoma*), 14 pcs., 1 oz.	85	0	22.0	0	0	5	1.0
Ginger, ground, 1 tsp.	6	.2	1.3	.1	0	1	.2
Ginger, pickled:							
(*Eden*), 1 tbsp.	15	0	3.0	0	0	340	1.0
Japanese, 1 oz.	10	.1	2.1	<.1	0	105	n.a.
sweet (*Shirakiku*), 1 tbsp.	5	0	1.0	0	0	55	0
Ginger drink (*Santa Cruz Hawaiian*), 8 fl. oz.	110	0	27.0	0	0	35	0
Ginkgo nut, shelled:							
raw, 1 oz.	52	1.2	10.7	.5	0	2	<1.0
canned, drained, 1 oz.	32	.6	6.3	.5	0	87	2.6

Food and Measure	cal.	prot. (gms)	carbo. (gms)	fat (gms)	chol. (mgs)	sod. (mgs)	fiber (gms)
dried, 1 oz.	99	2.9	20.6	.8	0	4	n.a.
Glacé, cake, see "Fruit, mixed, candied"							
Glaze, ham, see "Ham glaze"							
Glaze, pie, strawberry (*Smucker's*), 2 oz.	80	0	21.0	0	0	0	0
Gluten, see "Wheat flour"							
Goat, meat only, roasted, 4 oz.	162	30.7	0	3.4	85	98	0
Goat's milk, see "Milk, goat's"							
Godfather's Pizza, 1 slice:							
original crust, cheese:							
mini, ¼ pie	131	7.0	19.0	3.0	8	183	n.a.
medium, ⅛ pie	231	13.0	34.0	5.0	14	338	n.a.
large, ¹⁄₁₀ pie	258	15.0	36.0	6.0	18	396	n.a.
jumbo, ¹⁄₁₀ pie	382	22.0	53.0	9.0	27	580	n.a.
original crust, combo:							
mini, ¼ pie	176	10.0	21.0	7.0	16	382	n.a.
medium, ⅛ pie	306	17.0	36.0	11.0	27	660	n.a.
large, ¹⁄₁₀ pie	338	19.0	38.0	12.0	31	740	n.a.
jumbo, ¹⁄₁₀ pie	503	29.0	56.0	18.0	47	1096	n.a.
golden crust, cheese:							
medium, ⅛ pie	212	10.0	26.0	8.0	12	311	n.a.
large, ¹⁄₁₀ pie	242	12.0	28.0	9.0	14	363	n.a.
golden crust, combo:							
medium, ⅛ pie	271	13.0	28.0	12.0	22	562	n.a.
large, ¹⁄₁₀ pie	305	16.0	31.0	14.0	25	674	n.a.
Golden nugget squash (*Frieda's*), ¾ cup, 3 oz.	30	1.0	7.0	0	0	0	1.0
Goose, roasted:							
meat w/skin, 4 oz.	346	28.5	0	24.9	103	79	0
meat only, 4 oz.	270	32.9	0	14.4	109	86	0
Goose fat, 1 oz.	255	0	0	28.3	28	0	0
Goose liver, see "Liver" and "Pâté"							

Food and Measure	cal.	prot. (gms)	carbo. (gms)	fat (gms)	chol. (mgs)	sod. (mgs)	fiber (gms)
Gooseberry, fresh, ½ cup	34	.7	7.6	.4	0	1	3.2
Gooseberry, canned, ½ cup:							
in light syrup:							
(*Comstock/Wilderness*)	70	1.0	20.0	0	0	60	3.0
(*Oregon*)	90	<1.0	22.0	0	0	5	3.0
½ cup	93	.8	23.6	.3	0	3	3.0
Goulash seasoning mix (*Knorr*), 1 tbsp.	40	<1.0	6.0	1.5	0	530	0
Gourd, boiled, ½ cup:							
dishcloth, 1″ slices . . .	50	.6	12.8	.3	0	18	<1.0
white-flower, 1″ cubes	11	.4	2.7	<.1	0	1	<1.0
Grain, see specific listings							
Grain dishes, mix, 4, w/wild rice (*Fantastic Foods Healthy Complements*), ½ cup	160	5.0	35.0	1.0	0	480	2.0
Granadilla, see "Passion fruit"							
Granola, see "Cereal, ready-to-eat"							
Granola and cereal bar (see also "Snack bar"), 1 bar, except as noted:							
(*Kellogg's Rice Krispies Treats*)	90	1.0	18.0	2.0	0	100	0
(*Kudos M&M's*)	90	1.0	17.0	2.5	0	105	1.0
(*Kudos Snickers*)	100	1.0	16.0	3.5	0	110	0
all fruit varieties:							
(*Health Valley* Crispy Rice)	110	1.0	26.0	0	0	5	1.0
(*Health Valley* Granola)	140	2.0	35.0	0	0	5	3.0
(*Kellogg's Nutri-Grain*)	140	2.0	27.0	3.0	0	110	1.0

Food and Measure	cal.	prot. (gms)	carbo. (gms)	fat (gms)	chol. (mgs)	sod. (mgs)	fiber (gms)
apple:							
(*Barbara's Nature's Choice*)	110	2.0	27.0	0	0	90	2.0
(*Dolly Madison/ Hostess* Cereal)	120	1.0	25.0	1.5	0	90	1.0
(*Health Valley* Fruit Bar)	140	3.0	35.0	0	0	0	3.0
(*Health Valley Apple Bakes*)	70	2.0	19.0	0	0	30	2.0
(*Sun Ups*)	190	2.0	34.0	5.5	0	240	n.a.
apple cinnamon:							
(*Entenmann's*)	140	9.0	24.0	3.0	0	80	1.0
(*Health Valley Healthy Breakfast Bakes*)	110	2.0	26.0	0	0	25	3.0
(*Quaker* Fruit & Oatmeal Bar)	135	2.0	27.0	3.0	0	85	1.0
(*Quaker* Granola Low Fat)	105	1.0	21.0	2.0	0	70	1.0
(*Weight Watchers* Breakfast Bar) . . .	100	1.0	21.0	2.0	0	95	2.0
apple raisin (*Entenmann's*)	140	2.0	27.0	3.0	0	130	1.0
apricot (*Health Valley* Fruit Bar)	140	3.0	35.0	0	0	5	3.0
banana nut (*Hostess* Cereal)	120	2.0	25.0	2.0	0	80	2.0
berry:							
(*Quaker* Fruit & Oatmeal Bar)	135	2.0	27.0	3.0	0	80	1.0
triple (*Barbara's Nature's Choice Wheat Free*)	130	2.0	28.0	0	0	190	2.0
blueberry:							
(*Barbara's Nature's Choice*)	110	2.0	27.0	0	0	90	2.0
(*Dolly Madison/ Hostess* Cereal)	120	1.0	25.0	1.5	0	90	1.0
(*Entenmann's*)	140	1.0	25.0	3.0	0	90	1.0
(*Quaker* Fruit & Oatmeal Bar)	135	3.0	26.0	2.0	0	120	1.0

Food and Measure	cal.	prot. (gms)	carbo. (gms)	fat (gms)	chol. (mgs)	sod. (mgs)	fiber (gms)
Granola and cereal bar, blueberry *(cont.)*							
(*Weight Watchers Breakfast Bar*) . . .	100	1.0	21.0	2.0	0	90	2.0
filled, oat bran flakes w/ (*Health Valley Cereal Bar*)	110	2.0	26.0	0	0	25	3.0
mountain (*Health Valley Healthy Breakfast Bakes*)	110	2.0	26.0	0	0	25	3.0
brownie, fudge-filled (*Health Valley*)	110	3.0	26.0	0	0	30	4.0
carob chip (*Barbara's Nature's Choice* Granola)	80	2.0	16.0	2.0	0	5	2.0
cheesecake, all varieties (*Health Valley*)	160	3.0	34.0	1.5	0	30	3.0
cherry (*Barbara's Nature's Choice* Wheat Free*)	130	2.0	28.0	0	0	190	2.0
chocolate, creme-filled, all varieties (*Health Valley* Sandwich Bar)	150	3.0	35.0	0	0	30	3.0
chocolate chip:							
(*Health Valley* Granola Bar)	140	2.0	35.0	0	0	5	3.0
(*Kudos*)	120	2.0	19.0	4.5	5	80	1.0
(*Quaker Chewy*) . . .	80	1.0	13.0	2.5	0	45	1.0
raisin (*Entenmann's*)	140	2.0	28.0	3.0	0	110	1.0
squares (*Kellogg's Rice Krispies Treats*)	90	1.0	17.0	3.0	0	105	0
chocolate chunk (*Quaker Chewy*) . . .	110	2.0	22.0	2.0	0	80	1.0
chocolate fudge (*Kudos*)	120	1.0	19.0	4.5	5	75	1.0
cinnamon (*Nature Valley*), 2 bars	180	4.0	29.0	6.0	0	180	2.0

Food and Measure	cal.	prot. (gms)	carbo. (gms)	fat (gms)	chol. (mgs)	sod. (mgs)	fiber (gms)
cinnamon and raisin (*Barbara's Nature's Choice* Granola) ...	80	2.0	16.0	2.0	0	5	3.0
cookies and cream (*Quaker Chewy*) ...	115	2.0	22.0	2.5	0	80	1.0
cranberry (*Barbara's Nature's Choice*) ...	110	2.0	27.0	0	0	110	2.0
date: (*Health Valley* Fruit Bar)	140	3.0	34.0	0	0	5	3.0
(*Health Valley Date Bakes*)	70	2.0	19.0	0	0	30	2.0
marshmallow, all varieties (*Health Valley*)	90	1.0	22.0	0	0	20	1.0
oat bran, raisin cinnamon (*Health Valley* Fruit Bar)	160	3.0	34.0	1.0	0	10	2.0
oatmeal raisin (*Quaker Chewy* Low Fat) ...	110	2.0	22.0	2.0	0	70	1.0
oats 'n honey: (*Barbara's Nature's Choice* Granola)	80	2.0	15.0	2.0	0	5	2.0
(*Nature Valley*), 2 bars	180	4.0	29.0	6.0	0	180	2.0
peach (*Barbara's Nature's Choice*)	110	2.0	27.0	0	0	90	2.0
peanut butter: (*Barbara's Nature's Choice* Granola)	80	2.0	14.0	3.0	0	5	2.0
(*Kudos*)	130	2.0	18.0	5.0	5	85	1.0
(*Nature Valley*), 2 bars	190	5.0	29.0	6.0	0	180	2.0
peanut butter and chocolate chip (*Quaker Chewy*) ...	120	3.0	19.0	4.5	0	105	1.0
raisin: (*Health Valley* Fruit Bar)	140	2.0	35.0	0	0	5	3.0
(*Health Valley Raisin Bakes*)	70	2.0	19.0	0	0	30	2.0

Food and Measure	cal.	prot. (gms)	carbo. (gms)	fat (gms)	chol. (mgs)	sod. (mgs)	fiber (gms)
Granola and cereal bar *(cont.)*							
raisin apple-filled, raisin bran flakes w/ (*Health Valley* Cereal Bar)	110	2.0	26.0	0	0	25	3.0
raspberry:							
(*Entenmann's*)	140	1.0	25.0	3.0	0	100	1.0
(*Sun Ups*)	195	2.0	34.0	6.0	0	215	n.a.
(*Weight Watchers* Breakfast Bar)	100	1.0	21.0	2.0	0	90	2.0
red (*Health Valley Healthy Breakfast Bakes*)	110	2.0	26.0	0	0	25	3.0
raspberry or strawberry:							
(*Barbara's Nature's Choice*)	110	2.0	27.0	0	0	110	2.0
(*Dolly Madison/ Hostess* Cereal)	120	1.0	24.0	1.5	0	100	1.0
(*SnackWell's*)	130	1.0	29.0	1.0	0	95	n.a.
S'mores (*Quaker Chewy* Low Fat)	110	2.0	22.0	2.0	0	80	1.0
strawberry:							
(*Quaker* Fruit & Oatmeal Bar)	135	2.0	26.0	3.0	0	125	1.0
California (*Health Valley Healthy Breakfast Bakes*)	110	2.0	26.0	0	0	25	3.0
filled, fiber 7 flakes w/(*Health Valley* Cereal Bar)	110	2.0	26.0	0	0	25	3.0
Grape, fresh, 1/2 cup, except as noted:							
American type (slipskin):							
10 medium	15	.2	4.1	.1	0	tr.	.3
peeled and seeded	29	.3	7.9	.2	0	1	.6
champagne (*Frieda's*), 5 oz.	100	1.0	25.0	1.0	0	0	1.0

Food and Measure	cal.	prot. (gms)	carbo. (gms)	fat (gms)	chol. (mgs)	sod. (mgs)	fiber (gms)
European type (adherent skin):							
seeded, 1 lb.	287	2.7	72.0	2.3	0	7	2.7
seedless, 10 medium	36	.3	8.9	.3	0	1	.3
seedless or seeded	57	.5	14.2	.5	0	2	.5
Grape, canned, seedless, ½ cup:							
in light syrup (*Oregon* Thompson)	100	<1.0	23.0	0	0	0	1.0
in heavy syrup:							
(*Comstock*)	100	0	23.0	0	0	20	1.0
½ cup	94	.6	25.2	.1	0	7	.5
spiced (*Oregon* Thompson)	110	<1.0	27.0	0	0	5	1.0
Grape drink:							
(*Kool-Aid Bursts*), 6.75 fl. oz.	100	0	25.0	0	0	30	0
(*Snapple* Grapeade), 8 fl. oz.	120	0	29.0	0	0	10	0
(*Veryfine*), 8 fl. oz. . . .	120	0	31.0	0	0	7	0
(*Veryfine*), 10 fl. oz. . . .	160	0	39.0	0	0	10	0
(*Veryfine* Chillers Glacial), 8 fl. oz.	110	0	28.0	0	0	5	0
(*Veryfine* Chillers Glacial), 11.5 fl. oz. . . .	160	0	41.0	0	0	10	0
Grape drink blends, 8 fl. oz., except as noted:							
(*Fruitopia the Grape Beyond*)	119	0	31.0	0	0	58	0
(*Tropicana*), 11.5 fl. oz.	200	0	49.0	0	0	35	0
berry (*Tropicana Twister*)	130	<1.0	32.0	0	0	25	0
kiwi (*Arizona*)	120	0	29.0	0	0	20	0
watermelon (*Snapple* Squeeze)	120	0	30.0	0	0	10	0
Grape drink mix, 8 fl. oz.*:							
(*Kool-Aid*)	100	0	25.0	0	0	15	0

Food and Measure	cal.	prot. (gms)	carbo. (gms)	fat (gms)	chol. (mgs)	sod. (mgs)	fiber (gms)
Grape drink mix *(cont.)*							
(*Kool-Aid* Presweetened)	60	0	16.0	0	0	0	0
Grape juice, 8 fl. oz., except as noted:							
(*Juicy Juice*)	130	1.0	32.0	0	0	10	0
(*R.W. Knudsen*)	150	1.0	37.0	0	0	30	0
(*R.W. Knudsen* Aseptic)	140	1.0	35.0	0	0	30	0
(*R.W. Knudsen* Concord)	160	0	40.0	0	0	15	0
(*Season's Best*)	160	1.0	39.0	0	0	25	0
(*Veryfine*)	150	0	37.0	0	0	30	0
(*Veryfine*), 10 fl. oz.	190	0	47.0	0	0	35	0
(*Veryfine*), 11.5 fl. oz.	200	0	54.0	0	0	40	0
(*Veryfine* Juice-Up)	140	0	34.0	0	0	20	0
frozen* (*R.W. Knudsen* Organic)	150	1.0	37.0	0	0	30	0
sparkling (*After the Fall* Kosher Concord)	130	1.0	31.0	0	0	10	0
Grape leaves, in jars, (*Krinos*), 1 leaf	5	0	0	0	0	200	1.0
Grape leaves, stuffed (*Cedar's*), 6 pcs., 5 oz.	180	4.0	22.0	8.0	0	870	8.0
Grapefruit, fresh:							
(*Ocean Spray*), 2 oz.	50	1.0	14.0	0	0	0	6.0
pink or red, California or Arizona:							
1/2 medium, 3¾" ...	46	.6	11.9	.1	0	<1	1.4
sections w/juice, 1/2 cup	43	.6	11.1	.1	0	<1	1.3
pink or red, Florida:							
1/2 medium, 3¾" ...	37	.7	9.2	.1	0	<1	1.4
sections w/juice, 1/2 cup	34	.6	8.6	.1	0	<1	1.3
white, California:							
1/2 medium, 3¾" ...	43	1.0	10.7	.1	0	<1	1.3
sections w/juice, 1/2 cup	42	1.0	10.5	.1	0	<1	1.3

Food and Measure	cal.	prot. (gms)	carbo. (gms)	fat (gms)	chol. (mgs)	sod. (mgs)	fiber (gms)
white, Florida:							
½ medium, 3¾″ ...	38	.7	9.7	.1	0	<1	.2
sections w/juice,							
½ cup	38	.7	9.4	.1	0	<1	.2
Grapefruit, canned or chilled, ½ cup:							
in juice	46	.9	11.4	.1	0	9	.5
in juice, white or red (*Sunfresh Chilled*)	45	1.0	9.0	0	0	15	2.0
in extra-light syrup (*Sunfresh* Chilled)	80	1.0	19.0	0	0	10	2.0
in light syrup, white or red (*Sunfresh* Can)	70	1.0	17.0	0	0	0	1.0
Grapefruit, Chinese, see "Pummelo"							
Grapefruit drink, 8 fl. oz., except as noted:							
pink:							
(*Tropicana Twister*)	120	0	29.0	0	0	20	0
(*Tropicana Twister* Light)	40	0	10.0	0	0	100	0
ruby red:							
(*Ocean Spray*)	130	0	33.0	0	0	35	0
(*Season's Best*) ...	130	<1.0	33.0	0	0	30	0
(*Tropicana Twister*)	130	<1.0	33.0	0	0	30	0
(*Veryfine*)	140	0	34.0	0	0	40	0
(*Veryfine*), 10 fl. oz.	170	0	42.0	0	0	50	0
(*Veryfine*), 11.5 fl. oz.	200	0	49.0	0	0	60	0
Grapefruit drink blends, ruby red, 8 fl. oz.:							
and mango (*Ocean Spray*)	130	0	33.0	0	0	35	0
and tangerine:							
(*Ocean Spray*)	130	0	32.0	0	0	35	0
(*Twister*)	130	0	32.0	0	0	20	0
Grapefruit drink mix*, pink (*Crystal Light*), 8 fl. oz.	5	0	0	0	0	0	0

Food and Measure	cal.	prot. (gms)	carbo. (gms)	fat (gms)	chol. (mgs)	sod. (mgs)	fiber (gms)
Grapefruit juice, 8 fl. oz., except as noted:							
(*Goya*), 6 fl. oz.	60	2.0	13.0	0	0	15	0
(*R.W. Knudsen* Organic)	100	2.0	23.0	0	0	15	0
(*Veryfine*)	90	0	20.0	0	0	15	0
(*Veryfine*), 10 fl. oz.	110	0	25.0	0	0	20	0
(*Veryfine*), 11.5 fl. oz.	120	0	29.0	0	0	25	0
fresh, 6 fl. oz.	72	.9	17.0	.2	0	2	.2
golden (*Tropicana Pure Premium*)	90	1.0	22.0	0	0	0	0
pink:							
(*Minute Maid*)	124	0	34.0	0	0	32	0
(*Ocean Spray*)	110	0	28.0	0	0	35	0
(*Snapple*), 12 fl. oz.	190	0	47.0	0	0	20	0
pink or white (*R.W. Knudsen*)	100	2.0	23.0	0	0	35	0
red:							
(*R.W. Knudsen* Rio)	140	2.0	35.0	0	0	10	0
ruby (*Season's Best*)	90	<1.0	22.0	0	0	15	0
ruby (*Tropicana Pure Premium*)	100	1.0	23.0	0	0	0	0
white (*Ocean Spray*)	100	1.0	24.0	0	0	35	0
Grapefruit-orange juice blend (*Tropicana Pure Premium*), 8 fl. oz. . . .	110	2.0	26.0	0	0	0	0
Gravy, see specific listings							
Gravy seasoning (see also "Browning sauce") (*Kitchen Bouquet*), 1 tsp. . . .	15	0	3.0	0	0	10	0
Great northern bean, 1/2 cup:							
boiled	104	7.3	18.6	.4	0	2	6.2
canned:							
(*Allens*)	100	6.0	19.0	.5	0	310	7.0
(*Bush's Best*)	110	7.0	18.0	.5	0	400	7.0

Food and Measure	cal.	prot. (gms)	carbo. (gms)	fat (gms)	chol. (mgs)	sod. (mgs)	fiber (gms)
(*Green Giant/Joan of Arc*)	100	6.0	18.0	.5	0	290	6.0
(*Seneca*)	150	10.0	26.0	.5	0	520	3.0
w/liquid	150	9.7	27.6	.5	0	6	6.4
w/pork (*Bush's Best*)	110	6.0	17.0	1.5	5	460	6.0
w/sausage (*Trappey's*)	100	6.0	18.0	1.0	0	460	7.0
Green bean, fresh:							
raw, ½ cup	17	1.0	3.9	.1	0	3	1.9
boiled, drained, ½ cup	22	1.2	4.9	.2	0	2	2.0
Green bean, canned, ½ cup:							
(*Allens* Shell Outs) . . .	30	2.0	6.0	0	0	460	2.0
(*Green Giant Kitchen Sliced*)	20	<1.0	4.0	0	0	400	1.0
all styles:							
(*Seneca*)	25	<1.0	5.0	0	0	380	2.0
(*Seneca* No Salt) . . .	25	<1.0	5.0	0	0	10	2.0
except seasoned (*Del Monte*)	20	1.0	4.0	0	0	390	2.0
except seasoned (*Del Monte* No Salt)	20	1.0	4.0	0	0	10	2.0
whole (*Green Giant*)	25	<1.0	5.0	0	0	330	2.0
cut:							
(*Allens* No Salt)	15	0	3.0	0	0	10	2.0
(*Allens/Sunshine/ GaBelle/Alma/ Crest Top*)	30	0	6.0	.5	0	320	3.0
(*Bush's Best*)	25	1.0	5.0	0	0	430	2.0
(*Bush's Best* Blue Lake*)	25	1.0	5.0	0	0	430	2.0
(*Green Giant*)	20	<1.0	4.0	0	0	400	1.0
(*Green Giant* 50% Less Sodium) . . .	20	<1.0	4.0	0	0	200	1.0
French style:							
(*Allens*)	25	<1.0	4.0	0	0	300	2.0
(*Bush's Best*)	25	1.0	5.0	0	0	430	2.0
(*Green Giant*)	20	<1.0	4.0	0	0	390	1.0
Italian cut:							
(*Allens*)	35	1.0	7.0	.5	0	320	3.0

Food and Measure	cal.	prot. (gms)	carbo. (gms)	fat (gms)	chol. (mgs)	sod. (mgs)	fiber (gms)
Green bean, canned, Italian cut *(cont.)*							
(*Del Monte*)	30	1.0	6.0	0	0	390	3.0
w/potatoes (*Allens/ Sunshine*)	35	1.0	7.0	0	0	220	2.0
seasoned, French style (*Del Monte*)	20	1.0	4.0	0	0	360	2.0
and shelly beans (*Bush's Best*)	45	3.0	7.0	0	0	400	3.0
Green bean, dried:							
(*Mountain House*), ⅔ cup	25	1.0	5.0	0	0	0	2.0
almondine, French cut (*AlpineAire*), .9 oz.	100	4.0	13.0	3.0	0	560	5.0
Green bean, frozen:							
(*Seneca*), ¾ cup	30	1.0	6.0	0	0	0	3.0
whole:							
(*Birds Eye*), 21 pcs.	20	1.0	5.0	0	0	0	2.0
(*Birds Eye Farm Fresh*) Stir Fry), 1¾ cups	100	4.0	19.0	.5	0	30	2.0
(*Freshlike*), 1 cup	25	1.0	4.0	0	0	10	2.0
(*Freshlike* Stir Fry), 1 cup	30	1.0	5.0	0	0	20	2.0
(*Seabrook*), ¾ cup	25	1.0	4.0	0	0	10	2.0
cut:							
(*Birds Eye*), ½ cup	25	1.0	6.0	0	0	0	2.0
(*Cascadian Farm*), ⅔ cup	40	1.0	6.0	0	0	0	3.0
(*Freshlike*), ⅔ cup	25	1.0	4.0	0	0	10	2.0
(*Green Giant*), ¾ cup	25	1.0	5.0	0	0	0	2.0
(*Green Giant Harvest Fresh*), ⅔ cup	25	<1.0	5.0	0	0	95	2.0
(*McKenzie's*), ⅔ cup	25	1.0	4.0	0	0	10	2.0
Italian (*Birds Eye*), ½ cup	35	2.0	8.0	0	0	0	3.0
w/Szechuan sauce (*Cascadian Farm*), 1 cup	60	2.0	9.0	2.5	0	290	2.0

Food and Measure	cal.	prot. (gms)	carbo. (gms)	fat (gms)	chol. (mgs)	sod. (mgs)	fiber (gms)
Green bean combinations, frozen:							
(*Green Giant* Casserole), ²/₃ cup	130	2.0	10.0	9.0	15	510	2.0
w/almonds:							
(*Birds Eye*), ³/₄ cup	80	3.0	7.0	4.0	0	500	3.0
(*Cascadian Farm*), ³/₄ cup	70	3.0	10.0	3.0	0	115	3.0
(*Green Giant*), ²/₃ cup	60	2.0	5.0	3.0	0	95	2.0
mushroom casserole:							
(*Stouffer's* 36 oz.), ¹/₂ cup	130	3.0	12.0	8.0	2	450	2.0
w/mushroom garlic sauce (*Cascadian Farm*), ³/₄ cup ...	90	3.0	10.0	5.0	10	360	2.0
Green peas, see "Peas, green"							
Greens (see also specific listings), mixed, canned, ¹/₂ cup:							
(*Allens/Sunshine*)....	30	1.0	8.0	.5	0	10	4.0
(*Bush's Best*)	25	2.0	3.0	0	0	300	2.0
Grenadine syrup, 2 tbsp.:							
(*Rose's*)	90	0	22.0	0	0	10	0
(*Trader Vic's*)	90	0	23.0	0	0	15	0
Grilling sauce (see also specific listings), chili pepper spice or sweet 'n smoky (*Old El Paso*), 2 tbsp.	60	<1.0	5.0	0	0	380	0
Grits, see "Corn grits"							
Grog mixer (*Trader Vic's* Navy), 2 oz.	124	0	30.0	0	0	15	0
Ground cherry, ¹/₂ cup	37	1.3	7.8	.5	0	n.a.	2.0
Grouper, meat only:							
raw, 4 oz.	104	22.0	0	1.2	42	60	0
baked, broiled, or microwaved, 4 oz. ...	134	28.2	0	1.5	53	60	0

Food and Measure	cal.	prot. (gms)	carbo. (gms)	fat (gms)	chol. (mgs)	sod. (mgs)	fiber (gms)
Guacamole (see also "Avocado dip"), 2 tbsp.:							
(*Calavo*)	60	<1.0	3.0	5.0	0	160	0
(*Goya*)	57	1.0	3.0	5.0	0	147	2.0
dip, spicy (*Nalley*) . . .	120	1.0	2.0	12.0	10	170	0
Guanabana nectar, canned (*Goya*), 6 fl. oz.	110	0	27.0	0	0	20	<1.0
Guava:							
1 medium, 4 oz.	45	.7	10.7	.5	0	2	4.9
½ cup	42	.7	9.8	.5	0	2	4.5
strawberry, ½ cup . . .	85	.7	21.2	.7	0	45	7.8
Guava drink, 8 fl. oz.:							
(*Mauna La'i* Island)	130	0	32.0	0	0	35	0
(*Snapple* Guava Mania)	110	0	29.0	0	0	10	0
Guava juice (*After the Fall Guava Maya*), 8 fl. oz.	110	1.0	26.0	0	0	20	0
Guava nectar:							
(*Goya*), 6 fl. oz.	110	0	27.0	0	0	10	1.0
(*Kern's*), 8 fl. oz.	150	0	38.0	0	0	5	0
Guava sauce, ½ cup	43	.4	11.3	.2	0	4	4.3
Guavadilla, see "Passion fruit"							
Guinea hen, raw:							
meat w/skin, 4 oz. . . .	179	26.5	0	7.3	n.a.	n.a.	0
meat only, 4 oz.	125	23.4	0	2.8	71	n.a.	0
Gyro mix, dry (*Casbah*), .65 oz.	64	2.0	12.0	0	0	470	0

H

Food and Measure	cal.	prot. (gms)	carbo. (gms)	fat (gms)	chol. (mgs)	sod. (mgs)	fiber (gms)
Häagen-Dazs Ice Cream Shop, ½ cup, except as noted:							
ice cream:							
Baileys Irish Cream	270	5.0	23.0	17.0	115	85	0
Belgian chocolate mousse	330	5.0	29.0	21.0	85	60	3.0
butter pecan	310	5.0	20.0	23.0	110	160	<1.0
caramel, dulce de leche	290	5.0	28.0	17.0	100	110	0
cherry vanilla	240	4.0	23.0	15.0	100	75	0
chocolate	270	5.0	22.0	18.0	115	75	1.0
chocolate almond, Swiss	300	6.0	23.0	20.0	100	65	2.0
chocolate chip mint	300	5.0	25.0	20.0	95	65	1.0
chocolate chocolate chip	300	5.0	26.0	20.0	100	70	2.0
chocolate peanut butter, deep	350	8.0	26.0	24.0	80	100	4.0
coffee	270	5.0	21.0	18.0	120	85	0
coffee chip	290	5.0	25.0	19.0	100	75	<1.0
cookies and cream	270	5.0	23.0	17.0	110	115	0
macadamia brittle	300	4.0	25.0	20.0	110	120	0
macadamia nut	320	5.0	20.0	24.0	110	115	0
Midnight Cookies & Cream	300	5.0	29.0	18.0	90	140	1.0
mint chip	290	4.0	26.0	19.0	105	105	<1.0
pralines and cream	290	4.0	27.0	18.0	95	180	0
rum raisin	270	4.0	22.0	17.0	110	75	0
strawberry	250	4.0	23.0	16.0	95	80	<1.0
vanilla	270	5.0	21.0	18.0	120	85	0
vanilla chocolate chip	310	5.0	26.0	20.0	105	90	<1.0

Food and Measure	cal.	prot. (gms)	carbo. (gms)	fat (gms)	chol. (mgs)	sod. (mgs)	fiber (gms)
Häagen-Dazs, ice cream (cont.)							
vanilla coffee, French	270	5.0	21.0	18.0	120	85	0
vanilla Swiss almond	310	6.0	23.0	21.0	105	90	1.0
ice cream, *Exträas* :							
Brownies a la Mode	280	4.0	26.0	18.0	100	115	0
Cappuccino Commotion	310	5.0	25.0	21.0	100	105	1.0
Caramel Cone Explosion	310	5.0	27.0	20.0	95	130	<1.0
Cookie Cone Dynamo	300	4.0	29.0	19.0	95	140	0
Strawberry Cheesecake Craze	270	4.0	27.0	16.0	100	159	<1.0
ice cream, low fat:							
chocolate fudge brownie	190	7.0	34.0	2.5	30	110	1.0
coffee fudge	170	5.0	32.0	2.5	25	95	0
strawberry	150	5.0	28.0	2.0	15	40	0
vanilla caramel	180	6.0	32.0	2.5	20	120	0
ice cream bar, 1 pc.:							
chocolate and dark chocolate	350	5.0	28.0	24.0	85	60	2.0
coffee almond crunch	360	5.0	27.0	26.0	100	85	1.0
strawberry and white chocolate	320	4.0	24.0	23.0	70	75	0
vanilla and almonds	370	6.0	26.0	27.0	90	80	1.0
vanilla and milk chocolate	330	5.0	24.0	24.0	90	75	<1.0
ice cream bar, uncoated, 1 pc.:							
chocolate	200	4.0	16.0	13.0	85	55	<1.0
coffee or vanilla	190	3.0	15.0	13.0	85	65	0
ice cream sandwich, 1 pc.:							
vanilla	280	4.0	32.0	15.0	65	125	<1.0
vanilla and chocolate	270	4.0	32.0	14.0	65	120	1.0

Food and Measure	cal.	prot. (gms)	carbo. (gms)	fat (gms)	chol. (mgs)	sod. (mgs)	fiber (gms)
sorbet:							
chocolate	120	2.0	28.0	0	0	70	2.0
lemon, zesty	120	0	31.0	0	0	5	<1.0
mango	120	0	31.0	0	0	0	<1.0
Margarita	130	0	31.0	0	0	25	0
passion fruit	120	0	29.0	0	0	0	<1.0
raspberry	120	0	30.0	0	0	0	2.0
strawberry	130	0	32.0	0	0	0	<1.0
sorbet, soft serve:							
mango	100	0	25.0	0	0	0	<1.0
raspberry	100	0	25.0	0	0	0	2.0
sorbet bar, 1 pc.:							
chocolate	80	1.0	20.0	0	0	50	1.0
wild berry	90	0	22.0	0	0	5	<1.0
yogurt, frozen:							
cherry vanilla	140	6.0	30.0	0	<5	40	0
vanilla	140	6.0	29.0	0	<5	45	0
vanilla fudge	160	6.0	34.0	0	<5	100	0
vanilla raspberry swirl	130	4.0	28.0	0	<5	30	0
yogurt, frozen, soft serve:							
chocolate	110	4.0	23.0	0	0	65	<1.0
chocolate mousse	80	5.0	24.0	0	0	65	1.0
coffee	140	5.0	20.0	4.0	35	75	0
vanilla	110	5.0	22.0	0	<5	70	0
vanilla mousse	70	4.0	23.0	0	0	65	0
yogurt, frozen, soft serve mix:							
coffee, nonfat	110	5.0	22.0	0	<5	75	0
peach	120	4.0	26.0	0	0	65	0
piña colada	110	5.0	23.0	0	<5	70	0
strawberry	110	4.0	24.0	0	0	60	0
white chocolate	110	5.0	22.0	0	<5	75	0
yogurt bar, 1 pc.:							
banana-strawberry	90	2.0	20.0	0	0	15	0
chocolate-cherry . . .	100	3.0	21.0	0	0	40	<1.0
piña colada	100	3.0	19.0	1.0	15	45	0
raspberry-vanilla . . .	90	2.0	20.0	0	0	15	0
strawberry daiquiri	90	2.0	18.0	1.0	15.0	20	0

Food and Measure	cal.	prot. (gms)	carbo. (gms)	fat (gms)	chol. (mgs)	sod. (mgs)	fiber (gms)
Haddock, meat only:							
raw, 4 oz.	99	21.5	0	.8	65	78	0
baked, broiled, or microwaved, 4 oz. . . .	127	27.5	0	1.1	84	99	0
smoked, 4 oz.	132	28.6	0	1.1	87	865	0
Haddock, frozen, (*Frionor*), 4 oz.	90	20.0	0	1.0	60	70	0
Haddock entree, fillet, frozen:							
battered (*Van de Kamp's*), 2 pcs. . . .	260	13.0	18.0	16.0	30	530	0
breaded:							
(*Mrs. Paul's* Premium), 1 pc.	230	16.0	17.0	11.0	35	390	2.0
(*Van de Kamp's*), 2 pcs.	280	12.0	19.0	17.0	25	310	0
(*Van de Kamp's* Premium), 1 pc.	220	14.0	19.0	10.0	30	410	0
Hake, see "Whiting"							
Halibut, meat only:							
Atlantic and Pacific:							
raw, 4 oz.	124	23.6	0	2.6	37	61	0
baked, broiled, or microwaved, 4 oz.	159	30.3	0	3.3	46	78	0
Greenland:							
raw, 4 oz.	211	16.3	0	15.7	52	91	0
baked, broiled, or microwaved, 4 oz.	271	20.9	0	20.1	67	117	0
Halibut entree, frozen, fillet, battered (*Van de Kamp's*), 3 pcs.	300	13.0	20.0	21.0	20	520	0
Halvah, chocolate (*Joyva*), 1.75 oz.	340	4.0	16.0	22.0	0	105	2.0
Ham, fresh, meat only:							
whole leg, roasted:							
lean w/fat, 4 oz. . . .	333	28.4	0	23.5	105	67	0
lean w/fat, chopped or diced, 1 cup	411	35.0	0	29.0	131	83	0

Food and Measure	cal.	prot. (gms)	carbo. (gms)	fat (gms)	chol. (mgs)	sod. (mgs)	fiber (gms)
lean only, 4 oz.	249	32.1	0	12.5	107	73	0
lean only, chopped or diced, 1 cup	309	39.7	0	15.4	131	90	0
rump half, roasted:							
lean w/fat, 4 oz. . . .	311	30.2	0	20.2	108	69	0
lean only, 4 oz.	251	33.0	0	12.1	109	74	0
shank half, roasted:							
lean w/fat, 4 oz. . . .	344	27.6	0	25.1	104	66	0
lean only, 4 oz.	244	32.0	0	11.9	104	73	0
Ham, cured:							
whole leg, lean w/fat:							
unheated, 4 oz. . . .	279	21.0	.1	21.0	64	1456	0
roasted, 4 oz.	276	24.5	0	19.0	70	1346	0
roasted, chopped or diced, 1 cup	341	30.2	0	23.5	86	1661	0
whole leg, lean only:							
unheated, 4 oz. . . .	167	25.3	.1	6.5	59	1719	0
roasted, 4 oz.	178	28.4	0	6.2	62	1505	0
roasted, chopped or diced, 1 cup	219	35.1	0	7.7	78	1858	0
boneless (11% fat):							
unheated, 4 oz. . . .	206	19.9	3.5	12.0	65	1493	0
roasted, 4 oz.	202	25.7	0	10.2	67	1701	0
roasted, chopped or diced, 1 cup	249	31.7	0	12.6	83	2100	0
boneless, extra lean (5% fat):							
unheated, 4 oz. . . .	149	21.9	1.1	5.6	53	1620	0
roasted, 4 oz.	164	23.7	1.7	6.3	60	1364	0
roasted, chopped or diced, 1 cup	203	29.3	2.1	7.7	74	1684	0
Ham, refrigerated or canned, 3 oz., except as noted:							
(*Black Label* Refrigerator Can)	100	14.0	1.0	4.5	40	1020	0
(*Black Label* Shelf Can)	100	14.0	0	5.0	45	970	0
(*Cure 81*)	100	15.0	0	4.5	45	870	0
(*Curemaster*)	80	14.0	0	3.0	40	940	0
(*Hormel Always Tender*), 4 oz.	270	18.0	0	22.0	75	400	0

Food and Measure	cal.	prot. (gms)	carbo. (gms)	fat (gms)	chol. (mgs)	sod. (mgs)	fiber (gms)
Ham, refrigerated or canned *(cont.)*							
(*Jones Dairy Farm* Country Carved Family/Dainty/Country Club)	100	17.0	0	4.0	50	930	0
(*Jones Dairy Farm* Fully Cooked)	240	13.0	0	21.0	65	740	0
(*Jones Dairy Farm* Homestead)	140	16.0	0	8.0	55	750	0
(*Jones Dairy Farm* Old Fashioned)	220	15.0	0	18.0	65	1200	0
(*Jones Dairy Farm* Semi-Boneless)	180	16.0	0	13.0	60	800	0
(*Jones Dairy Farm* Skinless Shankless/ Spiral Sliced)	160	16.0	0	11.0	60	680	0
(*Spiral Cure 81*)	150	15.0	1.0	9.0	50	1090	0
chunk (*Hormel*), 2 oz.	90	9.0	0	6.0	30	600	0
honey (*Jones Dairy Farm* Country Carved Family)	100	16.0	0	4.0	45	950	0
maple (*Jones Dairy Farm* Country Carved Family)	100	15.0	1.0	4.0	45	810	0
slice:							
(*Boar's Head Sweet Slice*)	110	15.0	<1.0	5.0	40	780	0
(*Jones Dairy Farm* Lean Choice), 2 pcs., 1.6 oz.	50	9.0	0	1.5	30	420	0
(*Oscar Mayer*)	80	14.0	0	3.0	40	1010	0
steak:							
(*Jones Dairy Farm* Lean Choice)	100	15.0	1.0	4.0	50	960	0
(*Oscar Mayer*), 2 oz.	60	10.0	0	2.0	30	750	0
"Ham," vegetarian, frozen, sliced (*Worthington Wham*), 2 slices	80	7.0	1.0	5.0	0	430	0

Food and Measure	cal.	prot. (gms)	carbo. (gms)	fat (gms)	chol. (mgs)	sod. (mgs)	fiber (gms)
Ham entree, frozen, 1 pkg., except as noted:							
and cheese (*Healthy Choice Hearty Hand-fuls*), 6.1 oz.	320	19.0	50.0	5.0	25.0	590	4.0
croquette (*Goya*), 3 pcs., 3½ oz.	280	13.0	30.0	12.0	30	730	3.0
steak, honey-smoked, w/macaroni-cheese (*Marie Callender's*), 14 oz.	490	29.0	63.0	13.0	80	2310	5.0
Ham glaze:							
(*Boar's Head*), 2 tbsp.	120	0	30.0	0	0	95	0
(*Crosse & Blackwell*), 1 tbsp.	30	0	8.0	0	0	25	0
Ham lunch meat, 2 oz., except as noted:							
(*Black Bear* Lower Sodium)	50	10.0	1.0	1.0	25	420	0
(*Boar's Head* Deluxe)	60	9.0	2.0	1.0	25	590	0
(*Boar's Head* Deluxe Lower Sodium)	50	10.0	<1.0	1.0	20	460	0
(*Deli Delight*)	60	9.0	2.0	1.5	20	330	0
(*Hansel 'n Gretel* Deluxe)	65	9.0	1.0	2.0	25	560	0
(*Healthy Choice* Variety Pack), 1-oz. slice	30	5.0	1.0	1.0	10	240	0
(*Healthy Deli* Deluxe)	60	9.0	0	1.5	20	480	0
(*Healthy Deli* Tavern)	60	10.0	1.0	1.5	20	470	0
(*Hormel Light & Lean 97*), 1-oz. slice	25	4.0	0	1.0	15	340	0
(*Oscar Mayer* Lower Sodium), 3 slices, 2.2 oz.	70	10.0	2.0	2.5	30	530	0
baked:							
(*Healthy Choice*), 1-oz. slice	30	5.0	1.0	1.0	10	240	0

Food and Measure	cal.	prot. (gms)	carbo. (gms)	fat (gms)	chol. (mgs)	sod. (mgs)	fiber (gms)
Ham lunch meat, baked (cont.)							
(Healthy Choice Deli-Thin),							
6 slices, 1.9 oz.	60	9.0	1.0	1.5	20	470	0
(Oscar Mayer),							
3 slices, 2.2 oz.	70	11.0	2.0	2.5	30	790	0
(Oscar Mayer Free),							
3 slices, 1.7 oz.	35	7.0	1.0	0	20	540	0
Black Forest:							
(Boar's Head)	60	10.0	2.0	.5	30	580	0
(Healthy Deli)	60	10.0	1.0	1.5	20	480	0
boiled:							
(Oscar Mayer),							
3 slices, 2.2 oz.	60	10.0	0	2.5	30	820	0
(Oscar Mayer Deli-Thin), 4 slices,							
1.8 oz.	50	9.0	1.0	2.0	25	700	0
brown sugar cured							
(Healthy Choice Hearty Deli),							
3 slices, 2 oz.	70	10.0	3.0	1.5	30	480	0
cappicola:							
(Boar's Head Cappy)	60	10.0	3.0	1.5	15	530	0
(Hansel 'n Gretel Cappi)	60	9.0	2.0	1.5	20	280	0
(Healthy Deli Cappi)	60	9.0	2.0	1.5	20	480	0
chopped:							
(Black Label)	140	7.0	2.0	12.0	35	720	0
(Oscar Mayer), 1-oz. slice	50	4.0	1.0	3.0	15	340	0
cinnamon apple							
(Healthy Deli)	70	9.0	4.0	1.5	20	480	0
cooked:							
(Alpine Lace)	60	10.0	2.0	1.5	25	440	0
(Healthy Choice) . . .	60	9.0	1.0	1.5	25	410	0
(Healthy Choice),							
1-oz. slice	30	5.0	1.0	1.0	10	240	0
(Healthy Choice Deli-Thin),							
6 slices, 1.9 oz.	60	9.0	1.0	1.5	20	470	0
(Hormel Deli)	60	8.0	2.0	2.5	20	680	0

Food and Measure	cal.	prot. (gms)	carbo. (gms)	fat (gms)	chol. (mgs)	sod. (mgs)	fiber (gms)
(*Russer* Fat Free)	44	9.0	2.0	0	25	550	0
(*Russer Light*)	60	9.0	2.0	1.0	25	400	0
(*Russer Light* 97% Fat Free)	60	9.0	2.0	2.0	30	400	0
fresh, seasoned (*Boar's Head*)	80	14.0	0	3.0	35	310	0
glazed:							
(*Hansel 'n Gretel*)	60	10.0	2.0	1.5	20	620	0
(*Healthy Deli*)	60	10.0	2.0	1.5	20	480	0
honey:							
(*Alpine Lace*)	60	9.0	2.0	2.0	25	535	0
(*Healthy Choice*) ...	60	9.0	2.0	1.5	25	480	0
(*Healthy Choice*), 1-oz. slice	30	5.0	1.0	1.0	10	240	0
(*Healthy Choice* Deli-Thin Savory Selections), 6 slices, 1.9 oz.	60	10.0	2.0	1.5	20	470	0
(*Healthy Deli*)	60	9.0	2.0	1.5	20	480	0
(*Oscar Mayer* 96% Fat Free), 3 slices, 2.2 oz.	70	11.0	2.0	2.5	30	770	0
(*Oscar Mayer Free*), 3 slices, 1.7 oz.	35	7.0	2.0	0	20	570	0
(*Russer* Fat Free)	44	9.0	2.0	0	25	550	0
baked (*Healthy Choice* Hearty Deli), 3 slices, 2 oz.	70	10.0	3.0	1.5	30	480	0
maple (*Healthy Choice*)	60	9.0	3.0	1.5	20	480	0
maple (*Healthy Choice* Deli-Thin Savory Selec- tions), 6 slices, 1.9 oz.	60	10.0	3.0	1.5	20	400	0
mustard (*Healthy Choice* Deli-Thin Savory Selec- tions), 6 slices, 1.9 oz.	60	9.0	3.0	1.5	20	470	0

Food and Measure	cal.	prot. (gms)	carbo. (gms)	fat (gms)	chol. (mgs)	sod. (mgs)	fiber (gms)
Ham lunch meat *(cont.)*							
jalapeño (*Healthy Deli*)	60	8.0	3.0	1.5	15	480	0
loaf (*Diet Delight*)	150	9.0	3.0	11.0	30	400	0
maple:							
(*Healthy Deli* Vermont)	60	9.0	3.0	1.5	20	460	0
glazed (*Black Bear*)	60	9.0	2.0	1.5	30	450	0
glazed (*Boar's Head*)	60	10.0	3.0	1.0	20	570	0
minced, 1 oz.	75	4.6	.5	5.9	20	353	0
pepper:							
(*Boar's Head*)	60	10.0	2.0	1.0	20	610	0
(*Healthy Deli*)	60	9.0	2.0	1.5	20	470	0
prosciutto, see "Prosciutto"							
smoked:							
(*Healthy Choice*) ...	60	9.0	2.0	1.5	30	430	0
(*Healthy Choice*), 1-oz. slice	30	5.0	1.0	1.0	10	240	0
(*Healthy Choice* Deli-Thin), 6 slices, 1.9 oz.	60	8.0	2.0	1.5	20	470	0
(*Oscar Mayer* 96% Fat Free), 3 slices, 2.2 oz.	60	11.0	0	2.0	30	760	0
(*Oscar Mayer* Deli-Thin), 4 slices, 1.8 oz.	50	9.0	0	2.0	25	630	0
(*Oscar Mayer Free*), 3 slices, 1.7 oz.	35	7.0	1.0	0	15	550	0
double (*Healthy Deli*)	60	10.0	1.0	1.5	20	470	0
spiced (*Boar's Head*)	120	7.0	1.0	10.0	30	570	0
Virginia:							
(*Black Bear*)	50	9.0	2.0	1.0	25	580	0
(*Boar's Head*)	60	9.0	2.0	1.0	25	590	0
(*Deli Delight*)	70	9.0	3.0	1.5	20	330	0
(*Hansel 'n Gretel*)	65	10.0	2.0	2.0	25	600	0
(*Healthy Choice*) ...	60	9.0	2.0	1.5	25	420	0
oven-baked (*Healthy Deli*)	70	10.0	3.0	1.5	20	480	0

Food and Measure	cal.	prot. (gms)	carbo. (gms)	fat (gms)	chol. (mgs)	sod. (mgs)	fiber (gms)
smoked (*Russer* Fat Free)	48	9.0	3.0	0	25	550	0
smoked or regular (*Healthy Deli*) ...	60	9.0	2.0	1.5	20	480	0
Ham and cheese loaf:							
(*Hansel 'n Gretel*), 2 oz.	170	7.0	3.0	14.0	30	840	0
(*Oscar Mayer*), 1-oz. slice	70	4.0	1.0	5.0	20	350	0
Ham and cheese pocket, frozen, 1 pc.:							
(*Big Stuffs*), 5.4 oz.	420	19.0	50.0	16.0	50	1010	4.0
(*Deli Stuffs*), 4½ oz.	340	15.0	41.0	13.0	50	650	3.0
(*Hot Pockets*), 4½ oz.	320	14.0	39.0	12.0	40	620	3.0
cheddar:							
(*Croissant Pockets*), 4½ oz.	320	14.0	39.0	12.0	45	790	2.0
(*Lean Pockets*), 4½ oz.	270	13.0	40.0	7.0	30	670	2.0
melt (*Hot Pockets Toaster Breaks*), 2.1 oz.	180	4.0	22.0	8.0	10	330	1.0
Ham patty, 1 pc.:							
(*Hormel*)	180	7.0	1.0	16.0	40	620	0
and cheese (*Hormel*)	180	7.0	0	17.0	40	520	0
Ham spread, ¼ cup or 4 tbsp.:							
deviled:							
(*Hormel Cure 81*)	150	9.0	2.0	12.0	40	430	0
(*Underwood*)	160	8.0	0	14.0	45	440	0
honey (*Underwood*)	140	6.0	5.0	11.0	30	370	0
Ham-Swiss croissant, frozen (*Sara Lee*), 1 pc.	300	12.0	27.0	16.0	45	570	2.0
Hamburger, see "Beef sandwich"							
"Hamburger," vegetarian, see "Burger, vegetarian"							

Food and Measure	cal.	prot. (gms)	carbo. (gms)	fat (gms)	chol. (mgs)	sod. (mgs)	fiber (gms)
Hamburger entree mix, (*Hamburger Helper*), 1 cup*, except as noted:							
beef barbecue	320	21.0	37.0	10.0	55	760	1.0
beef pasta	270	20.0	26.0	10.0	50	910	1.0
beef Romanoff	280	20.0	27.0	10.0	50	890	0
beef stew	260	18.0	26.0	10.0	50	760	2.0
beef taco	280	19.0	31.0	10.0	50	960	2.0
beef teriyaki	290	18.0	34.0	10.0	50	990	2.0
cheddar'n bacon	330	23.0	27.0	15.0	65	980	2.0
cheddar and broccoli	350	22.0	33.0	15.0	60	830	0
cheddar melt	310	20.0	31.0	12.0	55	890	1.0
cheddar spirals, reduced sodium	300	20.0	27.0	13.0	55	590	0
cheese, nacho	320	22.0	30.0	13.0	55	930	<1.0
cheese, three	340	21.0	32.0	15.0	55	830	<1.0
cheeseburger macaroni	360	23.0	33.0	16.0	65	940	1.0
cheesy hashbrowns	400	21.0	39.0	19.0	60	530	2.0
cheesy Italian	320	22.0	28.0	14.0	60	920	1.0
cheesy shells	330	21.0	30.0	15.0	60	840	<1.0
chili macaroni	290	20.0	30.0	10.0	55	870	2.0
fettuccine Alfredo	300	20.0	26.0	13.0	55	860	0
Italian, zesty	300	20.0	32.0	10.0	55	880	2.0
Italian herb, reduced sodium	270	19.0	29.0	10.0	50	630	2.0
Italian Parmesan w/rigatoni	300	20.0	31.0	1.0	50	870	<1.0
lasagna	270	19.0	29.0	10.0	50	1000	2.0
lasagna, 4-cheese . . .	330	21.0	31.0	14.0	55	860	0
meat loaf, 1/6 loaf* . . .	270	24.0	11.0	14.0	110	580	0
meaty spaghetti and cheese	290	20.0	30.0	10.0	50	970	1.0
Mexican, zesty	280	19.0	31.0	10.0	50	690	2.0
mushroom and wild rice	310	20.0	30.0	12.0	55	880	2.0
Pizzabake, 1/6 pan* . . .	270	17.0	28.0	10.0	45	720	<1.0
pizza pasta	280	19.0	31.0	10.0	50	750	2.0
potato Stroganoff	250	17.0	23.0	11.0	50	870	2.0
potatoes au gratin . . .	280	18.0	25.0	13.0	55	730	2.0

Food and Measure	cal.	prot. (gms)	carbo. (gms)	fat (gms)	chol. (mgs)	sod. (mgs)	fiber (gms)
ravioli	280	20.0	30.0	10.0	50	840	1.0
ravioli w/cheese topping	310	20.0	34.0	10.0	50	960	1.0
rice Oriental	280	18.0	32.0	10.0	50	990	0
Salisbury	270	19.0	26.0	10.0	50	790	1.0
Southwestern beef, reduced sodium	300	20.0	32.0	10.0	50	620	2.0
spaghetti	270	19.0	27.0	10.0	50	940	1.0
Stroganoff	320	21.0	30.0	13.0	55	830	0
Swedish meatballs . . .	290	19.0	25.0	14.0	55	780	2.0
Hard sauce, brandied (*Crosse & Blackwell*), 2 tbsp.	180	0	24.0	9.0	25	20	0
Hardee's, 1 serving:							
breakfast:							
Big Country:							
bacon	820	33.0	62.0	49.0	535	1870	n.a.
sausage	1000	41.0	62.0	66.0	570	2310	n.a.
biscuit:							
Apple Cinnamon 'N' Raisin	200	2.0	30.0	8.0	0	350	n.a.
bacon and egg . . .	570	22.0	45.0	33.0	275	1400	n.a.
bacon, egg, cheese	610	24.0	45.0	37.0	280	1630	n.a.
Biscuit 'N' Gravy	510	10.0	55.0	28.0	15	1500	n.a.
ham	400	9.0	47.0	20.0	15	1340	n.a.
ham, country	430	15.0	45.0	22.0	25	1930	n.a.
ham, egg, cheese	540	20.0	48.0	30.0	285	1660	n.a.
jelly	440	6.0	57.0	21.0	0	1000	n.a.
Rise 'N' Shine . . .	390	6.0	44.0	21.0	0	1000	n.a.
sausage	510	14.0	44.0	31.0	25	1360	n.a.
sausage and egg	630	23.0	45.0	40.0	285	1480	n.a.
Ultimate Omelet	570	22.0	45.0	33.0	290	1370	n.a.
Frisco sandwich, ham	500	24.0	46.0	25.0	290	1370	n.a.
Hash Rounds, regular	230	3.0	24.0	14.0	0	560	n.a.
pancakes, 3 pcs.	280	8.0	56.0	2.0	15	890	n.a.
sandwiches:							
burger:							
hamburger	270	14.0	29.0	11.0	35	670	n.a.

Food and Measure	cal.	prot. (gms)	carbo. (gms)	fat (gms)	chol. (mgs)	sod. (mgs)	fiber (gms)
Hardee's, sandwiches (cont.)							
The Boss	570	27.0	42.0	33.0	85	910	n.a.
Frisco	720	33.0	43.0	46.0	95	1340	n.a.
Mushroom 'N'							
Swiss	490	28.0	39.0	25.0	80	1100	n.a.
The Works	270	25.0	41.0	30.0	80	1030	n.a.
cheeseburger:							
regular	310	16.0	30.0	14.0	40	890	n.a.
cravin' bacon	690	30.0	38.0	46.0	95	1150	n.a.
mesquite bacon	370	19.0	32.0	18.0	45	970	n.a.
1/4-lb. double	470	27.0	31.0	27.0	80	1290	n.a.
chicken, grilled	350	25.0	38.0	11.0	65	950	n.a.
chicken fillet	480	26.0	54.0	18.0	55	1280	n.a.
Fisherman's Fillet	560	26.0	54.0	27.0	65	1330	n.a.
Hot Ham 'N Cheese	310	16.0	34.0	12.0	50	1410	n.a.
roast beef, regular	320	17.0	26.0	16.0	43	820	n.a.
roast beef, big	460	26.0	35.0	24.0	70	1230	n.a.
chicken:							
breast	370	29.0	29.0	15.0	75	1190	n.a.
leg	170	13.0	15.0	7.0	45	570	n.a.
thigh	330	19.0	30.0	15.0	60	1000	n.a.
wing	200	10.0	23.0	8.0	30	740	n.a.
chicken sides:							
baked beans, 5 oz.	170	8.0	32.0	1.0	0	600	n.a.
cole slaw, 4 oz. . . .	240	2.0	13.0	20.0	10	340	n.a.
gravy, 1.5 oz.	20	<1.0	3.0	<1.0	0	260	n.a.
mashed potatoes,							
4 oz.	70	2.0	14.0	<1.0	0	330	n.a.
salads:							
garden	220	12.0	11.0	13.0	40	350	n.a.
grilled chicken	150	20.0	11.0	3.0	60	610	n.a.
side	25	1.0	4.0	<1.0	0	45	n.a.
salad dressing:							
French, fat free	70	0	17.0	0	0	580	0
ranch	290	1.0	6.0	29.0	25	510	0
Thousand Island . . .	250	1.0	9.0	23.0	35	540	0
fries:							
small	240	4.0	33.0	10.0	0	100	n.a.
medium	350	5.0	49.0	15.0	0	150	n.a.
large . . . . , . . .	430	6.0	59.0	18.0	0	190	n.a.
desserts/shakes:							
Big Cookie	280	4.0	41.0	12.0	15	150	n.a.

Food and Measure	cal.	prot. (gms)	carbo. (gms)	fat (gms)	chol. (mgs)	sod. (mgs)	fiber (gms)
cone:							
chocolate	180	5.0	34.0	2.0	15	110	0
Cool Twist	180	4.0	34.0	2.0	10	120	0
vanilla	170	4.0	34.0	2.0	10	130	0
peach cobbler, 6 oz.	310	2.0	60.0	7.0	0	360	n.a.
shake:							
chocolate	370	13.0	67.0	5.0	30	270	0
peach	390	10.0	77.0	4.0	25	290	0
strawberry......	420	11.0	83.0	4.0	20	270	0
vanilla	350	12.0	65.0	5.0	20	300	0
sundae:							
hot fudge........	290	7.0	51.0	6.0	20	310	n.a.
strawberry......	210	5.0	43.0	2.0	10	140	n.a.
Hash, see "Beef hash" and "Sausage hash"							
Hazelnut, see "Filbert"							
Hazelnut spread							
(*Nutella*), 2 tbsp.	160	2.0	19.0	9.0	0	30	0
Hazelnut syrup:							
(*Ferrara*), 2 oz.	130	0	32.0	0	0	12	0
(*Watkins*), 1 tbsp. ...	40	0	18.0	0	0	0	0
Head cheese:							
(*Boar's Head*), 2 oz.	99	10.0	<1.0	5.0	65	420	0
(*Hansel 'n Gretel*), 2 oz.	90	9.0	2.0	5.0	35	960	0
(*Oscar Mayer*), 1-oz. slice	50	5.0	0	4.0	25	360	0
Heart, braised or simmered, 4 oz.:							
beef	199	32.6	.5	6.4	219	71	0
chicken, broiler-fryer	210	30.0	.1	9.0	274	54	0
lamb..............	210	28.3	2.2	9.0	282	71	0
pork	168	26.8	.5	5.7	251	40	0
turkey	201	30.3	2.3	6.9	256	62	0
veal	211	33.0	.1	7.7	200	66	0
Herbs, see specific listings							
Herring, fresh:							
Atlantic, meat only:							
raw, 4 oz.	180	20.4	0	10.3	68	102	0

Food and Measure	cal.	prot. (gms)	carbo. (gms)	fat (gms)	chol. (mgs)	sod. (mgs)	fiber (gms)
Herring, Atlantic *(cont.)*							
baked, broiled, or							
microwaved,							
4 oz.	230	26.1	0	13.1	87	130	0
kippered, 4 oz.	246	27.9	0	14.0	93	1041	0
pickled, 4 oz.	297	16.1	10.9	20.4	15	987	0
lake, see "Cisco"							
Pacific, meat only:							
raw, 4 oz.	224	18.6	0	15.8	87	84	0
baked, broiled, or							
microwaved,							
4 oz.	284	23.8	0	20.2	112	108	0
Herring, canned, see							
"Sardine"							
Herring, in jars, fillet,							
¼ cup, except as							
noted:							
in dill sauce:							
(*Elf*)	100	7.0	7.0	5.0	25	540	0
(*Fish Market*)	100	7.0	7.0	5.0	25	540	0
(*Vita*)	100	7.0	7.0	5.0	25	540	0
slices (*Vita* Lunch),							
2 oz.	130	9.0	5.0	8.0	40	600	0
in sour cream:							
(*Elf*)	110	8.0	5.0	6.0	25	520	0
(*Fish Market*)	110	8.0	5.0	6.0	25	520	0
(*Vita*)	120	7.0	8.0	7.0	35	600	0
in wine sauce:							
(*Elf*)	100	8.0	8.0	4.0	25	360	0
(*Elf* Old Fashioned)	120	7.0	5.0	8.0	20	1100	0
(*Fish Market*)	100	8.0	8.0	4.0	25	360	0
(*Vita* Party Snacks							
Tastee Bits), 2 oz.	120	9.0	10.0	5.0	30	480	0
roll mops (*Elf*)	100	7.0	8.0	4.0	20	520	0
Herring oil, see "Oil"							
Herring salad:							
(*Blue Ridge Farms*),							
⅓ cup	150	9.0	17.0	6.0	50	250	1.0
(*Vita*), ¼ cup	110	4.0	15.0	4.0	20	600	0
Hickory nut, dried,							
shelled, 1 oz.	187	3.6	5.2	18.3	0	tr.	1.8

Food and Measure	cal.	prot. (gms)	carbo. (gms)	fat (gms)	chol. (mgs)	sod. (mgs)	fiber (gms)
Hiziki, see "Seaweed"							
Hoisin sauce (*House of Tsang*), 1 tsp.	15	0	4.0	0	0	120	0
Hollandaise sauce mix (*Knorr Classic Sauces*), 1 tsp.	10	0	2.0	0	0	85	0
Homestyle gravy mix* (*Pillsbury*), ¼ cup	15	0	3.0	0	0	270	0
Hominy, dry, white (*Goya*), ¼ cup	180	4.0	39.0	0	0	0	0
Hominy, canned, ½ cup:							
golden:							
(*Allens/Uncle William*)	120	2.0	27.0	.5	0	340	4.0
(*Bush's Best*)	60	1.0	13.0	.5	0	550	3.0
(*Van Camp's*)	80	1.0	17.0	1.0	0	540	1.0
Mexican (*Allens/Uncle William*)	120	2.0	25.0	1.0	0	340	3.0
w/peppers:							
golden (*Bush's Best*)	70	2.0	14.0	1.0	0	570	3.0
white (*Bush's Best*)	80	2.0	16.0	1.0	0	500	4.0
white:							
(*Allens/Uncle William*)	100	2.0	22.0	.5	0	340	4.0
(*Bush's Best* Pozole Blanco)	70	1.0	14.0	1.0	0	530	4.0
(*Van Camp's*)	80	1.0	16.0	1.0	0	530	1.0
Hominy grits, dry, see "Corn grits"							
Honey, 1 tbsp.:							
(*Aunt Sue's/ Grandma's/Sue Bee*)	60	0	17.0	0	0	0	0
(*Goya*)	60	0	17.0	0	0	0	0
Honey bun, see "Bun, sweet"							
Honey butter, see "Butter, flavored"							
Honey loaf, see "Lunch meat"							

Food and Measure	cal.	prot. (gms)	carbo. (gms)	fat (gms)	chol. (mgs)	sod. (mgs)	fiber (gms)
Honey mustard, see "Mustard"							
Honey mustard sauce:							
(*Rice Road*), 1 tbsp.	20	0	4.0	0	0	270	0
Dijon (*World Harbors* Mont St. Michel), 2 tbsp.	30	0	7.0	0	0	230	0
Honey roll sausage, beef, 1 oz.	52	5.3	.6	3.0	14	375	0
Honeycomb, strained (*Frieda's*), 1 oz. ...	86	.1	23.3	0	0	1	0
Honeydew:							
1/10 melon, 7″ x 2″	46	.6	11.8	.1	0	13	.8
pulp, cubed, 1/2 cup	30	.4	7.8	.1	0	9	.5
Horned melon (*Frieda's*), 3.5-oz. melon	25	0	0	0	0	0	1.0
Horseradish, fresh:							
leafy tips, 1/2 cup:							
raw, chopped	6	.9	.8	.1	0	1	.2
boiled, drained, chopped	13	1.1	2.3	.2	0	2	.4
pods, 1/2 cup:							
raw, sliced	19	1.1	4.3	.1	0	21	1.6
boiled, drained, sliced	21	1.2	4.8	.1	0	25	2.5
Horseradish, pre- pared, 1 tsp.:							
(*Boar's Head*)	5	0	0	0	0	30	0
(*Heluva* Good)	0	0	0	0	0	5	0
(*Kraft*)	0	0	0	0	0	50	0
w/beets (*Gold's*)	0	0	0	0	0	30	0
creamy (*Kraft*)	0	0	0	0	0	50	0
mustard (*Heluva* Good)	6	0	0	0	0	10	0
Horseradish root (*Frieda's*), 1 tbsp.	0	0	1.0	0	0	0	0
Horseradish sauce (*Sauceworks*), 1 tsp.	20	0	<1.0	1.5	<5	35	0

Food and Measure	cal.	prot. (gms)	carbo. (gms)	fat (gms)	chol. (mgs)	sod. (mgs)	fiber (gms)
Hot buttered rum, batter (*Trader Vic's*), 1 oz.	136	0	23.5	4.7	15	10	0
Hot dog, see "Frankfurter"							
Hot dog sauce, see "Chili sauce"							
Hot fudge sauce, see "Chocolate topping"							
Hot sauce, see "Pepper sauce" and specific listings							
Hubbard squash:							
raw (*Frieda's*), ¾ cup, 3 oz.	35	2.0	7.0	0	0	0	2.0
baked, cubed, ½ cup	51	2.5	11.0	.6	0	8	2.9
boiled, drained, mashed, ½ cup	35	1.8	7.6	.4	0	6	3.4
Hummus, 2 tbsp., except as noted:							
(*Athenos* Original) . . .	60	2.0	5.0	3.5	0	180	1.0
(*Cedar's* Hommus) . . .	50	3.0	5.0	2.0	0	120	3.0
(*Cedar's* Sports Dip Hommus)	34	2.0	4.0	1.0	0	130	2.0
(*Sabra* Chumus), 1 oz.	69	2.4	3.9	4.8	0	32	1.5
(*Vita* Original)	34	0	4.0	1.0	0	81	1.0
bagel, w/chives (*Vita*)	32	1.0	4.0	1.0	0	76	1.0
chili pepper (*Yorgo*)	50	2.0	4.0	3.0	0	105	1.0
cucumber dill (*Athenos*)	60	2.0	5.0	4.0	0	240	1.0
eggplant, see "Eggplant appetizer"							
garlic:							
extra or roasted (*Vita*)	35	1.0	5.0	1.0	0	74	1.0
extra (*Yorgo*)	35	1.0	3.0	2.0	0	60	1.0
roasted (*Athenos*)	50	1.0	5.0	3.0	0	190	1.0
jalapeño (*Vita* Hot! Hot!)	33	1.0	4.0	1.0	0	95	1.0
lemon pepper (*Yorgo*)	50	2.0	1.0	3.0	0	105	1.0

Food and Measure	cal.	prot. (gms)	carbo. (gms)	fat (gms)	chol. (mgs)	sod. (mgs)	fiber (gms)
Hummus *(cont.)*							
olive, black *(Athenos)*	50	2.0	5.0	3.0	0	230	1.0
pimiento and olive							
(Cedar's Hommus)	56	3.0	5.0	3.0	0	135	3.0
red pepper:							
(Cedar's)	50	3.0	5.0	3.0	0	120	3.0
roasted *(Athenos)*	60	2.0	6.0	3.5	0	210	1.0
roasted *(Vita)*	28	1.0	4.0	1.0	0	76	1.0
salsa *(Vita)*	33	1.0	4.0	1.0	0	95	1.0
scallion *(Athenos)* . . .	50	2.0	6.0	3.5	0	230	1.0
spinach and olive							
(Vita)	32	1.0	4.0	1.0	0	76	1.0
tahini:							
(Sabra), 1 oz.	80	2.6	1.3	7.0	0	67	.8
(Yorgo)	50	2.0	5.0	2.5	0	60	1.0
tomato basil *(Vita)* . . .	32	1.0	4.0	1.0	0	74	1.0
vegetable:							
(Vita)	32	1.0	4.0	1.0	0	74	1.0
tahini *(Yorgo)*	45	2.0	1.0	2.0	0	60	1.0
Hummus mix, dry:							
(Casbah), 1 oz.	160	5.0	14.0	8.0	0	180	1.0
(Fantastic Foods Dip),							
2 tbsp.	60	3.0	9.0	2.0	0	220	2.0
Hunter sauce mix							
(Knorr Classic),							
1 tbsp.	25	<1.0	4.0	.5	0	280	0
Hush puppy mix							
(Martha White),							
1/4 cup fried*	300	4.0	27.0	20.0	<5	620	1.0
Hyacinth beans,							
1/2 cup:							
fresh, boiled, drained	22	1.3	4.1	.1	0	1	n.a.
dried, boiled	114	7.9	20.1	.6	0	7	n.a.

I

Food and Measure	cal.	prot. (gms)	carbo. (gms)	fat (gms)	chol. (mgs)	sod. (mgs)	fiber (gms)
Ice:							
(*Good Humor* Snow Cone), 7 fl. oz.	60	0	14.0	0	0	5	0
cherry:							
(*Frozfruit Chill*), 4 fl. oz.	70	0	18.0	0	0	5	0
(*Frozfruit Chill*), 8 fl. oz.	150	0	39.0	0	0	35	0
(*Icee*), 3 fl. oz.	70	0	18.0	0	0	5	0
(*Luigi's*), 6 fl. oz.	110	0	27.0	0	0	20	0
(*Mama Tish's/Fruttuoso Sorbetto/ Premium Italian Ices*), 4 fl. oz. ...	90	0	22.0	0	0	5	0
chocolate:							
(*Mama Tish's/Fruttuoso Sorbetto/ Premium Italian Ices*), 4 fl. oz. ...	100	<1.0	25.0	0	0	115	1.0
fudge (*Luigi's*), 6 fl. oz.	160	0	40.0	0	0	25	<1.0
grape (*Luigi's*), 6 fl. oz.	110	0	27.0	0	0	20	0
lemon:							
(*Frozfruit Chill*), 4 fl. oz.	70	0	17.0	0	0	5	0
(*Frozfruit Chill*), 8 fl. oz.	130	0	34.0	0	0	15	0
(*Frozfruit Chill* No Sugar), 4 fl. oz.	60	0	14.0	0	0	10	0
(*Frozfruit Chill* No Sugar), 8 fl. oz.	120	0	29.0	0	0	15	0

Food and Measure	cal.	prot. (gms)	carbo. (gms)	fat (gms)	chol. (mgs)	sod. (mgs)	fiber (gms)
Ice, lemon *(cont.)*							
(*Luigi's*), 6 fl. oz.	100	0	26.0	0	0	20	0
(*Mama Tish's/Frut-tuoso Sorbetto/ Premium Italian Ices*), 4 fl. oz. ...	80	0	21.0	0	0	10	0
(*Mama Tish's/Frut-tuoso Sorbetto/ Premium Italian Ices No Sugar*), 4 fl. oz.	70	0	19.0	0	0	35	0
lemonade (*Minute Maid* cup), 12 fl. oz.	300	0	77.0	0	0	55	0
margarita:							
(*Frozfruit Chill*), 4 fl. oz.	70	0	17.0	0	0	5	0
(*Frozfruit Chill*), 8 fl. oz.	140	0	35.0	0	0	35	0
orange:							
(*Frozfruit Chill*), 4 fl. oz.	70	1.0	16.0	0	0	10	0
(*Frozfruit Chill*), 8 fl. oz.	150	0	38.0	0	0	30	0
(*Icee*), 3 fl. oz.	60	0	14.0	0	0	10	0
raspberry:							
(*Frozfruit Chill*), 4 fl. oz.	60	0	13.0	0	0	5	0
(*Frozfruit Chill*), 8 fl. oz.	150	0	39.0	0	0	40	0
(*Mama Tish's/Frut-tuoso Sorbetto/ Premium Italian Ices*), 4 fl. oz. ...	100	0	24.0	0	0	10	0
blue (*Icee*), 3 fl. oz.	70	0	18.0	0	0	5	0
strawberry:							
(*Frozfruit Chill*), 4 fl. oz.	60	0	15.0	0	0	5	0
(*Frozfruit Chill*), 8 fl. oz.	130	0	34.0	0	0	30	0
(*Icee*), 3 fl. oz.	60	0	14.0	0	0	10	0
(*Luigi's*), 6 fl. oz.	110	0	27.0	0	0	20	0

Food and Measure	cal.	prot. (gms)	carbo. (gms)	fat (gms)	chol. (mgs)	sod. (mgs)	fiber (gms)
(*Mama Tish's/Frut-tuoso Sorbetto/ Premium Italian Ices*), 4 fl. oz. ...	80	0	20.0	0	0	5	0
(*Mama Tish's/Frut-tuoso Sorbetto/ Premium Italian Ices* No Sugar), 4 fl. oz.	70	0	18.0	0	0	30	0
(*Minute Maid* cup), 12 fl. oz.	300	0	77.0	0	0	50	0
Ice bar (see also "Fruit bar, frozen"), 1 bar:							
(*Cool Creations* Pop)	50	0	13.0	0	0	5	0
(*Cool Creations Sur-prise* Pop)	60	0	14.0	0	0	5	0
(*Good Humor Bubble Play* Sports Bar) ...	110	n.a.	27.0	0	0	5	0
(*Good Humor Hyper Stripe*)	80	n.a.	21.0	0	0	0	0
(*Good Humor Jumbo Jet Star*)	80	n.a.	20.0	0	0	0	0
banana/chocolate (*Good Humor Ba-nana Bonanza*)	90	n.a.	20.0	0	0	15	0
cotton candy (*Froz-fruit*)	100	1.0	20.0	2.0	10	20	0
Ice cream, ½ cup,:							
almond:							
praline (*Edy's/ Dreyer's Grand*)	170	3.0	21.0	8.0	25	85	0
toast (*Dreyer's Grand*)	150	3.0	15.0	9.0	25	30	0
amaretto (*Häagen-Dazs DiSaronno*) ...	260	4.0	26.0	15.0	95	80	0
apple crisp (*Edy's Homemade*)	150	3.0	21.0	6.0	25	70	0
apple pie (*Edy's/ Dreyer's Grand* Lim-ited Edition)	140	2.0	18.0	7.0	25	45	0

Food and Measure	cal.	prot. (gms)	carbo. (gms)	fat (gms)	chol. (mgs)	sod. (mgs)	fiber (gms)
Ice cream *(cont.)*							
banana:							
cream pie (*Edy's/ Dreyer's* Home- made)	130	3.0	17.0	6.0	25	60	0
nut (*Blue Bell*)	170	4.0	18.0	9.0	30	60	0
pudding (*Blue Bell*)	190	3.0	24.0	9.0	35	60	0
split (*Blue Bell*)	170	3.0	22.0	8.0	30	60	0
split (*Blue Bell* Diet)	110	3.0	14.0	4.0	15	65	0
split (*Blue Bell* Light)	110	3.0	20.0	2.0	10	65	0
banana and chocolate (*Edy's/Dreyer's Grand* Light Chiquita)	110	2.0	13.0	5.0	15	40	0
banana chocolate chunk (*Healthy Choice*)	120	3.0	22.0	2.0	5	55	<2.0
(*Ben & Jerry's Cherry Garcia*)	260	5.0	26.0	16.0	70	60	0
(*Ben & Jerry's Chubby Hubby*)	350	6.0	33.0	21.0	55	250	1.0
(*Ben & Jerry's Chunky Monkey*)	310	5.0	32.0	19.0	55	55	3.0
(*Ben & Jerry's Dil- bert's World Totally Nuts*)	310	5.0	27.0	21.0	45	105	<1.0
(*Ben & Jerry's Phish Food*)	300	4.0	41.0	14.0	35	80	3.0
(*Ben & Jerry's Wavy Gravy*)	340	7.0	32.0	20.0	60	120	9.0
Black Forest:							
(*Healthy Choice*) . . .	120	3.0	23.0	2.0	5	50	1.0
cake (*Blue Bell*)	170	2.0	22.0	8.0	20	70	1.0
black walnut:							
(*Blue Bell*)	160	3.0	16.0	9.0	40	50	0
(*Edy's* Homemade)	160	4.0	16.0	9.0	30	65	0
blackberry: (*Ben & Jerry's* Cobbler Low Fat)	180	3.0	34.0	3.0	20	70	<1.0

Food and Measure	cal.	prot. (gms)	carbo. (gms)	fat (gms)	chol. (mgs)	sod. (mgs)	fiber (gms)
blueberry cheesecake:							
(*Blue Bell*)	160	3.0	20.0	8.0	30	120	0
New York (*Edy's/ Dreyer's Grand Limited Edition*)	130	2.0	18.0	6.0	20	35	0
brownie sundae							
(*Edy's/Dreyer's* Fat Free No Sugar)	110	3.0	25.0	0	0	70	0
butter almond							
(*Breyers*)	170	n.a.	15.0	11.0	35	120	0
butter pecan:							
(*Ben & Jerry's*)	330	6.0	22.0	25.0	65	140	2.0
(*Blue Bell* Buttered)	180	4.0	17.0	11.0	30	90	0
(*Blue Bell* Buttered Light)	150	5.0	22.0	5.0	10	120	0
(*Breyers*)	180	n.a.	14.0	12.0	35	115	0
(*Breyers Smucker's* Homemade)	170	n.a.	16.0	11.0	50	70	0
(*Edy's/Dreyer's* Homemade)	160	4.0	16.0	9.0	30	125	0
(*Edy's/Dreyer's* No Sugar)	110	3.0	12.0	5.0	10	55	0
(*Edy's/Dreyer's Grand*)	160	3.0	25.0	10.0	25	90	0
(*Edy's/Dreyer's Grand* Light)	120	3.0	16.0	5.0	20	100	0
(*Eskimo Pie* Reduced Fat)	140	4.0	16.0	7.0	15	25	1.0
(*Häagen-Dazs*)	310	5.0	20.0	23.0	110	160	<1.0
crunch (*Healthy Choice*)	120	3.0	22.0	2.0	<5	60	1.0
Butterfinger (*Edy's/ Dreyer's Grand* Limited Edition)	160	3.0	19.0	8.0	25	50	0
cappuccino chocolate chunk (*Healthy Choice*)	120	3.0	22.0	2.0	10	60	1.0
cappuccino mocha fudge (*Healthy Choice*)	120	3.0	22.0	2.0	<5	50	1.0

Food and Measure	cal.	prot. (gms)	carbo. (gms)	fat (gms)	chol. (mgs)	sod. (mgs)	fiber (gms)
Ice cream *(cont.)*							
caramel and cream (*Breyers Smucker's* Homemade)	160	n.a.	19.0	8.0	45	60	0
caramel cream, dreamy (*Edy's Grand* Light)	110	2.0	18.0	3.0	20	60	0
caramel crunch sundae (*Blue Bell*)	190	3.0	24.0	10.0	30	125	0
caramel praline:							
crunch (*Breyers*) . . .	180	n.a.	22.0	9.0	30	75	0
crunch (*Breyers* Fat Free)	120	n.a.	25.0	0	<5	90	0
crunch (*Edy's/ Dreyer's* Fat Free)	110	3.0	25.0	0	0	60	0
pecan (*Breyers* Light)	180	n.a.	30.0	4.5	15	90	0
cherry, black, vanilla swirl:							
(*Edy's* Fat Free)	100	3.0	22.0	0	0	45	0
(*Edy's/Dreyer's* No Sugar)	90	3.0	12.0	3.0	10	50	0
cherry amaretto cordial (*Blue Bell*)	170	3.0	20.0	8.0	30	50	0
cherry chocolate chip (*Edy's Grand*)	150	2.0	18.0	8.0	25	35	0
cherry chocolate chunk:							
(*Edy's/Dreyer's Grand*)	150	2.0	17.0	8.0	25	30	0
(*Healthy Choice*) . . .	110	3.0	19.0	2.0	<5	55	<1.0
cherry cobbler (*Edy's* Homemade)	150	3.0	20.0	6.0	25	60	0
cherry vanilla:							
(*Blue Bell*)	160	3.0	19.0	8.0	35	55	0
(*Breyers*)	150	n.a.	17.0	8.0	30	30	0
(*Häagen-Dazs*)	240	4.0	23.0	15.0	100	75	0
chocolate:							
(*Blue Bell* Decadence)	190	2.0	20.0	11.0	25	65	0
(*Breyers*)	160	n.a.	18.0	9.0	30	20	0

Food and Measure	cal.	prot. (gms)	carbo. (gms)	fat (gms)	chol. (mgs)	sod. (mgs)	fiber (gms)
(*Breyers* Fat Free)	90	n.a.	19.0	0	0	55	0
(*Edy's/Dreyer's* Grand)	150	3.0	16.0	8.0	25	30	0
(*Edy's/Dreyer's* Grand Mumbo Jumbo)	170	3.0	18.0	9.0	20	45	0
(*Häagen-Dazs*)	270	5.0	22.0	18.0	115	75	1.0
(*Newman's Own* Chocolate Mud Bath)	190	4.0	21.0	10.0	35	45	1.0
Dutch (*Blue Bell*) . . .	170	3.0	17.0	9.0	40	60	0
Dutch, double (*Blue Bell*)	140	3.0	23.0	4.0	15	100	0
French (*Breyers* Light)	150	n.a.	22.0	5.0	30	55	0
milk (*Blue Bell*)	190	4.0	21.0	10.0	40	75	0
triple (*Blue Bell*) . . .	180	3.0	21.0	9.0	35	60	0
triple (*Edy's/ Dreyer's* No Sugar)	100	3.0	13.0	3.5	10	60	0
triple (*Edy's/ Dreyer's Grand* Thunder Limited Edition)	160	2.0	18.0	9.0	25	40	0
chocolate almond: fudge (*Edy's/ Dreyer's Grand* Light)	120	3.0	16.0	5.0	20	45	0
marshmallow (*Blue Bell*)	190	3.0	23.0	10.0	30	85	0
chocolate brownie crunch (*Edy's/ Dreyer's* Fat Free)	110	3.0	25.0	0	0	55	0
chocolate chip:							
(*Blue Bell*)	170	3.0	18.0	10.0	35	65	0
(*Breyers*)	170	n.a.	17.0	10.0	35	35	0
(*Edy's/Dreyer's* Homemade)	170	3.0	19.0	9.0	30	70	0
(*Edy's/Dreyer's Grand* Chips!) . . .	170	3.0	18.0	9.0	25	35	0

Food and Measure	cal.	prot. (gms)	carbo. (gms)	fat (gms)	chol. (mgs)	sod. (mgs)	fiber (gms)
Ice cream, chocolate chip *(cont.)*							
chocolate (*Häagen-Dazs*)	300	5.0	26.0	20.0	100	70	2.0
cookie dough (*Ben & Jerry's*)	300	5.0	34.0	16.0	65	95	0
cookie dough (*Blue Bell*)	190	3.0	23.0	10.0	25	90	0
cookie dough (*Breyers*)	180	n.a.	20.0	10.0	35	50	0
mint (*Blue Bell*)	170	3.0	18.0	10.0	35	75	0
mint (*Breyers*)	170	n.a.	17.0	10.0	35	35	0
mint (*Breyers* Light)	140	n.a.	21.0	5.0	10	50	0
mint (*Breyers* No Sugar)	100	n.a.	12.0	5.0	25	50	0
mint (*Edy's/Dreyer's Grand* Chips!) . . .	170	3.0	18.0	9.0	25	35	0
mint (*Healthy Choice*)	120	3.0	21.0	2.0	<5	50	<1.0
chocolate chunk:							
chocolate (*Healthy Choice*)	120	3.0	21.0	2.0	<5	45	2.0
double (*Edy's/ Dreyer's* Home-made)	190	3.0	21.0	10.0	30	65	0
chocolate cream pie (*Blue Bell*)	180	4.0	21.0	9.0	50	75	1.0
chocolate fudge:							
(*Edy's/Dreyer's* Fat Free)	110	3.0	25.0	0	0	55	0
(*Edy's/Dreyer's* Fat Free No Sugar)	100	4.0	22.0	0	0	60	0
(*Edy's/Dreyer's Grand* Light)	110	3.0	17.0	5.0	20	50	0
brownie (*Ben & Jerry's*)	280	5.0	32.0	15.0	45	90	2.0
double (*Breyers* Homemade)	180	n.a.	23.0	9.0	40	50	0
mousse (*Edy's/ Dreyer's Grand*)	160	2.0	19.0	8.0	25	45	0
sundae (*Edy's Grand*)	170	3.0	19.0	9.0	20	50	0

Food and Measure	cal.	prot. (gms)	carbo. (gms)	fat (gms)	chol. (mgs)	sod. (mgs)	fiber (gms)
chocolate marshmallow (*Eskimo Pie* Reduced Fat)	130	4.0	23.0	4.0	15	10	1.0
chocolate peanut butter:							
(*Edy's* Homemade)	200	5.0	18.0	12.0	30	105	0
chunk (*Edy's/ Dreyer's* Fat Free)	120	4.0	26.0	0	0	65	0
chocolate pecan cheesecake (*Blue Bell*)	200	3.0	22.0	11.0	30	160	0
chocolate rainbow (*Breyers*)	120	n.a.	16.0	10.0	25	40	0
chocolate sundae (*Blue Bell*)	170	3.0	21.0	8.0	30	60	0
coconut almond fudge chip (*Ben & Jerry's*)	310	5.0	24.0	22.0	40	70	2.0
coconut cream pie (*Ben & Jerry's* Low Fat*)	160	4.0	29.0	2.5	15	75	0
coffee:							
(*Ben & Jerry's Coffee Coffee Buzz Buzz Buzz*)	290	4.0	27.0	18.0	65	90	1.0
(*Blue Bell*)	160	3.0	18.0	8.0	35	55	0
(*Breyers*)	150	n.a.	15.0	9.0	35	35	0
(*Edy's/Dreyer's Grand*)	140	2.0	16.0	8.0	25	35	0
(*Häagen-Dazs*)	270	5.0	21.0	18.0	120	85	0
(*Newman's Own Giddy Up Coffee*)	170	4.0	16.0	10.0	55	50	0
fudge (*Edy's/ Dreyer's* Fat Free)	110	3.0	24.0	0	0	55	0
fudge (*Edy's/ Dreyer's* Fat Free No Sugar)	100	3.0	22.0	0	0	60	0
mocha chip (*Häagen-Dazs*)	290	4.0	25.0	19.0	110	90	<1.0
cookie chunk (*Edy's/ Dreyer's* Fat Free)	110	3.0	25.0	0	0	70	0

Food and Measure	cal.	prot. (gms)	carbo. (gms)	fat (gms)	chol. (mgs)	sod. (mgs)	fiber (gms)
Ice cream *(cont.)*							
cookie creme de menthe (*Healthy Choice*)	130	3.0	24.0	2.0	<5	60	<1.0
cookie dough:							
(*Edy's/Dreyer's Grand*)	170	3.0	20.0	9.0	25	75	0
(*Edy's/Dreyer's Grand* Light)	130	3.0	18.0	5.0	20	75	0
cookie jar (*Edy's/ Dreyer's Grand* Limited Edition)	170	3.0	19.0	9.0	25	65	0
cookies and cream:							
(*Blue Bell*)	180	3.0	20.0	10.0	35	80	0
(*Blue Bell* Light) . . .	120	4.0	20.0	3.0	10	85	0
(*Breyers*)	170	n.a.	19.0	9.0	30	45	0
(*Edy's/Dreyer's Grand*)	160	3.0	19.0	8.0	25	65	0
(*Edy's/Dreyer's Grand* Light)	120	3.0	17.0	4.0	20	55	0
(*Häagen-Dazs*)	270	5.0	23.0	17.0	110	115	0
(*Healthy Choice*) . . .	120	3.0	21.0	2.0	<5	90	<1.0
mint (*Breyers* Fat Free)	100	n.a.	21.0	0	<5	75	0
mint (*Dreyer's Grand* Light)	120	3.0	17.0	4.0	20	70	0
cookies and fudge (*Edy's* Homemade)	160	3.0	21.0	7.0	25	80	0
cookies and sweet cream (*Ben & Jerry's* Low Fat) . . .	180	5.0	33.0	3.0	20	105	2.0
(*Edy's/Dreyer's Grand* I Scream Sandwich Limited Edition) . . .	160	3.0	19.0	8.0	25	75	0
(*Edy's/Dreyer's Grand Goo Goo Cluster* Limited Edition) . . .	170	2.0	22.0	8.0	25	60	0
espresso chip:							
(*Edy's Grand*)	150	2.0	17.0	8.0	25	30	0
fudge (*Dreyer's Grand* Light)	120	3.0	18.0	4.0	15	60	0

Food and Measure	cal.	prot. (gms)	carbo. (gms)	fat (gms)	chol. (mgs)	sod. (mgs)	fiber (gms)
French Silk (*Edy's/ Dreyer's Grand Light*)	120	3.0	19.0	4.0	15	55	0
fruit rainbow (*Breyers*)	140	n.a.	16.0	8.0	30	35	0
fudge:							
brownie (*Healthy Choice*)	120	3.0	22.0	2.0	5	55	<2.0
brownie, double (*Edy's/Dreyer's No Sugar*)	100	3.0	13.0	3.5	30	60	0
brownie, double (*Edy's/Dreyer's Grand*)	170	2.0	19.0	9.0	25	40	0
brownie hot (*Blue Bell*)	200	4.0	24.0	10.0	40	105	0
cake, turtle (*Healthy Choice*)	130	3.0	25.0	2.0	<5	60	2.0
chunk (*Ben & Jerry's* New York Super)	320	5.0	28.0	21.0	50	65	4.0
ripple (*Eskimo Pie Reduced Fat*)	120	4.0	19.0	4.0	15	20	0
vanilla caramel (*Ben & Jerry's*)	300	4.0	33.0	17.0	70	115	1.0
Irish cream (*Häagen-Dazs Baileys*)	270	5.0	23.0	17.0	115	85	0
lemon (*Blue Bell*)	150	2.0	19.0	7.0	30	60	0
macadamia nut brittle (*Häagen-Dazs*)	300	4.0	25.0	20.0	110	120	0
marble fudge:							
(*Edy's/Dreyer's* Fat Free)	110	3.0	24.0	0	0	55	0
(*Edy's/Dreyer's* No Sugar)	90	3.0	13.0	3.0	10	60	0
(*Milky Way* Lowfat)	130	3.0	22.0	3.0	10	85	0
mint:							
chip (*Häagen-Dazs*)	290	4.0	26.0	19.0	105	105	<1.0
chip (*Newman's Own Lovable Mint Chip*)	230	4.0	23.0	14.0	55	60	0

Food and Measure	cal.	prot. (gms)	carbo. (gms)	fat (gms)	chol. (mgs)	sod. (mgs)	fiber (gms)
Ice cream, mint *(cont.)*							
chocolate chip, see "chocolate chip," above							
chocolate cookie (*Ben & Jerry's*)	280	4.0	28.0	17.0	70	130	1.0
cookie, thin (*Edy's/ Dreyer's Grand Girl Scouts*)	170	2.0	18.0	10.0	25	60	0
fudge (*Dreyer's* Fat Free)	110	3.0	24.0	0	0	55	0
patty, vanilla and chocolate (*Ben & Jerry's* Low Fat)	170	5.0	32.0	3.0	10	75	2.0
mocha fudge:							
(*Edy's/Dreyer's* No Sugar)	90	3.0	13.0	3.0	10	60	0
almond (*Dreyer's* Grand)	170	3.0	18.0	9.0	25	40	0
almond (*Dreyer's* Grand Light)	120	3.0	16.0	5.0	20	50	0
mud pie (*Dreyer's* Grand)	160	2.0	19.0	8.0	25	65	0
Neapolitan:							
(*Blue Bell*)	160	3.0	17.0	9.0	40	55	0
(*Dreyer's Grand*)	140	2.0	16.0	7.0	25	30	0
(*Eskimo Pie* Re-duced Fat)	110	4.0	18.0	4.0	15	10	0
peach (*Breyers*)	130	n.a.	17.0	6.0	25	25	0
peach vanilla:							
(*Blue Bell* Home-made)	180	2.0	24.0	8.0	35	45	0
(*Blue Bell* Home-made Light)	140	3.0	24.0	3.0	15	50	0
peanut butter cup:							
(*Ben & Jerry's*)	380	7.0	32.0	25.0	65	130	2.0
(*Blue Bell*)	230	4.0	25.0	12.0	35	85	0
(*Edy's Grand* Light cups!)	130	3.0	17.0	5.0	20	55	0

Food and Measure	cal.	prot. (gms)	carbo. (gms)	fat (gms)	chol. (mgs)	sod. (mgs)	fiber (gms)
(Edy's/Dreyer's Grand Limited Edition)	170	3.0	18.0	9.0	25	60	0
pecan praline:							
(Newman's Own Pistol Packin' Praline Pecan)	200	3.0	22.0	11.0	30	125	0
and cream (Blue Bell)	200	3.0	23.0	11.0	35	80	0
peppermint:							
(Blue Bell)	160	3.0	20.0	8.0	35	60	0
(Edy's/Dreyer's Grand Limited Edition)	150	2.0	17.0	8.0	25	40	0
pistachio almond (Blue Bell)	170	4.0	17.0	10.0	30	80	0
praline and caramel or caramel cluster (Healthy Choice) ...	130	3.0	25.0	2.0	<5	70	<1.0
raspberry ribbon, wild (Healthy Choice) ...	110	3.0	20.0	2.0	5	45	1.0
raspberry vanilla swirl (Edy's/Dreyer's Fat Free No Sugar)	90	3.0	19.0	0	0	50	0
rocky road:							
(Blue Bell)	180	4.0	19.0	9.0	30	75	1.0
(Blue Bell Diet)	100	3.0	14.0	4.0	10	80	1.0
(Blue Bell Light) ...	110	3.0	18.0	3.0	5	75	1.0
(Breyers)	180	n.a.	24.0	9.0	25	25	0
(Edy's/Dreyer's Grand)	170	3.0	17.0	10.0	25	30	0
(Edy's/Dreyer's Grand Light)	120	3.0	17.0	4.0	20	45	0
(Healthy Choice) ...	140	3.0	28.0	2.0	<5	60	2.0
rum raisin (Häagen-Dazs)	270	4.0	22.0	17.0	110	75	0
S'mores:							
(Ben & Jerry's S'mores Low Fat)	190	5.0	35.0	2.0	15	85	1.0
(Blue Bell)	180	4.0	27.0	7.0	20	75	0
(Snickers)	220	5.0	26.0	11.0	25	85	0

Food and Measure	cal.	prot. (gms)	carbo. (gms)	fat (gms)	chol. (mgs)	sod. (mgs)	fiber (gms)
Ice cream (cont.)							
strawberry:							
(*Blue Bell*)	150	3.0	20.0	6.0	25	45	0
(*Breyers*)	130	n.a.	15.0	7.0	30	30	0
(*Edy's/Dreyer's* No Sugar)	80	3.0	11.0	3.0	10	50	0
(*Häagen-Dazs*)	250	4.0	23.0	16.0	95	80	<1.0
real (*Edy's/Dreyer's Grand*)	130	2.0	17.0	6.0	20	25	0
and vanilla (*Blue Bell* Homemade)	160	3.0	24.0	6.0	25	50	0
and vanilla (*Blue Bell* Homemade Light)	140	3.0	24.0	3.0	15	55	0
strawberry cheesecake (*Blue Bell*)	170	3.0	22.0	8.0	35	115	0
strawberry and cream:							
(*Breyers Smucker's* Homemade)	150	n.a.	18.0	8.0	45	50	0
(*Edy's/Dreyer's* Homemade)	130	3.0	17.0	6.0	25	55	0
Homemade	130	3.0	17.0	6.0	25	55	0
tin roof (*Blue Bell*) . . .	200	4.0	22.0	10.0	30	65	0
toffee crunch:							
coffee (*Ben & Jerry's Coffee Heath*)	310	4.0	32.0	18.0	65	125	0
vanilla (*Ben & Jerry's Vanilla Heath*)	310	4.0	30.0	19.0	70	135	0
vanilla:							
(*Ben & Jerry's World's Best*) . . .	250	4.0	22.0	16.0	75	60	0
(*Blue Bell* Country)	160	3.0	16.0	9.0	40	50	0
(*Blue Bell* Country Diet)	100	4.0	14.0	4.0	15	65	0
(*Blue Bell* French)	170	3.0	18.0	9.0	80	50	0
(*Blue Bell* Homemade)	180	4.0	20.0	9.0	40	70	0
(*Blue Bell* Homemade Light)	140	5.0	22.0	4.0	20	75	0
(*Breyers*)	150	n.a.	15.0	9.0	35	35	0

Food and Measure	cal.	prot. (gms)	carbo. (gms)	fat (gms)	chol. (mgs)	sod. (mgs)	fiber (gms)
(*Breyers* Fat Free)	90	n.a.	19.0	0	0	65	0
(*Breyers* Home-made)	150	n.a.	16.0	8.0	50	35	0
(*Breyers* Light)	120	n.a.	19.0	3.0	10	55	0
(*Breyers* No Sugar)	90	n.a.	11.0	4.5	25	45	0
(*Breyers* Soft 'n Creamy)	150	n.a.	19.0	7.0	30	35	0
(*Dreyer's Grand*)	150	2.0	14.0	10.0	35	30	0
(*Edy's Grand*)	140	2.0	15.0	8.0	25	30	0
(*Edy's/Dreyer's* Fat Free)	100	3.0	22.0	0	0	45	0
(*Edy's/Dreyer's* Fat Free No Sugar)	90	3.0	19.0	0	0	50	0
(*Edy's/Dreyer's* Homemade)	140	3.0	16.0	7.0	30	65	0
(*Edy's/Dreyer's* No Sugar)	80	3.0	11.0	3.0	10	55	0
(*Edy's/Dreyer's* Grand Light)	100	3.0	15.0	3.0	20	50	0
(*Edy's/Dreyer's* Grand Godzilla Limited Edition)	160	2.0	19.0	8.0	25	50	0
(*Eskimo Pie* Re-duced Fat)	110	4.0	17.0	4.0	15	10	0
(*Häagen-Dazs*)	270	5.0	21.0	18.0	120	85	0
(*Healthy Choice*) . . .	100	3.0	18.0	2.0	5	50	1.0
(*Newman's Own Ob-scene Vanilla Bean*)	170	4.0	17.0	10.0	60	50	0
bean (*Blue Bell*) . . .	190	4.0	20.0	10.0	40	55	0
bean (*Blue Bell* Diet)	100	5.0	21.0	0	0	85	0
bean (*Blue Bell* Light)	140	5.0	22.0	4.0	20	70	0
bean (*Edy's/Dreyer's* Grand)	140	2.0	15.0	8.0	25	35	0
French (*Breyers*) . . .	160	n.a.	15.0	10.0	n.a.	40	0
French (*Edy's/ Dreyer's Grand*)	160	2.0	16.0	10.0	55	30	0
vanilla and caramel: (*Edy's/Dreyer's* Fat Free No Sugar)	100	3.0	21.0	0	0	60	0

Food and Measure	cal.	prot. (gms)	carbo. (gms)	fat (gms)	chol. (mgs)	sod. (mgs)	fiber (gms)
Ice cream, vanilla and caramel (cont.)							
(Edy's/Dreyer's No Sugar)	90	3.0	13.0	3.0	10	60	0
vanilla chocolate:							
(Breyers Take Two)	160	n.a.	17.0	9.0	35	35	0
(Edy's Grand)	150	3.0	16.0	8.0	25	30	0
swirl (Edy's/Dreyer's Fat Free No Sugar)	100	4.0	20.0	0	0	50	0
vanilla chocolate chip (Häagen-Dazs)	310	5.0	26.0	20.0	105	90	<1.0
vanilla chocolate strawberry:							
(Breyers)	150	n.a.	16.0	8.0	30	30	0
(Breyers Fat Free)	90	n.a.	19.0	0	0	55	0
(Breyers Home- made)	150	n.a.	17.0	8.0	50	35	0
(Breyers Light)	120	n.a.	19.0	3.0	10	50	0
(Breyers No Sugar)	90	n.a.	11.0	2.5	25	45	0
(Breyers Soft 'n Creamy)	150	n.a.	19.0	7.0	30	35	0
(Edy's Grand)	140	2.0	16.0	7.0	25	30	0
vanilla fudge:							
(Häagen-Dazs)	290	5.0	26.0	18.0	100	110	0
twirl (Breyers)	160	n.a.	19.0	8.0	35	35	0
twirl (Breyers Fat Free)	100	n.a.	22.0	0	0	65	0
twirl (Breyers No Sugar)	100	n.a.	14.0	2.5	25	55	0
vanilla orange sherbet (Breyers Take Two)	130	n.a.	21.0	5.0	20	30	0
vanilla strawberry (Breyers Fat Free Take Two)	80	n.a.	19.0	0	<5	55	0
vanilla Swiss almond (Häagen-Dazs)	310	6.0	23.0	21.0	105	90	1.0
white chocolate al- mond (Blue Bell) ...	190	4.0	17.0	12.0	35	65	0
"Ice cream," nondairy, ½ cup:							
Better Pecan (Tofutti)	220	1.0	22.0	13.0	0	200	0

Food and Measure	cal.	prot. (gms)	carbo. (gms)	fat (gms)	chol. (mgs)	sod. (mgs)	fiber (gms)
cappuccino (*Rice Dream*)	150	0	23.0	6.0	0	100	1.0
cappuccino almond fudge (*Rice Dream Supreme*)	170	1.0	24.0	8.0	0	95	2.0
carob (*Rice Dream*)	150	1.0	24.0	6.0	0	100	2.0
carob almond (*Rice Dream*)	170	1.0	24.0	8.0	0	95	2.0
cherry chocolate chunk (*Rice Dream Supreme*)	170	1.0	27.0	7.0	0	85	1.0
cherry vanilla (*Rice Dream*)	150	0	24.0	6.0	0	90	1.0
chocolate:							
(*Rice Dream*)	150	1.0	24.0	7.0	0	100	2.0
(*Tofutti* Supreme)	180	3.0	18.0	11.0	0	180	0
chocolate almond chunk (*Rice Dream Supreme*)	170	2.0	25.0	8.0	0	95	2.0
chocolate chip (*Rice Dream*)	170	1.0	26.0	8.0	0	95	1.0
chocolate cookie crunch (*Tofutti*)	210	3.0	26.0	11.0	0	100	1.0
chocolate fudge brownie (*Rice Dream* Supreme)	170	1.0	28.0	7.0	0	95	2.0
cocoa marble fudge (*Rice Dream*)	150	1.0	25.0	6.0	0	100	2.0
cookie n' dream (*Rice Dream*)	170	1.0	26.0	7.0	0	100	1.0
espresso bean, double (*Rice Dream* Supreme)	160	1.0	24.0	7.0	0	95	1.0
mint carob chip (*Rice Dream*)	170	1.0	26.0	8.0	0	95	1.0
mint chocolate chip (*Rice Dream*)	170	1.0	26.0	8.0	0	95	1.0
mint chocolate cookie (*Rice Dream* Supreme)	170	1.0	26.0	8.0	0	100	1.0

Food and Measure	cal.	prot. (gms)	carbo. (gms)	fat (gms)	chol. (mgs)	sod. (mgs)	fiber (gms)
"Ice cream," nondairy *(cont.)*							
Neapolitan (*Rice Dream*)	150	1.0	24.0	6.0	0	100	2.0
orange vanilla swirl (*Rice Dream*)	150	0	23.0	6.0	0	100	1.0
peanut butter cup (*Rice Dream* Supreme)	180	2.0	25.0	8.0	0	105	2.0
pralines n' dream (*Rice Dream* Supreme)	180	1.0	24.0	9.0	0	95	1.0
strawberry (*Rice Dream*)	140	0	24.0	5.0	0	85	1.0
vanilla:							
(*Rice Dream*)	150	0	23.0	6.0	0	100	1.0
(*Tofutti*)	190	2.0	20.0	11.0	0	210	0
Vanilla Almond Bark (*Tofutti*)	210	3.0	21.0	13.0	0	130	0
vanilla fudge (*Tofutti*)	190	2.0	25.0	9.0	0	130	0
vanilla Swiss almond (*Rice Dream*)	180	1.0	25.0	8.0	0	95	1.0
wildberry (*Tofutti* Supreme)	190	2.0	24.0	9.0	0	190	0
Ice cream bar, 1 bar, except as noted:							
almond (see also "vanilla," below):							
(*Dove* 4-Pack)	280	5.0	23.0	19.0	30	110	1.0
(*Dove* Single)	350	6.0	29.0	24.0	40	140	1.0
(*Klondike*)	310	n.a.	26.0	21.0	25	90	n.a.
toasted (*Good Humor* Multipack)	180	n.a.	25.0	8.0	10	40	n.a.
toasted (*Good Humor* Single)	250	n.a.	34.0	12.0	15	35	n.a.
(*Ben & Jerry's Chunky Monkey*)	360	5.0	32.0	25.0	40	50	1.0
(*Ben & Jerry's Phish Stick*)	330	4.0	38.0	20.0	25	85	2.0
(*Ben & Jerry's Totally Nuts*)	370	6.0	24.0	29.0	30	115	1.0
(*Butterfinger*)	190	2.0	16.0	13.0	15	35	0

Food and Measure	cal.	prot. (gms)	carbo. (gms)	fat (gms)	chol. (mgs)	sod. (mgs)	fiber (gms)
cappuccino (*Klondike*)	290	n.a.	25.0	20.0	15	65	n.a.
candy center crunch (*Good Humor*)	300	n.a.	22.0	23.0	15	80	n.a.
caramel creme swirl w/toffee chips (*Dove* 4-Pack)...........	280	3.0	31.0	16.0	30	100	0
caramel crunch (*Klondike* Multi Pack) ...	300	n.a.	31.0	18.0	30	95	n.a.
chocolate:							
(*Good Humor Hershey's* Single) ...	240	n.a.	24.0	15.0	10	20	0
(*Nestlé Crunch*) ...	200	2.0	17.0	14.0	15	40	0
(*3 Musketeers* Single)	190	2.0	22.0	11.0	20	40	0
(*3 Musketeers* 6-Pack)	150	2.0	17.0	9.0	10	35	0
w/dark chocolate (*Dove* 4-Pack) ...	260	3.0	27.0	17.0	25	30	1.0
w/dark chocolate (*Dove* Single) ...	330	4.0	29.0	21.0	30	40	1.0
w/dark chocolate (*Häagen-Dazs* Multipack)......	290	4.0	23.0	20.0	70	45	2.0
w/dark chocolate (*Häagen-Dazs* Single)	350	5.0	28.0	24.0	85	60	2.0
w/dark chocolate (*Klondike* Multi Pack)..........	290	n.a.	24.0	20.0	30	75	n.a.
w/milk chocolate (*Klondike* Multi Pack)..........	290	n.a.	22.0	20.0	20	60	n.a.
w/milk chocolate (*Milky Way*).....	220	3.0	24.0	13.0	20	65	0
w/milk chocolate (*Milky Way* Reduced Fat)......	140	2.0	19.0	7.0	5	50	0
chocolate eclair:							
(*Good Humor* Multipack)...........	170	n.a.	21.0	9.0	10	60	0

Food and Measure	cal.	prot. (gms)	carbo. (gms)	fat (gms)	chol. (mgs)	sod. (mgs)	fiber (gms)
Ice cream bar, chocolate eclair *(cont.)*							
(*Good Humor* Single)	230	n.a.	29.0	11.0	10	85	0
chocolate fudge:							
(*Smart Ones Chocolate Treat*)	100	3.0	20.0	.5	0	25	1.0
chocolate mousse							
(*Smart Ones*)	40	2.0	9.0	1.0	5	20	1.0
coffee/almond crunch:							
(*Häagen-Dazs* Multipack)	310	4.0	23.0	22.0	80	70	<1.0
(*Häagen-Dazs* Single)	360	5.0	27.0	26.0	100	85	1.0
cookie dough (*Ben & Jerry's*)	420	5.0	44.0	25.0	55	130	<1.0
cookies and cream:							
(*Edy's/Dreyer's*) . . .	250	3.0	22.0	17.0	20	90	0
(*Oreo*)	180	2.0	18.0	12.0	20	95	0
fruit, w/cream, see "Fruit bar, frozen"							
(*Klondike* Krispy Krunch), 5 fl. oz.	300	n.a.	28.0	20.0	25	85	n.a.
(*Klondike* Krunch), 4 fl. oz.	270	n.a.	26.0	17.0	25	75	n.a.
(*Klondike* Original Multi Pack)	290	n.a.	25.0	20.0	30	70	n.a.
(*Klondike* Original Single)	290	n.a.	24.0	20.0	15	65	n.a.
mint, green, and chocolate fudge truffle swirl (*Dove* 4-Pack)	290	3.0	31.0	27.0	30	40	0
mint cookie, thin (*Edy's/Dreyer's Girl Scouts*)	280	3.0	23.0	19.0	20	80	0
mocha cashew crunch (*Dove* 4-Pack)	260	3.0	25.0	17.0	30	55	0
Neapolitan (*Klondike* Multi Pack)	280	n.a.	25.0	19.0	25	60	n.a.
(*Nestlé Crunch Crunch King*)	270	3.0	21.0	19.0	20	45	0

Food and Measure	cal.	prot. (gms)	carbo. (gms)	fat (gms)	chol. (mgs)	sod. (mgs)	fiber (gms)
(*Nestlé Crunch* Reduced Cal)	130	3.0	14.0	7.0	5	40	0
snack size, see "Ice cream nuggets"							
(*Snickers*)	200	4.0	19.0	13.0	15	55	0
strawberry shortcake:							
(*Good Humor* Multipack)	160	n.a.	20.0	8.0	10	60	0
(*Good Humor* Single)	220	n.a.	31.0	10.0	10	75	0
strawberry/white chocolate:							
(*Häagen-Dazs* Multipack)	270	4.0	20.0	19.0	60	60	0
(*Häagen-Dazs* Single)	320	4.0	24.0	23.0	70	75	0
toffee crunch (*Ben & Jerry's Vanilla Heath*)	330	4.0	33.0	22.0	65	105	<1.0
vanilla:							
(*Ben & Jerry's* Peace Pop)	330	4.0	29.0	23.0	75	55	<1.0
(*Klondike* Multi Pack)	290	n.a.	25.0	20.0	30	70	n.a.
(*Nestlé Crunch*) . . .	200	2.0	16.0	14.0	15	40	0
(*3 Musketeers* Single)	190	2.0	21.0	11.0	20	40	0
(*3 Musketeers* 6-Pack)	150	2.0	16.0	8.0	10	35	0
almonds (*Edy's/ Dreyer's*)	250	4.0	21.0	17.0	25	40	0
almonds (*Häagen-Dazs* Multipack)	320	5.0	22.0	23.0	75	65	1.0
almonds (*Häagen-Dazs* Single)	370	6.0	26.0	27.0	90	80	1.0
w/dark chocolate (*Dove* 4-Pack) . . .	260	3.0	26.0	17.0	30	30	0
w/dark chocolate (*Dove* Single) . . .	330	4.0	32.0	21.0	35	40	0
w/dark chocolate (*Eskimo Pie*)	160	2.0	14.0	11.0	15	35	0

Food and Measure	cal.	prot. (gms)	carbo. (gms)	fat (gms)	chol. (mgs)	sod. (mgs)	fiber (gms)
Ice cream bar, vanilla *(cont.)*							
w/dark chocolate (*Eskimo Pie* No Sugar)	120	3.0	13.0	8.0	10	40	0
w/dark chocolate (*Good Humor* Multipack)	200	n.a.	15.0	14.0	30	30	0
w/dark chocolate (*Häagen-Dazs* Multipack)	290	4.0	22.0	20.0	70	50	1.0
w/dark chocolate (*Häagen-Dazs* Single)	350	5.0	27.0	24.0	85	65	1.0
w/dark chocolate (*Milky Way*)	220	3.0	23.0	13.0	15	60	0
w/dark chocolate (*Milky Way* Reduced Fat)	140	2.0	19.0	7.0	5	50	0
w/milk chocolate (*Dove* 4-Pack) . . .	260	3.0	25.0	17.0	30	45	0
w/milk chocolate (*Dove* Single) . . .	330	4.0	31.0	21.0	40	55	0
w/milk chocolate (*Edy's/Dreyer's*)	250	3.0	22.0	17.0	25	45	n.a.
w/milk chocolate (*Eskimo Pie*)	160	2.0	12.0	12.0	10	30	0
w/milk chocolate (*Good Humor* Multipack)	190	n.a.	15.0	14.0	35	30	0
w/milk chocolate (*Häagen-Dazs* Multipack)	280	4.0	20.0	20.0	75	60	0
w/milk chocolate (*Häagen-Dazs* Single)	330	5.0	24.0	24.0	90	75	<1.0
w/milk chocolate w/crisps (*Eskimo Pie* No Sugar) . . .	120	3.0	13.0	8.0	10	40	0
w/milk chocolate w/toffee crunch (*Smart Ones*) . . .	110	2.0	12.0	6.0	5	25	1.0

Food and Measure	cal.	prot. (gms)	carbo. (gms)	fat (gms)	chol. (mgs)	sod. (mgs)	fiber (gms)
orange coated (*Smart Ones*) ...	40	2.0	10.0	.5	5	15	0
"Ice cream" bar, nondairy, 1 bar:							
carob coated:							
chocolate (*The Rice Dream Bar*)	270	2.0	32.0	15.0	0	95	2.0
strawberry (*The Rice Dream Bar*)	250	1.0	31.0	13.0	0	80	1.0
vanilla (*The Rice Dream Bar*)	270	1.0	33.0	14.0	0	95	1.0
chocolate (*Smart Ones* Treat)	100	3.0	20.0	.5	0	25	1.0
nut coated, chocolate or vanilla (*The Nutty Rice Dream Bar*) ...	260	4.0	23.0	18.0	0	55	2.0
Ice cream cake, 2.4-oz. slice, except as noted:							
(*Viennetta* Individuals), 1 pc.	240	n.a.	21.0	15.0	35	65	0
cappuccino (*Viennetta*)	190	n.a.	19.0	11.0	35	35	0
chocolate (*Viennetta*)	190	n.a.	18.0	12.0	25	40	0
vanilla (*Viennetta*) ...	190	n.a.	19.0	11.0	40	40	0
Ice cream cone, plain, unfilled, 1 pc.:							
bowl, waffle (*Keebler*)	50	<1.0	10.0	1.0	0	25	0
cone:							
fudge dip (*Keebler*)	35	0	6.0	1.5	0	20	0
sugar (*Keebler*)	50	<1.0	10.0	.5	0	15	0
waffle (*Keebler*) ...	50	<1.0	10.0	1.0	0	25	0
Ice cream cone, filled, 1 cone:							
(*Eskimo Pie* No Sugar)	210	3.0	24.0	12.0	15	30	0
(*Good Humor American Glory*)	230	n.a.	36.0	8.0	5	135	n.a.
(*Good Humor King Cone*)	300	n.a.	48.0	10.0	20	110	n.a.
(*Snickers*)	290	5.0	34.0	15.0	20	115	0

Food and Measure	cal.	prot. (gms)	carbo. (gms)	fat (gms)	chol. (mgs)	sod. (mgs)	fiber (gms)
Ice cream cone, filled *(cont.)*							
caramel:							
(*Klondike*)	310	n.a.	34.0	17.0	20	100	n.a.
(*Klondike* Kombo Kones)	320	n.a.	42.0	15.0	20	125	n.a.
chocolate (*Drumstick*)	320	6.0	36.0	17.0	25	90	2.0
chocolate dipped (*Drumstick*)	320	5.0	40.0	16.0	25	90	1.0
cookies 'n cream:							
(*Oreo*)	230	4.0	27.0	12.0	20	120	<1.0
sundae (*Edy's/ Dreyer's*)	250	4.0	31.0	12.0	20	75	n.a.
fudge (*Klondike* Kombo Kones)	320	n.a.	42.0	15.0	20	100	n.a.
sundae:							
(*Good Humor* Premium)	290	n.a.	33.0	14.0	20	85	n.a.
(*Good Humor* Variety Pack)	260	n.a.	35.0	12.0	15	80	n.a.
(*Good Humor* Hershey's)	290	n.a.	33.0	14.0	20	85	n.a.
vanilla (*Drumstick*) . . .	340	6.0	35.0	19.0	20	90	2.0
vanilla caramel (*Drumstick*)	360	6.0	38.0	20.0	25	100	2.0
vanilla fudge:							
(*Drumstick*)	360	5.0	39.0	20.0	20	100	2.0
sundae (*Edy's/ Dreyer's*)	240	4.0	31.0	11.0	20	60	n.a.
"Ice cream" cone, filled, nondairy, 1 cone:							
chocolate (*Rice Dream*)	270	3.0	37.0	14.0	0	140	2.0
vanilla (*Rice Dream*)	270	3.0	36.0	14.0	0	150	2.0
Ice cream cup, plain, unfilled (*Keebler*), 1 cup	15	0	4.0	0	0	20	0
Ice cream cup, filled: (*Klondike* Sundae), 6 fl. oz.	280	n.a.	27.0	18.0	40	65	n.a.

Food and Measure	cal.	prot. (gms)	carbo. (gms)	fat (gms)	chol. (mgs)	sod. (mgs)	fiber (gms)
chocolate:							
(*Carnation*), 3 fl. oz.	140	2.0	16.0	8.0	25	40	0
sundae (*Carnation*), 5 fl. oz.	210	2.0	30.0	9.0	30	55	1.0
strawberry:							
(*Carnation*), 3 fl. oz.	100	1.0	12.0	5.0	20	25	0
sundae (*Carnation*), 5 fl. oz.	200	2.0	29.0	8.0	30	55	0
vanilla:							
(*Carnation*), 3 fl. oz.	100	1.0	11.0	6.0	20	30	0
(*Carnation*), 5 fl. oz.	170	2.0	19.0	10.0	35	50	0
Ice cream malt, 12 fl. oz.:							
chocolate (*Carnation*)	270	7.0	48.0	6.0	20	130	1.0
vanilla (*Carnation*) . . .	260	6.0	48.0	5.0	20	130	0
Ice cream nuggets, 5 pcs., except as noted:							
(*Nestlé Crunch*), 8 pcs.	310	4.0	25.0	21.0	20	60	0
(*Snickers* Snack Size), 4 pcs.	390	7.0	37.0	25.0	25	105	0
cherry royale (*Dove Bite Size*)	340	3.0	35.0	21.0	30	35	0
chocolate:							
dark (*Bon-Bons*) . . .	190	2.0	16.0	13.0	15	55	0
dark (*Bon-Bons*), 8 pcs.	310	3.0	26.0	21.0	25	60	0
double (*Dove Bite Size*)	330	4.0	34.0	21.0	30	35	1.0
milk (*Bon-Bons*) . . .	200	2.0	17.0	14.0	10	35	0
milk (*Bon-Bons*), 8 pcs.	330	3.0	27.0	23.0	20	60	0
Irish creme cordial w/dark chocolate (*Dove Bite Size*) . . .	340	3.0	33.0	22.0	35	35	0
peppermint w/dark chocolate (*Dove Bite Size*)	360	3.0	39.0	22.0	30	35	0

Food and Measure	cal.	prot. (gms)	carbo. (gms)	fat (gms)	chol. (mgs)	sod. (mgs)	fiber (gms)
Ice cream nuggets *(cont.)*							
vanilla:							
classic (*Dove Bite*							
Size)	320	4.0	31.0	21.0	35	50	0
French (*Dove Bite*							
Size)	330	3.0	33.0	21.0	50	35	0
Ice cream pie or							
patty, see "Ice							
cream sandwich"							
Ice cream sandwich,							
1 pc.:							
(*Eskimo Pie* No Sugar)	160	4.0	27.0	4.0	10	135	<1.0
(*Frozfruit*), 4.5 oz. . . .	273	5.0	34.0	13.0	32	87	2.0
(*Frozfruit*), 10 oz. . . .	355	8.0	57.0	19.0	38	127	3.0
(*Good Humor* Pre-							
mium Cookie)	290	n.a.	44.0	11.0	20	210	n.a.
(*Good Humor* Variety							
Pack)	160	n.a.	25.0	5.0	15	140	n.a.
(*Good Humor* Ameri-							
can Glory)	70	n.a.	28.0	8.0	15	120	n.a.
(*Klondike* Big Bear Fat							
Free)	130	n.a.	25.0	0	0	110	n.a.
(*Klondike Choc Burger*							
Multi Pack)	320	n.a.	39.0	17.0	20	140	0
(*Klondike Choc Burger*							
Single)	350	n.a.	39.0	19.0	30	115	0
(*Klondike Choco Taco*)	310	n.a.	37.0	17.0	20	100	n.a.
(*Smart Ones*)	150	3.0	28.0	3.0	5	150	1.0
(*SnackWell's*)	90	2.0	18.0	1.5	5	85	1.0
chocolate chip:							
(*Frozfruit*)	273	5.0	34.0	13.0	32	87	2.0
cookie (*Hershey's*)	290	n.a.	44.0	11.0	20	210	n.a.
cookies and cream							
(*Cool Creations*) . . .	240	2.0	34.0	11.0	15	250	1.0
mini (*Cool Creations*)	110	1.0	16.0	5.0	10	70	0
mocha pie (*Frozfruit*)	300	5.0	43.0	14.0	15	55	4.0
Neapolitan (*Good Hu-*							
mor Giant)	260	n.a.	39.0	10.0	20	150	n.a.
nectar pie (*Frozfruit*)	310	5.0	42.0	15.0	10	15	3.0

Food and Measure	cal.	prot. (gms)	carbo. (gms)	fat (gms)	chol. (mgs)	sod. (mgs)	fiber (gms)
peanut butter:							
(*Reese's* Cup Multipack)	160	n.a.	14.0	11.0	10	45	0
(*Reese's* cup Single)	220	n.a.	20.0	16.0	10	65	0
vanilla:							
(*Good Humor* Giant)	240	n.a.	35.0	10.0	20	160	n.a.
(*Häagen-Dazs*)	260	4.0	32.0	13.0	65	125	0
w/fudge (*Eskimo Pie Arctic Madness*)	260	4.0	26.0	16.0	15	85	1.0
vanilla and chocolate (*Häagen-Dazs*)	260	4.0	31.0	13.0	65	120	1.0
"Ice cream" sandwich, nondairy, 1 pc.:							
chocolate or mint (*Rice Dream*)	320	3.0	39.0	18.0	0	80	2.0
mocha or vanilla (*Rice Dream*)	320	3.0	40.0	17.0	0	80	1.0
Ice cream and sorbet, see "Sorbet"							
Icing, cake, see "Frosting"							
Irish cream syrup (*Ferrara*), 2 oz.	130	0	32.0	0	0	12	0
Italian cut beans, see "'Green beans, canned"							
Italian sausage, see "Sausage"							
Italian seasoning, 1 tsp. . . . . :	3	.1	.6	.1	0	<1	.2

J

Food and Measure	cal.	prot. (gms)	carbo. (gms)	fat (gms)	chol. (mgs)	sod. (mgs)	fiber (gms)
Jack-in-the-Box,							
1 serving:							
breakfast items:							
Breakfast Jack	280	17.0	30.0	12.0	195	920	1.0
Country Crock							
Spread	25	0	0	2.5	0	45	0
croissant, sausage	690	21.0	37.0	51.0	240	1000	1.0
croissant, supreme	520	21.0	39.0	32.0	235	1240	1.0
grape jelly	40	0	10.0	0	0	0	0
hash browns	170	1.0	14.0	12.0	0	250	1.0
pancakes, w/bacon	370	12.0	59.0	9.0	30	1020	3.0
sandwich, sour-							
dough	440	20.0	36.0	24.0	355	1120	1.0
sandwich, ultimate	620	34.0	40.0	36.0	455	1800	2.0
syrup	130	0	30.0	0	0	5	0
burgers:							
cheeseburger:							
double	460	23.0	31.0	27.0	80	920	2.0
ultimate	1030	47.0	40.0	79.0	205	1370	4.0
ultimate, bacon	1150	53.0	41.0	89.0	230	1770	4.0
hamburger	280	12.0	30.0	12.0	45	560	2.0
hamburger							
w/cheese	320	14.0	30.0	16.0	60	760	2.0
Jumbo Jack	590	25.0	42.0	36.0	80	720	4.0
Jumbo Jack							
w/cheese	680	29.0	43.0	44.0	105	1180	4.0
Sourdough Jack ...	690	31.0	38.0	46.0	110	1180	3.0
sandwiches:							
chicken	450	16.0	39.0	26.0	45	1030	2.0
chicken, spicy							
crispy	560	25.0	55.0	27.0	50	1140	2.0
chicken Caesar	490	24.0	41.0	26.0	55	1050	3.0

Food and Measure	cal.	prot. (gms)	carbo. (gms)	fat (gms)	chol. (mgs)	sod. (mgs)	fiber (gms)
chicken fajita pita	280	24.0	25.0	9.0	75	840	3.0
chicken fillet, grilled	520	27.0	42.0	26.0	140	1240	4.0
chicken supreme	680	23.0	46.0	45.0	85	1500	4.0
Philly cheesesteak	520	33.0	41.0	25.0	155	1980	4.0
cheese slices:							
American, 1 slice	45	2.0	1.0	4.0	10	230	0
Swiss style, 1 slice	40	2.0	1.0	4.0	10	210	0
taco	170	7.0	12.0	10.0	20	460	2.0
taco, monster	270	12.0	19.0	17.0	30	670	4.0
finger foods:							
bacon cheddar po-							
tato wedges	800	20.0	49.0	58.0	55	1470	4.0
chicken breast,							
5 pcs.	360	27.0	24.0	17.0	80	970	1.0
chicken, 4 pcs., and							
fries	730	26.0	79.0	34.0	65	1690	5.0
dipping sauces,							
1 oz.:							
barbecue	45	1.0	11.0	0	0	310	0
buttermilk house	130	<1.0	3.0	13.0	10	240	<1.0
sweet and sour	45	<1.0	11.0	0	0	160	0
egg rolls, 3 pcs. . . .	440	15.0	40.0	24.0	35	1020	4.0
egg rolls, 5 pcs. . . .	730	25.0	67.0	41.0	60	1700	7.0
fish and chips	780	19.0	86.0	39.0	45	1740	6.0
jalapeños, stuffed:							
7 pcs.	530	14.0	46.0	31.0	60	1730	3.0
10 pcs.	750	20.0	65.0	44.0	80	2470	5.0
salsa, 1 oz.	10	0	2.0	0	0	200	0
sour cream, 1.1 oz.	60	1.0	1.0	6.0	20	30	0
salads:							
chicken teriyaki	670	26.0	128.0	4.0	15	1730	3.0
garden chicken	200	23.0	8.0	9.0	65	420	3.0
side salad	50	2.0	3.0	3.0	10	75	1.0
croutons	50	1.0	8.0	2.0	0	105	0
soy sauce	5	1.0	1.0	0	0	480	0
salad dressings:							
blue cheese	210	1.0	11.0	15.0	25	750	0
buttermilk house . . .	290	1.0	6.0	30.0	20	560	0
Italian, low-cal	25	0	2.0	1.5	0	670	0
Thousand Island . . .	250	1.0	10.0	24.0	35	570	0

Food and Measure	cal.	prot. (gms)	carbo. (gms)	fat (gms)	chol. (mgs)	sod. (mgs)	fiber (gms)
Jack-in-the-Box *(cont.)*							
sides:							
fries:							
regular	350	4.0	46.0	16.0	0	710	3.0
jumbo	430	4.0	58.0	20.0	0	890	4.0
super scoop	610	6.0	82.0	28.0	0	1250	5.0
fries, curly:							
seasoned.......	410	6.0	45.0	23.0	0	1010	4.0
chili cheese	650	14.0	65.0	41.0	25	1760	4.0
ketchup..........	10	0	3.0	0	0	105	0
onion rings	460	7.0	50.0	25.0	0	780	3.0
desserts/shakes:							
apple turnover, hot	340	4.0	41.0	18.0	0	510	2.0
carrot cake	370	3.0	54.0	16.0	40	340	2.0
cheesecake	320	7.0	32.0	18.0	65	220	<1.0
double fudge cake	300	3.0	50.0	10.0	50	320	1.0
shakes, regular:							
cappuccino	630	11.0	80.0	29.0	95	320	0
chocolate	630	11.0	85.0	27.0	85	330	<1.0
Oreo cookie	320	13.0	91.0	36.0	95	730	2.0
strawberry.......	640	10.0	85.0	28.0	85	300	0
vanilla	610	12.0	73.0	31.0	95	320	0
Jackfruit, trimmed, 1 oz.	27	.4	6.8	.1	0	1	.5
Jackfruit, dried (*Frieda's*), cup	120	2.0	30.0	0	0	0	1.0
Jackson wonder beans, dried (*Frieda's*), ½ cup	120	7.0	22.0	0	0	0	9.0
Jalapeño, see "Pepper, jalapeño"							
Jalapeño dip (see also "Cheese dip"), 2 tbsp.:							
(*Kraft*)	60	1.0	3.0	4.0	0	260	0
(*Old El Paso*)	30	1.0	4.0	1.0	<5	125	2.0
Jalapeño dip mix, dry (*Watkins*), 1 tsp.	10	0	2.0	0	0	120	0
Jalapeño relish (*Old El Paso*), 1 tbsp.	5	0	1.0	0	0	110	0

Food and Measure	cal.	prot. (gms)	carbo. (gms)	fat (gms)	chol. (mgs)	sod. (mgs)	fiber (gms)
Jalfrazzi entree, see "Vegetable entree, packaged"							
Jalfrezzi sauce, see "Curry sauce, cooking"							
Jam and preserves (see also "Fruit spread"), 1 tbsp., except as noted:							
all fruits (*Knott's Berry Farm*), 1 tsp.	18	0	4.0	0	0	0	0
all fruits (*Smucker's*)	50	0	13.0	0	0	0	0
grape (*Kraft*)	60	0	14.0	0	0	10	0
marmalade:							
lemon-pear, pineapple-orange, or 3-fruit (*Crosse & Blackwell*)	60	0	14.0	0	0	0	0
orange (*Crosse & Blackwell*)	50	0	13.0	0	0	0	0
plum, red (*Kraft*)	60	0	13.0	0	0	10	0
raspberry-cherry or twinberry (*Watkins*)	42	0	11.0	0	0	0	0
strawberry (*Kraft*) . . .	50	0	13.0	0	0	10	0
Java plum:							
medium, .4 oz.	5	.1	1.4	<.1	0	1	<1.0
seeded, ½ cup	41	.5	10.5	.2	0	9	<1.0
Jelly, 1 tbsp.:							
all fruits (*Smucker's*)	50	0	13.0	0	0	0	0
apple (*Kraft*)	60	0	14.0	0	0	10	0
apple-strawberry (*Kraft*)	50	0	13.0	0	0	10	0
blackberry (*Kraft*) . . .	50	0	13.0	0	0	10	0
grape (*Kraft*)	50	0	14.0	0	0	10	0
guava (*Goya*)	50	0	12.0	0	0	0	0
guava or red currant:							
(*Crosse & Blackwell*)	50	0	13.0	0	0	0	0
(*Kraft*)	50	0	13.0	0	0	10	0

Food and Measure	cal.	prot. (gms)	carbo. (gms)	fat (gms)	chol. (mgs)	sod. (mgs)	fiber (gms)
Jelly *(cont.)*							
mint (*Crosse & Blackwell*)	60	0	14.0	0	0	0	0
strawberry (*Kraft*) . . .	60	0	14.0	0	0	10	0
Jerk sauce (see also "Marinade"), 2 tbsp.:							
(*World Harbors Blue Mountain*)	70	0	18.0	0	0	200	0
dipping (*Helen's Tropical Exotics* Jamaican)	45	1.0	10.0	0	0	640	1.0
Jerk seasoning (*Helen's Tropical Exotics*), 1 tbsp.	30	1.0	7.0	0	0	210	1.0
Jerusalem artichoke: (*Frieda's* Sun Choke), ½ cup, 3 oz.	70	2.0	14.0	0	0	0	1.0
sliced, ½ cup	57	1.5	13.1	<.1	0	n.a.	1.2
Jicama, see "Yam bean tuber"							
Jujube:							
raw, seeded, 1 oz. . . .	22	.3	5.7	.1	0	1	n.a.
dried, 1 oz.	81	1.0	20.1	.3	0	3	n.a.
Jute, potherb:							
raw, ½ cup	5	.7	.8	<.1	0	1	n.a.
boiled, drained, ½ cup	16	1.6	3.1	.1	0	5	.9

K

Food and Measure	cal.	prot. (gms)	carbo. (gms)	fat (gms)	chol. (mgs)	sod. (mgs)	fiber (gms)
Kabocha squash							
(*Frieda's*), ³/₄ cup, 3 oz.	30	1.0	7.0	0	0	0	1.0
Kale, fresh, ¹/₂ cup:							
raw, chopped	17	1.1	3.4	.2	0	15	.7
boiled, drained, chopped	21	1.2	3.7	.3	0	15	1.3
Kale, canned, ¹/₂ cup:							
(*Allens/Sunshine*)	25	2.0	3.0	.5	0	20	2.0
(*Stubb's*)	25	2.0	3.0	.5	0	20	2.0
chopped (*Bush's Best*)	30	2.0	4.0	0	0	330	2.0
Kale, Chinese							
(*Frieda's* Gai Lan), 1 cup, 3 oz.	15	2.0	1.0	0	0	1	0
Kale, Scotch, ¹/₂ cup:							
raw, chopped	14	1.0	2.8	.2	0	24	<1.0
boiled, drained, chopped	18	1.2	3.7	.3	0	29	<2.0
Kamranga, see "Carambola"							
Kamut flakes, see "Cereal, ready-to-eat"							
Kamut flour (*Arrowhead Mills*), ¹/₄ cup	110	4.0	25.0	.5	0	0	4.0
Kasha, see "Buckwheat groats"							
Kelp, see "Seaweed"							
Ketchup, 1 tbsp., except as noted:							
(*Healthy Choice*)	10	0	2.0	0	0	100	0
(*Heinz*)	15	0	4.0	0	0	190	0

Food and Measure	cal.	prot. (gms)	carbo. (gms)	fat (gms)	chol. (mgs)	sod. (mgs)	fiber (gms)
Ketchup *(cont.)*							
(*Hunt's*)	15	0	3.5	0	0	200	0
(*Hunt's* No Salt)	15	0	4.0	0	0	10	0
(*Muir Glen*)	15	0	3.0	0	0	190	0
(*Smucker's*)	25	0	7.0	0	0	110	0
(*Uncle Dave's*), 1 tsp.	15	0	3.0	0	0	150	0
w/horseradish							
(*Gold's*), 1 tsp.	5	0	1.0	0	0	60	0
KFC, 1 serving:							
chicken, 1 pc.:							
Original Recipe:							
breast	400	29.0	16.0	24.0	135	1116	1.0
drumstick	140	13.0	4.0	9.0	75	422	0
thigh	250	16.0	6.0	18.0	95	747	1.0
whole wing	140	9.0	5.0	10.0	55	414	0
Extra Tasty Crispy:							
breast	470	31.0	25.0	28.0	80	930	1.0
drumstick	190	13.0	8.0	11.0	60	260	<1.0
thigh	370	19.0	18.0	25.0	70	540	2.0
whole wing	200	10.0	10.0	13.0	45	290	<1.0
Hot & Spicy:							
breast	180	32.0	23.0	35.0	110	1110	2.0
drumstick	190	13.0	10.0	11.0	50	300	<1.0
thigh	370	18.0	13.0	27.0	90	570	1.0
whole wing	210	10.0	9.0	15.0	50	340	<1.0
Tender Roast:							
breast, w/skin . . .	251	37.0	1.0	10.8	151	830	0
breast, w/out skin	169	31.4	<2.0	4.3	112	797	0
drumstick, w/skin	97	14.5	<1.0	4.3	85	271	0
drumstick, w/out							
skin	67	11.0	<1.0	2.4	63	259	0
thigh, w/skin	207	18.4	<1.0	12.0	120	504	0
thigh, w/out skin	106	12.9	<1.0	5.5	84	312	0
wing, w/skin	121	12.2	1.0	7.7	74	331	0
Chicken *Twister*	480	25.0	51.0	20.0	60	760	2.0
Crispy Strips, 3 pcs.:							
Colonel's	261	19.8	10.0	15.8	40	658	2.0
Spicy Buffalo	350	22.0	22.0	19.0	35	1110	2.0
Hot Wings, 6 pcs. . . .	471	27.0	18.0	33.0	150	1230	2.0
pot pie, chicken	770	29.0	69.0	42.0	70	2160	5.0

Food and Measure	cal.	prot. (gms)	carbo. (gms)	fat (gms)	chol. (mgs)	sod. (mgs)	fiber (gms)
sandwiches:							
Original Recipe	497	28.6	45.5	22.3	52	1213	3.0
BBQ-flavored, value	256	17.0	28.0	8.0	57	782	2.0
sides and vegetables:							
baked beans, BBQ	190	6.0	33.0	3.0	5	760	6.0
biscuit, 1 pc.	180	4.0	20.0	10.0	0	560	<1.0
cole slaw, 5 oz. . . .	180	2.0	21.0	9.0	5	280	3.0
corn on the cob	150	5.0	35.0	1.5	0	20	2.0
cornbread, 1 pc.	228	3.0	24.0	13.0	42	194	1.0
green beans	45	1.0	7.0	1.5	5	730	3.0
macaroni & cheese	180	7.0	21.0	8.0	10	860	2.0
Mean Greens	70	4.0	11.0	3.0	10	650	5.0
potato salad	230	4.0	23.0	14.0	15	540	2.0
potato wedges	280	5.0	28.0	13.0	5	750	5.0
potatoes, mashed, w/gravy	120	1.0	17.0	6.0	<1	440	2.0
Kidney beans, dry: (*Arrowhead Mills*),							
¼ cup	160	11.0	29.0	.5	0	0	10.0
boiled, ½ cup	112	7.6	20.1	.4	0	2	6.5
Kidney beans, canned (see also "Baked Beans"), ½ cup:							
red:							
(*Eden* Organic)	100	8.0	18.0	0	0	15	10.0
(*Progresso*)	110	7.0	20.0	.5	0	280	8.0
(*Seneca*)	120	7.0	20.0	0	0	220	7.0
(*Van Camp's* New Orleans)	90	7.0	20.0	.5	0	470	6.0
dark (*Allens/East Texas Fair/Trappey's*)	130	8.0	22.0	1.0	0	310	8.0
dark (*Bush's Best*)	130	8.0	21.0	1.0	0	260	7.0
dark (*Progresso*)	110	8.0	20.0	0	0	340	6.0
dark (*Van Camp's*)	90	6.0	20.0	0	0	760	6.0
dark or light (*Brooks*)	120	7.0	22.0	.5	0	500	8.0
dark or light (*Green Giant/Joan of Arc*)	110	8.0	20.0	0	0	340	6.0
light (*Allens/Trappey's*)	120	6.0	22.0	1.0	0	340	8.0

Food and Measure	cal.	prot. (gms)	carbo. (gms)	fat (gms)	chol. (mgs)	sod. (mgs)	fiber (gms)
Kidney beans, canned, red *(cont.)*							
light (*Bush's Best*)	110	7.0	20.0	0	0	260	7.0
light (*Van Camp's*)	90	6.0	20.0	0	0	390	6.0
w/bacon (*Trappey's New Orleans*) ...	110	6.0	20.0	1.0	0	410	6.0
w/chili gravy (*Trappey's*)	110	6.0	20.0	1.0	0	510	7.0
w/jalapeño, light (*Trappey's*)	110	6.0	19.0	1.0	0	420	6.0
w/liquid	108	6.7	20.0	.4	0	437	8.2
Spanish style (*Goya*)	110	6.0	18.0	1.0	0	620	5.0
white:							
(*Eden* Organic)	100	6.0	17.0	1.0	0	40	5.0
(*Progresso* Cannellini)	100	5.0	18.0	.5	0	270	5.0
Kidney beans, freeze-dried (*AlpineAire*), 1 oz.	110	7.0	19.0	0	0	0	5.0
Kidney beans, sprouted, raw, ½ cup	27	3.9	3.8	.5	0	n.a.	<1.0
Kidneys, braised:							
beef, 4 oz.	163	28.9	1.1	3.9	439	152	0
lamb, 4 oz.	155	26.8	1.1	4.1	641	171	0
pork, 4 oz.	171	28.8	0	5.3	544	91	0
pork, chopped, 1 cup	211	35.6	0	6.6	673	111	0
veal, 4 oz.	185	29.8	0	6.4	897	125	0
Kielbasa (see also "Polish sausage"), 2 oz.:							
(*Boar's Head*)	120	9.0	0	10.0	50	440	0
(*Healthy Choice* Polska)	70	7.0	2.0	1.5	20	480	0
(*Hormel*)	150	8.0	0	13.0	40	530	0
Kim chee (*Frieda's*), ¼ cup, 2 oz.	15	1.0	2.0	0	0	340	1.0
Kishka (*Hebrew National*), 2 oz.	160	5.0	10.0	11.0	15	430	2.0
Kiwi, fresh:							
(*Frieda's*), 5 oz.	90	1.0	21.0	.5	0	5	5.0
large, 3.7 oz.	55	.9	13.5	.4	0	4	3.1

Food and Measure	cal.	prot. (gms)	carbo. (gms)	fat (gms)	chol. (mgs)	sod. (mgs)	fiber (gms)
medium, 3.1 oz.	46	.8	11.3	.3	0	4	2.6
Kiwi, dried (*Sonoma*),							
7–8 pcs., 1 oz.	90	1.0	19.0	1.0	0	0	2.0
Kiwi drink blends,							
8 fl. oz., except as							
noted:							
(*Crazy Kiwi Passion*)	130	0	32.0	0	0	35	0
strawberry:							
(*Arizona*)	120	0	29.0	0	0	20	0
(*Chiquita* Cocktail)	120	0	31.0	0	0	10	0
(*Ocean Spray*)	120	0	31.0	0	0	35	0
(*Snapple* Cocktail)	110	0	28.0	0	0	10	0
(*Snapple* Diet)	20	0	5.0	0	0	10	0
(*Veryfine/Veryfine*							
Chiller)	170	0	43.0	0	0	20	0
(*Veryfine* Chiller),							
11.5 fl. oz.	200	0	49.0	0	0	20	0
(*Veryfine* Diet)	15	0	4.0	0	0	10	0
Kiwi juice (*After the*							
Fall Bear), 8 fl. oz.	100	1.0	24.0	0	0	15	0
Knish, potato, frozen							
(*Cohen's Famous*),							
1 pc.	200	4.0	38.0	4.0	0	530	2.0
Knockwurst, 1 link:							
(*Ball Park*), 4 oz.	360	12.0	4.0	33.0	80	1320	0
beef:							
(*Ball Park*), 4 oz.	340	13.0	1.0	32.0	75	1120	0
(*Boar's Head*), 4 oz.	310	15.0	1.0	27.0	50	950	0
(*Hebrew National*),							
3 oz.	260	10.0	1.0	24.0	55	670	0
(*Shofar*), 3 oz.	210	10.0	1.0	17.0	40	530	0
Kohlrabi, ½ cup, ex-							
cept as noted:							
raw:							
(*Frieda's*), cup,							
3 oz.	25	1.0	5.0	0	0	15	3.0
sliced	19	1.2	4.3	.1	0	14	2.5
boiled, drained, sliced	24	1.5	5.5	.1	0	17	.9
Kombu, see "Sea-							
weed"							

Food and Measure	cal.	prot. (gms)	carbo. (gms)	fat (gms)	chol. (mgs)	sod. (mgs)	fiber (gms)
Kumquat:							
(*Frieda's*), 5 oz.	90	1.0	23.0	0	0	10	9.0
medium, .7 oz.	12	.2	3.1	<.1	0	1	1.3
seeded, 1 oz.	18	.3	4.7	<.1	0	2	1.9
Kun choy, see "Celery, Chinese"							

L

Food and Measure	cal.	prot. (gms)	carbo. (gms)	fat (gms)	chol. (mgs)	sod. (mgs)	fiber (gms)
Lamb, choice, meat only, 4 oz., except as noted:							
cubed, leg/shoulder:							
braised or stewed	253	38.2	0	10.0	122	79	0
broiled	211	31.8	0	8.3	102	86	0
foreshank, braised:							
lean w/fat	276	32.2	0	15.3	120	82	0
lean only	212	35.2	0	6.8	118	84	0
ground:							
raw	320	18.8	0	26.5	83	67	0
broiled	321	28.1	0	22.3	110	92	0
broiled, 1 cup	328	28.7	0	23.1	113	94	0
leg, whole, roasted:							
lean w/fat	293	29.0	0	18.7	105	75	0
lean w/fat, 1 slice, 3″ diam. x ¼″ ...	73	7.2	0	4.7	26	19	0
lean only	217	32.1	0	8.8	101	77	0
lean only, 3″ slice	54	8.0	0	2.2	25	19	0
leg, shank, roasted:							
lean w/fat	255	29.9	0	14.1	102	74	0
lean w/fat, 1 slice, 3″ diam. x ¼″ ...	64	7.5	0	3.5	26	18	0
lean only	204	31.9	0	7.6	99	75	0
lean only, 3″ slice	51	8.0	0	1.9	25	19	0
leg, sirloin, roasted:							
lean w/fat	331	27.9	0	23.4	110	77	0
lean w/fat, 1 slice, 3″ diam. x ¼″ ...	83	7.0	0	5.9	27	19	0
lean only	231	32.1	0	10.4	104	81	0
lean only, 3″ slice	58	8.0	0	2.6	26	20	0

Food and Measure	cal.	prot. (gms)	carbo. (gms)	fat (gms)	chol. (mgs)	sod. (mgs)	fiber (gms)
Lamb *(cont.)*							
loin, roasted:							
lean w/fat	350	25.6	0	26.8	108	73	0
lean only	229	30.2	0	11.1	99	75	0
loin chop, broiled:							
lean w/fat, 2¼ oz.							
(4.2 oz. raw							
w/bone)	201	16.1	0	14.7	64	49	0
lean w/fat	358	28.5	0	26.2	113	87	0
lean only, 1.6 oz.							
(4.2 oz. raw							
w/bone and fat)	100	13.9	0	4.5	44	39	0
lean only	245	34.0	0	11.0	108	95	0
rib:							
broiled, lean w/fat	409	25.1	0	33.6	112	86	0
broiled, lean only	266	31.5	0	14.7	103	96	0
roasted, lean w/fat	407	24.0	0	33.8	110	83	0
roasted, lean only	263	29.7	0	15.1	100	92	0
shoulder, whole:							
braised, lean w/fat	390	32.5	0	27.8	132	85	0
braised, lean only	321	37.2	0	10.0	133	90	0
roasted, lean w/fat	313	25.5	0	22.6	104	75	0
roasted, lean only	231	28.3	0	12.2	99	77	0
Lamb, New Zealand,							
frozen, meat only,							
4 oz.:							
foreshank:							
braised, lean w/fat	293	30.6	0	18.0	116	53	0
braised, lean only	211	34.9	0	6.8	115	56	0
leg, whole:							
roasted, lean w/fat	279	28.1	0	17.6	115	49	0
roasted, lean only	205	31.4	0	7.9	113	51	0
loin chop:							
broiled, lean w/fat	357	26.6	0	27.1	127	56	0
broiled, lean only	226	33.2	0	9.3	129	62	0
rib:							
roasted, lean w/fat	386	21.5	0	32.6	113	49	0
roasted, lean only	222	27.7	0	11.5	107	54	0
shoulder:							
braised, lean w/fat	405	32.0	0	29.8	139	58	0
braised, lean only	323	38.6	0	17.6	144	64	0

Food and Measure	cal.	prot. (gms)	carbo. (gms)	fat (gms)	chol. (mgs)	sod. (mgs)	fiber (gms)
Lamb curry entree, frozen (*Curry Classics*), 10-oz. pkg.	480	37.0	16.0	29.0	95	1210	6.0
Lamb sausage, see "Sausage"							
Lamb's quarters, boiled, drained, chopped, ½ cup ...	29	2.9	4.5	.6	0	n.a.	1.9
Lard, pork, 1 tbsp.	115	0	0	12.8	12	<1	0
Lasagna entree, canned or packaged, 1 cup, except as noted:							
(*Dinty Moore American Classics*), 1 bowl...........	340	22.0	28.0	16.0	60	990	3.0
(*Hormel* Microwave cup)	210	9.0	31.0	6.0	20	840	2.0
(*Hormel Health Selections*)	170	9.0	29.0	1.5	15	470	3.0
(*Nalley*)	250	15.0	33.0	6.0	45	1070	6.0
(*Nalley*), 7½-oz. can cheese, three (*Nalley*),	200	10.0	26.0	6.0	25	990	5.0
7½-oz. can	180	11.0	21.0	6.0	35	840	5.0
w/meat sauce (*Chef Boyardee*)	270	9.0	41.0	8.0	30	830	2.0
Lasagna entree, dried (*Mountain House*), 1 cup	240	14.0	24.0	9.0	35	570	3.0
Lasagna entree, frozen, 1 pkg., except as noted:							
(*Amy's*), 10¼ oz.	310	19.0	37.0	11.0	35	680	6.0
(*Healthy Choice* Roma), 13½ oz. ...	400	26.0	59.0	7.0	35	580	9.0
Alfredo: (*Smart Ones*), 9 oz.	300	14.0	46.0	7.0	20	680	3.0
w/broccoli (*The Budget Gourmet Value Classics*), 8 oz.	310	11.0	41.0	11.0	15	620	3.0

Food and Measure	cal.	prot. (gms)	carbo. (gms)	fat (gms)	chol. (mgs)	sod. (mgs)	fiber (gms)
Lasagna entree, frozen *(cont.)*							
bake (*Stouffer's*), 10¼ oz.	370	18.0	47.0	12.0	30	900	6.0
cheese:							
(*Lean Cuisine* Casserole), 10 oz.	270	13.0	40.0	6.0	10	590	5.0
(*Lean Cuisine* Classic), 11½ oz. . . .	280	19.0	40.0	4.5	15	560	6.0
extra (*Marie Callender's*), 1 cup	350	16.0	36.0	16.0	20	720	4.0
five (*Lean Cuisine*), ¹⁄₁₂ of 96-oz. pkg.	210	14.0	30.0	3.5	25	590	3.0
five (*Stouffer's*), 10¾ oz.	360	21.0	40.0	13.0	35	960	6.0
three (*The Budget Gourmet*), 8½ oz.	310	15.0	34.0	12.0	30	700	2.0
chicken:							
(*Lean Cuisine*), 10 oz.	270	19.0	30.0	8.0	35	590	5.0
(*Lean Cuisine*), ¹⁄₁₂ of 96-oz. pkg. . . .	230	13.0	30.0	6.0	35	550	4.0
(*Stouffer's* 39 oz.), 1 cup	320	13.0	29.0	17.0	30	750	4.0
cheese, w/chicken scallopini (*Lean Cuisine Cafe Classics*), 10 oz.	290	21.0	33.0	8.0	30	590	3.0
Florentine (*Smart Ones*), 10½ oz. . . .	290	15.0	36.0	8.0	30	650	5.0
garden (*Smart Ones*), 11 oz.	270	14.0	36.0	7.0	30	610	5.0
meat (*Wolfgang Puck's*), 12 oz.	490	24.0	51.0	22.0	55	800	4.0
w/meat sauce:							
(*Banquet*), 9½ oz.	260	10.0	38.0	8.0	10	820	5.0
(*Banquet* Family), 1 cup	100	13.0	37.0	11.0	60	960	2.0
(*The Budget Gourmet* Low Fat), 8½ oz.	250	12.0	34.0	7.0	20	580	3.0

Food and Measure	cal.	prot. (gms)	carbo. (gms)	fat (gms)	chol. (mgs)	sod. (mgs)	fiber (gms)
(*The Budget Gourmet Value Classics*), 8 oz.	300	12.0	39.0	10.0	20	490	3.0
(*Freezer Queen*), 10 oz.	290	13.0	42.0	8.0	15	1530	5.0
(*Freezer Queen* Family), 1 cup	270	12.0	39.0	8.0	15	930	4.0
(*Lean Cuisine*), 10½ oz.	290	21.0	37.0	6.0	25	560	4.0
(*Marie Callender's*), 1 cup	370	17.0	34.0	18.0	35	740	4.0
(*Marie Callender's* Family), 1 cup . . .	350	17.0	32.0	16.0	50	770	3.0
(*Smart Ones*), 9 oz.	240	13.0	43.0	2.5	10	560	4.0
(*Smart Ones* Traditional), 10½ oz. . .	300	22.0	38.0	7.0	40	790	3.0
(*Stouffer's*), 10½ oz.	370	23.0	39.0	14.0	45	1050	4.0
(*Stouffer's* 21 oz.), 1 cup or ⅓ pkg.	250	17.0	28.0	8.0	30	720	3.0
(*Stouffer's* 40 oz.), 1 cup or ⅕ pkg.	270	16.0	28.0	10.0	30	620	3.0
(*Stouffer's* 96 oz.), 1 cup or ¹⁄₁₂ pkg.	300	20.0	29.0	11.0	35	710	3.0
mozzarella (*The Budget Gourmet Value Classics*), 8 oz. . . .	280	12.0	40.0	8.0	15	610	3.0
sausage, Italian:							
(*The Budget Gourmet*), 8½ oz. . . .	330	15.0	32.0	15.0	35	710	2.0a
(*Marie Callender's*), 15 oz.	710	26.0	70.0	36.0	30	1330	8.0
vegetable:							
(*Amy's*), 9½ oz. . . .	300	15.0	39.0	10.0	15	680	5.0
(*Amy's* Family Size), 7 oz.	200	10.0	27.0	8.0	10	480	4.0
(*Lean Cuisine*), 10½ oz.	260	15.0	35.0	7.0	20	590	5.0
(*Stouffer's*), 10½ oz.	440	21.0	43.0	20.0	35	1110	5.0

Food and Measure	cal.	prot. (gms)	carbo. (gms)	fat (gms)	chol. (mgs)	sod. (mgs)	fiber (gms)
Lasagna entree, frozen, vegetable *(cont.)*							
(*Stouffer's* 96 oz.),							
1 cup or ¹⁄₁₂ pkg.	330	13.0	36.0	15.0	15	770	4.0
tofu (*Amy's*),							
9¹⁄₂ oz.	300	18.0	41.0	10.0	0	630	6.0
zucchini (*Healthy*							
Choice), 13¹⁄₂ oz.	330	20.0	58.0	1.5	10	310	11.0
Leek:							
fresh:							
(*Frieda's*), 1 cup,							
3 oz.	50	1.0	12.0	0	0	15	2.0
raw, 9.9-oz. leek ...	76	1.9	17.6	.4	0	25	2.2
raw, chopped,							
¹⁄₂ cup	32	.8	7.4	.2	0	10	.9
boiled, drained,							
chopped, ¹⁄₂ cup	16	.4	4.0	.1	0	6	<1.0
freeze-dried, 1 tbsp.	1	<.1	.2	tr.	0	<1	<1.0
Lemon:							
2¹⁄₈″ lemon, 3.9 oz.	22	1.3	11.6	.3	0	3	n.a.
1 wedge, ¹⁄₄ medium	5	.3	2.9	.1	0	1	n.a.
peeled, 2¹⁄₈″ lemon ...	17	.6	5.4	.2	0	1	1.6
Lemon curd (*Crosse &*							
Blackwell), 1 tbsp.	50	0	13.0	0	0	0	0
Lemon herb sauce							
mix (*Knorr* Classic),							
1 tbsp.	30	<1.0	4.0	1.0	0	260	0
Lemon juice, fresh,							
1 tbsp.	4	.1	1.3	0	0	<1	.1
Lemon peel, fresh,							
1 tbsp.	-¹	.1	1.0	<.1	0	0	.6
Lemon peel, candied,							
diced (*Paradise/*							
White Swan),							
2 tbsp., 1 oz.	80	0	21.0	0	0	15	2.0
Lemon pepper:							
(*Lawry's*), ¹⁄₄ tsp.	0	0	0	0	0	80	0
1 tsp.	7	.2	1.5	0	0	425	.3
Lemon sauce, Oriental							
(*Ka•Me*), 1 tbsp.	45	0	11.0	0	0	125	0

¹ *Cannot be calculated; no digestibility value for fresh peel.*

Food and Measure	cal.	prot. (gms)	carbo. (gms)	fat (gms)	chol. (mgs)	sod. (mgs)	fiber (gms)
Lemon seasoning (*Old Bay Dash O' Lemon*), ¼ tsp. . . .	0	0	0	0	0	110	0
Lemon-dill oil, see "Oil"							
Lemonade, 8 fl. oz., except as noted:							
(*After the Fall*)	90	1.0	23.0	0	0	10	0
(*Arizona*)	110	0	27.0	0	0	25	0
(*Hood*)	110	0	28.0	0	0	5	0
(*R.W. Knudsen*)	120	0	29.0	0	0	35	0
(*R.W. Knudsen* Aseptic)	110	1.0	27.0	0	0	· 35	0
(*Santa Cruz* Organic)	120	0	29.0	0	0	35	0
(*Snapple*)	100	0	26.0	0	0	10	0
(*Sunkist*)	120	0	30.0	0	0	30	0
(*Sunkist* Diet)	0	0	0	0	0	85	0
(*Tropicana*)	140	0	35.0	0	0.	20	0
(*Tropicana Twister* Light)	35	0	9.0	0	0	95	0
(*Veryfine*), 10 fl. oz.	160	0	40.0	0	0	15	0
(*Veryfine* Chiller)	130	0	32.0	0	0	·15	0
(*Veryfine* Chiller), 11.5 fl. oz.	190	0	46.0	0	0	20	0
(*Veryfine* Chiller 20 oz.)	120	0	29.0	0	0	5	0
(*Welch's*)	110	0	29.0	0	0	140	0
pink:							
(*Arizona*)	110	0	28.0	0	0	25	0
(*Snapple*)	120	0	29.0	0	0	10	0
(*Snapple* Diet)	20	0	4.0	0	0	10	0
(*Tropicana Twister*)	120	0	29.0	0	0	35	0
(*Veryfine* Chiller), 11.5 fl. oz.	190	0	46.0	0	0	20	0
(*Veryfine* Diet)	15	0	4.0	0	0	10	0
frozen* (*R.W. Knudsen* Natural/Organic)	120	0	29.0	0	0	35	0
Lemonade fruit blends, 8 fl. oz., except as noted:							
berry (*Fruitopia*)	106	0	28.0	0	0	58	0

Food and Measure	cal.	prot. (gms)	carbo. (gms)	fat (gms)	chol. (mgs)	sod. (mgs)	fiber (gms)
Lemonade fruit blends *(cont.)*							
cherry:							
(*R.W. Knudsen*) . . .	120	0	29.0	0	0	35	0
(*Snapple*)	120	0	30.0	0	0	10	0
cranberry (*R.W. Knudsen*)	120	0	29.0	0	0	35	0
ginger (*R.W. Knudsen* Echinacea)	100	0	25.0	0	0	8	0
peach (*Snapple*)	120	0	29.0	0	0	10	0
strawberry:							
(*Santa Cruz* Organic)	120	0	29.0	0	0	35	0
(*Veryfine* Chiller) . . .	150	0	38.0	0	0	10	0
(*Veryfine* Chiller), 11.5 fl. oz.	170	0	43.0	0	0	20	0
Lemonade mix*, 8 fl. oz.:							
(*Country Time*)	70	0	17.0	0	0	15	0
(*Crystal Light*)	5	0	0	0	0	0	0
(*Kool-Aid*)	100	0	25.0	0	0	15	0
(*Kool-Aid* Presweetened)	70	0	17.0	0	0	0	0
pink:							
(*Country Time*)	70	0	17.0	0	0	10	0
(*Crystal Light*)	5	0	0	0	0	20	0
(*Kool-Aid*)	100	0	25.0	0	0	15	0
Lemon-lime drink (*Veryfine* Chiller Avalanche), 8 fl. oz.	120	0	29.0	0	0	5	0
Lemon-lime drink mix* (*Kool-Aid*), 8 fl. oz.	100	0	25.0	0	0	10	0
Lentil:							
dry, green or red (*Arrowhead Mills*), ¼ cup	150	11.0	27.0	0	0	15	9.0
cooked:							
½ cup	115	8.9	19.9	.4	0	2	7.8
dehydrated (*AlpineAire*), 1 oz.	80	7.0	0	6.0	0	0	6.0

Food and Measure	cal.	prot. (gms)	carbo. (gms)	fat (gms)	chol. (mgs)	sod. (mgs)	fiber (gms)
Lentil, sprouted, raw, ½ cup	40	3.4	8.4	.2	0	4	n.a.
Lentil dishes, canned, ½ cup:							
(*Eden* Organic)	90	8.0	13.0	0	0	210	4.0
dhal (*Patak's* Moong)	160	7.0	20.0	6.0	5	630	4.0
Lentil dishes, mix, dry:							
pilaf (*Casbah*), ¾ cup	240	9.0	38.0	.5	0	400	2.0
red, and bow ties (*Marrakesh Express* Terrazza), cup	240	13.0	42.0	2.0	40	390	5.0
Lentil entree, packaged, w/rice, 1 pkg.:							
creamy yellow, w/vegetables (*Tamarind Tree* Channa Dal Masala)	340	13.0	62.0	5.0	0	700	10.0
spicy (*Tamarind Tree* Dal Makhani)	330	14.0	55.0	6.0	5	670	14.0
Lentil rice loaf, frozen (*Natural Touch*), 3.2-oz. slice	170	8.0	14.0	9.0	0	370	4.0
Lentil salad, garden (*Cedar's*), 2 tbsp.	30	1.0	4.0	1.0	0	45	2.0
Lettuce:							
Bibb or Boston:							
1 head, 5″ diam.	21	2.1	3.8	.4	0	8	1.6
2 inner leaves	2	.2	.4	<.1	0	1	.5
butter (*Dole*), 1 head	21	2.0	4.0	.1	0	8	2.0
cos/romaine:							
1 inner leaf	2	.2	.2	<.1	0	1	.2
shredded, ½ cup . . .	4	.5	.7	.1	0	2	.7
shredded (*Dole*), 1½ cups	18	1.0	2.0	1.0	0	40	1.0
iceberg:							
head, 6″ diam.	70	5.4	11.3	1.0	0	48	7.5
leaf, .7 oz.	3	.2	.4	<.1	0	2	.3
precut (*Dole*), 3 oz.	15	1.0	3.0	0	0	15	1.0
leaf, shredded (*Dole*), 1½ cups	12	1.0	1.0	0	0	40	1.0

Food and Measure	cal.	prot. (gms)	carbo. (gms)	fat (gms)	chol. (mgs)	sod. (mgs)	fiber (gms)
Lettuce *(cont.)*							
looseleaf, shredded, ½ cup	5	.4	1.0	.1	0	3	.5
Lima beans, ½ cup, except as noted:							
fresh:							
raw, trimmed	88	5.3	15.7	.7	0	6	3.8
boiled, drained	104	5.8	20.1	.3	0	14	4.5
mature:							
(*Frieda's*), cup, 3 oz.	120	8.0	20.0	0	0	530	8.0
(*Frieda's* Christmas)	120	7.0	22.0	0	0	0	9.0
baby, boiled	115	7.3	21.2	.3	0	2	7.0
large, boiled	108	7.3	19.6	.4	0	2	6.6
Lima beans, canned, ½ cup:							
(*Green Giant/Joan of Arc* Butterbeans) . . .	90	6.0	16.0	0	0	450	4.0
(*Seneca*)	70	2.0	15.0	0	0	220	3.0
(*Stubb's* Butter Beans)	120	7.0	22.0	.5	0	460	6.0
(*Van Camp's* Butterbeans)	110	8.0	22.0	.5	0	430	7.0
baby:							
(*Allens* Butterbeans)	120	7.0	22.0	.5	0	460	6.0
(*Bush's Best* Butter Beans)	120	7.0	19.0	.5	0	510	5.0
green:							
(*Allens/East Texas Fair* Limas)	120	7.0	23.0	.5	0	370	8.0
(*Bush's Best* Butter Beans)	110	6.0	19.0	1.0	0	340	6.0
(*Bush's Best* Medium Lima)	110	6.0	17.0	1.0	0	310	5.0
(*Bush's Best* Small Lima)	100	5.0	16.0	1.0	0	320	5.0
(*Del Monte*)	80	4.0	15.0	0	0	390	4.0
(*Sunshine* Butterbeans)	120	7.0	23.0	.5	0	370	8.0
green and white (*Allens* Limas)	110	6.0	20.0	1.0	0	280	9.0

Food and Measure	cal.	prot. (gms)	carbo. (gms)	fat (gms)	chol. (mgs)	sod. (mgs)	fiber (gms)
large:							
(*Allens* Butterbeans)	120	7.0	20.0	.5	0	290	7.0
(*Bush's Best* Butter Beans)	100	6.0	18.0	.5	0	450	5.0
w/bacon, baby:							
green (*Trappey's* Limas)	120	6.0	22.0	1.0	0	330	6.0
white (*Trappey's* Limas)	130	8.0	21.0	1.5	0	350	6.0
w/sausage, large white (*Trappey's* Butterbeans)	110	6.0	21.0	1.0	0	300	6.0
speckled (*Bush's Best* Butter Beans)	110	6.0	19.0	.5	0	420	5.0
Lima beans, frozen, ½ cup, except as noted:							
(*Birds Eye* Butterbeans)	100	6.0	20.0	0	0	130	4.0
(*McKenzie's* Petite)	110	6.0	22.0	.5	0	140	5.0
(*McKenzie's* Speckled Butter Beans)	100	6.0	20.0	0	0	130	4.0
(*Seneca*), ⅔ cup	120	6.0	23.0	0	0	15	6.0
baby:							
(*Birds Eye*)	130	7.0	24.0	0	0	115	6.0
(*Freshlike*)	110	6.0	22.0	.5	0	140	5.0
(*Green Giant Harvest Fresh*)	80	4.0	15.0	0	0	130	4.0
(*Seabrook*)	110	6.0	22.0	0	0	140	5.0
in butter sauce (*Green Giant*), ⅔ cup	120	6.0	18.0	2.5	<5	330	6.0
Fordhook:							
(*Birds Eye*)	100	6.0	19.0	0	0	10	5.0
(*Freshlike*)	90	6.0	17.0	0	0	10	5.0
(*Seneca*), ⅔cup . . .	90	5.0	17.0	0	0	50	2.0
Lima beans w/ham, canned (*Nalley*), 1 cup	240	17.0	34.0	5.0	15	1070	15.0
Lime:							
2"-diam. lime	20	.5	7.1	.1	0	1	1.9

Food and Measure	cal.	prot. (gms)	carbo. (gms)	fat (gms)	chol. (mgs)	sod. (mgs)	fiber (gms)
Lime *(cont.)*							
peeled, seeded, 1 oz.	9	.2	3.0	.1	0	1	.8
Lime curd (*Crosse & Blackwell*), 1 tbsp.	50	0	13.0	0	0	0	0
Lime drink, 8 fl. oz.:							
(*After the Fall* Key West)	100	1.0	25.0	0	0	10	0
(*R.W. Knudsen* Cactus Cooler)	120	0	29.0	0	0	35	0
Lime juice:							
fresh, 1 tbsp.	4	.1	1.4	<.1	0	tr.	.1
sweetened (*Rose's*), 1 tsp.	10	0	2.0	0	0	0	0
Ling, meat only:							
raw, 4 oz.	99	21.5	0	.7	n.a.	153	0
baked, broiled, or microwaved, 4 oz. . . .	126	27.6	0	.9	n.a.	196	0
Lingcod, meat only:							
raw, 4 oz.	96	20.0	0	1.2	59	67	0
baked, broiled, or microwaved, 4 oz. . . .	124	25.7	0	1.5	76	86	0
Linguine:							
dry, see "Pasta"							
refrigerated:							
(*Contadina*), 1¼ cups	240	10.0	45.0	2.5	90	20	2.0
plain or herb (*Di Giorno*), 2.5 oz. . .	190	7.0	39.0	1.5		125	2.0
Linguine dishes, mix, 1 cup*:							
chicken and broccoli (*Pasta Roni*)	370	11.0	49.0	16.0	5	950	3.0
chicken Parmesan, creamy (*Pasta Roni*)	410	13.0	51.0	18.0	10	1090	3.0
garlic and butter (*Lipton* Pasta & Sauce)	260	7.0	40.0	9.0	5	850	2.0
Linguine entree, frozen, 8-oz. pkg.:							
w/clams and shrimp:							
(*The Budget Gourmet*)	280	12.0	43.0	8.0	25	510	2.0

Food and Measure	cal.	prot. (gms)	carbo. (gms)	fat (gms)	chol. (mgs)	sod. (mgs)	fiber (gms)
(*The Budget Gourmet* Low Fat)	260	12.0	38.0	6.0	45	410	3.0
w/tomatoes and sausage (*The Budget Gourmet Value Classics*)	280	9.0	38.0	10.0	20	500	3.0
Liquor[1], 1 fl. oz.:							
80 proof	65	0	tr.	0	0	tr.	0
90 proof	74	0	tr.	0	0	tr.	0
100 proof	83	0	tr.	0	0	tr.	0
Liver:							
beef, pan-fried, 4 oz.	246	30.3	8.9	9.1	547	120	0
chicken, simmered:							
4 oz.	178	27.6	1.0	6.2	716	58	0
chopped, 1 cup	219	34.1	1.2	7.6	883	71	0
duck, raw, 1 oz.	39	5.3	1.0	1.3	146	n.a.	0
goose, raw, 1 oz.	38	4.6	1.8	1.2	n.a.	40	0
lamb, pan-fried, 4 oz.	270	29.0	4.3	14.3	559	141	0
pork, braised, 4 oz.	187	29.5	4.3	5.0	403	56	0
turkey, raw (*Shady Brook Farms*), 4 oz.	160	23.0	n.a.	5.0	530	110	0
turkey, simmered:							
4 oz.	192	27.2	3.9	6.7	710	73	0
chopped, 1 cup	237	33.6	4.8	8.3	876	89	0
veal (calves'), braised, 4 oz.	187	24.5	3.1	7.8	636	60	0
Liver cheese (*Oscar Mayer*), 1.3-oz. slice	120	6.0	1.0	10.0	80	420	0
Liver pâté, see "Pâté"							
Liverwurst (see also "Braunschweiger"), 2 oz.:							
(*Boar's Head* Strassburger)	170	8.0	1.0	12.0	85	560	0
(*Hansel 'n Gretel*)	170	9.0	4.0	13.0	95	730	0
Liverwurst spread:							
(*Hormel*), 4 tbsp.	130	8.0	2.0	10.0	70	650	0
(*Underwood*), 2 oz.	170	7.0	3.0	14.0	65	380	1.0

[1] *Includes all pure distilled liquors: bourbon, brandy, gin, rum, Scotch, tequila, vodka, etc.*

Food and Measure	cal.	prot. (gms)	carbo. (gms)	fat (gms)	chol. (mgs)	sod. (mgs)	fiber (gms)
Lo bok, see "Radish, Chinese"							
Lobster, northern, meat only:							
raw, 4 oz.	102	21.3	.6	1.0	108	n.a.	0
boiled or steamed:							
4 oz.	111	23.2	1.5	.7	82	431	0
1 cup, 5.1 oz.	142	29.7	1.9	.9	104	551	0
"Lobster," imitation, frozen or refrigerated:							
chunk style, ½ cup:							
(*Captain Jac Lobster Tasties*)	90	8.0	12.0	1.0	10	470	0
(*Louis Kemp Lobster Delights*) . . .	80	8.0	12.0	0	10	600	0
salad (*Louis Kemp Lobster Delights*), ½ cup	80	8.0	12.0	0	10	600	0
tail, whole (*Captain Jac Lobster Tasties*), 4-oz. tail	120	11.0	17.0	0	10	620	0
Lobster, spiny, see "Spiny lobster"							
Lobster sauce (*Progresso*), ½ cup	100	3.0	6.0	7.0	5	430	2.0
Loganberry:							
fresh, 1 cup	89	1.4	21.5	.9	0	1	n.a.
canned, in light syrup (*Oregon*), ½ cup . . .	105	<1.0	25.0	.5	0	0	5.0
frozen, ½ cup	40	1.1	9.6	.2	0	1	3.6
Long beans (*Frieda's*), ¾ cup, 3 oz.	40	2.0	7.0	0	0	0	0
Long John Silver's:							
entrees:							
chicken plank, battered, 2-oz. pc.	130	7.0	10.0	7.0	15	380	n.a.
clams, breaded, 2.5 oz.	250	9.0	26.0	14.0	35	580	n.a.

Food and Measure	cal.	prot. (gms)	carbo. (gms)	fat (gms)	chol. (mgs)	sod. (mgs)	fiber (gms)
fish:							
battered, 3.4-oz. pc.	230	12.0	15.0	14.0	30	560	n.a.
battered, jr., 2-oz. pc.	140	6.0	10.0	9.0	15	360	n.a.
lemon crumb, 2 pcs., 5.3 oz.	240	23.0	10.0	12.0	55	790	n.a.
lemon crumb, à la carte, 2 pcs. w/rice	480	27.0	52.0	17.0	55	1490	n.a.
lemon crumb, Add-a-Piece, 1 pc. w/rice	150	12.0	9.0	7.0	30	460	n.a.
shrimp, battered, 1 pc.	35	1.0	2.0	2.0	10	75	0
meal, lemon crumb							
fish, 1 serving	730	31.0	89.0-	29.0	60	1720	n.a.
meals, everyday value:							
chicken plank:							
2, w/fries	600	18.0	57.0	33.0	35	1420	n.a.
1, w/3 shrimp, fries	550	14.0	51.0	32.0	45	1230	n.a.
fish, jr., w/fries:							
2 pcs.	620	15.0	57.0	37.0	30	1380	n.a.
1, w/chicken plank	610	17.0	57.0	35.0	30	1400	n.a.
1, w/3 shrimp ...	560	13.0	52.0	34.0	45	1210	n.a.
shrimp, 5, w/fries	500	10.0	47.0	30.0	50	1030	n.a.
sandwiches, 1 pc.:							
chicken, *Grab n Go*	330	13.0	40.0	13.0	20	820	n.a.
chicken, *Grab n Go* w/cheese	380	16.0	40.0	18.0	35	1070	n.a.
fish, *Grab n Go*	340	11.0	40.0	15.0	20	800	n.a.
fish, *Grab n Go* w/cheese	390	14.0	40.0	20.0	35	1050	n.a.
Ultimate Fish......	430	18.0	44.0	21.0	35	1340	3.0
wrap, 12.5 oz.	840	20.0	99.0	41.0	10	2180	n.a.
salads, 1 serving:							
chicken, grilled	140	20.0	10.0	2.5	45	260	n.a.
garden	45	3.0	9.0	0	0	25	n.a.
ocean chef	130	14.0	15.0	2.0	60	540	4.0
side.............	20	1.0	3.0	0	0	10	<1.0

Food and Measure	cal.	prot. (gms)	carbo. (gms)	fat (gms)	chol. (mgs)	sod. (mgs)	fiber (gms)
Long John Silver's *(cont.)*							
salad dressings, 1 pkt.:							
French, fat free	40	0	10.0	0	0	240	0
Italian	90	0	2.0	9.0	0	290	0
ranch	170	0	1.0	18.0	10	260	0
ranch, fat free	40	0	9.0	0	0	290	0
Thousand Island ...	120	0	5.0	10.0	15	290	0
sides and soup:							
broccoli cheese soup, 8-oz. bowl	180	5.0	13.0	12.0	15	1240	n.a.
cheese sticks, 5 pcs.	160	6.0	12.0	9.0	10	360	<1.0
coleslaw, 4 oz.	170	2.0	23.0	7.0	0	310	n.a.
corn cobbette, 1 pc.:							
plain	80	3.0	19.0	.5	0	0	0
w/butter	140	3.0	19.0	8.0	0	0	0
fries, regular, 3 oz.	250	3.0	28.0	15.0	0	500	3.0
fries, large, 5 oz.	420	5.0	46.0	24.0	0	830	n.a.
hushpuppy, 1 pc.	60	1.0	0	2.5	0	25	0
rice, 4 oz.	180	3.0	34.0	4.0	0	560	n.a.
sauces/condiments, 1 pkt.:							
honey mustard	20	0	5.0	0	0	60	0
ketchup..........	10	0	2.0	0	0	110	0
malt vinegar	0	0	0	0	0	15	0
shrimp sauce	15	0	3.0	0	0	180	0
sweet 'n' sour sauce	20	0	5.0	0	0	45	0
tartar sauce.......	40	0	2.0	3.5	5	105	0
dessert pie, 1 pc.:							
chocolate creme ...	280	4.0	29.0	17.0	15	125	n.a.
key lime creme cheese........	310	4.0	33.0	19.0	20	140	n.a.
lemon, double.....	350	6.0	41.0	18.0	40	180	n.a.
pecan	390	3.0	53.0	19.0	40	250	n.a.
pineapple creme cheesecake	310	4.0	36.0	17.0	5	105	n.a.
strawberries n' creme	280	4.0	32.0	15.0	15	130	n.a.
Longan, shelled:							
fresh, seeded, 1 oz.	17	.4	4.3	<.1	0	<1	.3

Food and Measure	cal.	prot. (gms)	carbo. (gms)	fat (gms)	chol. (mgs)	sod. (mgs)	fiber (gms)
dried, 1 oz.	81	1.4	21.0	.1	0	14	<1.0
Loquat:							
(*Frieda's*), 5 oz.	70	1.0	17.0	0	0	0	2.0
medium, .6 oz.	5	<.1	1.2	<.1	0	<1	.2
peeled, seeded, 1 oz.	13	.1	3.4	.1	0	<1	.5
Lotus root:							
(*Frieda's*), 1 cup, 3 oz.	50	2.0	15.0	0	0	35	4.0
raw, trimmed, 1 oz.	16	.7	4.9	<.1	0	11	1.4
boiled, drained, 4 oz.	75	1.8	18.2	.1	0	51	3.5
Lotus seed:							
raw, 1 oz.	25	1.2	4.9	.2	0	<1	n.a.
dried, 1 oz.	94	4.4	18.3	.6	0	1	n.a.
fried, 1 cup	106	4.9	20.6	.6	0	1	n.a.
Lox, see "Salmon, smoked"							
Lunch meat, loaf (see also specific listings), 2 oz., except as noted:							
(*Diet Delight* Deluxe)	160	7.0	7.0	6.0	25	390	0
barbecue (*Diet Delight*)	150	7.0	6.0	11.0	25	400	0
Dutch (*Diet Delight*)	160	8.0	4.0	12.0	30	400	0
honey (*Oscar Mayer*), 1-oz. slice	35	5.0	1.0	1.0	15	380	0
Italian (*Diet Delight*)	150	7.0	5.0	11.0	30	400	0
jalapeño (*Hansel 'n Gretel*)	150	5.0	6.0	12.0	30	910	0
macaroni and cheese (*Hansel 'n Gretel*)	160	7.0	8.0	12.0	30	890	0
mother's loaf, pork, 1 oz.	80	3.4	2.1	6.3	13	320	0
old-fashioned:							
(*Oscar Mayer*), 1-oz. slice	70	4.0	2.0	4.5	15	330	0
(*Russer Light*)	90	8.0	4.0	4.0	30	430	0
olive:							
(*Boar's Head*)	130	6.0	<1.0	12.0	20	639	0
(*Hansel 'n Gretel*)	180	6.0	7.0	14.0	35	850	0
(*Oscar Mayer*), 1-oz. slice	70	3.0	2.0	6.0	20	360	0

Food and Measure	cal.	prot. (gms)	carbo. (gms)	fat (gms)	chol. (mgs)	sod. (mgs)	fiber (gms)
Lunch meat *(cont.)*							
pepper (*Diet Delight*)	110	8.0	5.0	6.0	25	400	0
pickle (*Diet Delight*)	110	7.0	7.0	6.0	25	400	0
pickle and pimiento:							
(*Oscar Mayer*), 1-oz.							
slice	80	3.0	3.0	6.0	20	360	0
(*Russer Light* P&P)	100	8.0	4.0	6.0	30	430	0
spiced:							
(*Hansel 'n Gretel*)	180	7.0	6.0	15.0	40	840	0
(*Oscar Mayer*), 1-oz.							
slice	70	4.0	2.0	5.0	20	340	0
Lunch meat, canned,							
2 oz., except as							
noted:							
(*Celebrity*)	170	6.0	<1.0	16.0	50	810	0
(*Spam/Spam* Smoked)	170	7.0	0	16.0	40	750	0
(*Spam* Less Salt)	170	7.0	0	16.0	40	560	0
(*Spam* Lite)	110	9.0	0	8.0	45	560	0
(*Treet*)	130	6.0	3.0	11.0	50	740	0
spread (*Spam*),							
4 tbsp.	140	8.0	1.0	12.0	40	570	0
Lunch "meat," vege-							
tarian, canned							
(*Loma Linda*							
Nuteena), ³/₈" slice	160	6.0	6.0	13.0	0	120	2.0
Lupin, boiled, ½ cup	98	12.9	8.2	2.4	0	3	2.3
Lychee, shelled, 1 oz.:							
raw, seeded	19	.2	4.7	.1	0	<1	.4
dried.............	79	1.1	20.0	.3	0	1	1.3

M

Food and Measure	cal.	prot. (gms)	carbo. (gms)	fat (gms)	chol. (mgs)	sod. (mgs)	fiber (gms)
Macadamia nut:							
(*Frieda's*), 5 pcs., 1 oz.	210	2.0	4.0	22.0	0	0	3.0
(*Mauna Loa*), 1 oz.	220	2.0	3.0	22.0	0	60	2.0
(*Mauna Loa* Unsalted),							
1 oz.	220	2.0	3.0	22.0	0	0	2.0
dried, shelled:							
1 oz.	199	2.4	3.9	20.9	0	1	2.6
1 cup	940	11.1	18.4	98.8	0	6	12.5
honey-roasted (*Mauna*							
Loa), 1 oz.	210	2.0	6.0	21.0	0	35	2.0
oil-roasted, 1 oz.	204	2.1	3.7	21.7	0	2	n.a.
onion-garlic (*Mauna*							
Loa), 1.4-oz. pkg.	320	3.0	5.0	31.0	0	190	3.0
Macaroni (see also							
"Pasta"):							
uncooked:							
2 oz.	211	7.3	42.6	.9	0	4	1.4
elbow, 1 cup	389	13.4	78.4	1.7	0	8	2.5
cooked:							
4 oz.	160	5.4	32.1	.8	0	1	1.8
elbow, 1 cup	197	6.7	39.7	.9	0	1	2.2
small shells, 1 cup	162	5.5	32.6	.8	0	1	1.8
spirals, 1 cup	189	6.4	38.0	.9	0	1	2.1
vegetable (tri-color),							
4 oz.	145	5.1	30.2	.1	0	7	4.9
whole-wheat, 4 oz.	141	6.0	30.1	.6	0	3	5.0
Macaroni entree,							
canned or pack-							
aged, 1 cup, except							
as noted:							
and beef:							
(*Chef Boyardee*							
Beefaroni)	240	9.0	33.0	8.0	25	960	3.0

Food and Measure	cal.	prot. (gms)	carbo. (gms)	fat (gms)	chol. (mgs)	sod. (mgs)	fiber (gms)
Macaroni entree, canned or packaged, and beef *(cont.)*							
(*Chef Boyardee Beefaroni*), 7 oz.	190	8.0	30.0	5.0	20	720	3.0
(*Kid's Kitchen Beefy*)	190	11.0	23.0	6.0	25	800	2.0
(*Kid's Kitchen Cheezy*)	260	15.0	33.0	7.0	30	910	1.0
(*Nalley*)	220	12.0	7.0	4.0	0	1130	7.0
and cheese:							
(*Chef Boyardee*) ...	200	8.0	28.0	6.0	15	1090	1.0
(*Franco-American*)	210	8.0	29.0	7.0	10	1060	4.0
(*Hormel* Microwave Cup)	260	12.0	30.0	11.0	35	660	1.0
(*Kid's Kitchen*)	270	12.0	30.0	11.0	35	670	1.0
(*Nalley*), 7½ oz. ...	250	10.0	22.0	14.0	50	920	4.0
chili, see "Chili"							
Macaroni entree, frozen, 1 pkg., except as noted:							
and beef:							
(*Freezer Queen*), 9 oz.	230	12.0	32.0	6.0	15	650	4.0
(*Lean Cuisine*), 10 oz.	270	15.0	43.0	4.0	25	590	4.0
(*Stouffer's*), 11½ oz.	420	20.0	40.0	20.0	50	1530	5.0
and cheese:							
(*Amy's*), 9 oz.	390	17.0	50.0	14.0	40	550	4.0
(*Banquet*), 9½ oz.	320	11.0	44.0	11.0	20	970	4.0
(*Banquet* Family), 1 cup	210	8.0	33.0	5.0	10	1290	4.0
(*The Budget Gourmet* Side Dish), 5¾ oz.	260	8.0	31.0	11.0	35	540	1.0
(*The Budget Gourmet Value Classics* Homestyle), 8 oz.	320	12.0	43.0	11.0	20	740	2.0
(*Freezer Queen*), 8 oz.	350	15.0	46.0	11.0	25	720	4.0

Food and Measure	cal.	prot. (gms)	carbo. (gms)	fat (gms)	chol. (mgs)	sod. (mgs)	fiber (gms)
(*Freezer Queen* Family), 1 cup	240	9.0	40.0	5.0	5	770	2.0
(*Healthy Choice*), 9 oz.	320	15.0	50.0	7.0	25	580	4.0
(*Kid Cuisine* Magical), 10.8 oz. ...	410	10.0	72.0	13.0	15	870	4.0
(*Lean Cuisine*), 10 oz.	290	14.0	45.0	6.0	15	470	4.0
(*Marie Callender's*), 13½ oz.	510	22.0	65.0	18.0	35	2020	5.0
(*Marie Callender's* Family), 1 cup ...	300	15.0	41.0	9.0	25	1190	3.0
(*Smart Ones* Homestyle), 9 oz.	290	12.0	45.0	7.0	10	630	2.0
(*Stouffer's* 12 oz.), 1 cup or ½ pkg.	320	13.0	31.0	16.0	30	990	3.0
(*Stouffer's* 20 oz.), 1 cup	340	13.0	32.0	18.0	30	980	2.0
(*Stouffer's* 40 oz.), 1 cup	380	16.0	40.0	17.0	35	1020	2.0
(*Stouffer's* 76 oz.), 1 cup	360	15.0	37.0	17.0	30	940	2.0
w/broccoli (*Stouffers*), 10½ oz.	360	15.0	37.0	17.0	25	1050	5.0
cheddar (*The Budget Gourmet Value Classics* Low Fat), 8 oz.	270	10.0	45.0	6.0	10	520	2.0
four (*Wolfgang Puck's*), 12 oz.	610	27.0	51.0	33.0	90	720	2.0
three, bake (*Swanson Lunch & More*), 10 oz. ...	400	15.0	53.0	14.0	20	1580	3.0
and cheese, nondairy (*Amy's* Soy Cheeze), 9 oz.	360	16.0	42.0	14.0	0	500	4.0
and cheese pot pie (*Banquet*), 6½ oz.	200	7.0	36.0	3.0	10	750	1.0

Food and Measure	cal.	prot. (gms)	carbo. (gms)	fat (gms)	chol. (mgs)	sod. (mgs)	fiber (gms)
Macaroni entree mix, and cheese, dry:							
(*Kraft* Deluxe Original), 3½ oz.	320	14.0	44.0	10.0	25	730	1.0
(*Kraft* Original), 2½ oz.	260	11.0	47.0	2.5	10	560	1.0
(*Kraft Thick 'n Creamy*), 2½ oz.	260	11.0	48.0	2.5	10	560	2.0
three (*Knorr* Cup), 1 cont.	230	8.0	41.0	3.5	10	940	1.0
w/vegetables (*AlpineAire*), 3 oz. . . .	340	17.0	44.0	11.0	30	970	2.0
w/white cheddar (*Kraft*), 2½ oz.	260	11.0	47.0	3.0	10	560	1.0
Macaroni and cheese, see "Macaroni entree"							
Macaroni and cheese loaf, see "Lunch meat"							
Macaroni salad, refrigerated (*Shally Sherman Foods*), ¾ cup	240	4.0	32.0	11.0	5	110	3.0
Mace, ground, 1 tsp.	8	.1	.9	.6	0	1	.1
Mackerel, meat only:							
Atlantic, 4 oz.:							
raw	232	21.1	0	15.8	80	102	0
baked, broiled, or microwaved	297	27.0	0	20.2	85	94	0
king, 4 oz.:							
raw	119	23.0	0	2.3	61	179	0
baked, broiled, or microwaved	152	29.5	0	2.9	77	230	0
Pacific/jack, 4 oz.:							
raw	179	22.8	0	9.0	53	98	0
baked, broiled, or microwaved	228	29.2	0	11.5	68	125	0
Spanish, 4 oz.:							
raw	158	21.9	0	7.2	86	67	0

Food and Measure	cal.	prot. (gms)	carbo. (gms)	fat (gms)	chol. (mgs)	sod. (mgs)	fiber (gms)
baked, broiled, or microwaved	179	26.8	0	7.2	83	75	0
Mackerel, canned, boneless, drained, jack, 4 oz.	177	26.3	0	7.1	90	430	0
Mackerel, smoked (*Spence & Co.*), 2 oz.	180	13.0	0	15.0	30	840	0
Madras sauce, see "Curry sauce"							
Mahimahi, see "Dolphinfish"							
Mai Tai mixer (*Trader Vic's*), 4 fl. oz.	130	0	32.0	0	0	20	0
Malanga (*Frieda's*), cup, 3 oz.	90	1.0	23.0	0	0	10	3.0
Malt cooler (*Bartles & Jaymes*), 12 fl. oz.:							
original	190	0	29.0	0	0	0	0
berry	210	0	33.0	0	0	5	0
berry, Brazilian Mist	200	0	31.0	0	0	0	0
cherry, black	200	0	32.0	0	0	5	0
Fuzzy Navel	230	0	39.0	0	0	5	0
kiwi strawberry	214	0	39.0	0	0	4	0
Margarita	260	0	46.0	0	0	40	0
Oriental dragon fruit	200	0	31.0	0	0	0	0
peach	210	0	33.0	0	0	5	0
piña colada	270	0	48.0	0	0	5	0
strawberry daiquiri ...	220	0	36.0	0	0	5	0
tropical	230	0	37.0	0	0	5	0
Malt drink (*Goya*), 12 fl. oz.	280	1.0	50.0	0	0	80	0
Malted, ice cream, see "Ice cream malt"							
Malted milk powder: natural, 3 tbsp.:							
(*Carnation*)	90	3.0	15.0	2.0	5	85	<1.0
(*Kraft* Instant)	90	3.0	15.0	2.0	5	85	0

Food and Measure	cal.	prot. (gms)	carbo. (gms)	fat (gms)	chol. (mgs)	sod. (mgs)	fiber (gms)
Malted milk powder *(cont.)*							
chocolate, 3 tbsp.:							
(*Carnation*)	90	1.0	18.0	1.0	0	40	<1.0
(*Kraft* Instant)	80	1.0	17.0	1.0	0	40	<1.0
Mammy apple,							
peeled, seeded,							
1 oz.	14	.1	3.5	.1	0	4	.9
Mandioca, see "Yuca							
root"							
Mango, fresh:							
(*Frieda's*), 5 oz.	90	1.0	24.0	0	0	0	3.0
10.6-oz. fruit	135	1.1	35.2	.6	0	4	3.7
peeled, sliced, ½ cup	54	.4	14.0	.2	0	2	1.5
Mango, canned or							
chilled, ½ cup:							
in extra light syrup							
(*Sunfresh* Chilled)	100	0	25.0	.5	0	5	0
in light syrup (*Sun-*							
fresh Can)	90	0	22.0	0	0	0	0
Mango, dried:							
(*Frieda's*), 4 pcs.,							
1.4 oz.	130	0	32.0	1.0	0	35	0
(*Sonoma*), 6 pcs.,							
1.1 oz.	100	0	23.0	0	0	25	0
Mango drink, 8 fl. oz.							
(*Mango Mango!*)	130	0	33.0	0	0	35	0
(*Snapple* Mango Mad-							
ness Cocktail)	110	0	29.0	0	0	10	0
peach (*R.W. Knudsen*)	120	0	30.0	0	0	50	0
Mango drink mix*							
(*Tang*), 8 fl. oz.	100	0	25.0	0	0	0	0
Mango juice (*After the*							
Fall Mango Mon-							
tage), 8 fl. oz.	110	1.0	27.0	0	0	10	0
Mango nectar:							
(*Goya*), *6 fl. oz.*	110	<1.0	27.0	0	0	15	1.0
(*Kern's*), 8 fl. oz.	150	0	36.0	0	0	5	0
Mango relish, see							
"Chutney"							
Mango-orange nectar							
(*Kern's*), 8 fl. oz.	140	0	35.0	0	0	10	0

Food and Measure	cal.	prot. (gms)	carbo. (gms)	fat (gms)	chol. (mgs)	sod. (mgs)	fiber (gms)
Mango-pineapple-banana smoothie (*Del Monte* Blenders), 6.25 fl. oz.	180	1.0	44.0	0	0	10	1.0
Manicotti entree, frozen, 1 pkg., except as noted:							
cheese:							
(*Stouffer's*), 9 oz.	360	19.0	34.0	16.0	40	850	4.0
(*Stouffer's*), 1/12 of 61-oz. pkg.	160	8.0	17.0	7.0	20	480	2.0
marinara sauce (*The Budget Gourmet*), 8 1/2 oz.	290	12.0	33.0	14.0	40	720	3.0
three (*Healthy Choice*), 11 oz.	300	15.0	40.0	9.0	35	550	5.0
cheese and spinach (*Lean Cuisine Hearty Portions*), 15 1/2 oz.	370	25.0	50.0	8.0	35	850	8.0
Manioc, see "Yuca root"							
Maple syrup, 1/4 cup:							
(*Cary's/Maple Orchard's/MacDonald's*)	210	0	52.0	0	0	15	0
(*Maple Grove Farms*)	200	0	53.0	0	0	5	0
(*Russell Farms*)	200	0	53.0	0	0	7	0
Margarine, 1 tbsp.:							
(*Land O Lakes* Stick)	100	0	0	11.0	0	115	0
(*Land O Lakes* Tub)	100	0	0	11.0	0	105	0
(*Land O Lakes* Country Morning Blend Stick)	100	0	0	11.0	0	90	0
(*Land O Lakes* Country Morning Stick Unsalted)	100	0	0	11.0	0	0	0
(*Land O Lakes* Country Morning Blend Tub)	80	0	0	8.0	0	80	0
(*Nucoa No-Burn*)	100	0	0	11.0	0	160	0
(*Smart Balance*)	80	0	0	9.0	0	90	0

Food and Measure	cal.	prot. (gms)	carbo. (gms)	fat (gms)	chol. (mgs)	sod. (mgs)	fiber (gms)
Margarine (cont.)							
light:							
(Land O Lakes Country Morning Blend Stick)	50	0	0	6.0	10	110	0
(Land O Lakes Country Morning Blend Tub)	50	0	0	6.0	5	110	0
(Smart Balance) . . .	45	0	0	5.0	0	100	0
(Smart Beat Trans Fat Free)	20	0	0	2.0	0	105	0
unsalted (Smart Beat)	25	0	0	2.5	0	0	0
squeeze (Smart Beat)	5	0	1.0	0	0	100	0
soft:							
(Chiffon Tub)	100	0	0	11.0	0	105	0
(Parkay Tub)	100	0	0	11.0	0	105	0
(Parkay Diet Tub) . . .	50	0	0	6.0	0	110	0
spread:							
(Kraft Touch of Butter Stick)	90	0	0	10.0	0	110	0
(Kraft Touch of Butter Tub)	60	0	0	7.0	0	110	0
(Land O Lakes Spread with Sweet Cream Tub)	80	0	0	8.0	0	70	0
(Parkay Stick 53%)	70	0	0	7.0	0	120	0
(Parkay Stick 70%)	90	0	0	10.0	0	110	0
(Parkay Tub 50%)	60	0	0	7.0	0	110	0
(Parkay Light Tub 40%)	50	0	0	6.0	0	120	0
salted (Land O Lakes Spread with Sweet Cream Stick)	90	0	0	10.0	0	90	0
unsalted (Land O Lakes Spread with Sweet Cream Stick)	90	0	0	10.0	0	0	0

Food and Measure	cal.	prot. (gms)	carbo. (gms)	fat (gms)	chol. (mgs)	sod. (mgs)	fiber (gms)
squeeze (*Kraft Touch of Butter*)	80	0	0	9.0	0	115	0
squeeze (*Parkay* 64%)	80	0	0	9.0	0	120	0
whipped:							
(*Chiffon*)	70	0	0	7.0	0	70	0
(*Parkay*)	70	0	0	7.0	0	70	0
Margarita mixer, 4 fl. oz., except as noted:							
bottled:							
(*Holland House*) . . .	130	0	29.0	0	0	40	0
(*Major Peters'*), 5.8 fl. oz.	190	0	47.0	0	0	15	0
peach (*Daily's*)	190	0	48.0	0	0	75	2.0
raspberry (*Daily's*)	180	0	46.0	0	0	75	2.0
strawberry (*Trader Vic's*)	160	0	40.0	0	0	20	0
frozen (*Bacardi*), 2 fl. oz.	90	0	25.0	0	0	0	0
Marinade (see also "Salad dressing," "Stir-fry sauce," and specific listings), 1 tbsp., except as noted:							
(*House of Tsang Mandarin*)	25	0	6.0	0	0	680	0
(*Stubb's* Moppin' Sauce)	30	0	1.0	3.0	0	320	0
Cajun, spicy (*Cardini's*)	10	0	2.0	0	0	350	0
citrus grill (*Lawry's* 30-Minute), 2 tbsp.	15	0	3.0	0	0	210	0
citrus lime dill (*Cardini's*)	20	0	4.0	0	0	410	0
garlic and herb (*Cardini's*)	10	0	2.0	0	0	430	0
Hawaiian (*Lawry's* 30-Minute), 2 tbsp.	20	0	4.0	0	0	250	0

Food and Measure	cal.	prot. (gms)	carbo. (gms)	fat (gms)	chol. (mgs)	sod. (mgs)	fiber (gms)
Marinade *(cont.)*							
herb and garlic							
(*Lawry's 30-Min-*							
ute), 2 tbsp.	10	0	2.0	0	0	400	0
hickory (*Lawry's*							
30-Minute), 2 tbsp.	20	0	5.0	0	0	420	0
honey Dijon (*Cardini's*)	20	0	4.0	0	0	430	0
honey hickory (*World*							
Harbors Ember							
Wisp), 2 tbsp.	45	0	10	0	0	230	0
jerk:							
(*Helen's Tropical Ex-*							
otics)	10	0	1.0	.5	0	30	0
Caribbean (*Lawry's*							
30-Minute),							
2 tbsp.	25	0	6.0	0	0	430	0
lemon pepper:							
(*Cardini's* Zesty) . . .	15	0	4.0	0	0	340	0
(*Lawry's* 30-Min-							
ute), 2 tbsp.	10	0	2.0	0	0	380	0
and garlic (*World*							
Harbors Acadia),							
2 tbsp.	35	0	8.0	0	0	140	0
mesquite:							
(*Lawry's* 30-Min-							
ute), 2 tbsp.	5	0	1.0	0	0	350	0
fajita (*Cardini's*) . . .	10	0	2.0	0	0	270	0
red wine:							
(*Cardini's*)	10	0	3.0	0	0	460	0
(*Lawry's* 30-Min-							
ute), 2 tbsp.	20	0	4.0	0	0	250	0
seasoned (*Lawry's*)	10	<1.0	2.0	0	0	680	0
teriyaki:							
(*Lawry's* 30-Min-							
ute), 2 tbsp.	25	0	6.0	0	0	570	0
tangy (*Cardini's*) . . .	20	1.0	4.0	0	0	550	0
Thai ginger (*Lawry's*							
30-Minute), 2 tbsp.	10	0	2.0	0	0	400	0
Marjoram, dried,							
1 tsp.	2	.1	.4	<.1	0	<1	.1

Food and Measure	cal.	prot. (gms)	carbo. (gms)	fat (gms)	chol. (mgs)	sod. (mgs)	fiber (gms)
Marmalade, see "Jam and preserves"							
Marrow beans, dried (*Frieda's*), ½ cup	120	7.0	22.0	0	0	0	9.0
Marrow squash, raw, trimmed, 1 oz.	4	.2	1.0	<.1	0	n.a.	<1.0
Marshmallow, see "Candy"							
Marshmallow topping, 2 tbsp.:							
(*Kraft* Creme)	40	0	10.0	0	0	10	0
(*Marshmallow Fluff*)	60	0	15.0	0	0	10	0
(*Smucker's*)	120	0	29.0	0	0	0	0
Masa, see "Cornmeal"							
Masala sauce, see "Curry sauce, cooking"							
Matzo, see "Cracker"							
Mayonnaise, 1 tbsp.:							
in jars:							
(*Hellmann's/Best Foods*)	100	0	0	11.0	5	80	0
(*Hellmann's/Best Foods* Light)	50	.1	1.0	5.1	9	122	0
(*Hellmann's/Best Foods* Ultra Low Fat)	24	.1	4.3	.8	1	135	0
(*Kraft*)	100	0	0	11.0	10	75	0
(*Nalley* Cholesterol Free)	40	0	2.0	4.0	0	85	0
(*Nalley* Light)	50	0	1.0	5.0	10	100	0
(*Nalley* Real)	100	0	0	11.0	5	85	0
(*Smart Beat* Fat Free)	10	0	3.0	0	0	135	0
refrigerated:							
(*Delouis Fils*)	110	0	0	12.0	30	70	0
garlic (*Delouis Fils* Aioli)	102	0	0	11.2	27	97	0
Mayonnaise dressing, 1 tbsp.:							
(*Kraft* Fat Free)	10	0	2.0	0	0	105	0

Food and Measure	cal.	prot. (gms)	carbo. (gms)	fat (gms)	chol. (mgs)	sod. (mgs)	fiber (gms)
Mayonnaise dressing *(cont.)*							
(*Kraft Light*)	50	0	1.0	5.0	0	110	0
(*Miracle Whip*)	70	0	2.0	7.0	5	85	0
(*Miracle Whip Free*)	15	0	3.0	0	0	120	0
(*Miracle Whip Light*)	40	0	3.0	3.0	0	120	0
(*Nalley* Whip)	60	0	3.0	5.0	10	110	0
(*Spin Blend*)	60	0	3.0	5.0	5	110	0
(*Spin Blend* Fat Free)	15	0	3.0	0	0	110	0
tofu:							
(*Nayonaise*)	35	0	1.0	3.0	0	105	0
(*Nayonaise* Fat Free)	10	0	2.0	0	0	120	0
McDonald's, 1 serving:							
breakfast bagel:							
plain	310	12.0	63.0	1.0	0	530	2.0
ham, egg, and cheese	550	26.0	54.0	26.0	265	1530	2.0
Spanish omelet	690	27.0	56.0	39.0	280	1560	3.0
steak, egg, and cheese	630	37.0	55.0	28.0	290	1290	3.0
breakfast biscuit:							
plain	290	5.0	34.0	15.0	0	780	1.0
bacon, egg, cheese	470	18.0	36.0	28.0	235	1250	1.0
sausage	470	11.0	35.0	31.0	35	1080	1.0
sausage and egg . . .	550	18.0	35.0	37.0	245	1160	1.0
breakfast burrito . . .	320	13.0	23.0	20.0	195	600	2.0
breakfast dishes:							
eggs, scrambled . . .	160	13.0	1.0	11.0	425	170	0
2 hash browns	130	1.0	14.0	8.0	0	330	1.0
hotcakes:							
plain	310	9.0	53.0	7.0	15	610	2.0
w/syrup, margarine	570	9.0	100.0	16.0	15	750	2.0
sausage	170	6.0	0	16.0	35	290	0
breakfast muffins:							
Egg McMuffin	290	17.0	27.0	12.0	235	790	1.0
English	140	4.0	25.0	2.0	0	210	1.0
Sausage McMuffin	360	13.0	26.0	23.0	45	740	1.0
Sausage McMuffin, w/egg	440	19.0	27.0	28.0	255	890	1.0

Food and Measure	cal.	prot. (gms)	carbo. (gms)	fat (gms)	chol. (mgs)	sod. (mgs)	fiber (gms)
Danish and muffin:							
apple bran muffin, low fat	300	6.0	61.0	3.0	0	380	3.0
apple Danish	360	5.0	51.0	16.0	40	290	1.0
cheese Danish	410	7.0	47.0	22.0	70	340	0
cinnamon roll	390	6.0	50.0	18.0	65	310	1.0
sandwiches:							
Arch Deluxe	550	28.0	39.0	31.0	90	1010	4.0
Arch Deluxe, w/bacon	590	32.0	39.0	34.0	100	1150	4.0
Big Mac	560	26.0	45.0	31.0	85	1070	3.0
cheeseburger	320	15.0	35.0	13.0	40	820	2.0
Crispy Chicken Deluxe	500	26.0	43.0	25.0	55	1100	4.0
Filet-O-Fish	450	16.0	42.0	25.0	50	870	2.0
Fish Filet Deluxe	560	23.0	54.0	28.0	60	1060	4.0
Grilled Chicken Deluxe	440	27.0	38.0	20.0	60	1040	4.0
Grilled Chicken Deluxe, w/out mayo	300	27.0	38.0	5.0	50	930	4.0
hamburger	260	13.0	34.0	9.0	30	580	2.0
Quarter Pounder	420	23.0	37.0	21.0	70	820	2.0
Quarter Pounder, w/cheese	530	28.0	38.0	30.0	95	1290	2.0
Chicken McNuggets:							
4 pcs.	190	12.0	10.0	11.0	40	340	0
6 pcs.	290	18.0	15.0	17.0	60	510	0
9 pcs.	430	27.0	23.0	26.0	90	770	0
***McNuggets* sauce pkt.:**							
barbeque	45	0	10.0	0	0	250	0
honey	45	0	12.0	0	0	0	0
honey mustard	50	0	3.0	4.5	10	85	0
hot mustard	60	1.0	7.0	3.5	5	240	<1.0
mayonnaise, light	40	0	1.0	4.0	5	85	0
sweet and sour	50	0	11.0	0	0	140	0
french fries:							
small	210	3.0	26.0	10.0	0	135	2.0
large	450	6.0	57.0	22.0	0	290	5.0
Super Size	540	8.0	68.0	26.0	0	350	6.0

Food and Measure	cal.	prot. (gms)	carbo. (gms)	fat (gms)	chol. (mgs)	sod. (mgs)	fiber (gms)
McDonald's (cont.)							
salads:							
chicken, grilled	120	21.0	7.0	1.5	45	240	3.0
garden	35	2.0	7.0	0	0	20	3.0
croutons, 1 pkt. . . .	50	2.0	7.0	1.5	0	80	0
salad dressing, 1 pkt.:							
Caesar	160	2.0	7.0	14.0	20	450	0
ranch	230	1.0	10.0	21.0	20	550	0
red French, reduced							
calorie	160	0	23.0	8.0	0	490	0
vinaigrette, herb . . .	50	0	11.0	0	0	330	0
desserts and shakes:							
baked apple pie	260	3.0	34.0	13.0	0	200	<1.0
chocolate chip							
cookie	170	2.0	22.0	10.0	20	120	1.0
McDonaldland							
Cookies, 1 pkg.	180	3.0	32.0	5.0	0	190	1.0
McFlurry:							
Butterfinger	620	16.0	90.0	22.0	70	260	<1.0
M&M	630	16.0	90.0	23.0	75	210	1.0
Nestlé Crunch . . .	630	16.0	89.0	24.0	75	230	<1.0
Oreo	570	15.0	82.0	20.0	70	280	<1.0
shake, small:							
chocolate	360	11.0	60.0	9.0	40	250	0
strawberry	360	11.0	60.0	9.0	40	180	0
vanilla	360	11.0	59.0	9.0	40	250	0
sundae, hot caramel	360	7.0	61.0	10.0	35	180	0
sundae, hot fudge	340	8.0	52.0	12.0	30	170	1.0
sundae, strawberry	290	7.0	50.0	7.0	30	95	<1.0
sundae nuts	40	2.0	2.0	3.5	0	2	<1.0
vanilla cone, re-							
duced fat	150	4.0	23.0	4.5	20	75	0
Meat, see specific list-							
ings							
"Meat," ground, veg-							
etarian (see also							
"Burger, vegetar-							
ian"), frozen							
(Morningstar Farms							
Ground Meatless),							
½ cup	60	10.0	4.0	0	0	260	2.0

Food and Measure	cal.	prot. (gms)	carbo. (gms)	fat (gms)	chol. (mgs)	sod. (mgs)	fiber (gms)
Meat, lunch, see "Lunch meat" and specific listings							
Meat, potted, see "Meat spread"							
Meat loaf dinner, frozen, 1 pkg.:							
(*Banquet Extra Helping*), 16 oz.	610	29.0	34.0	40.0	110	1940	6.0
(*Healthy Choice* Traditional), 12 oz.	320	15.0	52.0	5.0	35	460	6.0
(*Swanson Hungry Man*), 16½ oz.	630	25.0	64.0	30.0	50	1600	6.0
Meat loaf entree, frozen, 1 pkg., except as noted:							
(*Banquet*), 9½ oz. . . .	280	12.0	23.0	16.0	60	1020	3.0
(*Stouffer's* Homestyle), 9 oz.	390	22.0	28.0	21.0	90	840	3.0
in gravy (*Stouffer's*), ⅙ of 33-oz. pkg.	190	15.0	10.0	10.0	50	550	0
w/gravy, mashed potato:							
(*Marie Callender's*), 14 oz.	540	23.0	42.0	30.0	95	1570	6.0
(*Marie Callender's Family*), 1 patty, ½ cup potato	300	12.0	26.0	16.0	70	1000	3.0
(*Stouffer's Hearty Portions*), 17 oz.	480	23.0	46.0	23.0	90	1580	8.0
gravy, savory, and (*Banquet* Family), 1 patty, w/gravy . . .	190	10.0	7.0	13.0	35	750	1.0
tomato sauce and:							
(*Freezer Queen* Family), ⅙ pkg.	150	11.0	10.0	7.0	21	480	2.0
w/potatoes, peas (*Freezer Queen*), 9½ oz.	260	13.0	23.0	13.0	20	810	5.0

Food and Measure	cal.	prot. (gms)	carbo. (gms)	fat (gms)	chol. (mgs)	sod. (mgs)	fiber (gms)
Meat loaf entree *(cont.)*							
w/whipped potato:							
(*Lean Cuisine American Favorites*),							
9⅜ oz.	250	18.0	30.0	6.0	50	590	4.0
(*Stouffer's*), ⅙ of							
69-oz. pkg.	380	22.0	33.0	18.0	70	950	4.0
"Meat" loaf mix, vegetarian (*Natural Touch*), 4 tbsp.	100	14.0	12.0	.5	0	700	7.0
Meat seasoning (see also specific listings), ¼ tsp.:							
(*Aromat*)	0	0	0	0	0	230	0
(*Chef Paul Prudhomme's Magic Seasoning Blends* Magic)	0	0	0	0	0	135	0
Meat spread (see also specific listings):							
(*Oscar Mayer*), 2 oz.	130	4.0	8.0	10.0	25	460	0
potted (*Hormel*), 4 tbsp., 2 oz.	100	7.0	0	8.0	50	610	0
Meat tenderizer (*Tone's*), 1 tsp.	7	0	1.2	.2	0	1760	tr.
Meatball, refrigerated, w/barbecue sauce (*Lloyd's*), 6 pcs. w/sauce	250	12.0	27.0	15.0	25	300	1.0
"Meatball," vegetarian, w/gravy, canned (*Loma Linda Tender Rounds*), 6 pcs.	120	14.0	5.0	5.0	0	330	3.0
Meatball entree, frozen, 1 pkg.:							
Italian style:							
(*Healthy Choice Hearty Handfuls*), 6.1 oz.	320	18.0	51.0	5.0	15	590	6.0

Food and Measure	cal.	prot. (gms)	carbo. (gms)	fat (gms)	chol. (mgs)	sod. (mgs)	fiber (gms)
and vegetables (*The Budget Gourmet*), 8½ oz.	280	10.0	25.0	15.0	25	580	4.0
Swedish:							
(*The Budget Gourmet*), 10 oz.	550	18.0	42.0	34.0	155	1030	3.0
(*Healthy Choice*), 9.1 oz.	280	14.0	35.0	6.0	50	590	3.0
(*Marie Callender's*), 12½ oz.	520	28.0	44.0	26.0	65	1020	3.0
(*Smart Ones*), 9.1 oz.	290	18.0	34.0	7.0	30	600	3.0
(*Stouffer's*), 10¼ oz.	470	23.0	45.0	22.0	65	970	2.0
w/pasta (*Lean Cuisine*), 9 oz.	290	21.0	38.0	6.0	45	580	3.0
Meatball pocket, w/mozzarella, frozen (*Hot Pockets*), 1 pc.	320	15.0	39.0	11.0	30	620	4.0
Meatball stew, canned (*Dinty Moore*), 1 cup	250	13.0	17.0	15.0	40	1120	2.0
Melon balls, frozen, cantaloupe/honeydew, ½ cup	28	.7	6.9	.2	0	27	.6
Melon drink, 8 fl. oz.:							
(*Mega Melon*).......	130	0	33.0	0	0	35	0
(*Snapple* Melonberry Cocktail)	120	0	29.0	0	0	10	0
Melon salad, chilled, in extra light syrup (*Sunfresh* Lite), ½ cup	45	0	10	0	0	15	2.0
Menudo spice mix (*Gebhardt*), ¼ tsp.	0	<1	0	0	0	50	0
Mexican beans (see also "Chili beans" and "Pinto beans"), canned, ½ cup:							
(*Allens/Brown Beauty* Chili)	120	6.0	22.0	1.0	0	300	8.0

Food and Measure	cal.	prot. (gms)	carbo. (gms)	fat (gms)	chol. (mgs)	sod. (mgs)	fiber (gms)
Mexican beans *(cont.)*							
(*El Rio*)	110	6.0	20.0	.5	0	430	6.0
(*Old El Paso* Mexe) . . .	110	7.0	19.0	0	0	630	7.0
w/jalapeño:							
(*Brown Beauty*)	120	7.0	21.0	1.0	0	370	7.0
(*Trappey's* Mexi-							
Beans)	130	7.0	22.0	1.5	0	460	8.0
Mexican dinner (see							
also specific list-							
ings), frozen, 1 pkg.:							
(*Patio* Fiesta), 12 oz.	350	11.0	53.0	11.0	25	1760	7.0
(*Patio* Ranchers),							
13 oz.	470	13.0	55.0	22.0	35	2670	9.0
style:							
(*Patio*), 13¼ oz. . . .	470	15.0	59.0	19.0	30	2210	10.0
(*Swanson*),							
13¼ oz.	470	18.0	59.0	18.0	25	1610	5.0
Mexican dinner mix							
(see also specific							
listings), 2 pcs.*:							
nacho cheese flavor							
(*Old El Paso One*							
Skillet Mexican Kit)	490	24.0	55.0	19.0	65	1470	2.0
salsa flavor (*Old El*							
Paso One Skillet							
Mexican Kit)	460	23.0	57.0	16.0	55	1390	3.0
taco flavor (*Old El*							
Paso One Skillet							
Mexican Kit)	460	23.0	55.0	16.0	60	1220	2.0
Mexican entree, see							
specific listings							
Mexican seasoning							
mix (*Chi-Chi's*),							
1 tsp.	10	0	2.0	0	0	290	0
Milk, 8 fl. oz.:							
buttermilk:							
cultured, nonfat							
(*Hood*)	90	9.0	13.0	0	<5	220	0
cultured	99	8.1	11.7	2.2	9	257	0
light (*Friendship*)	120	9.0	12.0	4.0	15	125	0

Food and Measure	cal.	prot. (gms)	carbo. (gms)	fat (gms)	chol. (mgs)	sod. (mgs)	fiber (gms)
whole:							
(*Hood*)	150	8.0	12.0	8.0	35	125	0
(*Parmalat*)	160	9.0	13.0	8.0	35	130	0
3.3% fat	150	8.0	11.4	8.2	33	120	0
reduced/low fat:							
2% fat (*Hood*)	130	8.0	13.0	5.0	20	125	0
2% fat (*Parmalat*)	130	9.0	13.0	5.0	20	130	0
2% fat	121	8.1	11.7	4.7	18	122	0
2% fat, protein forti-							
fied	137	9.7	13.5	4.9	19	145	0
1% fat (*Hood*)	110	8.0	13.0	2.5	15	125	0
1% fat (*Parmalat*)	110	9.0	13.0	2.5	15	135	0
1% fat	102	8.0	11.7	2.6	10	123	0
1% fat, fortified							
(*Hood Nuform*)	120	10.0	15.0	2.5	15	150	0
1% fat, protein forti-							
fied	119	9.7	13.6	2.9	10	143	0
skim/fat free:							
(*Hood*)	80	8.0	13.0	0	<5	125	0
(*Parmalat*)	90	8.0	13.0	.3	5	130	0
8 fl. oz.	86	8.4	11.9	.4	4	126	0
Milk, canned, 2 tbsp.:							
condensed, sweet-							
ened: (*Carnation*)	130	3.0	22.0	3.0	10	45	0
evaporated:							
(*Carnation*)	40	2.0	3.0	2.0	10	30	0
(*Carnation* Fat Free)	25	2.0	4.0	0	0	40	0
(*Carnation* Lowfat)	25	2.0	3.0	.5	5	35	0
(*Jerzee*)	40	2.0	3.0	2.0	10	30	0
(*Pet*)	40	2.0	3.0	2.0	10	30	0
filled (*Jerzee*)	35	2.0	3.0	2.0	5	35	0
skim (*Jerzee*)	25	2.0	4.0	0	0	40	0
skim (*Pet*)	25	2.0	4.0	0	0	40	0
Milk, chocolate, see							
"Chocolate milk"							
Milk, dry:							
buttermilk:							
sweet cream, 1 cup	464	41.2	58.8	6.9	83	621	0
sweet cream,							
1 tbsp.	25	2.2	3.2	.4	5	34	0
whole, 1 oz.	141	7.5	10.9	7.6	27	105	0

Food and Measure	cal.	prot. (gms)	carbo. (gms)	fat (gms)	chol. (mgs)	sod. (mgs)	fiber (gms)
Milk, dry *(cont.)*							
whole, 1 cup	635	33.7	49.2	34.2	124	475	0
nonfat:							
regular, 1 cup	435	43.4	62.4	.9	24	642	0
instant, 3.2-oz. pkt.	244	23.9	35.5	.5	12	373	0
(*Carnation*), ⅓ cup	80	8.0	12.0	0	<5	125	0
Milk, goat's, 1 cup:							
(*Meyenberg*)	140	8.0	11.0	7.0	25	115	0
fresh	168	8.7	10.9	10.1	28	122	0
"Milk," nondairy (see also "Soy beverage"), 8 fl. oz.:							
(*EdenBlend* Original)	120	7.0	18.0	3.0	0	85	0
(*Grainaissance Amazake* Original)	150	3.0	34.0	0	0	20	4.0
(*Rice Dream* Original)	120	1.0	25.0	2.0	0	90	0
(*Vitamite*)	110	3.0	14.0	5.0	0	120	0
(*Vitamite* Nonfat)	90	1.0	21.0	0	0	70	0
flavored:							
(*Grainaissance Amazake* Gimme Green)	190	5.0	37.0	2.5	0	35	4.0
almond shake, cocoa almond, hazelnut, sesame, vanilla pecan (*Grainaissance Amazake*)	200	4.0	36.0	4.0	0	20	5.0
apricot (*Grainaissance Amazake*)	160	3.0	35.0	0	0	20	4.0
banana (*Grainaissance Amazake*)	160	3.0	35.0	0	0	20	4.0
carob (*Rice Dream*)	150	1.0	32.0	2.5	0	100	0
chocolate (*Rice Dream*)	170	1.0	36.0	3.0	0	115	2.0
coffee (*Grainaissance Amazake*)	170	3.0	34.0	2.0	0	75	3.0
mocha java (*Grainaissance Amazake*)	180	3.0	37.0	2.0	0	20	4.0

Food and Measure	cal.	prot. (gms)	carbo. (gms)	fat (gms)	chol. (mgs)	sod. (mgs)	fiber (gms)
rice nog (*Grainaissance Amazake*)	190	3.0	39.0	2.0	0	65	4.0
vanilla (*Rice Dream*)	130	1.0	28.0	2.0	0	90	0
mix*:							
(*Vitamite*)	110	3.0	14.0	5.0	0	120	0
chocolate							
(*Chocomite*)	120	1.0	24.0	3.5	0	240	1.0
Milk, sheep's, 1 cup	264	14.7	13.1	17.2	n.a.	108	0
Milkfish, meat only:							
raw, 4 oz.	168	23.3	0	7.6	59	n.a.	0
baked, broiled, or microwaved, 4 oz. . . .	215	29.8	0	9.8	76	n.a.	0
Millet:							
raw, 1 oz.	107	3.1	20.7	1.2	0	1	2.4
cooked, 4 oz.	135	4.0	26.8	1.1	0	2	1.5
hulled (*Arrowhead Mills*), ¼ cup	150	5.0	34.0	1.5	0	0	3.0
Millet flour (*Arrowhead Mills*), ¼ cup	110	4.0	26.0	1.0	0	0	2.0
Mincemeat, see "Pie filling"							
Mint sauce (*Crosse & Blackwell*), 1 tsp.	5	0	1.0	0	0	0	0
Miso, soy, 1 tbsp., except as noted:							
(*Eden/Eden* Organic Hacho)	35	3.0	2.0	1.5	0	600	1.0
1 oz.	58	3.3	7.9	1.7	0	1034	1.5
½ cup	284	16.3	38.6	8.4	0	5032	7.6
w/barley (*Eden* Organic Mugi)	25	2.0	3.0	1.0	0	760	1.0
w/brown rice (*Eden* Organic Genmai) . . .	25	2.0	3.0	1.0	0	810	<1.0
rice w/soy (*Eden* Organic Shiro)	35	2.0	5.0	1.0	0	410	1.0
Mocha syrup (*Ferrara*), 2 oz.	130	0	32.0	0	0	12	0
Mochi (*Grainaissance*), 1½ oz.:							
plain, organic	110	2.0	24.0	1.0	0	0	2.0
cashew-date	110	2.0	24.0	2.0	0	35	2.0

Food and Measure	cal.	prot. (gms)	carbo. (gms)	fat (gms)	chol. (mgs)	sod. (mgs)	fiber (gms)
Mochi *(cont.)*							
mugwort-wheatgrass	110	2.0	24.0	1.0	0	0	2.0
raisin-cinnamon	120	2.0	25.0	1.0	0	35	3.0
pizza flavor	110	2.0	24.0	1.0	0	65	2.0
sesame-garlic.	110	2.0	23.0	1.5	0	20	2.0
Molasses, blackstrap *(New Morning),*							
1 tbsp.	60	<1.0	13.0	0	0	20	0
Monkfish, meat only:							
raw, 4 oz.	86	16.4	0	1.7	29	21	0
baked, broiled, or microwaved, 4 oz. . . .	110	21.0	0	2.2	36	26	0
Monosodium glutamate *(Tone's),*							
1 tsp.	0	0	0	0	0	638	0
Mortadella, 2 oz.:							
(Cinghiale)	160	9.0	0	14.0	30	560	0
w/pistachios *(Cinghiale)*	170	9.0	3.0	14.0	30	560	0
Moth beans, boiled, 4 oz.	133	8.9	23.8	.6	0	11	n.a.
Mousse mix, dry:							
chocolate, dark:							
(Alsa), 2 tbsp.	80	0	8.0	4.0	0	40	0
(Nestlé European Style), ¼ pkg. . . .	90	3.0	13.0	2.5	0	15	3.0
chocolate, milk:							
(Alsa), 2 tbsp.	80	0	10.0	4.0	0	40	0
(Nestlé European Style), ¼ pkg. . . .	90	0	14.0	2.5	0	30	2.0
chocolate, white *(Alsa),* 2 tbsp.	70	0	8.0	3.5	0	40	0
chocolate raspberry truffle *(Nestlé European Style),* ¼ pkg.	90	0	14.0	2.5	0	30	2.0
Irish crème *(Nestlé European Style),* ¼ pkg.	90	0	14.0	2.5	0	30	2.0
mocha *(Nestlé European Style),* ¼ pkg.	90	1.0	15.0	2.0	0	20	1.0

Food and Measure	cal.	prot. (gms)	carbo. (gms)	fat (gms)	chol. (mgs)	sod. (mgs)	fiber (gms)
Mudslide drink mixer							
(*Daily's*), 4 fl. oz.	300	0	69.0	3.0	0	70	0
Muffin, 1 pc., except as noted:							
apple:							
(*Awrey's*), 1½ oz.	130	2.0	18.0	6.0	20	220	0
(*Awrey's*), 2½ oz.	250	2.0	28.0	14.0	55	100	0
spice (*Hostess* Loaf)	430	3.0	61.0	18.0	80	350	1.0
banana:							
bran (*Hostess* Low Fat)	240	4.0	47.0	3.0	0	270	2.0
mini (*Awrey's*), 2 pcs.	200	2.0	22.0	10.0	30	150	0
nut (*Awrey's* Grande)	400	7.0	46.0	22.0	90	440	2.0
nut (*Dolly Madison* Mega)	620	8.0	78.0	31.0	75	540	2.0
nut (*Hostess* Hearty)	620	8.0	78.0	31.0	75	540	2.0
nut (*Hostess* Loaf)	460	4.0	63.0	20.0	60	300	0
walnut, mini (*Hostess*), 3 pcs.	160	2.0	16.0	9.0	25	100	0
blueberry:							
(*Awrey's*), 1½ oz.	130	2.0	19.0	5.0	10	180	<1.0
(*Awrey's*), 2½ oz.	210	3.0	30.0	9.0	20	280	1.0
(*Awrey's* Grande)	340	5.0	43.0	16.0	90	310	1.0
(*Awrey's* Muffin Top)	210	3.0	31.0	8.0	20	290	1.0
(*Dolly Madison* Mega/*Hostess* Hearty)	590	8.0	78.0	28.0	80	590	1.0
(*Entenmann's*)	120	2.0	27.0	0	0	230	<1.0
(*Hostess* Loaf)	440	5.0	62.0	19.0	80	460	2.0
(*Hostess* Low Fat)	230	4.0	47.0	2.5	0	350	1.0
mini (*Awrey's*), 2 pcs.	180	2.0	22.0	9.0	30	140	0
mini (*Hostess*), 3 pcs.	150	1.0	18.0	8.0	25	110	0
carrot raisin (*Awrey's* Grande)	360	6.0	59.0	11.0	60	370	2.0
cheese streusel (*Awrey's* Grande)	380	8.0	48.0	17.0	95	380	1.0

Food and Measure	cal.	prot. (gms)	carbo. (gms)	fat (gms)	chol. (mgs)	sod. (mgs)	fiber (gms)
Muffin *(cont.)*							
chocolate chip:							
(*Dolly Madison* Mega/*Hostess* Hearty)	620	8.0	78.0	29.0	80	580	2.0
chocolate (*Awrey's* Grande)	460	6.0	51.0	26.0	100	450	1.0
chocolate (*Hostess* Loaf)	400	5.0	58.0	17.0	45	330	2.0
mini (*Hostess*), 3 pcs.	160	2.0	17.0	9.0	20	100	0
cinnamon, mini (*Hostess* Bites), 3 pcs.	130	1.0	18.0	6.0	15	110	0
cinnamon apple, mini (*Hostess*), 3 pcs.	160	1.0	16.0	9.0	25	110	0
corn:							
(*Awrey's*), 1½ oz.	130	2.0	20.0	5.0	15	270	0
(*Awrey's*), 2½ oz.	220	4.0	33.0	8.0	25	430	<1.0
(*Entenmann's*)	210	3.0	30.0	9.0	15	300	<1.0
cranberry:							
nut (*Awrey's*)	120	2.0	20.0	4.0	10	210	0
orange (*Dolly Madison* Mega/Hostess Hearty)	590	6.0	79.0	28.0	90	580	1.0
cream cheese (*Dolly Madison* Mega/Hostess Hearty) ...	620	7.0	73.0	33.0	90	630	1.0
English:							
(*Awrey's*)	140	5.0	28.0	1.0	0	230	2.0
(*Pepperidge Farm*)	130	5.0	26.0	1.0	0	250	2.0
(*Thomas'*)	120	4.0	25.0	1.0	0	200	1.0
(*Thomas'* Sandwich)	190	7.0	38.0	2.0	0	280	2.0
(*Wonder*)	130	4.0	25.0	1.0	0	290	1.0
cinnamon raisin (*Pepperidge Farm*)	140	5.0	28.0	1.0	0	230	2.0
cinnamon raisin (*Thomas'*)	140	4.0	30.0	1.0	0	180	1.0
cinnamon raisin (*Wonder*)	140	5.0	26.0	1.5	0	260	2.0
oat bran (*Thomas'*)	130	4.0	26.0	1.0	0	210	2.0

Food and Measure	cal.	prot. (gms)	carbo. (gms)	fat (gms)	chol. (mgs)	sod. (mgs)	fiber (gms)
seven grain (*Pepperidge Farm*) ...	130	5.0	26.0	1.0	0	230	2.0
sourdough (*Pepperidge Farm*)	130	5.0	26.0	1.0	0	250	2.0
sourdough (*Thomas'*)	120	4.0	25.0	1.0	0	190	1.0
sourdough (*Wonder*)	130	4.0	25.0	1.0	0	290	1.0
lemon poppyseed:							
(*Awrey's*)	170	2.0	19.0	10.0	35	65	0
(*Awrey's* Grande)	390	5.0	41.0	23.0	85	280	<1.0
mini (*Awrey's*), 2 pcs.	160	2.0	24.0	6.0	10	160	0
oat bran (*Hostess*) ...	160	2.0	21.0	8.0	0	150	1.0
raisin bran:							
(*Awrey's*), 1½ oz.	110	2.0	18.0	4.0	15	170	1.0
(*Awrey's* Grande)	340	5.0	47.0	16.0	90	310	4.0
(*Awrey's/Awrey's* Muffin Top), 2½ oz.	190	3.0	30.0	7.0	20	280	2.0
raspberry (*Hostess* Loaf)	440	5.0	62.0	19.0	80	460	2.0
rocky road, mini (*Hostess*), 3 pcs.	160	1.0	18.0	6.0	15	110	0
Muffin, frozen, 1 pc.:							
apple oatmeal (*Pepperidge Farm Wholesome Choice*)	160	4.0	28.0	3.5	0	190	3.0
banana (*Weight Watchers*)	170	3.0	41.0	0	0	310	3.0
blueberry:							
(*Pepperidge Farm Wholesome Choice*)	140	3.0	27.0	2.5	0	190	2.0
(*Sara Lee*)	220	3.0	27.0	11.0	15	170	<1.0
(*Weight Watchers*)	160	3.0	38.0	0	0	290	2.0
bran w/raisins (*Pepperidge Farm Wholesome Choice*)	150	4.0	30.0	2.5	0	260	4.0
chocolate chip (*Weight Watchers*)	190	3.0	39.0	2.0	0	350	4.0

Food and Measure	cal.	prot. (gms)	carbo. (gms)	fat (gms)	chol. (mgs)	sod. (mgs)	fiber (gms)
Muffin, frozen *(cont.)*							
corn:							
(*Pepperidge Farm Wholesome Choice*)	150	4.0	27.0	3.0	0	190	1.0
(*Sara Lee*)	260	3.0	30.0	14.0	25	220	1.0
Muffin mix, 1 pc.*, except as noted:							
apple cinnamon:							
(*Betty Crocker*)	170	3.0	24.0	7.0	35	220	0
(*Martha White/ Mother's Best*)	170	3.0	31.0	4.0	<5	350	<1.0
(*Martha White* Low Fat)	160	2.0	34.0	2.0	0	200	<1.0
(*Pillsbury*)	180	3.0	31.0	5.0	5	190	<1.0
(*Sweet Rewards*)	140	2.0	29.0	2.0	20	200	0
(*Sweet Rewards* Fat Free)	120	2.0	29.0	0	0	200	0
apple streusel (*Betty Crocker*)	210	3.0	35.0	7.0	20	210	1.0
banana nut:							
(*Betty Crocker* Box)	170	3.0	28.0	6.0	20	250	1.0
(*Betty Crocker* Pouch)	170	3.0	22.0	7.0	35	250	0
(*Martha White*)	210	3.0	24.0	11.0	35	250	<1.0
(*Pillsbury*)	170	3.0	27.0	6.0	5	230	<1.0
blackberry (*Martha White/Mother's Best*)	170	3.0	31.0	4.0	<5	350	<1.0
blueberry:							
(*Betty Crocker*)	160	3.0	25.0	6.0	35	220	0
(*Duncan Hines*)	160	2.0	28.0	5.0	15	270	0
(*Duncan Hines* Bakery Style)	190	2.0	32.0	6,0	15	260	0
(*Martha White/ Mother's Best*)	170	3.0	31.0	4.0	<5	350	<1.0
(*Martha White* Low Fat)	160	2.0	34.0	2.0	0	200	<1.0
(*Pillsbury*)	180	3.0	31.0	5.0	5	190	0
(*Pillsbury* Low Fat)	160	2.0	34.0	2.0	0	210	<1.0

Food and Measure	cal.	prot. (gms)	carbo. (gms)	fat (gms)	chol. (mgs)	sod. (mgs)	fiber (gms)
double (*Martha White*)	180	3.0	31.0	5.0	30	320	1.0
twice (*Betty Crocker*)	140	2.0	25.0	4.0	20	180	0
wild (*Betty Crocker*)	170	2.0	29.0	5.0	20	220	0
wild (*Sweet Rewards*)	120	2.0	27.0	0	0	200	0
bran (*Mother's Best*)	190	4.0	29.0	6.0	15	420	2.0
caramel nut (*Betty Crocker*)	170	3.0	24.0	7.0	35	230	0
chocolate, double (*Betty Crocker*)	200	2.0	31.0	7.0	20	220	0
chocolate chip:							
(*Betty Crocker*)	170	3.0	23.0	8.0	35	240	0
(*Duncan Hines*)	190	2.0	30.0	8.0	10	250	1.0
(*Pillsbury*)	190	3.0	31.0	6.0	5	190	<1.0
chocolate (*Martha White*)	200	3.0	23.0	11.0	35	210	2.0
cinnamon:							
(*Martha White*)	190	3.0	34.0	5.0	5	210	<1.0
(*Pillsbury*)	160	3.0	27.0	4.0	5	170	<1.0
swirl (*Duncan Hines*)	200	3.0	33.0	6.0	20	250	0
corn:							
(*Betty Crocker*)	160	3.0	25.0	6.0	35	270	0
(*Gladiola*)	180	4.0	24.0	8.0	55	360	<1.0
yellow (*Martha White*)	180	3.0	32.0	4.0	<5	290	<1.0
honey:							
bran (*Martha White*)	200	4.0	26.0	9.0	40	290	3.0
pecan (*Martha White*)	180	4.0	22.0	8.0	35	250	4.0
lemon poppyseed:							
(*Betty Crocker* Box)	190	3.0	30.0	7.0	20	220	0
(*Betty Crocker* Pouch)	180	3.0	25.0	8.0	35	190	0
(*Martha White*)	210	3.0	26.0	10.0	40	240	<1.0
oat bran (*Arrowhead Mills*), dry, 1/3 cup	160	2.0	33.0	2.5	0	240	4.0

Food and Measure	cal.	prot. (gms)	carbo. (gms)	fat (gms)	chol. (mgs)	sod. (mgs)	fiber (gms)
Muffin mix *(cont.)*							
raspberry:							
(*Martha White/ Mother's Best*)	170	3.0	31.0	4.0	<5	290	<1.0
swirl (*Duncan Hines*)	160	2.0	27.0	4.5	15	260	0
strawberry:							
(*Martha White/ Mother's Best*)	170	3.0	31.0	4.0	<5	350	<1.0
(*Martha White* Low Fat)	160	2.0	34.0	2.0	0	200	<1.0
(*Pillsbury*)	180	3.0	31.0	5.0	5	190	0
whole grain (*Arrowhead Mills*), dry, ⅓ cup	150	7.0	26.0	2.0	0	160	7.0
Muffin sandwich, see "Breakfast sandwich"							
Mulberry:							
10 berries, ½ oz.	7	.2	1.5	.1	0	2	.3
½ cup.............	31	1.0	6.9	.3	0	7	1.2
Mullet, striped, meat only:							
raw, 4 oz.	133	22.0	0	4.3	56	74	0
baked, broiled, or microwaved, 4 oz. ...	170	28.1	0	5.5	71	81	0
Multigrain chips, see "Snack chips and crisps"							
Mung beans:							
dry (*Arrowhead Mills*), ¼ cup	160	11.0	28.0	.5	0	0	9.0
boiled, ½ cup	107	7.1	19.3	.4	0	2	7.7
Mung beans, sprouted:							
raw, 1 oz.	9	.9	1.7	.1	0	2	.5
boiled, drained, ½ cup	13	1.3	2.6	.1	0	6	.9
Mungo beans, boiled, ½ cup	95	6.8	16.5	.5	0	7	5.8
Mushroom, ½ cup:							
fresh:							
raw, pcs.	9	.7	1.6	.2	0	1	.4

Food and Measure	cal.	prot. (gms)	carbo. (gms)	fat (gms)	chol. (mgs)	sod. (mgs)	fiber (gms)
boiled,							
drained, pcs. ...	21	1.7	4.0	.4	0	2	1.7
canned:							
all styles:							
(*BinB*)	30	3.0	1.0	0	0	460	2.0
(*Green Giant*) ...	30	3.0	1.0	0	0	440	2.0
w/garlic (*BinB*)	35	3.0	1.0	0	0	410	1.0
Mushroom, chanterelle, dried							
(*Frieda's*), 2 pcs.	15	1.0	2.0	0	0	0	1.0
Mushroom, enoki, fresh:							
(*Frieda's*), 4 oz.	40	2.0	7.0	0	0	0	3.0
trimmed, 1 oz.	10	.4	2.2	.1	0	1	<1.0
large, 4⅛" long	2	.1	.4	<.1	0	<1	<1.0
Mushroom, morel, dried (*Frieda's*),							
3 pcs.	15	1.0	2.0	0	0	0	0
Mushroom, oyster, fresh (*Frieda's*),							
3 oz.	20	2.0	4.0	0	0	0	1.0
Mushroom, padi straw, dried							
(*Frieda's*), 6 pcs.	15	1.0	2.0	0	0	0	0
Mushroom, porcini, dried (*Frieda's*),							
5 pcs.	15	1.0	2.0	0	0	0	1.0
Mushroom, portobello, dried							
(*Frieda's*), 7 pcs.	5	0	1.0	0	0	5	0
Mushroom, shiitake:							
fresh:							
raw (*Frieda's*), 3 oz.	20	2.0	4.0	0	0	0	1.0
cooked, 4 medium							
or ½ cup pcs. ...	40	1.1	10.4	.2	0	3	1.5
dried, 4 medium,							
½ oz.	44	1.4	11.3	.2	0	2	1.7
frozen (*Seneca*),							
½ cup	20	1.0	4.0	0	0	490	3.0
Mushroom, wood ear, fresh (*Frieda's*), 3 oz.	20	2.0	4.0	0	0	0	1.0

Food and Measure	cal.	prot. (gms)	carbo. (gms)	fat (gms)	chol. (mgs)	sod. (mgs)	fiber (gms)
Mushroom, Yamabiko honshimeji, fresh (*Frieda's*), ¼ cup, 1 oz.	10	1.0	1.0	0	0	0	1.0
Mushroom blends:							
pasta, soup, or steak (*Frieda's*), 6 pcs.	15	1.0	2.0	0	0	0	1.0
poultry, sauce, or stir-fry (*Frieda's*), 4 pcs.	15	1.0	2.0	0	0	0	0
Mushroom gravy, in jars, ¼ cup:							
(*Franco-American*) . . .	20	1.0	3.0	1.0	<5	300	0
(*Heinz* Homestyle Fat Free)	10	0	3.0	0	0	300	0
creamy (*Franco-American*)	20	1.0	4.0	1.0	<5	310	0
rich (*Heinz* Homestyle)	20	1.0	3.0	.5	0	370	0
Mushroom gravy mix:							
(*Knorr* Classic), 2 tsp.	20	<1.0	2.0	1.0	0	200	0
(*Knorr* Classic Hunter), 1 tbsp. . . .	25	<1.0	4.0	.5	0	20	0
(*Loma Linda Gravy Quik*), ¼ cup*	15	<1.0	3.0	0	0	300	<1.0
Mushroom sauce mix (*Knorr* Classic Sauces), 2 tsp.	20	<1.0	2.0	1.0	0	200	0
Mussel, blue, meat only:							
raw, 4 oz.	98	13.5	4.2	2.5	32	324	0
raw, 1 cup	129	17.9	5.5	3.4	42	429	0
boiled or steamed, 4 oz.	195	27.0	8.4	5.1	64	418	0
Mussel entree, frozen, in tomato sauce (*Plumpy*), 3 oz. . . .	100	12.0	6.0	2.5	30	410	<1.0
Mustard, prepared, 1 tsp.:							
(*Boar's Head* Delicatessen Style)	0	0	0	0	0	40	0
(*French's Classic Yellow*)	0	0	0	0	0	55	0

Food and Measure	cal.	prot. (gms)	carbo. (gms)	fat (gms)	chol. (mgs)	sod. (mgs)	fiber (gms)
(French's Hearty Deli)	5	0	0	0	0	80	0
(Gulden's Spicy Brown)	5	0	0	0	0	50	0
(Hunt's)	5	0	.5	0	0	65	0
(Jack Daniels Old No. 7)	5	0	0	0	0	70	0
(Kraft)	0	0	0	0	0	60	0
(Nance's Sharp & Creamy)	15	0	2.0	1.0	0	95	0
Dijon:							
(French's)	5	0	0	0	0	115	0
(Grey Poupon)	5	<1.0	<1.0	0	0	120	0
hickory smoke (Jack Daniels)	5	0	0	0	0	125	0
honey:							
(Boar's Head)	10	0	2.0	0	0	25	0
(French's)	5	0	1.0	0	0	40	0
(Nance's)	15	0	3.0	0	0	100	0
(Watkins)	15	0	2.0	.5	0	110	0
honey Dijon (Jack Daniels)	10	0	2.0	0	0	70	0
horseradish:							
(French's)	0	0	0	0	0	85	0
(Jack Daniels)	5	0	0	0	0	75	0
(Kraft)	0	0	0	0	0	55	0
(Watkins)	10	0	1.0	0	0	120	0
hot:							
(Eden Organic)	0	0	<1.0	0	0	65	0
(Nance's)	15	0	2.0	1.0	0	90	0
jalapeño (Watkins) ...	10	0	1.0	0	0	150	0
sweet onion (French's)	10	0	2.0	0	0	70	0
Mustard blend (Dijonnaise), 1 tbsp.	20	.3	2.4	.9	1	211	0
Mustard cabbage, see "Cabbage, mustard"							
Mustard greens, fresh:							
chopped, raw, 1 oz. or ½ cup	7	.8	1.4	.1	0	7	.6
boiled, drained, ½ cup	11	1.6	1.5	.2	0	11	1.4

Food and Measure	cal.	prot. (gms)	carbo. (gms)	fat (gms)	chol. (mgs)	sod. (mgs)	fiber (gms)
Mustard greens, canned, ½ cup:							
(*Allens/Sunshine*)	30	1.0	5.0	.5	0	10	3.0
(*Stubb's*)	30	1.0	5.0	.5	0	10	3.0
chopped (*Bush's Best*)	25	2.0	3.0	0	0	400	2.0
Mustard greens, frozen, chopped (*Birds Eye*), 1 cup	30	2.0	2.0	0	0	20	2.0
Mustard powder, 1 tsp.	9	.5	.3	.6	0	<1	<1.0
Mustard sauce (*Heluva* Good), 1 tsp.	6	0	0	0	0	100	0
Mustard seeds, 1 tsp.	15	.8	1.2	1.0	0	<1	<1.0
Mustard spinach:							
raw, chopped, ½ cup	17	1.7	2.9	.2	0	n.a.	n.a.
boiled, drained, chopped, ½ cup . . .	14	1.5	2.5	.2	0	n.a.	n.a.
Mustard tallow, 1 tbsp.	115	0	0	12.8	13	0	0

N

Food and Measure	cal.	prot. (gms)	carbo. (gms)	fat (gms)	chol. (mgs)	sod. (mgs)	fiber (gms)
Nacho dip, see "Cheese dip"							
Nacho snack, stuffed, frozen, 6 pcs.:							
(*Totino's* Grande)	210	6.0	25.0	9.0	10	510	2.0
cheese:							
and beef (*Totino's*)	220	7.0	25.0	10.0	10	590	1.0
jalapeño (*Totino's*)	200	6.0	25.0	8.0	10	670	1.0
nacho (*Totino's*) ...	220	7.0	26.0	10.0	15	710	1.0
three (*Totino's*)	210	7.0	25.0	9.0	10	690	1.0
chicken and cheese (*Totino's*)	200	7.0	25.0	8.0	10	630	1.0
taco (*Totino's*)	220	7.0	25.0	10.0	15	610	1.0
Name yam (*Frieda's*), 3 oz.	100	1.0	24.0	0	0	10	3.0
Natto, ½ cup	187	15.6	12.6	9.7	0	6	4.8
Navy beans, boiled, ½ cup	129	7.9	24.0	.5	0	1	3.3
Navy beans, canned, ½ cup:							
(*Allens*)	110	6.0	19.0	1.0	0	380	6.0
(*Bush's Best*)	110	5.0	19.0	.5	0	450	6.0
(*Eden* Organic)	110	7.0	20.0	.5	0	15	7.0
w/bacon or bacon and jalapeño (*Trappey's*)	110	6.0	17.0	1.5	0	420	7.0
w/liquid	148	9.9	26.8	.6	0	587	6.7
Navy beans, dehydrated (*AlpineAire*), 1 oz.	100	10.0	17.0	1.0	0	0	8.0
Navy beans, sprouted, raw, ½ cup	35	3.2	6.8	.4	0	n.a.	n.a.

Food and Measure	cal.	prot. (gms)	carbo. (gms)	fat (gms)	chol. (mgs)	sod. (mgs)	fiber (gms)
Nectarine:							
1 medium, 2½″ diam.	67	1.3	16.0	.6	0	<1	2.2
sliced, ½ cup	34	.7	8.1	.3	0	<1	1.1
New England sausage							
(*Oscar Mayer*),							
2 slices, 1.6 oz. ...	60	8.0	1.0	2.5	25	570	0
Newburg sauce mix							
(*Knorr* Classic							
Sauces), 1 tbsp. ...	35	1.0	5.0	1.0	0	350	0
Noodle, Chinese:							
cellophane or long							
rice, dry, 2 oz.	199	.1	48.8	<.1	0	6	<1.0
chow mein:							
(*Chun King/La*							
Choy), ½ cup ...	140	3.0	18.0	6.5	0	210	1.0
(*Frieda's*), 4 oz. ...	270	10.0	40.0	1.0	0	550	4.0
½ cup	119	1.9	13.0	6.9	0	99	.9
crispy wide (*La Choy*),							
½ cup	150	3.0	15.0	8.5	0	275	4.0
rice (*La Choy*), ½ cup	120	2.0	21.0	3.0	0	380	0
Noodle, egg, dry:							
(*Borden* Enriched),							
1 cup	210	8.0	39.0	2.5	55	20	1.0
(*Kluski* Enriched),							
1 cup	220	8.0	40.0	3.0	55	210	1.0
(*Manischewitz*),							
1¾ cups	210	8.0	40.0	1.0	0	20	2.0
fettuccine, 2 oz.:							
(*Al Dente*)	220	8.0	41.0	2.0	40	20	2.0
basil, curry, dill, red							
chili, squid ink,							
tarragon, or 3-							
pepper (*Al Dente*)	210	8.0	42.0	1.5	33	15	2.0
fennel–bell pepper							
(*Al Dente*)	210	8.0	42.0	1.5	33	15	2.0
fiesta (*Al Dente*) ...	210	8.0	42.0	1.5	28	25	2.0
garlic-parsley (*Al*							
Dente)	220	8.0	41.0	2.0	33	15	2.0
lemon-chive (*Al*							
Dente)	220	8.0	42.0	1.5	33	15	2.0

Food and Measure	cal.	prot. (gms)	carbo. (gms)	fat (gms)	chol. (mgs)	sod. (mgs)	fiber (gms)
mushroom, wild (*Al Dente*)	210	8.0	42.0	2.0	33	15	2.0
sesame, spicy (*Al Dente*)	220	8.0	40.0	3.0	33	15	2.0
spinach (*Al Dente*)	210	8.0	42.0	1.5	26	30	3.0
tomato (*Al Dente*)	210	7.0	42.0	1.5	17	20	3.0
wheat (*Al Dente*) ...	220	8.0	42.0	1.5	33	20	2.0
linguine, 2 oz.:							
(*Al Dente*)	210	8.0	41.0	2.0	40	20	2.0
spinach (*Al Dente*)	220	8.0	42.0	1.5	26	30	3.0
spaetzel (*Maggi*), 1/6 pkg.	180	7.0	33.0	1.5	35	460	2.0
yolk-free (*Borden*), 1 cup	210	8.0	41.0	1.0	0	25	1.0
Noodle, egg, cooked:							
1 cup	212	7.6	39.7	2.4	53	11	1.8
spinach, 1 cup	211	8.1	38.8	2.5	52	20	3.7
Noodle, egg-free (*Borden* Eggless Enriched), 2 oz.	210	7.0	42.0	1.0	0	0	2.0
Noodle, Japanese, dry:							
(*Nasoya* Natural), uncooked, 1 cup, 2¾ oz.	210	8.0	43.0	.5	0	440	2.0
soba, uncooked, 2 oz.:							
(*Eden* Organic Traditional)	200	8.0	38.0	1.5	0	80	3.0
(*Eden* Traditional)	190	8.0	37.0	1.0	0	490	3.0
buckwheat (*Eden*)	200	5.0	41.0	1.5	0	30	3.0
lotus root (*Eden*) ...	190	9.0	37.0	1.0	0	470	4.0
mugwort (*Eden*) ...	190	8.0	37.0	.5	0	550	2.0
wild yam (*Eden* Jinenjo)	190	9.0	37.0	.5	0	510	2.0
soba, cooked, 1 cup	113	5.8	24.4	.1	0	40	n.a.
somen:							
uncooked, 2 oz.	203	6.5	42.2	.5	0	1049	2.4
cooked, 1 cup	230	7.0	48.5	.3	0	284	n.a.
udon, uncooked, 2 oz.:							
(*Eden*)	190	8.0	37.0	1.5	0	660	3.0

Food and Measure	cal.	prot. (gms)	carbo. (gms)	fat (gms)	chol. (mgs)	sod. (mgs)	fiber (gms)
Noodle, Japanese, udon, uncooked *(cont.)*							
(*Eden* Organic Traditional)	200	8.0	38.0	1.5	0	80	2.0
brown rice (*Eden*)	190	8.0	38.0	1.0	0	510	2.0
brown rice (*Eden* Organic Traditional)	200	8.0	38.0	2.0	0	80	3.0
udon, cooked, 4 oz.	115	2.8	23.0	.6	0	51	n.a.
Noodle dinner, frozen, Asian stir-fry (*Amy's*), 10 oz. ...	240	12.0	41.0	4.5	0	680	6.0
Noodle dishes, mix, 1 cup*:							
Alfredo:							
(*Lipton* Noodles & Sauce).........	330	12.0	42.0	14.0	80	1040	2.0
broccoli (*Lipton* Noodles & Sauce)	340	12.0	43.0	14.0	80	970	2.0
beef (*Lipton* Noodles & Sauce).........	280	8.0	43.0	9.5	60	910	2.0
butter (*Lipton* Noodles & Sauce).........	310	8.0	41.0	14.0	70	870	2.0
butter and herb (*Lipton* Noodles & Sauce)	300	9.0	42.0	13.0	65	780	2.0
cheddar cheese:							
(*Kraft*)	430	12.0	46.0	21.0	70	780	1.0
chicken:							
(*Kraft*)	330	10.0	45.0	12.0	60	1430	1.0
(*Lipton* Noodles & Sauce).........	290	8.0	42.0	10.5	65	830	2.0
broccoli (*Lipton* Noodles & Sauce)	310	11.0	44.0	11.0	70	840	2.0
creamy (*Lipton* Noodles & Sauce) ...	320	11.0	42.0	13.0	75	810	2.0
Parmesan (*Lipton* Noodles & Sauce)	330	14.0	40.0	15.0	75	850	2.0
sour cream and chives (*Lipton* Noodles & Sauce)	310	10.0	41.0	14.0	70	870	2.0

Food and Measure	cal.	prot. (gms)	carbo. (gms)	fat (gms)	chol. (mgs)	sod. (mgs)	fiber (gms)
Stroganoff (*Lipton* Noodles & Sauce)	300	13.0	40.0	11.0	70	950	2.0
tetrazzini (*Lipton* Noodles & Sauce)	300	10.0	41.0	11.5	70	950	2.0
Noodle entree, canned or packaged, 1 cup, except as noted:							
and beef (*Hunt's*)	150	10.0	22.0	4.0	15	1240	5.0
and chicken:							
(*Hormel* Microwave Cup)	200	8.0	20.0	9.0	40	1140	1.0
(*Hunt's*)	175	12.0	21.0	6.0	35	1280	2.0
(*Nalley* Dinner)	190	11.0	21.0	7.0	30	1320	1.0
rings (*Kid's Kitchen*)	150	10.0	17.0	4.0	30	1110	1.0
w/vegetables (*Nalley*)	160	9.0	19.0	6.0	15	1240	2.0
w/vegetables (*Nalley*), 7½ oz.	140	9.0	19.0	3.0	20	930	2.0
Noodle entree, frozen, 1 pkg., except as noted:							
w/beef (*Freezer Queen* Family), 1 cup	190	9.0	31.0	3.0	20	1080	3.0
escalloped, and chicken:							
(*Marie Callender's*), 1 cup	420	13.0	44.0	21.0	45	1010	3.0
(*Marie Callender's Family*), 1 cup ...	260	8.0	22.0	16.0	30	670	1.0
escalloped, and turkey (*The Budget Gourmet Value Classics*), 8 oz.	320	10.0	32.0	17.0	50	620	2.0
Japanese noodles and vegetables (*Cascadian Farm Veggie Bowl*)	180	9.0	29.0	2.5	0	630	4.0

Food and Measure	cal.	prot. (gms)	carbo. (gms)	fat (gms)	chol. (mgs)	sod. (mgs)	fiber (gms)
Noodle entree, frozen *(cont.)*							
kung pao, and vegetables (*Smart Ones*),							
10 oz.	250	8.0	37.0	8.0	5	650	5.0
Romanoff (*Stouffer's*),							
½ of 12-oz. pkg.	240	8.0	27.0	11.0	25	610	2.0
soufflé, sweet (*Melrose*), ½ cup	210	4.0	37.0	5.0	45	135	1.0
Nopales, see "Cactus pads"							
Nori, see "Seaweed"							
Nut filling, see "Pastry filling"							
Nut topping, see specific nut listings							
Nutmeg, ground,							
1 tsp.	12	.1	1.1	.8	0	tr.	.1
Nuts, see specific listings							
Nuts, mixed (see also "Snack mix"), 1 oz., except as noted:							
(*Planters*)	170	6.0	6.0	15.0	0	115	2.0
(*Planters* Deluxe)	170	5.0	6.0	16.0	0	110	2.0
w/peanuts:							
(*Paradise/White Swan*), ¼ cup, 1.2 oz.	210	7.0	6.0	18.0	0	40	4.0
(*River Queen* 70% Peanuts)	160	6.0	5.0	14.0	0	140	2.0
(*River Queen* 70% Peanuts Unsalted)	160	7.0	5.0	15.0	0	0	2.0
(*River Queen* Premium)	170	6.0	5.0	15.0	0	140	2.0
(*River Queen* Premium Unsalted)	170	6.0	5.0	15.0	0	5	2.0
w/out peanuts:							
(*Paradise/White Swan* Fancy), ¼ cup, 1.2 oz.	220	6.0	7.0	18.0	0	60	4.0
(*River Queen* Fancy)	170	5.0	6.0	16.0	0	140	2.0

Food and Measure	cal.	prot. (gms)	carbo. (gms)	fat (gms)	chol. (mgs)	sod. (mgs)	fiber (gms)
(*River Queen* Fancy Unsalted)	170	5.0	6.0	16.0	0	0	2.0
dry-roasted:							
(*River Queen* Unsalted)	160	5.0	7.0	14.0	0	0	2.0
w/peanuts	169	4.9	7.2	14.6	0	3	2.6
w/peanuts, salted	169	4.9	7.2	14.6	0	190	2.6
oil-roasted:							
w/peanuts	175	4.8	6.1	16.0	0	3	2.8
w/peanuts, salted	175	4.8	6.1	16.0	0	185	2.8

O

Food and Measure	cal.	prot. (gms)	carbo. (gms)	fat (gms)	chol. (mgs)	sod. (mgs)	fiber (gms)
Oat (see also "Cereal, ready-to-eat"):							
flakes, rolled (*Arrowhead Mills*), cup ...	130	5.0	23.0	2.5	0	0	4.0
rolled or oatmeal:							
dry, 1 oz.	109	4.5	19.0	1.8	0	1	2.9
cooked, 1 cup	145	6.0	25.2	2.4	0	1	n.a.
steel cut (*Arrowhead Mills*), ¼ cup	170	6.0	29.0	3.0	0	0	5.0
whole-grain, 1 oz. ...	110	4.8	18.8	2.0	0	1	n.a.
Oat bran, dry:							
(*Arrowhead Mills*), ⅓ cup	150	8.0	23.0	2.5	0	0	7.0
1 oz.	70	4.9	18.8	2.0	0	1	4.5
Oat flour (*Arrowhead Mills*), ⅓ cup	120	5.0	20.0	2.0	0	0	4.0
Oat groats (*Arrowhead Mills*), ¼ cup	160	6.0	29.0	3.0	0	0	4.0
Ocean perch, Atlantic, meat only:							
raw, 4 oz.	107	21.1	0	1.9	48	85	0
baked, broiled, or microwaved, 4 oz. ...	137	27.1	0	2.4	61	109	0
Ocean perch entree, frozen, breaded fillet (*Van de Kamp's*), 2 pcs., 4 oz.	300	12.0	19.0	20.0	25	480	0
Octopus, meat only:							
raw, 4 oz.	93	16.9	2.5	1.2	55	n.a.	0
boiled or steamed, 4 oz.	186	33.8	5.0	2.4	109	n.a.	0
Octopus, canned:							
(*Goya*), ¼ cup	140	11.0	3.0	9.0	25	410	0

Food and Measure	cal.	prot. (gms)	carbo. (gms)	fat (gms)	chol. (mgs)	sod. (mgs)	fiber (gms)
spiced, in red sauce							
(*Reese*), 2 oz.	120	7.0	4.0	8.0	0	430	0
Oheloberry, ½ cup	20	.3	4.8	.2	0	1	n.a.
Oil, 1 tbsp., except as noted:							
(*Arrowhead Mills* Essential Balance) ...	130	0	0	14.0	0	0	0
(*House of Tsang Mongolian Fire*), 1 tsp.	45	0	0	5.0	0	0	0
almond, canola, cocoa butter, corn, cottonseed, hazelnut, oat, palm, or poppyseed	120	0	0	13.6	0	0	0
avocado or mustard	124	0	0	14.0	0	0	0
basil, garlic, garlic-ginger, lemon-dill, or onion (*Watkins* Liquid Spice)	120	0	0	14.0	0	0	0
butter oil............	112	<.1	0	12.7	33	n.a.	0
coconut	117	0	0	13.6	0	0	0
cod liver	123	0	0	13.6	78	n.a.	0
curry (*House of Tsang Singapore*), 1 tsp.	45	0	0	5.0	0	0	0
flax seed (*Arrowhead Mills*)	130	0	0	14.0	0	0	0
grapeseed, flavored, all varieties (*Watkins*)	120	0	0	14.0	0	0	0
herring	123	0	0	13.6	104	n.a.	0
olive, peanut, safflower, sesame, soybean, sunflower, vegetable, or walnut	120	0	0	14.0	0	0	0
salmon	123	0	0	13.6	66	n.a.	0
sardine	123	0	0	13.6	97	n.a.	0
sesame:							
hot pepper (*Eden*)	130	0	0	14.0	0	0	0
pure or hot chili (*House of Tsang*), 1 tsp.	45	0	0	5.0	0	0	0

Food and Measure	cal.	prot. (gms)	carbo. (gms)	fat (gms)	chol. (mgs)	sod. (mgs)	fiber (gms)
Oil, sesame *(cont.)*							
toasted *(Eden)*	120	0	0	14.0	0	0	0
wok *(House of Tsang)*	130	0	0	14.0	0	0	0
Okra, fresh:							
raw, sliced, ½ cup ...	19	1.0	3.8	.1	0	4	1.3
boiled, drained,							
8 pods, 3″ x ⅝″ ...	27	1.6	6.1	.1	0	5	2.1
boiled, drained, sliced,							
½ cup	25	1.5	5.8	.1	0	4	2.0
Okra, canned, ½ cup:							
cut:							
(Allens/Trappey's)	25	1.0	6.0	0	0	400	3.0
(Stubb's)	25	1.0	6.0	0	0	400	3.0
gumbo *(Trappey's* Cre-							
ole)	35	2.0	6.0	0	0	290	3.0
w/tomatoes *(Allens/*							
Trappey's)	25	1.0	5.0	0	0	380	3.0
w/tomatoes and corn							
(Allens/Trappey's)	30	<1.0	6.0	0	0	280	4.0
Okra, frozen:							
whole *(Birds Eye/*							
Freshlike), 9 pods	25	1.0	5.0	0	0	35	3.0
cut, ¾ cup:							
(Birds Eye/Freshlike)	25	1.0	5.0	0	0	35	3.0
(McKenzie's)	25	1.0	5.0	0	0	35	3.0
boiled, drained, sliced,							
½ cup	34	1.9	7.5	.3	0	3	2.6
Old-fashioned loaf,							
see "Lunch meat"							
Olive, pickled:							
black, see "ripe," be-							
low							
Calamata:							
(Krinos), 3 pcs.,							
½ oz.	45	0	2.0	4.0	0	230	0
(Zorba), 5 pcs.,							
½ oz.	90	1.0	2.0	9.0	0	260	0
Greek, black:							
(Krinos), 2 pcs.,							
½ oz.	35	0	2.0	3.0	0	240	0

Food and Measure	cal.	prot. (gms)	carbo. (gms)	fat (gms)	chol. (mgs)	sod. (mgs)	fiber (gms)
(*Krinos* Alfonso), 2 pcs., ½ oz.	35	0	1.0	3.0	0	380	0
(*Krinos* Napflion), 5 pcs., ½ oz.	20	0	2.0	1.5	0	260	0
(*Zorba*), 1 pc.	60	0	6.0	4.0	0	540	0
10 medium	65	.4	1.7	6.9	0	631	0
10 extra large	89	.6	2.3	9.5	0	868	0
pitted, 1 oz.	96	.6	2.5	10.2	0	932	0
green, w/pits:							
10 small	33	.4	.4	3.6	0	686	.7
10 large	45	.5	.5	4.9	0	926	1.0
10 giant	76	.9	.9	8.3	0	1572	1.7
green, cracked (*Krinos*), 2 pcs., ½ oz.	20	0	2.0	1.0	0	220	0
green, pitted, 1 oz. . . .	33	.4	.4	3.6	0	680	.7
green, Spanish (*Zorba*), 2 pcs., ½ oz.	25	<1.0	1.0	2.0	0	230	0
ripe, pitted:							
(*Lindsay*), 6 small, 5 medium, 4 large, or 1⅓ tbsp. chopped	25	0	1.0	2.5	0	115	0
(*Lindsay*), 6 extra large or 1 colossal	25	0	1.0	2.5	0	110	0
(*Lindsay*), 1 jumbo	25	0	1.0	2.0	0	135	0
(*Lindsay*), 1 super colossal	15	0	1.0	1.0	0	75	0
sliced (*Lindsay*), 2 tbsp.	25	0	1.0	2.5	0	125	0
wedged (*Lindsay*), 2 tbsp.	30	0	1.0	3.0	0	140	0
ripe, w/pits: (*Lindsay*), 5 medium or 4 large	25	0	0	2.5	0	125	0
stuffed:							
w/almonds (*Reese*), 4 pcs., ½ oz.	35	0	<1.0	3.5	0	310	0
w/minced anchovies (*Reese*), 4 pcs., ½ oz.	25	0	<1.0	2.0	0	220	0
queen (*Goya*), 1 pc.	20	0	1.0	1.5	0	160	0

Food and Measure	cal.	prot. (gms)	carbo. (gms)	fat (gms)	chol. (mgs)	sod. (mgs)	fiber (gms)
Olive Garden Garden Fare, 1 serving:							
lunch entrees:							
capellini pomodoro	380	13.0	60.0	10.0	5	1030	n.a.
capellini primavera	350	14.0	58.0	7.0	10	820	n.a.
capellini primavera w/chicken	510	39.0	59.0	13.0	45	1550	n.a.
chicken giardino . . .	360	23.0	47.0	9.0	50	900	n.a.
linguine alla marinara	330	10.0	57.0	6.0	0	710	n.a.
shrimp primavera	410	26.0	62.0	6.0	125	830	n.a.
minestrone soup, 6 fl. oz.	100	5.0	18.0	1.0	0	670	n.a.
breadstick, plain, 1 pc.	140	5.0	26.0	1.5	0	270	n.a.
dinner entrees:							
capellini pomodoro	620	22.0	98.0	16.0	10	1620	n.a.
capellini primavera	600	23.0	99.0	12.0	10	1450	n.a.
capellini primavera w/chicken	760	48.0	101.0	18.0	50	2190	n.a.
chicken giardino . . .	550	42.0	71.0	11.0	85	1000	n.a.
grilled chicken Capri	550	58.0	52.0	12.0	70	1660	n.a.
linguine alla marinara	530	17.0	94.0	9.0	0	1100	n.a.
shrimp primavera	730	50.0	106.0	12.0	255	1590	n.a.
dessert, apple caramellina . . . . . : .	570	7.0	130.0	2.5	10	230	n.a.
Olive loaf, see "Lunch meat"							
Olive oil, see "Oil"							
Olive salad (*Progresso*), 2 tbsp.	25	0	1.0	2.5	0	360	<1.0
Omelet, see "Egg breakfast"							
Ong choy, see "Spinach, water"							
Onion, fresh/stored:							
raw:							
(*Frieda's* Boiler/Cipolline), 3 pcs., 3 oz.	30	1.0	7.0	0	0	0	2.0

Food and Measure	cal.	prot. (gms)	carbo. (gms)	fat (gms)	chol. (mgs)	sod. (mgs)	fiber (gms)
(*Frieda's* Maui),							
⅓ cup, 3 oz.	10	0	3.0	0	0	0	1.0
(*Frieda's* Pearl),							
⅔ cup, 3 oz.	30	1.0	7.0	0	0	0	2.0
1 oz.	11	.3	2.4	<.1	0	1	.5
chopped, ½ cup . . .	30	.9	6.9	0.1	0	2	1.4
chopped, 1 tbsp.	4	.1	.9	<.1	0	tr.	.2
boiled, drained,							
chopped, ½ cup . . .	47	1.4	10.7	.2	0	3	1.5
Onion, cocktail, see							
"Onion, in jars"							
Onion, in jars:							
whole, ½ cup:							
(*Green Giant*)	35	<1.0	8.0	0	0	410	1.0
(*Hanover*)	25	1.0	6.0	0	0	420	1.0
cocktail, 1 tbsp.:							
(*Boar's Head Sweet*							
Vidalia)	10	0	2.0	0	0	15	0
(*Crosse & Black-*							
well)	0	0	1.0	0	0	250	0
pickled, sour (*London*							
Pub), ¼ cup,							
1.1 oz.	10	2.0	2.0	0	0	130	0
Onion, frozen:							
(*Seneca*), cup	30	4.0	7.0	0	0	0	3.0
diced (*Birds Eye*),							
⅔ cup	30	<1.0	6.0	0	0	30	1.0
small whole (*Birds*							
Eye), 7 pcs.	30	1.0	7.0	0	0	10	1.0
chopped:							
(*Ore-Ida*), ¾ cup . . .	20	1.0	5.0	0	0	15	1.0
boiled, drained,							
1 tbsp.	4	.1	1.0	<.1	0	2	.2
in cream sauce (*Birds*							
Eye Side Orders),							
½ cup	60	2.0	8.0	2.0	10	280	1.0
rings, see "Onion							
rings"							
Onion, dried:							
flakes, 1 tbsp.	16	.5	4.2	<.1	0	1	.5

Food and Measure	cal.	prot. (gms)	carbo. (gms)	fat (gms)	chol. (mgs)	sod. (mgs)	fiber (gms)
Onion, dried *(cont.)*							
french-fried							
(*French's*), 2 tbsp.	45	0	3.0	3.5	0	60	0
minced, 1 tsp.	7	.2	1.9	0	0	<1	.2
Onion, green (scal-lion), raw, trimmed, w/top:							
chopped, ½ cup	16	.9	3.7	.1	0	8	1.3
chopped, 1 tbsp.	2	.1	.4	<.1	0	1	.2
Onion, Welsh, 1 oz.	10	.5	1.8	.1	0	n.a.	<1.0
Onion dip, 2 tbsp.:							
creamy (*Kraft* Pre-mium)	45	<1.0	2.0	4.0	10	160	0
French:							
(*Breakstone's*)	50	1.0	2.0	4.0	20	160	0
(*Frito-Lay's*)	60	1.0	4.0	5.0	15	230	0
(*Heluva* Good)	60	1.0	2.0	5.0	20	170	0
(*Heluva* Good Fat Free)	25	1.0	3.0	0	0	200	0
(*Knudsen*)	50	1.0	2.0	4.0	20	160	0
(*Kraft*)	60	1.0	4.0	4.0	0	230	0
(*Kraft* Premium) . . .	50	<1.0	2.0	4.0	10	160	0
(*Nalley*)	100	1.0	3.0	10.0	15	250	0
(*Ruffles*)	70	1.0	4.0	5.0	0	240	1.0
(*Ruffles* Lowfat) . . .	40	2.0	6.0	1.0	0	230	<1.0
(*Sealtest*)	50	1.0	2.0	4.0	20	160	0
green (*Kraft*)	60	1.0	4.0	4.0	0	190	0
sour cream and:							
(*T. Marzetti's* Veggie Dip)	130	1.0	2.0	13.0	25	220	0
(*T. Marzetti's* Veggie Dip Fat Free)	35	1.0	6.0	0	0	300	0
toasted (*Breakstone's*)	50	1.0	2.0	4.0	20	180	0
Onion dip mix:							
and chive (*Knorr*), ½ tsp.	5	0	<1.0	0	0	110	0
French (*Hidden Val-ley*), 2 tbsp.*	70	<1.0	2.0	6.0	15	160	0
Onion gravy, zesty (*Heinz* Home Style), ¼ cup	25	1.0	3.0	1.0	0	350	0

Food and Measure	cal.	prot. (gms)	carbo. (gms)	fat (gms)	chol. (mgs)	sod. (mgs)	fiber (gms)
Onion gravy mix:							
(*Knorr* Lyonnaise), 2 tsp.	20	<1.0	4.0	.5	0	370	0
(*Loma Linda Gravy Quik*), 1 tbsp.	20	<1.0	3.0	0	0	230	<1.0
Onion oil, see "Oil"							
Onion powder:							
(*Tone's*), ¼ tsp.	5	0	1.0	0	0	0	0
1 tsp.	10	.3	2.4	0	0	2	.2
Onion rings, frozen:							
(*Bland Farms Vidalia O's*), 6 pcs., 3 oz.	200	3.0	26.0	9.0	0	260	<1.0
(*Moore's*), 7 pcs., 3.2 oz.	200	3.0	28.0	11.0	0	220	2.0
(*Ore-Ida Onion Ringers*), 6 pcs., 3.2 oz.	220	3.0	25.0	12.0	0	350	3.0
Onion salt: (*Tone's*), 1 tsp.	1	.1	.4	tr.	0	1599	<.1
Onion sauce, in jars (*Boar's Head* Vidalia), 1 tbsp.	10	0	2.0	0	0	15	0
Onion snack chips, see "Snack chips and crisps"							
Opo squash (*Frieda's*), ⅔ cup, 3 oz.	10	1.0	3.0	0	0	0	0
Opossum, meat only, roasted, 4 oz.	251	34.2	0	11.6	n.a.	n.a.	0
Orange, fresh:							
blood (*Frieda's*), 5 oz.	70	1.0	16.0	0	0	0	3.0
California navel:							
2⅞" orange	65	1.4	16.3	.1	0	1	3.4
sections w/out membrane, ½ cup	38	.9	9.6	.1	0	1	2.0
California Valencia:							
2⅝" orange	59	1.3	14.4	.4	0	0	2.9
sections w/out membrane, ½ cup	44	.9	10.7	.3	0	0	2.2
Florida:							
2¹¹⁄₁₆" orange	69	1.1	17.4	.3	0	1	3.6

Food and Measure	cal.	prot. (gms)	carbo. (gms)	fat (gms)	chol. (mgs)	sod. (mgs)	fiber (gms)
Orange, Florida *(cont.)*							
sections w/out							
membrane, ½ cup	42	.7	10.7	.2	0	1	2.2
Orange, canned, in							
light syrup (*Sun-*							
fresh), ½ cup	80	1.0	18.0	0	0	0	2.0
Orange, mandarin,							
see "Tangerine"							
Orange drink, 8 fl. oz.,							
except as noted:							
(*Snapple* Tropic)	120	0	30.0	0	0	30	0
(*Veryfine*), 10 fl. oz.	130	0	33.0	0	0	70	0
(*Veryfine* Natural)	0	0	0	0	0	5	0
(*Veryfine/Veryfine Arc-*							
tic Chiller)	130	0	32.0	0	0	10	0
(*Whipper Snapple*							
Dream), 10 fl. oz.	150	0	36.0	0	0	60	0
Orange drink blends,							
8 fl. oz., except as							
noted:							
cranberry:							
(*Tropicana Twister*)	120	<1.0	30.0	0	0	45	0
(*Tropicana Twister*							
Light)	30	0	7.0	0	0	20	0
guava, nectar (*Kern's*)	150	0	36.0	0	0	10	0
peach:							
(*Tropicana Twister*)	120	0	31.0	0	0	20	0
strawberry (*Tropi-*							
cana Twister)	130	0	32.0	0	0	20	0
pineapple (*Tropicana*),							
11.5 fl. oz.	180	0	45.0	0	0	35	0
punch (*Kool-Aid*							
Bursts), 6.75 fl. oz.	100	0	24.0	0	0	30	0
raspberry:							
(*Tropicana Twister*)	120	0	31.0	0	0	20	0
(*Tropicana Twister*							
Light)	35	0	9.0	0	0	20	0
strawberry banana:							
(*Tropicana Twister*)	130	<1.0	32.0	0	0	45	0
(*Tropicana Twister*							
Light)	35	1.0	9.0	0	0	20	0

Food and Measure	cal.	prot. (gms)	carbo. (gms)	fat (gms)	chol. (mgs)	sod. (mgs)	fiber (gms)
strawberry guava (*Tropicana Twister*)	120	0	29.0	0	0	20	0
Orange drink mix, 8 fl. oz.*, except as noted:							
(*Kool-Aid*)	100	0	25.0	0	0	15	0
(*Kool-Aid* Presweetened)	60	0	16.0	0	0	5	0
(*Tang*)	100	0	24.0	0	0	0	0
creamy (*Watkins* Cooler), 5 tbsp. ...	25	0	4.0	1.0	0	10	0
Orange juice, 8 fl. oz., except as noted:							
(*After the Fall 24 Karrot Orange*)	120	1.0	29.0	0	0	45	0
(*Apple & Eve*), 10 fl. oz.	130	3.0	32.0	0	0	5	0
(*Hood*)	120	0	30.0	0	0	20	0
(*Minute Maid*)	114	0	27.0	0	0	26	0
(*Ocean Spray*)	120	0	31.0	0	0	35	0
(*R.W. Knudsen*)	100	2.0	23.0	0	0	35	0
(*Season's Best*)	110	1.0	27.0	0	0	15	0
(*Snapple* Grove), 12 fl. oz.	170	0	44.0	0	0	20	0
(*Tropicana Pure Premium*)	110	1.0	26.0	0	0	0	0
(*Tropicana Pure Premium* w/Calcium)	110	2.0	26.0	0	0	0	0
(*Veryfine*)	120	0	30.0	0	0	10	0
(*Veryfine*), 10 fl. oz.	150	0	37.0	0	0	10	0
(*Veryfine*), 11.5 fl. oz.	170	0	42.0	0	0	10	0
fresh, 6 fl. oz.	83	1.3	19.3	.4	0	2	.4
frozen* (*R.W. Knudsen*)	100	2.0	23.0	0	0	35	0
Orange juice blends, 8 fl. oz.:							
(*Minute Maid*)	124	0	32.0	0	0	33	0
(*Tropicana Bursters*)	110	2.0	25.0	0	0	0	0
kiwi passion (*Tropicana Pure Tropics*)	100	<1.0	26.0	0	0	15	0

Food and Measure	cal.	prot. (gms)	carbo. (gms)	fat (gms)	chol. (mgs)	sod. (mgs)	fiber (gms)
Orange juice blends *(cont.)*							
mango (*R.W. Knud-sen*)	120	0	30.0	0	0	50	0
peach mango:							
(*Dole*)	120	1.0	28.0	0	0	35	0
(*Tropicana Pure Tropics*)	110	<1.0	28.0	0	0	15	0
pineapple:							
(*Season's Best*) . . .	120	1.0	27.0	0	0	15	0
(*Tropicana Pure Tropics*)	110	<1.0	27.0	0	0	15	0
punch (*Juicy Juice*)	120	0	30.0	0	0	10	0
strawberry banana:							
(*Chiquita* Cocktail)	120	0	30.0	0	0	10	0
(*Dole*)	120	1.0	28.0	0	0	30	0
(*Tropicana Pure Tropics*)	110	<1.0	27.0	0	0	5	0
Orange peel, fresh, 1 tbsp.	[1]	.1	1.5	<.1	0	0	.2
Orange peel, can-died, diced (*Para-dise/White Swan*), 2 tbsp., 1.1 oz.	90	0	23.0	0	0	15	2.0
Orange sauce, Orien-tal (*Ka•Me* Manda-rin), 2 tbsp.	80	0	21.0	0	0	430	0
Oregano, dried, 1 tsp.	3	.1	.5	0	0	0	.1
Oriental 5-spice (*Tone's*), 1 tsp.	9	.3	1.9	.3	0	2	.5
Oriental sauce (see also "Stir-fry sauce" and specific list-ings): (*House of Tsang* Imperial), 1 tbsp.	25	0	5.0	0	0	410	0
Orzo pasta mix, mint-garlic (*Casbah*), ¾ cup	210	8.0	40.0	.5	0	390	.5

[1] *Cannot be calculated; no digestibility value for peel.*

Food and Measure	cal.	prot. (gms)	carbo. (gms)	fat (gms)	chol. (mgs)	sod. (mgs)	fiber (gms)
Oyster, meat only, 4 oz., except as noted:							
Eastern, wild:							
raw, 1 lb.	310	32.0	17.7	11.1	238	957	0
raw, 6 medium, 3 oz.	57	5.9	3.3	2.1	44	177	0
baked, broiled, or microwaved	82	9.4	5.4	2.2	56	277	0
steamed or poached	155	16.0	8.9	5.6	119	478	0
Eastern, farmed:							
raw	67	5.9	6.3	1.8	29	202	0
baked, broiled, or microwaved	90	7.9	8.3	2.4	43	185	0
Pacific:							
raw	93	10.7	5.6	2.6	n.a.	120	0
raw, boiled, or steamed, 1 medium	41	4.7	2.5	1.2	n.a.	53	0
boiled or steamed	185	21.4	11.2	5.2	n.a.	240	0
Oyster, canned:							
Eastern, wild:							
w/liquid, 4 oz.	78	8.0	4.4	2.8	62	127	0
w/liquid, 1 cup	170	17.5	9.7	6.1	136	277	0
smoked:							
(*Bumble Bee*), 2 oz.	120	10.0	6.0	7.0	35	210	0
(*Chicken of the Sea*), 3-oz. can	190	14.0	9.0	11.0	55	340	0
medium (*Reese*), 2 oz.	110	8.0	6.0	6.0	50	220	0
Oyster plant, see "Salsify"							
Oyster sauce, flavor (*Ka•Me*), 1 tbsp.	10	0	3.0	0	0	260	0
Oyster stew, see "Soup"							

P

Food and Measure	cal.	prot. (gms)	carbo. (gms)	fat (gms)	chol. (mgs)	sod. (mgs)	fiber (gms)
Palm, hearts of, in jars:							
(*Haddon House*), 4½ oz.	20	2.0	3.0	0	0	450	2.0
(*Sunfresh*), 3 pcs., 4.4 oz.	20	2.0	3.0	0	0	450	2.0
Pancake, frozen, 3 pcs.:							
(*Aunt Jemima* Home- style)	210	6.0	40.0	3.5	20	560	2.0
(*Aunt Jemima* Lowfat)	150	5.0	30.0	1.5	<5	530	8.0
(*Eggo*)	270	7.0	44.0	8.0	15	610	1.0
blueberry (*Aunt Je- mima*)	210	6.0	40.0	3.5	20	560	2.0
buttermilk (*Aunt Je- mima*)	210	6.0	40.0	3.5	20	600	2.0
Pancake batter, fro- zen, ½ cup:							
(*Aunt Jemima*)	250	7.0	50.0	3.5	40	850	2.0
blueberry (*Aunt Je- mima*)	290	6.0	55.0	5.0	40	850	2.0
buttermilk (*Aunt Je- mima*)	260	7.0	51.0	3.5	40	870	2.0
Pancake breakfast, frozen, w/sausage (*Swanson Great Starts*), 1 pkg.	490	14.0	52.0	25.0	90	950	3.0
Pancake mix, ⅓ cup dry, except as noted:							
(*Aunt Jemima* Origi- nal)	150	5.0	34.0	.5	0	745	1.0

Food and Measure	cal.	prot. (gms)	carbo. (gms)	fat (gms)	chol. (mgs)	sod. (mgs)	fiber (gms)
(*Aunt Jemima* Complete)	160	5.0	32.0	2.0	10	475	1.0
(*Betty Crocker* Original Complete), 1/3 cup or 3 cakes*	200	6.0	39.0	3.0	10	540	1.0
(*Bisquick Shake 'N Pour* Original), 3 cakes*	210	5.0	39.0	4.0	0	710	<1.0
(*Gladiola*), 1/2 cup	240	6.0	41.0	6.0	0	860	2.0
(*Hungry Jack* Original)	150	3.0	32.0	1.5	0	640	<1.0
(*Hungry Jack Extra Lights*)	160	3.0	33.0	1.5	0	590	<1.0
(*Hungry Jack Extra Lights* Complete)	150	4.0	30.0	2.0	0	600	<1.0
(*Martha White Flapstax*), 1/2 cup	240	5.0	45.0	4.0	35	600	<1.0
blue corn (*Arrowhead Mills*)	150	4.0	28.0	2.0	0	130	3.0
blueberry:							
(*AlpineAire*), 31/4 oz.	340	13.0	52.0	9.0	120	1280	7.0
(*Bisquick Shake 'N Pour*), 3 cakes*	210	6.0	40.0	3.5	0	640	1.0
buckwheat:							
(*Arrowhead Mills*)	140	8.0	25.0	1.5	0	220	5.0
(*Aunt Jemima*), 1/4 cup	100	4.0	23.0	1.0	0	580	4.0
buttermilk:							
(*Arrowhead Mills*), 1/4 cup	120	5.0	25.0	.5	<5	350	2.0
(*Aunt Jemima* Complete)	160	5.0	30.0	2.5	15	460	1.0
(*Aunt Jemima* Complete Reduced Cal)	130	7.0	28.0	1.5	15	630	5.0
(*Betty Crocker* Complete Box), 1/3 cup or 3 cakes*	200	5.0	39.0	2.5	10	540	1.0
(*Betty Crocker* Pouch)	180	5.0	31.0	3.5	0	510	1.0
(*Betty Crocker* Pouch), 3 cakes*	230	8.0	35.0	6.0	60	560	1.0

Food and Measure	cal.	prot. (gms)	carbo. (gms)	fat (gms)	chol. (mgs)	sod. (mgs)	fiber (gms)
Pancake mix, buttermilk *(cont.)*							
(*Bisquick Shake 'N Pour*), 3 cakes*	200	7.0	38.0	3.0	0	680	1.0
(*Hungry Jack*)	160	4.0	33.0	1.5	0	650	<1.0
(*Hungry Jack* Complete)	160	4.0	32.0	1.5	<5	570	<1.0
gluten-free (*Arrowhead Mills*), ¼ cup	130	4.0	24.0	2.0	0	180	5.0
kamut (*Arrowhead Mills*), ¼ cup	130	7.0	26.0	1.0	0	330	4.0
multigrain:							
(*Arrowhead Mills*), ¼ cup	120	5.0	24.0	.5	0	260	3.0
5 grain (*AlpineAire*), 1.2 oz.	120	3.0	22.0	3.0	0	210	1.0
oat bran (*Arrowhead Mills*)	140	7.0	25.0	1.5	0	160	6.0
whole grain (*Arrowhead Mills*), ¼ cup	120	5.0	24.0	.5	0	260	4.0
whole wheat (*Aunt Jemima*), ¼ cup	120	4.0	26.0	.5	0	625	3.0
wild rice (*Arrowhead Mills*)	140	3.0	30.0	1.0	0	65	0
Pancake syrup (see also "Maple syrup"), ¼ cup:							
(*Aunt Jemima/Aunt Jemima* Country Rich)	210	0	53.0	0	0	120	0
(*Aunt Jemima* Country Rich Lite)	100	0	26.0	0	0	230	0
(*Country Kitchen*)	200	0	53.0	0	0	110	0
(*Country Kitchen* Lite)	100	0	26.0	0	0	160	0
(*Hungry Jack*)	210	0	52.0	0	0	90	0
(*Hungry Jack* Lite) . . .	100	0	24.0	0	0	180	0
(*Log Cabin*)	200	0	52.0	0	0	60	0
(*Log Cabin* Lite)	100	0	26.0	0	0	180	0
(*Vermont Maid* Light)	100	0	26.0	0	0	100	0
butter flavor:							
(*Aunt Jemima* Butter Rich)	210	0	52.0	0	0	170	0

Food and Measure	cal.	prot. (gms)	carbo. (gms)	fat (gms)	chol. (mgs)	sod. (mgs)	fiber (gms)
(*Aunt Jemima* Butterlite)	100	0	26.0	0	0	180	0
(*Country Kitchen*)	200	0	53.0	0	0	200	0
(*Hungry Jack*)	210	0	52.0	0	0	90	0
(*Hungry Jack* Lite)	100	0	24.0	0	0	180	0
Pancreas, braised:							
beef, 4 oz.	307	30.7	0	19.5	n.a.	68	0
lamb, 4 oz.	265	25.9	0	17.1	454	59	0
pork, 4 oz.	248	32.3	0	12.2	357	48	0
veal (calf), 4 oz.	290	33.0	0	16.6	n.a.	n.a.	0
***Papa John's* Pizza,** 1 slice of 14″ pie, except as noted:							
original crust pizza:							
All the Meats	410	21.0	42.0	18.0	35	1040	3.0
cheese	286	14.0	37.0	9.0	18	540	2.0
Garden Special	298	14.0	36.0	11.0	20	570	3.0
pepperoni	310	15.0	35.0	13.0	25	570	2.0
sausage	340	15.0	40.0	13.0	25	910	2.0
The Works	369	18.0	37.0	17.0	29	840	3.0
thin crust pizza:							
All the Meats	330	15.0	23.0	20.0	39	919	2.0
cheese	220	9.0	22.0	11.0	18	480	2.0
Garden Special	238	9.0	23.0	12.0	19	540	3.0
pepperoni	266	11.0	22.0	15.0	24	580	2.0
sausage	270	12.0	22.0	15.0	29	730	2.0
The Works	319	14.0	24.0	19.0	35	760	3.0
sides:							
breadstick, 1 pc.	170	6.0	27.0	3.0	0	270	<1.0
cheesesticks, 2 pcs.	160	7.0	21.0	6.0	10	290	<1.0
garlic sauce, 1 tbsp.	75	0	2.0	8.5	0	115	0
nacho cheese, 1 tbsp.	30	1.5	0	2.0	8	113	0
pizza sauce, 1 tbsp.	10	0	1.0	.5	0	60	<1.0
Papaya, fresh:							
1-lb., 3½″ x 5⅛″	117	1.9	29.8	.4	0	8	5.5
peeled, cubed, ½ cup	27	.4	6.9	.1	0	2	1.3
Papaya, chilled, in extra light syrup (*Sunfresh*), ½ cup	70	1.0	17.0	0	0	5	1.0

Food and Measure	cal.	prot. (gms)	carbo. (gms)	fat (gms)	chol. (mgs)	sod. (mgs)	fiber (gms)
Papaya, creamed							
(*R.W. Knudsen*),							
2 fl. oz.	40	0	10.0	0	0	10	0
Papaya, dried:							
(*Frieda's*), 1/3 cup,							
1.4 oz.	140	0	29.0	2.5	0	40	4.0
(*Sonoma*), 2 pcs.,							
2 oz.	200	0	41.0	4.0	0	60	6.0
Papaya, frozen,							
(*Goya*), 1/3 pkg.	50	1.0	11.0	0	0	12	2.0
Papaya drink, 8 fl. oz.,							
except as noted:							
(*Snapple* Colada)	110	0	29.0	0	0	10	0
nectar:							
(*Kern's/Libby's*),							
11.5 fl. oz.	210	<1.0	51.0	0	0	10	0
(*R.W. Knudsen*) . . .	130	0	34.0	0	0	35	0
(*Santa Cruz* Or-							
ganic)	110	0	28.0	0	0	35	0
punch (*Veryfine*),							
10 fl. oz.	160	0	39.0	0	0	25	0
Papaya juice (*After*							
the Fall Pele's Pa-							
paya Nectar),							
8 fl. oz.	100	1.0	25.0	0	0	15	0
Pappadum (*Patak's*),							
3 pcs., 1 oz.	80	6.0	13.0	.5	0	819	3.0
Paprika:							
(*McCormick*), 1/4 tsp.	2	.1	.3	.1	0	<1	.2
1 tsp.	6	.3	1.2	.3	0	1	.6
Parfait, frozen, 1 pc.:							
double fudge brownie							
(*Weight Watchers*)	190	6.0	39.0	2.5	5	170	2.0
strawberry royale							
(*Weight Watchers*)	180	5.0	35.0	2.0	10	100	0
Parsley:							
fresh:							
10 sprigs	4	.3	.6	.1	0	6	.3
chopped, 1/2 cup . . .	11	.9	1.9	.2	0	17	1.0
dried:							
(*McCormick*),							
1/4 tsp.	<1	0	0	0	0	<1	0

Food and Measure	cal.	prot. (gms)	carbo. (gms)	fat (gms)	chol. (mgs)	sod. (mgs)	fiber (gms)
1 tsp.	1	.1	.2	.1	0	1	.2
freeze-dried, 1 tbsp.	1	.1	.2	<.1	0	2	.2
Parsley root:							
(*Frieda's*), ⅔ cup, 3 oz.	10	2.0	2.0	.5	0	70	1.0
1 oz.	3	.8	.7	.2	0	28	.4
Parsnip:							
raw, sliced, ½ cup . . .	50	.8	12.1	.2	0	7	3.3
boiled, drained:							
1 medium, 9″	130	2.1	31.3	.5	0	17	6.4
sliced, ½ cup	63	1.0	15.2	.2	0	8	3.1
Passion fruit:							
(*Frieda's*), 5 oz.	140	3.0	33.0	1.0	0	40	15.0
fresh, purple:							
1 medium	18	.4	4.2	.1	0	n.a.	1.9
trimmed, 1 oz.	27	.6	6.6	.2	0	n.a.	2.9
frozen, chunks (*Goya*),							
⅓ pkg.	70	2.0	15.0	0	0	35	2.0
Passion fruit juice:							
fresh:							
purple, 6 fl. oz.	95	.7	25.2	.1	0	n.a.	.4
yellow, 6 fl. oz.	111	1.2	26.8	.3	0	11	.4
bottled (*After the Fall Passion of the Islands*), 8 fl. oz.	100	1.0	26.0	0	0	10	0
Passion fruit juice drink:							
(*Mauna La'i* Paradise), 8 fl. oz.	130	0	32.0	0	0	35	0
(*Snapple* Supreme), 10 fl. oz.	160	0	39.0	0	0	20	0
Passion fruit syrup (*Trader Vic's*), 1 fl. oz.	80	0	21.0	0	0	15	0
Pasta, dry (see also "Macaroni" and specific pasta listings), uncooked, 2 oz., except as noted:							
(*Eden* Organic Extra Fine)	210	9.0	40.0	1.5	0	0	3.0

Food and Measure	cal.	prot. (gms)	carbo. (gms)	fat (gms)	chol. (mgs)	sod. (mgs)	fiber (gms)
Pasta *(cont.)*							
plain	211	7.3	42.6	.9	0	4	1.4
all styles:							
(*Delverde*)	200	7.0	41.0	.5	0	0	1.0
except spinach linguine, tomato-basil fusilli, and tricolor rotelle (*Contadina*)	210	12.0	36.0	1.5	0	0	3.0
alphabets, vegetable (*Eden* Organic)	200	8.0	40.0	1.0	0	0	3.0
angel hair:							
(*Al Dente Selecta*)	200	8.0	40.0	.5	0	0	5.0
(*DeBoles*)	210	7.0	41.0	1.0	0	0	1.0
garlic parsley (*DeBoles*)	210	7.0	41.0	1.0	0	5	2.0
w/Jerusalem ar- tichoke (*DeBoles*)	210	7.0	41.0	1.0	0	0	1.0
w/rice (*DeBoles*), ¼ pkg.	210	4.0	46.0	0	0	0	1.0
tomato-basil (*DeBoles*)	210	7.0	41.0	1.0	0	0	2.0
tomato–lemon pep- per (*DeBoles*), ¼ pkg.	200	7.0	41.0	.5	0	0	2.0
tomato-pesto (*DeBoles*), ¼ pkg.	200	8.0	41.0	.5	0	0	2.0
w/egg, see "Noodle, egg"							
elbow:							
(*DeBoles*), ¼ pkg.	200	7.0	41.0	.5	0	0	2.0
w/corn (*DeBoles*), ⅙ pkg.	200	4.0	43.0	2.0	0	15	5.0
pasta and cheese (*DeBoles*), ½ cup	190	8.0	35.0	1.5	15	230	1.0
plain or hot pepper (*Eden* Organic)	210	8.0	41.0	1.0	0	0	4.0
spelt (*Vita Spelt*) . . .	190	8.0	40.0	1.5	0	0	5.0

Food and Measure	cal.	prot. (gms)	carbo. (gms)	fat (gms)	chol. (mgs)	sod. (mgs)	fiber (gms)
fettuccine:							
garlic, roasted (*Al Dente Selecta*) . . .	220	8.0	42.0	2.0	15	10	2.0
garlic-parsley, tomato-pesto, or spinach (*DeBoles*), ¼ pkg.	200	8.0	41.0	.5	0	15	2.0
w/Jerusalem artichoke (*DeBoles*)	210	7.0	41.0	1.0	0	0	1.0
w/rice (*DeBoles*), ¼ pkg.	210	4.0	46.0	0	0	0	1.0
tomato-basil or tomato–lemon pepper (*DeBoles*), ¼ pkg.	200	7.0	41.0	.5	0	0	2.0
finbows, parsley garlic (*Eden* Organic)	210	8.0	41.0	1.0	0	0	4.0
fusilli, tomato-basil (*Contadina*)	210	12.0	36.0	1.5	0	35	3.0
kuzu, sweet potato, and kiri (*Eden*)	190	0	47.0	0	0	0	0
lasagna (*DeBoles*), ¼ pkg.	200	7.0	41.0	.5	0	0	2.0
linguine:							
(*DeBoles*)	210	7.0	41.0	1.0	0	0	1.0
w/Jerusalem artichoke (*DéBoles*)	210	7.0	41.0	1.0	0	0	1.0
spinach (*Contadina*)	210	12.0	36.0	1.5	0	25	3.0
mung bean (*Eden* Harusame)	190	0	47.0	0	0	5	0
penne:							
(*DeBoles*)	210	7.0	41.0	1.0	0	0	1.0
garlic-parsley (*DeBoles*), ¼ pkg.	200	7.0	41.0	.5	0	5	2.0
w/rice (*DeBoles*), ¼ pkg.	210	4.0	46.0	0	0	0	1.0
tomato-basil (*DeBoles*), ¼ pkg.	200	7.0	41.0	.5	0	0	2.0

Food and Measure	cal.	prot. (gms)	carbo. (gms)	fat (gms)	chol. (mgs)	sod. (mgs)	fiber (gms)
Pasta *(cont.)*							
ribbon:							
(*DeBoles*)	210	7.0	41.0	1.0	0	0	1.0
all varieties, except							
kluski and spinach							
(*Eden* Organic)	210	9.0	40.0	1.5	0	0	3.0
eggless (*DeBoles*),							
¼ pkg.	200	7.0	41.0	.5	0	0	2.0
kluski or spinach							
(*Eden* Organic)	210	8.0	41.0	1.0	0	0	4.0
eggless (*DeBoles*),							
¼ pkg.	200	7.0	41.0	.5	0	0	2.0
spelt (*Vita Spelt*) . . .	190	8.0	40.0	1.5	0	0	5.0
whole wheat							
(*DeBoles*)	210	7.0	40.0	2.0	0	0	5.0
rice (*Eden* Bifun)	200	5.0	44.0	.5	0	5	0
rigatoni:							
(*Al Dente Selecta*)	200	2.0	47.0	.5	0	0	1.0
(*DeBoles*)	210	7.0	41.0	1.0	0	0	1.0
garlic-parsley							
(*DeBoles*),							
¼ pkg.	200	7.0	41.0	.5	0	5	2.0
tomato-basil							
(*DeBoles*),							
¼ pkg.	200	7.0	41.0	.5	0	0	2.0
rotelle:							
roasted garlic and							
herb (*Mueller's*)	210	7.0	41.0	1.0	0	330	2.0
tricolor (*Contadina*)	210	12.0	36.0	1.5	0	15	3.0
rotini:							
(*Al Dente Selecta*)	200	8.0	40.0	.5	0	0	5.0
(*DeBoles*), ¼ pkg.	200	7.0	41.0	.5	0	0	2.0
garlic-parsley							
(*DeBoles*)	210	7.0	41.0	1.0	0	5	2.0
primavera (*DeBoles*)	210	7.0	41.0	1.0	0	0	1.0
tomato-basil							
(*DeBoles*)	210	7.0	41.0	1.0	0	0	2.0
shells:							
(*DeBoles*), ¼ pkg.	200	7.0	41.0	.5	0	0	2.0
and cheddar							
(*DeBoles*), ½ cup	190	8.0	35.0	1.5	15	230	1.0

Food and Measure	cal.	prot. (gms)	carbo. (gms)	fat (gms)	chol. (mgs)	sod. (mgs)	fiber (gms)
vegetable (*Eden Organic*)	200	8.0	40.0	1.0	0	0	3.0
spaghetti:							
(*DeBoles*)	210	7.0	41.0	1.0	0	0	1.0
(*Eden* Organic)	200	8.0	40.0	1.0	0	0	3.0
w/corn (*DeBoles*), ¼ pkg.	200	4.0	43.0	2.0	0	15	5.0
garlic-parsley (*DeBoles*), ¼ pkg.	200	8.0	41.0	.5	0	5	2.0
w/Jerusalem artichoke (*DeBoles*), ¼ pkg.	210	7.0	41.0	1.0	0	0	1.0
kamut (*Eden* Organic)	190	10.0	33.0	1.5	0	0	6.0
parsley garlic (*Eden* Organic)	210	8.0	41.0	1.0	0	0	4.0
w/rice (*DeBoles*), ¼ pkg.	210	7.0	41.0	1.0	0	70	1.0
w/spinach (*DeBoles*), ¼ pkg.	200	8.0	41.0	.5	0	15	2.0
tomato-basil (*DeBoles*), ¼ pkg.	200	7.0	41.0	.5	0	0	2.0
whole grain (*Eden* Organic)	210	10.0	40.0	1.5	0	0	6.0
spirals:							
kamut (*Eden* Organic)	190	10.0	33.0	1.5	0	0	6.0
w/rice (*DeBoles*), ¼ pkg.	210	4.0	46.0	0	0	0	1.0
rye (*Eden*)	200	6.0	44.0	0	0	10	8.0
sesame rice (*Eden* Organic)	200	9.0	37.0	2.0	0	0	6.0
spinach (*Eden* Organic)	210	8.0	41.0	1.0	0	0	4.0
vegetable (*Eden* Organic)	200	8.0	40.0	1.0	0	0	3.0
tricolor (*Borden*)	210	7.0	42.0	1.0	0	20	1.0

Food and Measure	cal.	prot. (gms)	carbo. (gms)	fat (gms)	chol. (mgs)	sod. (mgs)	fiber (gms)
Pasta *(cont.)*							
tubes, endless (*Eden Organic*)	210	8.0	41.0	1.0	0	0	4.0
twisted pair, kamut-quinoa (*Eden Organic*)	210	8.0	40.0	2.0	0	0	5.0
twists, pesto (*Eden Organic*)	200	8.0	40.0	1.0	0	0	3.0
whole wheat, all styles, except ribbon (*DeBoles*)	210	9.0	40.0	2.0	0	0	5.0
ziti (*DeBoles*)	210	7.0	41.0	1.0	0	0	1.0
Pasta, cooked, 1 cup:							
plain	197	6.7	39.7	.9	0	1	2.4
corn	176	3.7	39.1	1.0	0	1	3.4
spinach	183	6.4	36.6	.9	0	20	n.a.
whole wheat	174	7.5	37.2	.6	0	4	6.3
Pasta, refrigerated (see also specific pasta listings), plain:							
uncooked:							
w/egg, 2 oz.	163	6.4	31.0	1.3	41	15	2.0
spinach, w/egg, 2 oz.	164	6.4	31.6	1.2	41	15	n.a.
cooked:							
w/egg, 4 oz.	149	5.8	28.3	1.2	37	7	n.a.
spinach, w/egg, 4 oz.	147	5.7	28.4	1.1	37	7	n.a.
Pasta dinner, frozen (see also specific pasta listings), w/beef and broccoli (*Marie Callender's*), 15-oz. pkg.	570	35.0	73.0	15.0	70	1160	6.0
Pasta dishes, frozen (see also "Pasta entree, frozen"), 2 cups, except as noted:							
Alfredo (*Green Giant Pasta Accents*)	210	9.0	25.0	8.0	15	480	4.0

Food and Measure	cal.	prot. (gms)	carbo. (gms)	fat (gms)	chol. (mgs)	sod. (mgs)	fiber (gms)
cheddar:							
(*Freshlike Pasta Combo's* Classic)	200	6.0	24.0	9.0	10	500	2.0
creamy (*Green Giant Pasta Accents*), 2⅓ cups	250	9.0	36.0	8.0	15	700	5.0
white (*Birds Eye Pasta Secrets*) ...	240	7.0	30.0	10.0	10	560	2.0
white (*Green Giant Pasta Accents*), 1¾ cups	270	9.0	37.0	9.0	10	750	3.0
cheese, three (*Birds Eye Pasta Secrets*)	230	9.0	31.0	8.0	5	590	2.0
Florentine (*Green Giant Pasta Accents*)	310	13.0	44.0	9.0	20	910	5.0
garden herb seasoning (*Green Giant Pasta Accents*)	230	9.0	32.0	7.0	15	750	7.0
garlic:							
(*Green Giant Pasta Accents*)	260	7.0	36.0	10.0	15	640	3.0
herb (*Freshlike Pasta Combo's*)	260	7.0	33.0	11.0	5	330	2.0
zesty (*Birds Eye Pasta Secrets*) ...	240	7.0	31.0	10.0	5	310	2.0
herb, Italian (*Freshlike Pasta Combo's*), 2⅓ cups	240	9.0	32.0	9.0	5	700	2.0
lasagna style (*Green Giant Pasta Accents*)	260	9.0	33.0	10.0	10	540	4.0
marinara (*Cascadian Farm Veggie Bowl*), 9 oz.	180	11.0	30.0	3.0	0	600	3.0
Oriental style (*Green Giant Pasta Accents*), 2½ cups ...	260	8.0	35.0	10.0	20	580	4.0
pepper, roasted (*Freshlike Pasta Combo's*), 1 cup ...	310	7.0	32.0	16.0	25	460	2.0

Food and Measure	cal.	prot. (gms)	carbo. (gms)	fat (gms)	chol. (mgs)	sod. (mgs)	fiber (gms)
Pasta dishes, frozen *(cont.)*							
peppercorn:							
(*Freshlike Pasta Combo's*),							
2¼ cups	320	8.0	33.0	17.0	25	510	3.0
creamy (*Birds Eye Pasta Secrets*),							
2 cups	300	7.0	29.0	15.0	25	460	2.0
pesto, Italian (*Birds Eye Pasta Secrets*),							
2 cups	240	9.0	32.0	9.0	5	700	2.0
primavera:							
(*Birds Eye Pasta Secrets*), 2 cups	230	9.0	26.0	10.0	10	430	3.0
(*Cascadian Farm Veggie Bowl*),							
9 oz.	270	11.0	37.0	8.0	6	620	2.0
(*Green Giant Pasta Accents*),							
2¼ cups	290	12.0	39.0	9.0	5	530	4.0
creamy (*Freshlike Pasta Combo's*),							
2¼ cups	230	9.0	27.0	10.0	10	450	2.0
salad, no dressing:							
w/seafood (*Fitness First*), 1 cup	110	6.0	21.0	.5	0	200	2.0
w/shrimp (*Fitness First*), 1 cup	110	6.0	20.0	.5	15	170	2.0
vegetarian (*Fitness First*), 1 cup	100	4.0	19.0	0	0	25	3.0
w/white turkey (*Fitness First*), 1 cup	110	6.0	20.0	1.0	5	190	2.0
Pasta dishes, mix							
(see also specific pasta listings), 1 cup*, except as noted:							
broccoli:							
(*Pasta Roni*)	330	10.0	40.0	15.0	5	910	2.0

Food and Measure	cal.	prot. (gms)	carbo. (gms)	fat (gms)	chol. (mgs)	sod. (mgs)	fiber (gms)
au gratin (*Pasta Roni*)	280	10.0	39.0	10.0	5	900	2.0
and mushroom (*Pasta Roni*)	450	11.0	49.0	24.0	5	1130	2.0
butter and herb (*Lipton* Pasta & Sauce)	270	7.0	40.0	9.5	5	830	2.0
cheddar:							
broccoli (*Lipton* Pasta & Sauce)	340	11.0	49.0	10.5	15	970	1.0
mild (*Lipton* Pasta & Sauce)	290	10.0	41.0	10.0	10	930	<1.0
mild (*Pasta Roni*)	290	10.0	39.0	11.0	10	89	1.0
chicken:							
(*Pasta Roni*)	320	10.0	41.0	13.5	5	1020	2.0
(*Pasta Roni* Home-style)	230	7.0	39.0	6.0	0	930	3.0
and garlic (*Pasta Roni* Low Fat) . . .	210	8.0	39.0	3.0	5	990	2.0
herb Parmesan (*Lipton* Pasta & Sauce)	280	8.0	43.0	9.0	5	910	2.0
stir-fry (*Lipton* Pasta & Sauce)	270	8.0	43.0	8.0	0	900	2.0
garlic, creamy:							
(*Fantastic Foods Ready, Set, Pasta!* Cup), 2.2 oz.	240	10.0	42.0	3.5	10	590	1.0
(*Lipton* Pasta & Sauce)	350	10.0	50.0	13.0	15	980	1.0
garlic, roasted:							
chicken (*Lipton* Pasta & Sauce)	290	9.0	43.0	9.5	10	880	<1.0
and olive oil w/tomato (*Lipton* Pasta & Sauce)	270	8.0	42.0	8.5	0	880	2.0
hamburger, see "Hamburger entree mix"							
herb:							
and butter (*Pasta Roni*)	430	10.0	43.0	25.0	5	910	2.0

Food and Measure	cal.	prot. (gms)	carbo. (gms)	fat (gms)	chol. (mgs)	sod. (mgs)	fiber (gms)
Pasta dishes, mix, herb *(cont.)*							
savory, w/garlic (*Lipton* Pasta & Sauce)	280	8.0	52.0	9.0	5	890	2.0
mushroom, creamy (*Lipton* Pasta & Sauce)	320	10.0	46.0	10.5	15	870	0
Oriental stir-fry (*Pasta Roni*)	290	7.0	38.0	12.0	0	890	2.0
Parmesan:							
(*Pasta Roni* Parmesano)	390	12.0	49.0	17.0	5	950	2.0
smoke (*Fantastic Foods Ready, Set, Pasta!* Cup), 2.1 oz.	230	10.0	42.0	3.0	10	590	1.0
Romanoff (*Pasta Roni*)	400	11.0	46.0	20.0	10	1070	2.0
salad, ¾ cup*, except as noted:							
Caesar (*Suddenly Salad*)	220	5.0	30.0	9.0	0	580	1.0
Caesar (*Suddenly Salad* Low Fat)	170	5.0	30.0	3.0	0	580	1.0
Caesar, creamy (*Kraft*)	350	7.0	30.0	22.0	15	650	2.0
classic (*Suddenly Salad*)	250	7.0	8.0	38.0	0	910	2.0
classic (*Suddenly Salad* Lower Fat)	210	7.0	38.0	3.5	0	910	2.0
garden, Italian (*Suddenly Salad*)	140	5.0	28.0	1.0	0	520	2.0
garden primavera (*Kraft*)	280	8.0	34.0	12.0	<5	730	2.0
Italian (*Kraft* Light)	190	8.0	34.0	2.0	<5	660	2.0
Italian pepperoni (*Suddenly Salad*), 1 cup*	190	6.0	35.0	4.0	0	680	2.0
Italian pepperoni (*Suddenly Salad* Low Fat), 1 cup*	180	6.0	35.0	2.0	0	680	2.0

Food and Measure	cal.	prot. (gms)	carbo. (gms)	fat (gms)	chol. (mgs)	sod. (mgs)	fiber (gms)
Parmesan pepper-corn (*Kraft*)	360	8.0	28.0	25.0	20	610	2.0
ranch and bacon (*Kraft*)	360	7.0	30.0	23.0	15	500	2.0
ranch and bacon (*Suddenly Salad*)	330	7.0	30.0	20.0	15	480	1.0
ranch and bacon (*Suddenly Salad Low Fat*)	180	7.0	30.0	2.0	<5	530	1.0
spicy Thai (*Fantastic Foods Ready, Set, Pasta!* cup), 1.9 oz.	200	7.0	40.0	2.0	0	540	2.0
Stroganoff (*Pasta Roni*)	360	12.0	48.0	14.0	10	1020	2.0
Pasta entree, canned or packaged (see also specific listings), 1 cup:							
and chicken (*Hormel Health Selections*)	120	7.0	21.0	1.0	25	530	1.0
w/meat sauce, twists (*Franco-American Superiore*)	250	9.0	41.0	5.0	10	1160	2.0
w/meatballs: (*Chef Boyardee Junior* Dinosaurs)	290	8.0	39.0	11.0	35	990	2.0
in tomato sauce (*Franco-American Garfield*)	260	11.0	31.0	11.0	20	1150	5.0
tomato-cheese sauce (*Chef Boyardee Junior* ABC's/123's)	200	5.0	43.0	.5	<5	900	2.0
Pasta entree, dried, 1 serving: (*AlpineAire* Pasta Roma)	340	17.0	46.0	10.0	25	730	3.0
primavera (*Mountain House*)	220	10.0	32.0	6.0	20	690	4.0
stew, whole wheat (*AlpineAire*)	260	11.0	50.0	1.5	0	600	6.0

Food and Measure	cal.	prot. (gms)	carbo. (gms)	fat (gms)	chol. (mgs)	sod. (mgs)	fiber (gms)
Pasta entree, frozen (see also "Pasta dishes, frozen" and specific pasta listings), 1 pkg., except as noted:							
Alfredo, primavera (*Lean Cuisine*), 10 oz.	290	11.0	46.0	7.0	10	570	3.0
cheddar, w/beef and tomatoes (*Stouffer's*), 11 oz.	500	26.0	44.0	24.0	40	1200	2.0
w/cheddar and broccoli (*Banquet*), 9½ oz.	330	11.0	48.0	11.0	15	810	5.0
w/Italian sausage: (*Banquet* Family), 1 cup	340	12.0	28.0	20.0	35	920	3.0
and peppers (*Banquet*), 9½ oz. . . .	300	10.0	39.0	12.0	15	760	6.0
primavera: (*Amy's*), 9½ oz. . . .	320	15.0	39.0	12.0	65	680	3.0
Parmesan (*The Budget Gourmet Value Classics* Low Fat), 8 oz.	230	9.0	34.0	6.0	10	540	4.0
and spinach Romano (*Smart Ones*), 10.4 oz.	260	12.0	35.0	8.0	15	510	4.0
stuffed, trio (*Marie Callender's*), 10½ oz.	380	18.0	40.0	16.0	50	950	5.0
w/tomato-basil sauce (*Smart Ones*), 9.6 oz.	260	10.0	40.0	7.0	10	360	3.0
vegetable Italiano (*Healthy Choice*), 10 oz.	240	9.0	48.0	1.5	5	480	6.0
in wine-mushroom sauce (*The Budget Gourmet* Low Fat), 8½ oz.	270	13.0	39.0	7.0	25	770	4.0

Food and Measure	cal.	prot. (gms)	carbo. (gms)	fat (gms)	chol. (mgs)	sod. (mgs)	fiber (gms)
wraps, 12 oz.:							
beef Bolognese (*Wolfgang Puck's*)	530	26.0	70.0	17.0	100	730	6.0
chicken and spinach (*Wolfgang Puck's*)	460	22.0	68.0	11.0	100	540	6.0
sausage, Italian (*Wolfgang Puck's*)	700	36.0	67.0	29.0	160	1010	6.0
Pasta flour, see "Semolina flour"							
Pasta salad, see "Pasta dishes, mix"							
Pasta sauce, tomato (see also "Tomato sauce" and specific listings), ½ cup:							
(*Del Monte* Traditional)	60	2.0	15.0	.5	0	590	3.0
(*Eden* Organic Spaghetti)	80	3.0	12.0	2.5	0	320	3.0
(*Eden* Organic Spaghetti No Salt)	80	3.0	12.0	2.5	0	10	3.0
(*Healthy Choice* Traditional)	50	2.0	10.0	0	0	380	2.0
(*Hunt's* Original)	65	2.0	11.0	2.0	0	475	3.0
(*Muir Glen* Chunky)	80	2.0	13.0	2.0	0	300	3.0
(*Prego* Extra Chunky Tomato Supreme)	130	2.0	22.0	4.0	0	480	3.0
(*Prego* No Salt)	110	2.0	11.0	6.0	0	25	3.0
(*Prego* Traditional) ...	140	2.0	23.0	4.5	0	610	2.0
(*Progresso* Spaghetti)	100	3.0	12.0	4.5	<5	620	2.0
(*Ragú Old World Traditional*)	80	2.0	10.0	3.0	0	820	3.0
basil:							
(*Classico* Di Napoli)	50	2.0	9.0	1.0	0	390	2.0
(*Del Monte*)	70	2.0	16.0	1.0	0	600	3.0
(*Prego*)	110	2.0	19.0	3.0	0	420	3.0
(*Ragú* Light)	50	2.0	11.0	0	0	390	2.0
(*Ragú* Light No Sugar)	60	3.0	9.0	1.5	0	390	3.0

Food and Measure	cal.	prot. (gms)	carbo. (gms)	fat (gms)	chol. (mgs)	sod. (mgs)	fiber (gms)
Pasta sauce, basil *(cont.)*							
summer (*Five Brothers*)	60	2.0	10.0	1.5	0	470	3.0
beef:							
ground (*Aunt Millie's* Chunky)	100	3.0	16.0	2.5	<5	670	2.0
sautéed (*Ragú* Hearty)	120	3.0	18.0	4.0	<5	530	3.0
cheese, see "Cheese sauce, cooking"							
w/cheese:							
(*Hunt's* Classic) . . .	45	3.0	7.5	1.0	<5	545	1.5
four (*Classico* Di Parma)	80	2.0	8.0	4.0	<5	500	1.0
four (*Del Monte*) . . .	70	2.0	15.0	1.5	0	680	3.0
three (*Prego*)	100	3.0	18.0	2.0	5	460	3.0
eggplant, grilled, w/Parmesan (*Five Brothers*)	100	3.0	13.0	3.0	0	540	3.0
garden combination:							
(*Prego* Extra Chunky)	100	2.0	19.0	2.0	0	480	3.0
(*Ragú* Chunky Garden)	110	2.0	18.0	3.5	0	540	3.0
chunky (*Ragú* Light)	50	2.0	11.0	0	0	390	3.0
garlic (*Prego* Extra Chunky Supreme)	140	2.0	23.0	4.5	0	520	3.0
garlic, roasted:							
(*Classico* Di Sorrento)	60	2.0	9.0	1.5	0	390	2.0
(*Healthy Choice*) . . .	50	2.0	11.0	0	0	295	3.0
(*Muir Glen*)	50	2.0	9.0	0	0	350	2.0
(*Ragú* Hearty)	120	2.0	21.0	3.0	0	570	3.0
and herb (*Prego*)	110	2.0	17.0	3.5	0	520	3.0
and onion (*Hunt's* Classic)	60	1.0	12.5	1.0	0	525	2.0
Parmesan (*Prego* Extra Chunky) . . .	120	3.0	23.0	1.5	5	550	3.0
garlic and herb:							
(*Del Monte* Chunky)	60	2.0	11.0	1.5	0	490	<1.0
(*Healthy Choice*) . . .	50	2.0	10.0	0	0	340	2.0

Food and Measure	cal.	prot. (gms)	carbo. (gms)	fat (gms)	chol. (mgs)	sod. (mgs)	fiber (gms)
(*Hunt's* Classic) . . .	40	2.0	8.0	.5	0	560	3.0
garlic and mushroom (*Healthy Choice* Garlic Lover's)	45	2.0	10.0	0	0	360	2.0
garlic and onion:							
(*Contadina*)	80	3.0	12.0	2.0	0	690	3.0
(*Del Monte*)	80	2.0	16.0	1.0	0	490	2.0
(*Muir Glen*)	50	2.0	11.0	0	0	300	3.0
(*Ragú* Chunky Garden)	120	2.0	19.0	3.5	0	550	3.0
oven roasted (*Five Brothers*)	70	2.0	10.0	1.5	0	530	3.0
garlic and sun-dried tomato (*Healthy Choice*)	50	2.0	11.0	0	0	360	3.0
green pepper and mushroom:							
(*Del Monte*)	80	2.0	16.0	1.0	0	490	3.0
(*Muir Glen*)	70	2.0	10.0	2.0	0	360	4.0
hamburger (*Prego*)	120	3.0	17.0	4.0	10	580	3.0
herb:							
(*Ragú* Hearty)	110	3.0	18.0	3.0	0	580	3.0
Italian (*Del Monte* Chunky)	60	2.0	12.0	1.0	0	520	<1.0
Italian (*Muir Glen*)	60	2.0	13.0	0	0	300	2.0
and olive oil (*Ragú* Pasta Toss)	120	2.0	11.0	8.0	0	900	2.0
Italian, cooking (*Ragú* Traditional)	60	2.0	8.0	2.0	0	550	3.0
leek and sun-dried tomato (*Al Dente* Luscious)	100	2.0	9.0	7.0	0	370	1.0
marinara:							
(*Aunt Millie's* Chunky)	90	2.0	18.0	1.5	0	640	2.0
(*Aunt Millie's* Traditional)	70	2.0	9.0	3.0	0	320	2.0
(*Contadina*)	80	2.0	14.0	3.0	0	440	1.0
(*Prego*)	110	2.0	12.0	6.0	0	670	3.0
(*Prince* Chunky) . . .	70	2.0	13.0	1.5	0	610	2.0
(*Prince* Traditional)	50	2.0	9.0	.5	0	570	2.0

Food and Measure	cal.	prot. (gms)	carbo. (gms)	fat (gms)	chol. (mgs)	sod. (mgs)	fiber (gms)
Pasta sauce, marinara *(cont.)*							
(*Progresso*)	80	2.0	8.0	4.5	<5	480	2.0
(*Progresso* Authentic)	100	4.0	12.0	4.0	<5	590	3.0
(*Ragú* Old World)	80	2.0	9.0	4.5	0	820	3.0
cabernet (*Muir Glen*)	50	2.0	9.0	0	0	350	2.0
w/pizza paste (*Aunt Millie's*)	70	2.0	9.0	2.5	0	330	3.0
meat/meat flavor:							
(*Aunt Millie's* Traditional)	80	3.0	9.0	3.0	<5	330	2.0
(*Del Monte*)	60	3.0	14.0	1.0	<5	720	3.0
(*Hunt's*)	60	2.0	10.0	1.0	0	600	3.0
(*Prego*)	140	3.0	21.0	6.0	5	500	3.0
(*Prince* Chunky) . . .	90	2.0	13.0	3.0	<5	620	2.0
(*Prince* Traditional)	50	3.0	7.0	1.5	<5	620	2.0
(*Progresso*)	100	4.0	12.0	4.5	5	610	3.0
(*Ragú* Old World)	80	2.0	9.0	3.5	<5	820	3.0
mushroom:							
(*Aunt Millie's* Traditional)	70	2.0	10.0	2.0	0	330	2.0
(*Del Monte*)	60	2.0	16.0	1.0	0	490	2.0
(*Healthy Choice*) . . .	50	2.0	11.0	0	0	380	2.0
(*Hunt's*)	50	2.0	9.0	<1.0	0	605	2.5
(*Prego* Extra Chunky Supreme)	130	3.0	21.0	4.5	5	490	3.0
(*Prego* Made With Mushrooms)	150	2.0	23.0	5.0	0	670	3.0
(*Prince* Chunky) . . .	70	2.0	13.0	1.5	0	670	2.0
(*Prince* Traditional)	50	2.0	9.0	.5	0	580	2.0
(*Ragú* Old World)	80	2.0	10.0	3.0	0	820	3.0
and diced tomatoes (*Prego* Extra Chunky)	110	2.0	19.0	3.0	0	510	3.0
w/extra spice (*Prego* Extra Chunky) . . .	120	2.0	19.0	4.0	0	510	3.0
and garlic (*Prego*)	110	2.0	20.0	2.0	0	500	3.0
and garlic, chunky (*Ragú* Light)	50	3.0	11.0	0	0	390	2.0
and green pepper (*Contadina*)	80	3.0	12.0	2.0	0	690	3.0

Food and Measure	cal.	prot. (gms)	carbo. (gms)	fat (gms)	chol. (mgs)	sod. (mgs)	fiber (gms)
and green pepper (*Prego* Extra Chunky)	120	2.0	18.0	4.5	5	430	6.0
and green pepper (*Ragú* Chunky Garden)	110	2.0	18.0	3.5	0	570	3.0
and herb (*Muir Glen*)	45	2.0	10.0	0	0	360	2.0
and olives (*Classico Di Sicilia*)	70	2.0	11.0	1.5	0	430	2.0
and onion (*Ragú* Chunky Garden)	120	2.0	19.0	3.5	0	560	3.0
Parmesan (*Prego*)	130	3.0	23.0	3.5	10	480	2.0
portobello (*Classico Di Toscana*)	70	2.0	11.0	1.5	0	420	2.0
portobello (*Muir Glen*)	60	2.0	10.0	2.0	0	380	2.0
sautéed (*Five Brothers*)	70	2.0	10.0	3.0	0	440	3.0
super (*Ragú* Chunky Garden)	120	3.0	19.0	3.5	0	530	2.0
and sweet pepper (*Healthy Choice*)	40	2.0	9.0	0	0	310	2.0
olive and caper (*Al Dente* Outrageous)	90	1.0	8.0	7.0	0	450	1.0
olive and garlic (*Ragú* Chunky Garden) ...	120	2.0	18.0	4.5	0	600	3.0
onion and garlic: (*Prego* Extra Chunky)	110	2.0	19.0	3.5	0	480	3.0
diced (*Prego*)	120	2.0	18.0	4.5	0	520	3.0
sautéed (*Ragú* Hearty)	120	2.0	18.0	4.0	0	510	4.0
onion and mushroom (*Ragú* Hearty)	110	2.0	17.0	3.5	0	540	3.0
Parmesan: (*Prego*)	140	3.0	23.0	3.5	5	500	3.0
and Romano (*Ragú* Hearty)	120	4.0	18.0	3.5	<5	570	3.0

Food and Measure	cal.	prot. (gms)	carbo. (gms)	fat (gms)	chol. (mgs)	sod. (mgs)	fiber (gms)
Pasta sauce *(cont.)*							
peppers, sweet, and Italian sausage (*Aunt Millie's* Traditional)	60	3.0	8.0	2.0	5	350	2.0
peppers and onions (*Classico* Di Salerno)	60	2.0	9.0	2.0	0	410	2.0
pepperoni (*Prego*) ...	120	3.0	18.0	4.5	10	570	3.0
pizza (*Eden* Organic)	80	3.0	12.0	2.5	0	320	3.0
primavera (*Contadina*)	60	2.0	9.0	2.0	0	260	1.0
red pepper:							
(*Jacques Pépin's Kitchen* Pasta & Seafood)	50	1.0	7.0	2.5	5	330	1.0
roasted (*Muir Glen*)	60	1.0	10.0	1.5	0	380	2.0
roasted, and garlic (*Five Brothers*)	90	3.0	13.0	3.0	0	520	3.0
roasted, and garlic (*Prego*)	110	2.0	18.0	3.5	0	530	3.0
roasted, and onion (*Ragú* Chunky Garden)	120	2.0	18.0	3.5	0	530	2.0
spicy (*Classico* Di Roma Arrabbiata)	60	2.0	6.0	2.5	0	270	2.0
spicy (*Ragú* Hearty)	110	2.0	21.0	1.5	0	510	3.0
red wine and herbs (*Ragú* Hearty)	100	2.0	16.0	3.0	0	550	3.0
Romano:							
(*Muir Glen*)	90	2.0	14.0	2.5	0	300	4.0
w/garlic (*Five Brothers*)	90	3.0	10.0	4.0	<5	570	3.0
peccorino and herb (*Classico* Di Palermo)	80	4.0	8.0	3.0	<5	410	2.0
sausage, Italian:							
(*Hunt's* Chunky) ...	65	2.5	9.5	1.5	<5	540	3.0
and fennel (*Classico* D'Abruzzi)	90	4.0	7.0	5.0	10	470	2.0
and garlic (*Prego*)	120	3.0	16.0	5.0	10	500	3.0

Food and Measure	cal.	prot. (gms)	carbo. (gms)	fat (gms)	chol. (mgs)	sod. (mgs)	fiber (gms)
spinach and cheese:							
(*Ragú* Chunky Garden)	120	2.0	18.0	3.5	0	550	3.0
Florentine (*Classico* Di Firenze)	80	3.0	8.0	4.5	<5	490	2.0
sun-dried tomato:							
(*Muir Glen*)	45	1.0	8.0	0	0	350	2.0
and olive (*Classico* Di Capri)	80	2.0	8.0	4.0	0	430	2.0
sweet pepper and onion:							
(*Muir Glen*)	40	2.0	8.0	0	0	300	1.0
(*Ragú* Chunky Garden)	110	2.0	19.0	3.5	0	570	2.0
tomato:							
bits (*Angelia Mia*)	50	1.5	11.0	<1.0	0	610	2.5
fire-roasted, and garlic (*Classico* Di Siena)	60	2.0	10.0	1.0	0	390	2.0
Mediterranean roasted (*Five Brothers*)	90	3.0	12.0	3.0	0	520	3.0
Provençale (*Jacques Pépin's Kitchen* Pasta & Chicken)	80	1.0	8.0	5.0	0	460	<1.0
spicy and pesto (*Classico* Di Genoa)	90	3.0	9.0	5.0	0	530	2.0
vegetables:							
(*Healthy Choice* Chunky)	40	2.0	9.0	0	0	300	2.0
(*Hunt's* Chunky)	60	1.5	13.0	1.0	0	530	2.0
(*Prego* Extra Chunky Supreme)	120	2.0	18.0	4.0	10	500	3.0
garden (*Contadina*)	60	2.0	9.0	2.0	0	260	1.0
garden (*Muir Glen*)	60	1.0	9.0	3.0	0	370	1.0
garden, primavera (*Five Brothers*)	70	2.0	11.0	2.0	0	490	3.0
super, primavera (*Ragú* Chunky Garden)	110	2.0	17.0	3.5	0	480	4.0

Food and Measure	cal.	prot. (gms)	carbo. (gms)	fat (gms)	chol. (mgs)	sod. (mgs)	fiber (gms)
Pasta sauce, refrigerated, tomato, ½ cup, except as noted:							
cheese, four (*Di Giorno*), ¼ cup	200	5.0	2.0	19.0	45	410	0
marinara:							
(*Contadina*)	80	2.0	9.0	4.0	0	550	2.0
(*Di Giorno*)	100	3.0	12.0	4.5	<5	530	3.0
garlic, roasted (*Contadina*)	60	2.0	10.0	2.0	0	550	1.0
mushroom (*Contadina*)	70	2.0	11.0	2.5	0	480	3.0
meat (*Di Giorno* Traditional)	120	6.0	12.0	6.0	15	610	3.0
olive oil–garlic, w/cheeses (*Di Giorno*), ¼ cup	370	9.0	3.0	36.0	20	540	0
tomato:							
chunky, w/basil (*Di Giorno Light Varieties*)	70	2.0	16.0	0	0	290	2.0
herb Parmesan (*Contadina*)	140	3.0	12.0	9.0	10	720	4.0
plum, and mushroom (*Di Giorno*)	70	2.0	15.0	0	0	310	2.0
vegetable, garden (*Contadina*)	40	1.0	9.0	0	0	540	2.0
Pasta sauce mix (see also specific sauce listings):							
(*Knorr* Parma Rosa Pasta Sauces), 2 tbsp.	60	2.0	8.0	2.5	<5	550	0
garlic herb (*Knorr* Pasta Sauces), 2 tbsp.	70	1.0	8.0	3.5	0	860	0
sun-dried tomato (*Knorr* Pasta Sauces), 1 tbsp. . . .	45	1.0	9.0	.5	0	840	1.0

Food and Measure	cal.	prot. (gms)	carbo. (gms)	fat (gms)	chol. (mgs)	sod. (mgs)	fiber (gms)
Pasta seasoning, see "Pizza seasoning"							
Pasta wrap, see "Pasta entree, frozen"							
Pastrami, 2 oz., except as noted:							
(*Boar's Head* First Cut)	90	12.0	2.0	4.0	30	620	0
(*Boar's Head* Red Round)	80	12.0	1.0	3.0	35	460	0
(*Boar's Head* Round)	70	12.0	<1.0	2.5	30	530	0
(*Healthy Choice*)	60	10.0	1.0	1.5	30	410	0
(*Healthy Choice* Deli-Thin Savory Selections), 6 slices, 1.9 oz.	70	11.0	2.0	1.5	25	400	0
(*Healthy Deli*)	80	11.0	3.0	3.0	30	480	0
(*Hebrew National* Deli Thin Sliced), 4 slices, 2 oz.	90	6.0	5.0	4.0	35	500	0
(*Hebrew National* Thin Sliced), 4 slices, 2 oz.	90	13.0	1.0	4.0	35	500	0
turkey, see "Turkey pastrami"							
Pastry, see specific listings							
Pastry filling (see also "Pie filling"), canned, 2 tbsp.:							
almond (*Solo*)	120	1.0	23.0	2.5	0	45	2.0
apple, Dutch (*Solo*)	80	0	20.0	0	0	45	1.0
apricot (*Solo*)	80	0	17.0	0	0	20	1.0
blueberry (*Solo*)	80	0	17.0	0	0	25	1.0
cherry (*Solo*)	80	0	20.0	0	0	25	1.0
date (*Solo*)	100	0	22.0	0	0	40	3.0
nut, fancy (*Solo*)	140	1.0	25.0	5.0	0	55	5.0
pecan (*Solo*)	130	1.0	24.0	4.0	0	50	1.0
pineapple (*Solo*)	80	0	19.0	0	0	20	1.0
poppy seed (*Solo*) ...	140	2.0	30.0	4.0	0	30	3.0
prune plum (*Solo*) ...	70	0	18.0	0	0	25	1.0

Food and Measure	cal.	prot. (gms)	carbo. (gms)	fat (gms)	chol. (mgs)	sod. (mgs)	fiber (gms)
Pastry filling *(cont.)*							
raspberry (*Solo*)	80	0	19.0	0	0	25	1.0
strawberry (*Solo*)	70	0	18.0	0	0	20	1.0
Pastry flour, see "Wheat flour"							
Pastry shell (see also "Pie crust"):							
puff:							
patty shell (*Pepperidge Farm*), 1 pc.	230	3.0	23.0	14.0	0	135	2.0
sheet (*Pepperidge Farm*), ⅙ sheet	200	3.0	23.0	11.0	0	135	3.0
tart, 3″ shell:							
(*Oronoque*)	140	2.0	12.0	9.0	0	140	0
(*Pet-Ritz*)	130	1.0	13.0	8.0	0	170	0
Pâté, canned (see also "Liverwurst"):							
1 oz.	90	4.0	.4	7.9	n.a.	198	0
1 tbsp.	41	1.9	.2	3.6	n.a.	91	0
chicken liver:							
1 oz.	57	3.8	1.9	3.7	n.a.	n.a.	0
1 tbsp.	26	1.8	.9	1.7	n.a.	n.a.	0
goose liver:							
smoked, 1 oz.	131	3.2	1.3	12.4	43	n.a.	0
smoked, 1 tbsp. . . .	60	1.5	.6	5.7	20	n.a.	0
Pâté, refrigerated (*Charcuterie de Bretagne* de Campagne), 2 oz.	200	6.0	2.0	18.0	60	300	0
Pea pods, see "Peas, edible-podded"							
Peach, fresh:							
2½″ peach, 4 per lb.	37	.6	9.7	.1	0	tr.	1.7
sliced, ½ cup	37	.6	9.4	.1	0	1	1.7
Peach, canned, halves or slices, ½ cup, except as noted:							
in juice:							
(*Del Monte* Fruit Naturals)	60	0	15.0	0	0	10	1.0

Food and Measure	cal.	prot. (gms)	carbo. (gms)	fat (gms)	chol. (mgs)	sod. (mgs)	fiber (gms)
(*Del Monte* Fruit Naturals cup), 4 oz.	50	0	13.0	0	0	10	<1.0
(*Libby's* Lite)	60	1.0	13.0	0	0	10	1.0
in extra light syrup:							
(*Del Monte* Lite Cling)	60	0	15.0	0	0	10	1.0
(*Del Monte* Lite cup), 4 oz.	50	0	13.0	0	0	10	<1.0
(*Del Monte* Lite Freestone)	60	0	14.0	0	0	10	1.0
in light syrup:							
(*Del Monte* Orchard Select)	80	<1.0	20.0	0	0	10	<1.0
diced (*Del Monte* Cut-Ups), 4-oz. cup	80	<1.0	20.0	0	0	10	<1.0
diced (*Del Monte* Fruit Express), 6-oz. cup	110	1.0	29.0	0	0	10	2.0
w/cinnamon (*Del Monte* Chunky Cut)	80	0	20.0	0	0	10	1.0
in heavy syrup:							
(*Del Monte/Del Monte* Melba) . . .	100	0	24.0	0	0	10	1.0
diced (*Del Monte* Cup), 4 oz.	80	0	20.0	0	0	10	<1.0
spiced, whole (*Del Monte*)	100	0	24.0	0	0	10	<1.0
in pear juice, wildberry flavor (*Del Monte* Fruit Express), 6-oz. cup	110	1.0	29.0	0	0	10	2.0
raspberry flavor, natural (*Del Monte*)	80	<1.0	20.0	0	0	10	<1.0
raspberry flavor, wild, in light syrup (*Del Monte* Fruit Rageous), 4-oz. cup	80	<1.0	20.0	0	0	10	<1.0

Food and Measure	cal.	prot. (gms)	carbo. (gms)	fat (gms)	chol. (mgs)	sod. (mgs)	fiber (gms)
Peach, canned *(cont.)*							
raspberry gel, diced (*Del Monte* Cut-Ups), 4-oz. cup	90	0	23.0	0	0	60	<1.0
in sauce (*Del Monte* Fruit Rageous Peachy Pie), 4-oz. cup	80	<1.0	21.0	0	0	10	<1.0
spice (*Del Monte* Natural Harvest)	80	<1.0	21.0	0	0	10	<1.0
Peach, dried:							
(*Sonoma* Organic), 4 pcs., 1.4 oz.	130	2.0	31.0	0	0	0	3.0
(*Sun•Maid*), ¼ cup	100	2.0	25.0	0	0	0	3.0
freeze-dried, diced (*AlpineAire*), .4 oz. ...	40	1.0	9.0	0	0	0	0
sulfured:							
halves, ½ cup	192	2.9	49.1	.6	0	6	6.6
halves, 4.6 oz.	311	4.7	79.7	1.0	0,	9	10.7
Peach, frozen, sliced, sweetened, ½ cup	118	.8	30.0	.2	0	8	1.8
Peach butter (*Smucker's*), 1 tbsp.	45	0	11.0	0	0	10	0
Peach drink blends:							
(*Fruitopia* Peachberry Quencher), 8 fl. oz.	112	0	30.0	0	0	58	0
mango (*Whipper Snapple*), 10 fl. oz.	150	0	39.0	0	0	60	0
Peach dumpling, frozen (*Pepperidge Farm*), 3-oz. pc. ...	300	3.0	47.0	11.0	0	150	6.0
Peach juice:							
(*After the Fall Georgia Peach*), 8 fl. oz. ...	100	1.0	27.0	0	0	20	0
(*Dole* Orchard), 8 fl. oz.	140	0	34.0	0	0	35	0
(*Snapple* Dixie), 12 fl. oz.	170	0	42.0	0	0	25	0
Peach nectar:							
(*Goya*), 6 fl. oz.	110	<1.0	27.0	0	0	30	1.0

Food and Measure	cal.	prot. (gms)	carbo. (gms)	fat (gms)	chol. (mgs)	sod. (mgs)	fiber (gms)
(*Kern's*), 11.5 fl. oz.	210	1.0	52.0	0	0	5	0
(*R.W. Knudsen*),							
8 fl. oz.	120	0	30.0	0	0	25	0
Peach salsa, see							
"Salsa"							
Peach-raspberry							
smoothie (*Del*							
Monte Blenders),							
5.5 fl. oz.	160	1.0	40.0	0	0	10	3.0
Peanut, shelled, 1 oz.,							
except as noted:							
(*Beer Nuts* Classic) . . .	170	7.0	7.0	14.0	0	80	2.0
(*Beer Nuts* Old Fash-							
ioned)	185	8.0	6.0	15.0	0	60	2.0
(*Paradise/White Swan*							
Fancy), ¼ cup,							
1½ oz.	270	11.0	7.0	22.0	0	135	5.0
(*River Queen* Salted),							
3 tbsp., 1 oz.	150	7.0	5.0	13.0	0	140	2.0
(*River Queen* Un-							
salted), 3 tbsp. or							
1 oz.	160	7.0	5.0	13.0	0	0	2.0
unroasted	159	7.2	4.5	13.8	0	5	2.5
boiled, salted	90	3.8	6.0	6.2	0	213	2.5
Cajun (*River Queen*),							
3 tbsp., .9 oz.	150	7.0	5.0	12.0	0	300	2.0
cocktail:							
(*Planters*)	170	7.0	6.0	14.0	0	115	2.0
(*Planters* Lightly							
Salted)	170	7.0	5.0	15.0	0	55	2.0
(*Planters* Unsalted)	170	7.0	6.0	14.0	0	0	2.0
dry-roasted:							
(*Arrowhead Mills*							
Valencia), ¼ cup	190	8.0	7.0	16.0	0	240	3.0
(*Frito-Lay*), 1.1 oz.	200	7.0	5.0	16.0	0	180	2.0
(*Planters* Lightly							
Salted)	170	8.0	5.0	14.0	0	95	3.0
(*Planters* Unsalted)	160	8.0	6.0	14.0	0	0	2.0
(*River Queen*)	160	7.0	6.0	13.0	0	250	2.0
(*River Queen* Un-							
salted)	160	7.0	6.0	14.0	0	0	2.0

Food and Measure	cal.	prot. (gms)	carbo. (gms)	fat (gms)	chol. (mgs)	sod. (mgs)	fiber (gms)
Peanut, dry-roasted *(cont.)*							
½ cup	428	17.3	15.7	36.3	0	4	5.8
honey mustard (*Beer Nuts*), ¼ cup, .9 oz.	140	4.0	19.0	5.0	0	55	1.0
honey-roasted:							
(*Frito-Lay*), 1.6 oz.	270	10.0	10.0	21.0	0	80	3.0
(*Planters*)	160	6.0	8.0	13.0	0	95	2.0
(*River Queen*), 3 tbsp., .9 oz. . . .	150	6.0	7.0	12.0	0	70	2.0
(*Weight Watchers*), .7 oz.	100	7.0	7.0	5.0	0	100	2.0
dry-roasted (*Planters*)	150	7.0	8.0	12.0	0	95	2.0
hot:							
(*Beer Nuts* Cajun Devil), ¼ cup, .9 oz.	140	4.0	16.0	6.0	0	140	1.0
(*Frito-Lay*), 1.1 oz.	190	7.0	6.0	16.0	0	250	2.0
oil-roasted, ½ cup . . .	419	19.0	13.6	35.5	0	4	6.6
w/sesame seeds (*Beer Nuts*), ¼ cup, .9 oz.	130	4.0	15.0	6.0	0	90	2.0
Spanish (*River Queen*), 3 tbsp., 1 oz.	150	7.0	5.0	13.0	0	140	2.0
sweetened, salted (*River Queen* Pub Nuts), ¼ cup, 1.2 oz.	190	7.0	10.0	15.0	0	160	2.0
Peanut butter, 2 tbsp.:							
(*Jif* Reduced Fat)	190	8.0	15.0	12.0	0	250	2.0
(*Teddie* Unsalted)	190	8.0	7.0	16.0	0	0	3.0
chunky or creamy:							
(*Arrowhead Mills*)	200	9.0	6.0	15.0	0	0	1.0
(*Arrowhead Mills* Easy Spread)	200	8.0	7.0	15.0	0	100	2.0
(*Laura Scudder's* Old Fashioned)	200	8.0	6.0	16.0	0	110	2.0
(*Laura Scudder's* Old Fashioned Unsalted)	200	8.0	6.0	16.0	0	5	2.0

Food and Measure	cal.	prot. (gms)	carbo. (gms)	fat (gms)	chol. (mgs)	sod. (mgs)	fiber (gms)
(*Laura Scudder's* Reduced Fat)	200	9.0	12.0	12.0	0	120	2.0
(*Peter Pan/Peter Pan Plus*)	190	8.0	6.0	16.0	0	120	2.0
(*Smucker's* Natural)	200	7.0	7.0	16.0	0	120	2.0
(*Smucker's* Natural No Salt)	200	7.0	7.0	2.0	0	0	2.0
(*Smucker's* Reduced Fat Natural)	200	9.0	12.0	12.0	0	120	2.0
honey-roasted (*Peter Pan*)	190	8.5	6.0	16.0	0	n.a.	2.0
chunky/crunchy:							
(*Adams*)	200	10.0	5.0	16.0	0	90	1.0
(*Adams* No Stir)	200	10.0	4.0	16.0	0	120	2.0
(*Adams* Unsalted)	200	10.0	5.0	16.0	0	5	2.0
(*Jif* Reduced Fat)	190	8.0	15.0	12.0	0	200	2.0
(*Simply Jif*)	190	8.0	7.0	16.0	0	50	2.0
extra (*Jif*)	190	8.0	7.0	16.0	0	130	2.0
super (*Teddie*)	190	6.0	7.0	16.0	0	130	2.0
super (*Teddie* Old Fashioned)	190	8.0	7.0	16.0	0	100	3.0
creamy/smooth:							
(*Adams*)	200	10.0	4.0	16.0	0	115	1.0
(*Adams* No Stir) . . .	210	10.0	4.0	17.0	0	160	2.0
(*Adams* Unsalted)	200	10.0	5.0	15.0	0	0	2.0
(*Jif*)	190	8.0	7.0	16.0	0	150	2.0
(*Peter Pan* Whipped)	140	6.0	5.0	12.0	0	110	2.0
(*Simply Jif*)	190	8.0	6.0	16.0	0	65	2.0
(*Teddie*)	190	6.0	7.0	17.0	0	160	2.0
(*Teddie* Old Fashioned)	190	8.0	7.0	16.0	0	125	3.0
(*Teddie* Spread 25% Less Fat)	190	9.0	13.0	12.0	0	140	2.0
(*Teddie* Unsalted No Sugar)	190	7.0	7.0	17.0	0	0	3.0
Peanut butter sprinkles (*Reese's*), 2 tbsp.	150	2.0	19.0	7.0	<5	50	0
Peanut butter–jelly (*Goober's*), 3 tbsp.	230	7.0	24.0	13.0	0	160	2.0

Food and Measure	cal.	prot. (gms)	carbo. (gms)	fat (gms)	chol. (mgs)	sod. (mgs)	fiber (gms)
Peanut flour, 1 cup:							
defatted	196	31.3	20.8	.3	0	9	n.a.
defatted, salted	196	31.3	20.8	.3	0	108	n.a.
low fat	257	20.3	18.8	13.1	0	0	n.a.
Peanut sauce, Thai satay (*Ka•Me*), 2 tbsp.	80	2.0	9.0	4.0	0	340	0
Peanut topping (see also specific listings), 2 tbsp.:							
(*Teddie*)	200	5.0	7.0	17.0	0	125	2.0
peanut butter caramel (*Smucker's*)	150	3.0	24.0	4.5	0	125	<1.0
Pear, fresh, w/peel:							
Bartlett, 1 medium, 2½ per lb.	98	.7	25.1	.7	0	1	4.0
sliced, ½ cup	49	.3	12.5	.3	0	1	2.0
Pear, Asian:							
(*Frieda's*), 5 oz.	60	1.0	15.0	0	0	0	5.0
medium, 2¼″ x 2½″ diam.	51	.6	13.0	.3	0	0	4.4
Pear, canned, halves or slices, ½ cup, except as noted:							
in juice:							
(*Del Monte* Fruit Naturals)	60	0	15.0	0	0	10	1.0
(*Libby's* Lite)	60	0	13.0	0	0	10	1.0
in extra light syrup:							
(*Del Monte* Lite)	60	0	15.0	0	0	10	1.0
(*Del Monte* Lite cup), 4 oz.	50	0	13.0	0	0	10	<1.0
in light syrup, Bartlett (*Del Monte* Orchard Select)	80	<1.0	20.0	0	0	10	2.0
in heavy syrup:							
(*Del Monte*)	100	0	24.0	0	0	10	1.0
diced (*Del Monte* cup), 4 oz.	80	0	20.0	0	0	10	<1.0

Food and Measure	cal.	prot. (gms)	carbo. (gms)	fat (gms)	chol. (mgs)	sod. (mgs)	fiber (gms)
cinnamon flavor, in light syrup (*Del Monte* Halves)	80	0	21.0	0	0	10	1.0
ginger flavor, natural (*Del Monte*)	90	0	22.0	0	0	10	1.0
Pear, dried:							
(*Sonoma* Organic), 4 pcs., 1.4 oz.	140	1.0	32.0	0	0	0	7.0
2 oz.	149	1.1	39.5	.4	0	4	4.3
halves, ½ cup	236	1.7	62.7	.6	0	5	6.8
Pear juice, 8 fl. oz.:							
(*After the Fall*)	100	0	22.0	0	0	30	0
(*After the Fall* Rouge River)	100	1.0	24.0	0	0	20	0
(*R.W. Knudsen* Organic)	120	0	30.0	0	0	25	0
Pear nectar:							
(*Goya*), 12 fl. oz.	240	1.0	59.0	0	0	20	2.0
(*Kern's/Libby's*), 11.5 fl. oz.	220	0	54.0	0	0	5	3.0
(*Libby's*), 8 fl. oz. ...	150	0	38.0	0	0	0	2.0
(*Santa Cruz* Organic), 8 fl. oz.	120	0	30.0	0	0	30	0
canned, 6 fl. oz.	112	.2	29.6	<.1	0	7	1.1
Peas, see specific listings							
Peas, black-eyed, see "Black-eyed peas"							
Peas, cream, canned, ½ cup:							
(*Bush's Best*)	110	7.0	18.0	1.0	0	500	5.0
(*East Texas Fair*)	100	6.0	17.0	1.0	0	460	5.0
Peas, crowder, ½ cup:							
canned:							
(*Allens/East Texas Fair/Homefolks*)	110	6.0	19.0	1.0	0	460	8.0
(*Bush's Best*)	110	7.0	18.0	1.0	0	500	5.0
frozen (*Mckenzie's*)	120	8.0	22.0	1.0	0	10	4.0

Food and Measure	cal.	prot. (gms)	carbo. (gms)	fat (gms)	chol. (mgs)	sod. (mgs)	fiber (gms)
Peas, edible podded, fresh:							
raw:							
(*Frieda's* Snow), 1 cup, 3 oz.	35	2.0	6.0	0	0	0	2.0
(*Frieda's* Sugar Snap), cup, 3 oz.	35	2.0	6.0	0	0	0	2.0
½ cup	30	2.0	5.4	.1	0	3	1.9
boiled, drained, ½ cup	34	2.6	5.6	.2	0	3	2.2
Peas, edible podded, frozen:							
(*Birds Eye Farm Fresh* Sugar Snap Stir Fry), ¾ cup	35	1.0	5.0	0	0	20	1.0
(*Birds Eye Sugar Snap* Deluxe), ½ cup	90	2.0	2.0	0	0	10	2.0
(*Freshlike* Snow Pea), 1 cup	50	2.0	6.0	0	0	10	2.0
(*Freshlike* Snow Pea Stir Fry), 2 cups . . .	100	4.0	6.0	.5	0	35	3.0
(*Freshlike* Sugar Snap), ⅔ cup	45	2.0	6.0	0	0	10	2.0
(*Freshlike* Sugar Snap Stir Fry), ¾ cup	35	1.0	5.0	0	0	20	1.0
(*Green Giant* Sugar Snap), ¾ cup	35	2.0	7.0	0	0	0	3.0
(*Green Giant Harvest Fresh* Sugar Snap), ⅔ cup	50	3.0	10.0	0	0	95	3.0
(*Seneca* Snap), ⅔ cup	45	2.0	8.0	0	0	0	3.0
boiled, drained, ½ cup	42	2.8	7.2	.3	0	4	2.4
pods and water chestnuts (*Freshlike*), 1¼ cups	50	2.0	7.0	0	0	10	2.0
Peas, field, canned, (see also "Peas, crowder" and "Peas, purple hull"), ½ cup:							
(*Bush's Best*)	110	7.0	18.0	1.0	0	500	5.0

Food and Measure	cal.	prot. (gms)	carbo. (gms)	fat (gms)	chol. (mgs)	sod. (mgs)	fiber (gms)
fresh shell:							
(*Sunshine*)	120	7.0	21.0	1.0	0	350	6.0
w/snaps (*Allens/ East Texas Fair/ Homefolks*)	120	6.0	21.0	1.0	0	300	6.0
dry:							
w/bacon (*Trappey's*)	90	6.0	15.0	1.0	0	380	5.0
w/bacon and snaps (*Trappey's*)	110	6.0	19.0	1.0	0	380	4.0
w/snaps (*Bush's Best*)	110	7.0	17.0	.5	0	550	5.0
Peas, field, frozen, w/snaps (*Birds Eye* Southern), cup	130	9.0	24.0	1.0	0	15	4.0
Peas, green, fresh:							
raw:							
in pod, 1 lb.	140	9.3	24.9	.7	0	8	8.8
shelled, ½ cup	58	3.9	10.4	.3	0	3	3.7
boiled, drained, ½ cup	67	4.3	12.5	.2	0	2	4.4
Peas, green, canned, ½ cup:							
(*Del Monte*)	60	3.0	13.0	0	0	390	4.0
(*Del Monte* No Salt)	60	3.0	11.0	0	0	10	4.0
(*Seneca*)	70	4.0	12.0	0	0	310	5.0
(*Seneca* No Salt)	70	4.0	13.0	0	0	10	4.0
early or sweet:							
(*Bush's Best*)	80	5.0	12.0	1.0	0	340	4.0
(*Bush's Best* Small)	70	4.0	11.0	1.0	0	340	3.0
(*Green Giant*)	60	4.0	11.0	0	0	390	4.0
(*Green Giant* 50% Less Sodium) ...	60	4.0	11.0	0	0	195	4.0
(*LeSueur*)	60	4.0	12.0	0	0	380	3.0
(*LeSueur* 50% Less Sodium)	60	4.0	11.0	0	0	190	4.0
very young, small:							
(*Del Monte*)	60	3.0	10.0	0	0	360	4.0
Peas, green, dried:							
(*Frieda's*), ⅓ cup, 3 oz.	130	9.0	22.0	0	0	290	9.0
freeze-dried (*Al-pineAire*), ¾ oz. ...	80	5.0	14.0	0	0	115	5.0

Food and Measure	cal.	prot. (gms)	carbo. (gms)	fat (gms)	chol. (mgs)	sod. (mgs)	fiber (gms)
Peas, green, frozen, 2/3 cup, except as noted:							
(*Birds Eye*), 1/2 cup . . .	70	5.0	4.0	0	0	125	5.0
(*Seneca*)	80	5.0	14.0	0	0	30	6.0
baby:							
early (*Green Giant Harvest Fresh Le-Sueur*)	70	4.0	13.0	0	0	220	4.0
sweet (*Birds Eye Farm Fresh* Blend)	70	5.0	4.0	.5	0	105	4.0
early June (*LeSueur*)	60	5.0	11.0	0	0	150	5.0
garden:							
(*Cascadian Farm*)	70	4.0	12.0	0	0	55	5.0
(*Freshlike*)	70	5.0	12.0	.5	0	105	4.0
sweet:							
(*Green Giant*)	70	4.0	13.0	0	0	135	4.0
(*Green Giant Harvest Fresh*)	60	4.0	12.0	0	0	200	4.0
baby (*LeSueur Harvest Fresh*)	70	4.0	13.0	0	0	220	4.0
tiny:							
(*Freshlike*)	70	5.0	12.0	.5	0	105	4.0
(*John Cope's*)	70	5.0	12.0	0	0	n.a.	4.0
(*Seabrook*)	70	5.0	12.0	.5	0	105	4.0
tender (*Birds Eye Deluxe*), 1/2 cup	60	5.0	4.0	0	0	125	6.0
in butter sauce, 3/4 cup:							
baby, early (*LeSueur*)	100	5.0	16.0	2.0	<5	370	4.0
sweet (*Green Giant*)	100	4.0	16.0	2.0	<5	400	5.0
Peas, green, combinations, canned, 1/2 cup:							
and carrots:							
(*Del Monte*)	60	2.0	11.0	0	0	360	2.0
(*Green Giant*)	50	2.0	11.0	0	0	410	3.0
(*Seneca*)	60	3.0	11.0	0	0	300	4.0
w/mushrooms and onions (*LeSueur*)	60	3.0	11.0	0	0	380	2.0
w/pearl onions (*Green Giant*)	60	4.0	11.0	0	0	520	4.0

Food and Measure	cal.	prot. (gms)	carbo. (gms)	fat (gms)	chol. (mgs)	sod. (mgs)	fiber (gms)
w/pearl onions (*S&W*)	40	3.0	11.0	0	0	530	3.0
Peas, green, combinations, frozen, ⅔ cup, except as noted:							
baby (*Birds Eye Farm Fresh* Blend), ¾ cup	40	2.0	7.0	0	0	40	2.0
and carrots:							
(*Birds Eye* Southern)	50	3.0	9.0	0	0	65	3.0
(*Cascadian Farm*)	50	5.0	9.0	0	0	160	0
(*Seneca*)	50	3.0	9.0	0	0	45	4.0
w/mushrooms (*Le-Sueur*), ¾ cup	60	4.0	10.0	0	·0	105	4.0
w/onions:							
(*Seneca*)	70	5.0	12.0	0	0	55	5.0
pearl (*Birds Eye Side Orders*)	90	5.0	6.0	.5	0	520	5.0
pearl (*Cascadian Farm*), ¾ cup . . .	60	4.0	11.0	0	0	130	4.0
pearl (*Green Giant*)	60	4.0	12.0	0	0	125	4.0
pearl (*Green Giant Harvest Fresh*), ½ cup	50	3.0	10.0	0	0	170	3.0
w/potatoes in cream sauce (*Birds Eye Side Orders*), ½ cup	90	4.0	4.0	2.5	10	350	2.0
Peas, lady, canned, ½ cup:							
(*Sunshine*)	100	6.0	17.0	1.0	0	460	5.0
w/snaps (*East Texas Fair*)	100	7.0	17.0	1.0	0	420	4.0
Peas, pepper, canned (*East Texas Fair*), ½ cup	120	6.0	22.0	1.0	0	580	6.0
Peas, pigeon, canned, green (*Goya*), 8 oz.	110	10.0	26.0	0	0	560	8.0
Peas, w/pork, see "Baked beans" and specific bean listings							

Food and Measure	cal.	prot. (gms)	carbo. (gms)	fat (gms)	chol. (mgs)	sod. (mgs)	fiber (gms)
Peas, purple hull, ½ cup:							
canned:							
(*Allens/East Texas Fair/Homefolks*)	120	7.0	21.0	1.0	0	350	6.0
(*Bush's Best*)	110	7.0	18.0	1.0	0	500	5.0
(*Stubb's*)	120	6.0	21.0	1.0	0	300	6.0
frozen:							
(*Birds Eye*)	110	7.0	21.0	.5	0	10	4.0
(*Mckenzie's*)	110	7.0	21.0	.5	0	10	4.0
Peas, split, see "Split peas"							
Peas, sprouted:							
raw, ½ cup	77	5.3	17.0	.4	0	12	n.a.
boiled, drained, 4 oz.	134	8.0	24.8	.6	0	3	3.7
Peas, sugar snap or snow, see "Peas, edible podded"							
Peas, sweet, see "Peas, green"							
Peas, white acre, canned (*East Texas Fair*), ½ cup	100	6.0	17.0	1.0	0	460	5.0
Peas and carrots or onions, see "Peas, green, combinations"							
Pecan, shelled:							
(*Paradise/White Swan* Halves/Pieces), ¼ cup, 1 oz.	200	4.0	5.0	18.0	0	0	3.0
dried:							
1 oz.	190	2.2	5.2	19.2	0	<1	2.2
halves, 1 cup	721	8.4	19.7	73.1	0	1	8.2
chopped, 1 cup	794	9.2	21.7	80.5	0	1	9.0
dry-roasted, salted, 1 oz.	187	2.3	6.3	18.4	0	221	n.a.
oil-roasted, salted, 1 oz.	195	2.0	4.6	20.2	0	214	n.a.
Pecan filling, see "Pastry filling"							

Food and Measure	cal.	prot. (gms)	carbo. (gms)	fat (gms)	chol. (mgs)	sod. (mgs)	fiber (gms)
Pecan flour, 1 oz. ...	93	9.1	14.4	.4	0	tr.	n.a.
Pecan topping, 2 tbsp.:							
praline sauce (*Trader Vic's*)	120	1.0	21.0	5.0	0	50	0
in syrup (*Smucker's*)	170	1.0	20.0	10.0	0	0	0
Pectin, see "Fruit pectin"							
Penne, plain, see "Pasta"							
Penne dishes, mix, dry:							
Alfredo sauce (*Annie's*), ²/₃ cup	270	12.0	46.0	4.5	10	500	2.0
w/spicy sauce (*Al Dente*), ½ cup	240	9.0	46.0	1.5	0	500	2.0
w/sun-dried tomato Parmesan sauce (*Knorr*), ½ cup	270	9.0	50.0	3.5	<5	660	3.0
tomato marinara (*Fantastic Foods Healthy Compliments*), ½ cup	200	8.0	42.0	1.5	0	320	3.0
Penne entree, frozen, 1 pkg.:							
(*Smart Ones*), 10 oz.	300	11.0	43.0	8.0	15	560	3.0
w/beef ragout (*Wolfgang Puck's*), 12 oz.	410	23.0	38.0	18.0	95	610	4.0
w/chicken (*Weight Watchers Main Street Bistro Pollo*), 10 oz.	290	22.0	38.0	6.0	55	590	3.0
w/meat sauce (*Freezer Queen*), 9 oz.	250	9.0	40.0	6.0	10	870	4.0
and pepperoni (*Marie Callender's*), 15 oz.	800	29.0	74.0	43.0	30	1780	11.0
spicy, w/ricotta (*Smart Ones*), 10.2 oz. ...	280	11.0	45.0	6.0	`5	400	4.0
w/tomato sauce: (*Healthy Choice*), 8 oz.	230	9.0	36.0	5.0	10	490	5.0

Food and Measure	cal.	prot. (gms)	carbo. (gms)	fat (gms)	chol. (mgs)	sod. (mgs)	fiber (gms)
Penne entree, w/tomato sauce *(cont.)*							
basil (*Lean Cuisine*), 10 oz.	270	8.0	52.0	4.0	0	350	5.0
w/tomatoes, chunky (*The Budget Gourmet Value Classics Low Fat*), 8 oz.	270	10.0	46.0	6.0	10	410	3.0
Pepper, seasoning:							
black:							
ground, 1 tsp.	6	.3	1.7	.1	0	1	.7
whole, 1 tsp.	8	.3	1.9	0	0	1	.8
chili, 1 tsp.	9	.3	1.2	.3	0	<1	.7
red or cayenne, 1 tsp.	6	.2	1.0	.3	0	1	.7
seasoned (*Lawry's*), 1/4 tsp.	0	0	1.0	0	0	0	0
white, 1 tsp.	7	.3	1.7	.1	0	0	.2
Pepper, banana, 1 oz.:							
hot or mild (*Vlasic*) ...	5	0	1.0	0	0	480	0
mild (*Nalley*), 2 pcs.	5	0	1.0	0	0	360	0
Pepper, bell, see "Pepper, sweet"							
Pepper, cherry:							
(*Progresso Hot*), 1 oz.	10	0	2.0	0	0	150	<1.0
(*Progresso So Hot/ Sliced*), 2 tbsp. ...	25	0	2.0	2.0	0	30	1.0
sweet (*Nalley*), 2 pcs., 1 oz.	10	0	2.0	0	0	330	0
Pepper, chili, fresh:							
all varieties (*Frieda's Cucina*), 1-oz. pc.	10	1.0	3.0	0	0	0	0
green and red:							
1 medium, 1.6 oz.	18	.9	4.3	.1	0	3	.7
chopped, 1/2 cup ...	30	1.5	7.1	.2	0	5	1.1
Pepper, chili, in jars:							
whole, green:							
(*Chi-Chi's*), 3/4 pc.	10	0	1.0	0	0	15	0
(*Nalley*, 5 pcs., 1 oz.	10	0	2.0	0	0	340	0
(*Old El Paso Peeled*), 1 pc. ...	10	0	2.0	0	0	230	1.0

Food and Measure	cal.	prot. (gms)	carbo. (gms)	fat (gms)	chol. (mgs)	sod. (mgs)	fiber (gms)
(*Rosarita*), 2 tbsp.	5	0	1.0	0	0	75	<1.0
chopped:							
green (*Old El Paso*), 2 tbsp.	5	0	1.0	0	0	110	1.0
hot (*B&G Sandwich Toppers*), 1 tbsp.	5	0	1.0	0	0	120	0
w/liquid, ½ cup	17	.6	4.2	.1	0	n.a.	1.3
diced, green, 2 tbsp.:							
(*Chi-Chi's*), ¾ pc.	10	0	1.0	0	0	20	0
(*Pancho Villa*)	5	0	1.0	0	0	110	1.0
(*Rosarita*)	5	0	1.5	0	0	85	<1.0
strips, green (*Rosarita*), ¼ cup	5	0	1.0	<1.0	0	75	<1.0
Pepper, chili, relish, pickle (*Patak's*), 1 tbsp.	45	0	1.0	4.0	0	590	<1.0
Pepper, green or red, sweet, see "Pepper, sweet"							
Pepper, jalapeño:							
(*La Victoria* Marinated), 1.1 oz.	10	0	2.0	0	0	290	<1.0
(*La Victoria* Pickled), 1.1 oz.	10	0	2.0	0	0	115	<1.0
whole:							
(*Nalley*), 2 pcs., 1 oz.	5	0	1.0	0	0	360	0
(*Old El Paso* Peeled), 2 pcs., 1 oz.	5	0	1.0	0	0	200	0
(*Old El Paso* Pickled), 3 pcs., 1 oz.	5	0	1.0	0	0	200	1.0
w/escabeche (*Rosarita*), ¼ cup	10	<1.0	1.5	0	0	430	1.0
diced (*La Victoria*), 1.1 oz.	10	0	2.0	0	0	190	0
sliced:							
(*La Victoria* Nacho), 1.1 oz.	0	0	<1.0	0	0	370	<1.0
(*Nalley*), 13 pcs., 1 oz.	5	0	1.0	0	0	320	0

Food and Measure	cal.	prot. (gms)	carbo. (gms)	fat (gms)	chol. (mgs)	sod. (mgs)	fiber (gms)
Pepper, jalapeño, sliced *(cont.)*							
(*Old El Paso*),							
2 tbsp.	10	0	3.0	0	0	400	1.0
(*Rosarita*), 2 tbsp.	5	0	1.0	0	0	120	1.0
Pepper, roasted, see "Pepper, sweet, in jars"							
Pepper, serrano							
(*Stubb's*), 5 pcs.,							
1 oz.	5	0	1.0	0	0	330	0
Pepper, stuffed, entree, frozen:							
(*Stouffer's*), 10 oz.	200	11.0	27.0	5.0	20	820	3.0
(*Stouffer's*), 1/2 of							
1/2-oz. pkg.	180	8.0	20.0	7.0	25	530	2.0
(*Stouffer's*), 1/4 of							
32-oz. pkg.	190	9.0	23.0	7.0	25	910	2.0
Pepper, sweet, fresh:							
green and red:							
raw, 1 medium, 3¾"							
x 3"	20	.7	4.8	.1	0	1	1.3
raw, chopped,							
1/2 cup	13	.4	3.2	.1	0	1	.9
boiled, drained,							
1 medium	20	.7	4.9	.1	0	1	.9
boiled, drained,							
chopped, 1/2 cup	19	.6	4.6	.1	0	1	.8
yellow, raw:							
1 large, 5" x 3"	50	1.9	11.8	.4	0	3	n.a.
10 strips, 1.8 oz.	14	.5	3.3	.1	0	1	n.a.
Pepper, sweet, frozen:							
(*Freshlike* Stir Fry),							
1 cup	25	1.0	5.0	0	0	15	2.0
chopped, 1 oz.	6	.3	1.3	.1	0	1	.5
green, diced (*Birds Eye Southern*),							
3/4 cup	20	1.0	1.0	0	0	10	2.0
red (*Seneca*), 3/4 cup	25	1.0	4.0	0	0	0	2.0
stir-fry (*Birds Eye Farm Fresh*), 1 cup	25	1.0	5.0	0	0	15	2.0

Food and Measure	cal.	prot. (gms)	carbo. (gms)	fat (gms)	chol. (mgs)	sod. (mgs)	fiber (gms)
Pepper, sweet, in jars (see also "Pimiento"):							
fried w/onions (*Progresso*), 2 tbsp.	20	0	2.0	1.5	0	130	1.0
rings (*Vlasic*), 1 oz.	25	0	6.0	0	0	170	0
roasted:							
(*Krinos*), 1.7-oz. pc.	10	0	3.0	0	0	30	0
(*Progresso*), 2 pcs., 1 oz.	10	0	3.0	0	0	55	0
fire, w/garlic, oil (*Paesana*), 2 tbsp.	20	0	2.0	1.0	0	125	0
in olive oil (*Haddon House*), 2 tbsp.	20	1.0	5.0	0	0	180	1.0
salad, w/oregano, garlic (*B&G*), 1 oz. . . .	10	0	3.0	0	0	240	0
Pepper, sweet, marinated, sun-dried (*Antica Italia*), 1 oz.	170	0	2.0	18.0	0	5	1.0
Pepper loaf, see "Lunch meat"							
Pepper salad:							
(*B&G*), 1 oz.	10	0	3.0	0	0	240	0
drained (*Progresso*), 2 tbsp.	15	0	1.0	1.0	0	160	<1.0
Pepper sauce, hot (see also specific listings), 1 tsp., except as noted:							
(*Frank's RedHot*)	0	0	0	0	0	230	0
(*Frank's RedHot* Hotter)	0	0	0	0	0	210	0
(*Gebhardt*)	0	0	0	0	0	100	0
(*Helen's Tropical Exotics*)	0	0	1.0	0	0	40	0
(*Louisiana*)	0	0	0	0	0	240	0
(*Tabasco*)	0	0	0	0	0	30	0
(*Tabasco* Hababero)	5	0	0	0	0	140	0
(*Watkins* Calypso) . . .	10	0	3.0	0	0	25	0

Food and Measure	cal.	prot. (gms)	carbo. (gms)	fat (gms)	chol. (mgs)	sod. (mgs)	fiber (gms)
Pepper sauce *(cont.)*							
(*Watkins* Inferno),							
2 tbsp.	35	0	8.0	0	0	930	0
balsamic (*Roland*),							
1 tbsp.	10	0	2.0	0	0	120	0
w/garlic (*Tabasco*) . . .	0	0	0	0	0	95	0
jalapeño:							
(*Tabasco*), 3.5 oz.	15	<1.0	3.0	0	0	3200	<1.0
(*Watkins*)	0	0	0	0	0	70	0
Pepper steak, see "Beef entree, frozen"							
Peppercorn sauce mix (*Knorr* Classic),							
2 tsp.	25	<1.0	3.0	1.0	0	380	0
Pepperoncini:							
(*Krinos*), ¼ cup	5	0	2.0	0	0	950	0
(*Nalley*), 3 pcs., 1 oz.	5	0	1.0	0	0	310	0
(*Progresso* Tuscan),							
3 pcs., 1 oz.	10	0	1.0	0	0	450	0
(*Zorba*), 5 pcs.,							
1.1 oz.	15	1.0	2.0	0	0	450	0
Pepperoni:							
(*Bridgford*), 16 slices,							
1 oz.	130	6.0	0	12.0	25	500	0
(*Hansel 'n Gretel*),							
2 oz.	240	12.0	2.0	20.0	50	860	0
(*Hormel* Chunk or							
Sliced), 1 oz.	140	5.0	0	13.0	35	470	0
(*Hormel* Twin), 1 oz.	140	5.0	0	13.0	35	500	0
(*Hormel Pillow Pack*),							
16 slices, 1 oz.	140	5.0	0	13.0	35	470	0
(*Oscar Mayer*),							
15 slices, 1.1 oz.	140	6.0	0	13.0	25	550	0
turkey, see "Turkey pepperoni"							
Perch, meat only:							
raw, 4 oz.	103	22.0	0	1.1	102	70	0
baked, broiled, or microwaved, 4 oz. . . .	133	28.2	0	1.3	130	90	0

Food and Measure	cal.	prot. (gms)	carbo. (gms)	fat (gms)	chol. (mgs)	sod. (mgs)	fiber (gms)
ocean, see "Ocean perch"							
Persimmon, fresh:							
(*Frieda's*), 5 oz.	100	1.0	26.0	0	0	0	5.0
Japanese, 1 medium	118	1.0	31.2	.3	0	3	6.0
native, 1 medium, 1.1 oz.	32	.2	8.4	.1	0	<1	n.a.
Persimmon, dried:							
(*Frieda's* Fuyu), cup, 1.4 oz.	140	1.0	35.0	0	0	10	3.0
(*Sonoma*), 7 pcs., 1.4 oz.	140	1.0	35.0	0	0	10	3.0
Japanese, 1 oz.	78	.4	20.8	.2	0	1	4.1
Pesto sauce, in jars, ¼ cup, except as noted:							
(*Sonoma*)	110	3.0	6.0	9.0	2	125	1.0
black (*Cora* Gourmet)	200	2.0	5.0	26.0	0	1050	1.0
creamy (*Five Brothers*)	110	2.0	3.0	10.0	40	430	0
Genovese (*Italia In Talola*), 2 tbsp.	160	2.0	4.0	16.0	0	370	<1.0
green (*Cora* Gourmet)	140	3.0	2.0	13.0	0	460	2.0
red (*Cora* Gourmet), 2 tbsp.	190	2.0	3.0	20.0	0	240	1.0
white (*Cora* Gourmet)	120	1.0	1.0	12.0	0	260	0
Pesto sauce, refrigerated, ¼ cup:							
(*Di Giorno*)	320	8.0	3.0	31.0	15	500	0
w/basil (*Contadina*)	290	6.0	12.0	24.0	20	580	3.0
w/basil (*Contadina* Reduced Fat)	230	6.0	11.0	18.0	15	560	2.0
basil and garlic (*Christopher Ranch*)	230	4.0	4.0	23.0	0	325	3.0
w/sun-dried tomato (*Contadina*)	250	3.0	8.0	23.0	5	510	2.0
Pesto sauce mix, dry:							
(*Knorr* Pasta Sauces), 2 tsp.	15	<1.0	2.0	0	0	480	0
creamy (*Knorr* Pasta Sauces), 1 tbsp. . . .	25	<1.0	3.0	1.0	0	450	0

Food and Measure	cal.	prot. (gms)	carbo. (gms)	fat (gms)	chol. (mgs)	sod. (mgs)	fiber (gms)
Pesto sauce mix *(cont.)*							
red bell pepper (*Knorr* Pasta Sauces), tbsp.	25	<1.0	4.0	.5	0	510	<1.0
sun-dried tomato (*Knorr* Pasta Sauces), 1 tbsp. ...	35	1.0	6.0	.5	0	530	1.0
Pheasant, raw:							
meat w/skin, 4 oz. ...	205	25.7	0	10.5	n.a.	45	0
meat only:							
4 oz.	151	26.7	0	4.1	n.a.	42	0
½ breast, 6.4 oz.	243	44.4	0	5.9	n.a.	60	0
1 leg, 3.8 oz.	143	23.8	0	4.6	n.a.	48	0
Phyllo, see "Fillo pastry"							
Picante sauce (see also "Salsa"), 2 tbsp.:							
all styles:							
(*Muir Glen*)	10	0	2.0	0	0	180	0
(*Pace*)	10	0	2.0	0	0	220	0
hot:							
(*Chi-Chi's*)	10	0	2.0	0	0	270	0
(*Old El Paso* Thick 'n Chunky)	10	0	2.0	0	0	160	0
jalapeño:							
hot (*Rosarita* Zesty)	10	0	2.0	0	0	235	0
medium or mild (*Rosarita* Zesty)	10	0	2.0	0	0	225	0
medium:							
(*Chi-Chi's*)	10	0	2.0	0	0	200	0
(*Gracias* Superba)	10	0	2.0	0	0	170	0
(*Old El Paso* Thick 'n Chunky)	10	0	2.0	0	0	140	0
mild:							
(*Chi-Chi's*)	10	0	2.0	0	0	210	0
(*Gracias* Superba)	5	0	1.0	0	0	140	0
(*Old El Paso* Thick 'n Chunky)	10	0	2.0	0	0	130	0

Food and Measure	cal.	prot. (gms)	carbo. (gms)	fat (gms)	chol. (mgs)	sod. (mgs)	fiber (gms)
Pickle, cucumber, 1 oz., except as noted:							
bread and butter:							
(*Claussen*), 4 slices, 1 oz.	20	0	4.0	0	0	170	0
(*Claussen* Sandwich), 2 slices, 1.2 oz.	25	0	5.0	0	0	210	0
(*Mrs. Fannings*), 3 pcs. or 1 oz. . . .	25	0	6.0	0	0	190	0
(*Nalley* Banquet Chunks), 2½ pcs., 1 oz.	25	0	6.0	0	0	200	0
(*Nalley* Snackin' Slices), 3 pcs., 1 oz.	25	0	6.0	0	0	220	0
chips:							
(*Nalley*), 4½ pcs., 1 oz.	35	0	9.0	0	0	135	0
dill (*Nalley* Banquet), 4½ pcs., 1 oz.	5	0	1.0	0	0	350	0
w/honey (*Pickle Eater's*), 6 pcs., 1 oz.	25	0	7.0	0	0	0	0
cornichons (*Italica*), 7 pcs., 1.1 oz.	0	0	0	0	0	330	0
dill:							
(*Nalley* Banquet), 1 pc., 1 oz.	5	0	1.0	0	0	290	0
(*Nalley* Country), ½ pc., 1 oz.	5	0	1.0	0	0	270	0
(*Nalley* Dilliest), ½ pc., 1 oz.	5	0	1.0	0	0	330	0
(*Nalley* Tiny Banquet), 2½ pcs., 1 oz.	5	0	1.0	0	0	270	0
baby (*Nalley* Banquet), 1 pc., 1 oz.	5	0	1.0	0	0	280	0
baby (*Pickle Eater's*)	0	0	0	0	0	310	0

Food and Measure	cal.	prot. (gms)	carbo. (gms)	fat (gms)	chol. (mgs)	sod. (mgs)	fiber (gms)
Pickle, dill *(cont.)*							
garlic (*Ba-Tampte*)	0	0	<1.0	0	0	180	0
garlic (*Nalley*), ½ pc., 1 oz.	5	0	1.0	0	0	280	0
garlic (*Nalley* Tiny), 2½ pcs., 1 oz. . . .	5	0	1.0	0	0	290	0
halves (*Del Monte*), ¼ pickle, 1 oz.	5	0	1.0	0	0	370	<1.0
hamburger (*Claussen*), 10 slices, 1.1 oz.	5	0	0	0	0	410	0
hamburger chips (*Del Monte*), 5½ chips	5	0	0	0	0	300	0
w/onion (*Nalley* Walla Walla), ½ pc., 1 oz.	5	0	1.0	0	0	280	0
whole (*Del Monte*), 1½ pcs., 1 oz. . . .	5	0	1.0	0	0	370	<1.0
dill, kosher:							
(*Nalley*), ½ pc., 1 oz.	5	0	1.0	0	0	370	0
(*Nalley* Fresh Pack), ½ pc., 1 oz.	5	0	1.0	0	0	280	0
(*Pickle Eater's* Deli)	0	0	0	0	0	360	0
(*Pickle Eater's* No Salt)	0	0	0	0	0	5	0
chips (*Claussen*), 4 pcs., 1 oz.	5	0	1.0	0	0	320	0
halves (*Claussen*), ½ pc.	5	0	1.0	0	0	330	0
mini (*Claussen*), .8-oz. pc.	5	0	1.0	0	0	300	0
slices (*Claussen* Sandwich), 2 slices, 1.2 oz.	5	0	1.0	0	0	440	0
spears (*Claussen*), 1 pc., 1.2 oz.	5	0	1.0	0	0	320	0
spears (*Pickle Eater's*)	0	0	0	0	0	330	0

Food and Measure	cal.	prot. (gms)	carbo. (gms)	fat (gms)	chol. (mgs)	sod. (mgs)	fiber (gms)
whole (*Claussen*), ½ pc., 1 oz.	5	0	1.0	0	0	330	0
whole, tiny (*Del Monte*), 1½ pcs., 1 oz.	5	0	1.0	0	0	250	<1.0
garlic, hearty:							
(*Claussen* Deli Style), ½ pc., 1 oz.	5	0	1.0	0	0	260	0
(*Claussen* Sandwich), 2 slices, 1.2 oz.	5	0	1.0	0	0	320	0
sour, half:							
(*Ba-Tampte*)	0	0	<1.0	0	0	240	0
(*Claussen*)	5	0	1.0	0	0	260	0
sweet:							
(*Nalley*), 1½ pcs., 1 oz.	30	0	8.0	0	0	200	0
(*Nalley* Nubbins), 1 pc., 1 oz.	25	0	6.0	0	0	190	0
all varieties (*Del Monte*)	40	0	10.0	0	0	210	<1.0
all varieties (*Vlasic*)	40	0	10.0	0	0	170	0
gherkins (*Nalley*), about 1 pc., 1 oz.	25	0	7.0	0	0	110	0
midget (*Nalley*), about 3 pcs., 1 oz.	30	0	8.0	0	0	160	0
Pickle dip, dill (*Nalley*), 2 tbsp.	70	0	5.0	5.0	15	260	0
Pickle loaf, see "Lunch meat"							
Pickle relish (see also specific listings), cucumber, 1 tbsp.:							
(*Crosse & Blackwell* Branston)	25	0	6.0	0	0	125	0
dill, chunky (*Nalley*)	0	0	0	0	0	140	0
hamburger:							
(*Del Monte*)	20	0	6.0	0	0	220	<1.0
(*Heinz*)	10	0	3.0	0	0	180	0

Food and Measure	cal.	prot. (gms)	carbo. (gms)	fat (gms)	chol. (mgs)	sod. (mgs)	fiber (gms)
Pickle relish, hamburger *(cont.)*							
(*Nalley*)	15	0	3.0	0	0	110	0
hot dog:							
(*Del Monte*)	15	0	4.0	0	0	140	<1.0
(*Heinz*)	15	0	4.0	0	0	100	0
(*Nalley*)	15	0	3.0	0	0	120	0
India (*Heinz*)	20	0	5.0	0	0	100	0
piccalilli, tomato							
(*Pickle Eater's*)	10	0	2.0	0	0	75	0
red hot:							
(*Nalley*)	15	0	4.0	0	0	100	0
(*Ron's*)	15	0	4.0	0	0	100	0
sweet:							
(*B&G* Unsalted) . . .	20	0	5.0	0	0	0	0
(*Claussen*)	15	0	3.0	0	0	85	0
(*Del Monte*)	20	0	5.0	0	0	125	0
(*Nalley*)	20	0	4.0	0	0	125	0
honey (*Pickle Eater's*)	15	0	4.0	0	0	90	0
Pickled vegetables, see "Vegetables, mixed, pickled" and specific listings							
Pickling spice (*Tone's*), 1 tsp.	10	.3	1.2	.6	n.a.	1	.3
Pico de gallo, see "Salsa"							
Pie, 1/5 pie, except as noted:							
apple (*Entenmann's* Homestyle), 1/6 pie	340	2.0	56.0	12.0	0	330	2.0
coconut custard (*Entenmann's*)	340	7.0	37.0	18.0	135	300	1.0
pecan (*Entenmann's*)	550	6.0	67.0	30.0	130	350	2.0
pumpkin, custard (*Entenmann's*)	310	6.0	38.0	15.0	105	320	1.0
Pie, frozen (see also "Cobbler"):							
apple:							
(*Amy's*), 4 oz.	220	2.0	35.0	8.0	25	130	2.0
(*Mrs. Smith's*), 1/8 pie	310	2.0	44.0	14.0	0	380	1.0

Food and Measure	cal.	prot. (gms)	carbo. (gms)	fat (gms)	chol. (mgs)	sod. (mgs)	fiber (gms)
(*Sara Lee* Home-style), ⅛ pie	340	3.0	46.0	16.0	0	310	1.0
(*Sara Lee* Reduced Fat), ⅙ pie	290	4.0	51.0	8.0	<5	400	2.0
deep dish (*Mrs. Smith's* Special Recipe), 1/12 pie	330	2.0	46.0	15.0	0	360	2.0
apple, Dutch:							
(*Sara Lee* Home-style), ⅛ pie	350	3.0	53.0	15.0	0	320	2.0
crumb (*Mrs. Smith's*), ⅛ pie	350	3.0	53.0	14.0	0	300	1.0
banana cream:							
(*Mrs. Smith's*), ¼ pie	290	2.0	38.0	15.0	0	190	1.0
(*Pet-Ritz*), ⅓ pie . . .	350	3.0	44.0	18.0	5	300	2.0
blueberry (*Sara Lee* Homestyle), ⅛ pie	360	3.0	54.0	15.0	0	340	2.0
Boston cream, see "Cake, frozen"							
cherry:							
(*Mrs. Smith's*), ⅛ pie	310	3.0	45.0	14.0	0	400	1.0
deep dish (*Mrs. Smith's Special Recipe*), 1/12 pie	330	3.0	48.0	14.0	0	320	1.0
cherry-berry (*Mrs. Smith's Special Recipe*), 1/10 pie	360	3.0	53.0	15.0	0	400	1.0
chocolate, French silk (*Mrs. Smith's Restaurant Classics*), 1/9 pie	560	4.0	48.0	40.0	75	330	2.0
chocolate cream:							
(*Mrs. Smith's*), ¼ pie	330	2.0	42.0	17.0	0	220	1.0
(*Pet-Ritz*), ⅓ pie . . .	340	3.0	44.0	17.0	5	300	2.0
coconut cream:							
(*Mrs. Smith's*), ¼ pie	340	2.0	40.0	19.0	0	260	0
(*Pet-Ritz*), ⅓ pie . . .	350	3.0	44.0	18.0	5	300	2.0

Food and Measure	cal.	prot. (gms)	carbo. (gms)	fat (gms)	chol. (mgs)	sod. (mgs)	fiber (gms)
Pie, frozen, coconut cream *(cont.)*							
(*Sara Lee*), ⅕ pie	480	4.0	47.0	31.0	0	430	2.0
cookies and cream (*Mrs. Smith's Restaurant Classics*), ⅑ pie	390	4.0	49.0	20.0	0	230	2.0
fudge vanilla cream (*Pet-Ritz*), ⅓ pie . . .	350	3.0	44.0	18.0	5	300	2.0
key lime:							
(*Mrs. Smith's Restaurant Classics*), ⅑ pie	420	7.0	56.0	19.0	0	210	<1.0
cream (*Pet-Ritz*), ⅓ pie	350	3.0	44.0	18.0	5	300	2.0
lemon cream:							
(*Mrs. Smith's*), ¼ pie	300	2.0	41.0	15.0	0	180	0
(*Pet-Ritz*), ⅓ pie . . .	350	3.0	44.0	18.0	5	300	2.0
lemon meringue:							
(*Mrs. Smith's*), ⅕ pie	300	2.0	55.0	8.0	65	220	0
(*Sara Lee* Homestyle), ⅙ pie	350	2.0	59.0	11.0	0	460	5.0
mince/mincemeat (*Sara Lee* Homestyle), ⅛ pie	390	3.0	56.0	17.0	0	450	3.0
Mississippi mud (*Weight Watchers*), 2.4-oz. pc.	160	4.0	26.0	5.0	5	120	1.0
peach:							
(*Sara Lee* Homestyle), ⅛ pie	320	3.0	46.0	14.0	0	250	2.0
deep dish (*Mrs. Smith's Special Recipe*), 1/12 pie	300	2.0	41.0	14.0	0	330	2.0
peanut butter:							
chocolate cream (*Pet-Ritz*), ⅓ pie	370	3.0	44.0	20.0	5	300	2.0
cream (*Mrs. Smith's*), ¼ pie	360	4.0	39.0	21.0	0	250	0

Food and Measure	cal.	prot. (gms)	carbo. (gms)	fat (gms)	chol. (mgs)	sod. (mgs)	fiber (gms)
silk (*Mrs. Smith's Restaurant Classics*), 1/9 pie	600	8.0	51.0	41.0	55	330	2.0
pecan (*Sara Lee* Homestyle), 1/8 pie	520	5.0	70.0	24.0	45	480	3.0
pumpkin:							
(*Mrs. Smith's Hearty*), 1/8 pie . . .	240	5.0	38.0	8.0	45	330	2.0
(*Mrs. Smith's Special Recipe* Home-made), 1/10 pie . . .	280	5.0	40.0	11.0	40	340	2.0
(*Sara Lee* Home-style), 1/8 pie	260	4.0	37.0	11.0	30	460	2.0
cream (*Pet-Ritz*), 1/3 pie	350	3.0	44.0	18.0	5	300	2.0
pumpkin custard (*Mrs. Smith's*), 1/8 pie	230	17.0	36.0	8.0	45	320	1.0
raspberry, red (*Sara Lee* Homestyle), 1/8 pie	380	3.0	48.0	19.0	<5	330	2.0
Pie, mix, 1/6 pie*:							
cheesecake, see "Cake, mix"							
chocolate silk (*Jell-O* No Bake)	310	5.0	38.0	16.0	5	490	<1.0
coconut cream (*Jell-O* No Bake)	330	4.0	37.0	19.0	5	410	1.0
Pie, snack (see also "Tart"), 4 1/2-oz. pc., except as noted:							
apple:							
(*Dolly Madison*) . . .	480	3.0	67.0	22.0	15	390	2.0
(*Entenmann's*), 5 oz.	350	3.0	42.0	19.0	0	350	2.0
regular or French (*Hostess*)	480	3.0	67.0	22.0	15	390	2.0
blackberry (*Hostess*)	520	3.0	79.0	21.0	15	400	2.0
blueberry:							
(*Dolly Madison*) . . .	480	3.0	70.0	21.0	20	460	2.0
(*Entenmann's*), 5 oz.	420	3.0	59.0	19.0	0	340	2.0

Food and Measure	cal.	prot. (gms)	carbo. (gms)	fat (gms)	chol. (mgs)	sod. (mgs)	fiber (gms)
Pie, snack, blueberry *(cont.)*							
(*Hostess*)	480	3.0	70.0	20.0	20	460	2.0
cherry:							
(*Dolly Madison*) . . .	470	3.0	65.0	22.0	20	470	1.0
(*Entenmann's*),							
5 oz.	410	4.0	58.0	19.0	0	310	1.0
(*Hostess*)	470	3.0	65.0	22.0	20	470	1.0
chocolate pudding							
(*Dolly Madison*) . . .	530	4.0	71.0	24.0	30	410	1.0
lemon:							
(*Dolly Madison*) . . .	500	3.0	68.0	24.0	20	430	0
(*Entenmann's*),							
5 oz.	430	4.0	60.0	20.0	20	400	<1.0
(*Hostess*)	500	3.0	66.0	24.0	20	430	0
peach:							
(*Dolly Madison*) . . .	480	3.0	68.0	21.0	25	460	1.0
(*Entenmann's*),							
5 oz.	380	3.0	49.0	19.0	0	330	2.0
(*Hostess*)	480	3.0	68.0	21.0	25	460	1.0
pecan:							
(*Dolly Madison 3"*							
Pan), 3 oz.	360	3.0	44.0	19.0	70	320	1.0
fried (*Dolly Madi-*							
son)	530	4.0	80.0	21.0	10	430	1.0
pineapple:							
(*Dolly Madison*) . . .	460	4.0	62.0	21.0	15	340	1.0
(*Entenmann's*),							
5 oz.	400	3.0	55.0	19.0	0	350	1.0
(*Hostess*)	460	4.0	62.0	21.0	15	340	1.0
strawberry (*Hostess*)	510	3.0	71.0	23.0	15	360	2.0
Pie crust:							
chocolate cookie:							
(*Oreo*), 1/6 crust	140	1.0	18.0	7.0	0	170	1.0
(*Ready Crust*), 1/8							
crust	110	1.0	14.0	5.0	0	100	<1.0
graham:							
(*Honey Maid*),							
1/6 crust	140	1.0	18.0	7.0	0	125	<1.0
(*Ready Crust 9"*),							
1/8 crust	110	1.0	14.0	5.0	0	135	<1.0

Food and Measure	cal.	prot. (gms)	carbo. (gms)	fat (gms)	chol. (mgs)	sod. (mgs)	fiber (gms)
(*Ready Crust* 10″), ¹/₁₀ crust	130	1.0	17.0	6.0	0	170	<1.0
(*Ready Crust* Low Fat 9″), ⅛ crust	100	1.0	16.0	3.0	0	95	<1.0
mini (*Ready Crust*), .8-oz. crust	120	1.0	15.0	6.0	0	150	<1.0
shortbread (*Ready Crust* 9″), ⅛ crust	100	1.0	15.0	4.5	0	95	<1.0
vanilla cookie (*Nilla*), ⅙ crust	140	1.0	18.0	8.0	<5	65	0
Pie crust, frozen or refrigerated (see also "Pastry shell"), crust, except as noted:							
(*Oronoque* 6″), ¼ crust	110	2.0	10.0	7.0	0	115	0
(*Oronoque* 9″)	80	1.0	7.0	6.0	0	90	0
(*Pet-Ritz* 9″)	80	<1.0	9.0	4.5	<5	60	0
(*Pet Ritz* 9⅝″)	120	1.0	13.0	7.0	5	95	0
(*Pillsbury* All Ready)	120	<1.0	13.0	7.0	5	100	0
deep dish:							
(*Oronoque* 9″)	100	1.0	8.0	6.0	0	100	0
(*Oronoque* 10″) ...	120	2.0	11.0	8.0	0	130	0
(*Pet-Ritz* 9″)	90	1.0	11.0	5.0	<5	75	0
graham (*Oronoque*)	110	1.0	13.0	6.0	0	120	<1.0
vegetable shortening:							
(*Pet-Ritz* 9″)	80	1.0	10.0	4.5	0	75	0
deep dish (*Pet-Ritz*)	90	1.0	11.0	5.0	0	80	0
Pie crust mix:							
(*Betty Crocker*), ⅛ of 9″ crust	110	1.0	9.0	8.0	0	150	0
(*Flako*), ¼ cup dry ...	130	2.0	13.0	8.0	5	170	1.0
(*Pillsbury*), ⅛ of 9″ crust	100	1.0	10.0	6.0	0	150	0
Pie filling (see also "Pastry filling," "Pudding," and "Pudding, and pie filling mix"),							

Food and Measure	cal.	prot. (gms)	carbo. (gms)	fat (gms)	chol. (mgs)	sod. (mgs)	fiber (gms)
Pie filling *(cont.)*							
canned, cup, except as noted:							
apple:							
(*Comstock* Original)	100	0	25.0	0	0	10	2.0
(*Comstock* More Fruit/Orchard) ...	80	0	20.0	0	0	40	1.0
apple cinnamon:							
(*Comstock* Original Cinnamon 'n Spice)	100	0	26.0	0	0	60	1.0
(*Comstock* 25% More Fruit Cinnamon 'n Spice) ...	110	0	27.0	0	0	60	1.0
apple cranberry (*Comstock*)	90	1.0	22.0	0	0	50	1.0
apricot (*Comstock*)	100	0	23.0	0	0	5	1.0
banana cream (*Comstock*)	100	1.0	20.0	1.5	0	280	1.0
berry, triple (*Crosse & Blackwell*)	120	0	30.0	0	0	15	2.0
blackberry (*Comstock*)	110	1.0	26.0	0	0	20	3.0
blueberry:							
(*Comstock* Original)	100	0	25.0	0	0	15	1.0
(*Comstock* 25% More Fruit)	80	0	21.0	0	0	45	1.0
blueberry cranberry (*Comstock*)	100	0	25.0	0	0	15	1.0
cherry:							
(*Comstock* Original)	90	0	23.0	0	0	25	1.0
(*Comstock* Original Light)	60	0	15.0	0	0	15	1.0
(*Comstock* 25% More Fruit Light)	50	0	13.0	0	0	30	0
dark sweet (*Comstock* Original) ...	100	0	24.0	0	0	15	1.0
red tart, in water (*Oregon*), 2/3 cup	60	1.0	14.0	0	0	10	2.0
ruby red (*Comstock* Original)	90	0	23.0	0	0	25	0

Food and Measure	cal.	prot. (gms)	carbo. (gms)	fat (gms)	chol. (mgs)	sod. (mgs)	fiber (gms)
ruby red (*Comstock* 25% More Fruit)	90	0	23.0	0	0	70	0
cherry blackberry (*Crosse & Blackwell*)	100	0	26.0	0	0	15	0
cherry cranberry (*Comstock*)	90	1.0	22.0	0	0	30	0
chocolate cream (*Comstock* Original)	120	2.0	24.0	1.5	0	250	3.0
coconut creme (*Comstock* Original)	110	1.0	20.0	3.0	0	330	2.0
lemon (*Comstock* No Bake)	130	0	28.0	1.5	0	120	0
mince/mincemeat:							
(*Comstock* Original)	170	1.0	40.0	0	0	70	1.0
(*Crosse & Blackwell*), ¼ cup	180	<1.0	43.0	0	0	220	0
(*None Such*)	190	0	45.0	.5	0	230	0
w/brandy and rum (*Crosse & Blackwell*), ¼ cup	180	<1.0	43.0	0	0	230	0
w/brandy and rum (*None Such*)	200	0	47.0	1.0	0	250	0
condensed (*None Such*), 4 tsp.	150	0	36.0	.5	0	230	1.0
peach (*Comstock* 25% More Fruit)	80	1.0	19.0	0	0	15	1.0
pineapple, tropical (*Comstock*)	110	0	27.0	0	0	50	1.0
pumpkin, mix:							
(*Comstock*)	90	1.0	24.0	0	0	290	2.0
(*Libby's*)	90	<1.0	20.0	.5	0	115	2.0
raisin, California (*Comstock*)	120	1.0	29.0	0	0	25	3.0
raspberry (*Comstock* Royal)	100	1.0	25.0	0	0	45	3.0
strawberry (*Comstock* Berry Patch)	100	0	23.0	0	0	25	1.0
strawberry-rhubarb (*Lucky Leaf*)	90	0	23.0	0	0	35	1.0

Food and Measure	cal.	prot. (gms)	carbo. (gms)	fat (gms)	chol. (mgs)	sod. (mgs)	fiber (gms)
Pie filling mix, see "Pudding and pie filling mix"							
Pie glaze, see "Glaze"							
Pierogi, frozen, 3 pcs.:							
potato cheese:							
(*Mrs. T's*)	180	7.0	34.0	2.5	10	430	2.0
(*Old Fashioned Kitchen*)	185	5.0	33.0	3.0	45	175	0
potato onion:							
(*Giorgio*)	230	6.0	42.0	3.0	0	380	3.0
(*Old Fashioned Kitchen*)	182	4.0	35.0	3.0	36	195	.5
Pig's feet:							
simmered, 4 oz.	220	21.8	0	14.1	113	n.a.	0
pickled:							
cured, 1 oz.	58	3.8	<.1	4.6	26	n.a.	0
(*Hormel*), 2 oz.	80	7.0	0	6.0	45	530	0
Pigeon peas, 1/2 cup, except as noted:							
fresh:							
raw	105	5.5	18.4	1.3	0	4	3.2
boiled, drained	86	4.6	15.0	1.1	0	3	2.5
canned:							
dried (*El Jib*)	80	5.0	18.0	0	0	490	0
green (*Tupi*)	70	4.0	14.0	0	0	390	4.0
dried:							
(*Goya*), 1/4 cup	140	8.0	24.0	.5	0	10	3.0
boiled	102	5.7	19.5	.3	0	5	3.9
Pignolia nut, see "Pine nut"							
Pike:							
northern, meat only:							
raw, 4 oz.	100	21.8	0	.8	44	44	0
baked, broiled, or microwaved, 4 oz.	128	28.0	0	1.0	57	56	0
walleye, meat only, raw, 4 oz.	105	21.7	0	1.4	98	58	0

Food and Measure	cal.	prot. (gms)	carbo. (gms)	fat (gms)	chol. (mgs)	sod. (mgs)	fiber (gms)
baked, broiled, or microwaved, 4 oz.	135	27.8	0	1.8	125	74	0
Pili nuts, dried:							
shelled, 1 oz.	204	3.1	1.1	22.6	0	4	<1.0
shelled, 1 cup	863	13.0	4.8	95.5	0	4	3.4
Pimiento, drained (*S&W*), 2¼ oz.	20	1.0	3.0	0	0	180	0
Piña colada drink, see "Pineapple drink blends"							
Piña colada drink mix, dry (*Watkins Cooler*), 5 tbsp. . . .	25	0	4.0	1.0	0	10	0
Piña colada mixer:							
canned or bottled:							
(*Daily's*), 3 fl. oz.	160	0	37.0	2.0	0	115	1.0
(*Goya*), ⅓ cup	120	1.0	20.0	4.0	0	30	0
(*Mr & Mrs T*), 4.5 fl. oz.	180	0	43.0	0	0	130	0
(*Roland*), 3 fl. oz.	120	1.0	17.0	6.0	0	30	0
frozen (*Bacardi*), 2 fl. oz.	170	0	35.0	4.0	0	20	0
Pine nut, dried:							
pignolia:							
(*Frieda's*), ¼ cup, 1 oz.	150	7.0	4.0	15.0	0	0	1.0
(*Krinos*), .5 oz.	90	5.0	0	7.5	0	5	1.0
(*Progresso*), 1-oz. jar	170	10.0	2.0	13.0	0	0	0
1 oz.	146	6.8	4.0	14.4	0	1	1.3
1 tbsp.	51	2.4	1.4	5.1	0	<1	.5
pinyon:							
1 oz.	161	3.3	5.5	17.3	0	20	3.0
10 kernels	6	.1	.2	.6	0	1	.1
Pineapple:							
fresh:							
(*Frieda's* Sugar Loaf), ¾ cup, 3 oz.	30	1.0	7.0	0	0	0	1.0
diced, ½ cup	39	.3	9.6	.3	0	<1	.9

Food and Measure	cal.	prot. (gms)	carbo. (gms)	fat (gms)	chol. (mgs)	sod. (mgs)	fiber (gms)
Pineapple, fresh *(cont.)*							
sliced (*Dole*),							
2 slices	90	1.0	21.0	1.0	0	10	2.0
canned, see "Pineapple, canned"							
dried (*Sonoma*),							
1.4 oz.	140	0	30.0	2.0	0	30	2.0
frozen, sweetened,							
chunks, ½ cup	104	.5	27.1	.1	0	2	1.3
Pineapple, candied:							
(*Paradise/White*							
Swan), 6 pcs., 1 oz.	90	0	22.0	0	0	10	0
assorted (*Paradise/*							
White Swan),							
2 tbsp., 1 oz.	90	0	22.0	0	0	15	1.0
and cherries, see							
"Cherry, candied"							
green (*Paradise/White*							
Swan), 7 pcs., 1 oz.	90	0	22.0	0	0	15	1.0
red (*Paradise/White*							
Swan), 8 pcs.,							
1.1 oz.	100	0	24.0	0	0	15	1.0
Pineapple, canned,							
½ cup, except as							
noted:							
in juice:							
all varieties, except							
sliced (*Del Monte*)	70	0	17.0	0	0	10	1.0
crushed (*Dole*)	70	1.0	17.0	0	0	10	1.0
sliced (*Del Monte*),							
2 slices, 4 oz. . . .	60	0	16.0	0	0	10	1.0
sliced (*Dole*),							
2 slices, 4 oz. . . .	60	0	15.0	0	0	10	1.0
spears or wedges							
(*Del Monte*)	70	0	17.0	0	0	10	1.0
tidbits (*Del*							
Monte cup), 4 oz.	50	0	15.0	0	0	10	<1.0
tidbits or chunks							
(*Dole*)	60	0	15.0	0	0	10	1.0
in extra light syrup							
(*Sunfresh* Chilled)	80	1.0	17.0	0	0	65	0

Food and Measure	cal.	prot. (gms)	carbo. (gms)	fat (gms)	chol. (mgs)	sod. (mgs)	fiber (gms)
in light syrup:							
all varieties, except							
sliced (*Dole*)	80	1.0	20.0	0	0	10	1.0
sliced (*Dole*), 3½							
slices, 4 oz.	60	0	16.0	0	0	10	1.0
w/mandarin orange							
(*Dole*)	80	0	19.0	<1.0	0	10	1.0
in heavy syrup:							
4 oz.	88	.4	22.9	.1	0	1	.8
all varieties, except							
sliced (*Dole*)	90	1.0	24.0	0	0	10	1.0
chunks, tidbits, or							
crushed	100	.5	25.8	.1	0	2	.9
crushed or chunks							
(*Del Monte*)	90	0	24.0	0	0	10	1.0
sliced (*Del Monte*),							
2 slices	90	0	23.0	0	0	10	1.0
sliced (*Dole*),							
2 slices	90	1.0	23.0	0	0	10	1.0
in extra-heavy syrup:							
crushed (*Dole*)	110	0	29.0	0	0	10	1.0
cubes (*Dole*)	200	1.0	50.0	0	0	10	1.0
Pineapple, dried:							
(*Sonoma Organic*),							
¼ cup, 1.4 oz.	110	1.0	25.0	0	0	0	2.0
freeze-dried, chunks							
(*AlpineAire*), .4 oz.	45	0	10.0	0	0	0	1.0
Pineapple drink							
blends, 8 fl. oz., ex-							
cept as noted:							
coconut:							
(*Arizona* Piña Co-							
lada)	140	0	34.0	1.0	0	30	0
(*Farmer's Market*)	120	0	29.0	0	0	15	0
nectar (*Kern's*)	200	<1.0	36.0	6.0	0	40	2.0
nectar (*Kern's*),							
11.5 fl. oz.	290	1.0	52.0	8.0	0	55	3.0
guava nectar (*Goya*)	150	1.0	37.0	0	0	30	3.0
orange:							
(*Veryfine*), 10 fl. oz.	160	0	39.0	0	0	20	0

Food and Measure	cal.	prot. (gms)	carbo. (gms)	fat (gms)	chol. (mgs)	sod. (mgs)	fiber (gms)
Pineapple drink blends, orange *(cont.)*							
(*Veryfine*), 11.5 fl. oz.	180	0	46.0	0	0	15	0
(*Whipper Snapple*), 10 fl. oz.	160	0	41.0	0	0	60	0
passion fruit nectar (*Goya*), 6 fl. oz. ...	120	1.0	28.0	0	0	20	n.a.
Pineapple drink mix, 8 fl. oz.*:							
(*Kool-Aid*)	100	0	25.0	0	0	10	0
(*Kool-Aid* Presweetened)	60	0	17.0	0	0	0	0
Pineapple juice, 8 fl. oz., except as noted:							
(*Del Monte*), 6 fl. oz.	80	<1.0	20.0	0	0	5	0
(*Del Monte*)	130	1.0	32.0	0	0	10	1.0
(*Del Monte* Not From Concentrate)	110	1.0	29.0	0	0	15	2.0
(*Dole*)	130	2.0	29.0	0	0	20	0
(*Goya*), 6 fl. oz. ...	90	1.0	21.0	0	0	25	<1.0
(*Minute Maid*)	130	0	32.0	0	0	25	0
Pineapple juice blends, 8 fl. oz.:							
coconut (*R.W. Knudsen*)	130	0	32.0	0	0	50	0
guava (*Chiquita* Cocktail)	120	0	31.0	0	0	10	0
orange:							
(*Dole*)	120	2.0	27.0	0	0	20	0
(*Tropicana*)	110	1.0	26.0	0	0	10	0
orange-banana (*Dole*)	120	2.0	29.0	0	0	20	0
orange-strawberry (*Dole*)	130	0	32.0	0	0	20	0
Pineapple nectar blends, see "Pineapple drink blends"							
Pineapple topping, 2 tbsp.:							
(*Kraft*)	110	0	28.0	0	0	15	0

Food and Measure	cal.	prot. (gms)	carbo. (gms)	fat (gms)	chol. (mgs)	sod. (mgs)	fiber (gms)
(*Smucker's*)	110	0	28.0	0	0	0	0
Pineapple-banana-or-ange smoothie (*Del Monte Blenders*), 5.5 fl. oz.	170	1.0	44.0	0	0	10	<1.0
Pink beans, boiled, ½ cup	125	7.6	23.5	.4	0	2	4.5
Pinto beans:							
dry (*Arrowhead Mills*), ¼ cup	150	10.0	27.0	.5	0	0	8.0
boiled, ½ cup	117	7.0	21.8	.4	0	1	7.3
Pinto beans, canned, ½ cup, except as noted.							
(*Allens East Texas Fair/Brown Beauty*)	110	5.0	20.0	.5	0	290	7.0
(*Bush's Best*)	110	6.0	18.0	.5	0	430	6.0
(*Chi-Chi's*)	100	6.0	18.0	.5	0	540	3.0
(*Eden* Organic)	100	6.0	18.0	0	0	15	6.0
(*Gebhardt*)	90	6.5	17.5	1.0	0	505	7.0
(*Green Giant/Joan of Arc*)	110	6.0	20.0	.5	0	280	5.0
(*Old El Paso*)	100	6.0	19.0	.5	0	420	7.0
(*Progresso*)	110	7.0	18.0	1.0	0	250	7.0
(*Stokely*)	110	6.0	19.0	.5	0	350	3.0
w/bacon:							
(*Bush's Best*)	110	6.0	18.0	1.0	0	540	6.0
(*Trappey's*)	120	6.0	20.0	1.0	0	270	7.0
w/bacon and jalape-ños:							
(*Bush's Best*)	110	7.0	17.0	1.5	5	550	6.0
(*Trappey's Jalapinto*)	120	6.0	22.0	1.0	0	540	8.0
w/liquid	93	5.5	17.5	.4	0	499	4.2
w/pork (*Bush's Best*)	120	6.0	17.0	2.5	5	530	6.0
Spanish style (*Goya*), 7.5 oz.	140	11.0	31.0	1.0	0	860	10.0
spicy, see "Chili beans"							
Pinto beans, dehy-drated (*AlpineAire*), 1 oz.	100	6.0	18.0	0	0	0	6.0

Food and Measure	cal.	prot. (gms)	carbo. (gms)	fat (gms)	chol. (mgs)	sod. (mgs)	fiber (gms)
Pinto beans, **sprouted,** boiled, drained, 4 oz.	25	2.1	4.6	.4	0	58	<2.0
Pistachio nut, shelled, except as noted:							
dried:							
in shell (*Dole*), 1 oz.	90	3.0	3.0	7.0	0	250	n.a.
in shell (*River* *Queen*), ½ cup, 1 oz. edible	170	4.0	8.0	15.0	0	210	3.0
1 oz.	164	5.8	7.1	13.7	0	2	3.1
(*Dole*), 1 oz.	163	6.0	7.0	14.0	0	n.a.	n.a.
(*Sonoma*), ¼ cup, 1.1 oz.	190	6.0	9.0	14.0	0	220	3.0
dry-roasted, in shell:							
(*Planters*), ½ cup, 1 oz. edible nuts . . .	160	5.0	7.0	14.0	0	180	3.0
dry-roasted:							
(*Planters*), 1 oz. . . .	160	5.0	7.0	14.0	0	220	3.0
1 oz.	172	4.2	7.8	15.0	0	2	3.1
1 cup	776	19.1	35.2	67.6	0	8	13.8
Pita, see "Bread"							
Pitanga:							
1 medium, .3 oz.	2	.1	.5	<.1	0	<1	<1.0
½ cup	29	.7	6.5	.3	0	3	<1.0
Pizza, frozen, 1 pie, except as noted:							
(*Totino's Pizza Party* Zesty Italiano), ½ pie	390	14.0	36.0	21.0	15	900	2.0
artichoke heart (*Wolf-* *gang Puck's*), ½ pie	340	15.0	34.0	17.0	25	450	3.0
bacon burger (*Totino's* *Pizza Party*), ½ pie	380	14.0	34.0	21.0	15	870	2.0
Canadian bacon:							
(*Jeno's Crisp 'n* *Tasty*)	440	17.0	50.0	19.0	15	1160	2.0
(*Tombstone* Original 12"), ¼ pie	360	20.0	36.0	15.0	40	920	2.0
(*Totino's Pizza* *Party*), ½ pie	330	13.0	35.0	15.0	10	910	2.0

Food and Measure	cal.	prot. (gms)	carbo. (gms)	fat (gms)	chol. (mgs)	sod. (mgs)	fiber (gms)
cheese:							
(*Amy's*), 13 oz. ...	310	13.0	39.0	11.0	15	490	2.0
(*Celeste* Large), ¼ pie	320	14.0	32.0	16.0	25	590	3.0
(*Celeste* Large Premium), ¼ pie ...	350	15.0	33.0	18.0	30	710	2.0
(*Celeste* for One) ...	420	18.0	42.0	20.0	35	830	3.0
(*Jeno's Crisp 'n Tasty*)	460	19.0	52.0	19.0	20	860	2.0
(*Tombstone For One* ½ Less Fat)	360	23.0	45.0	10.0	15	920	3.0
(*Totino's* Family Size), ⅓ pie	370	16.0	39.0	16.0	20	720	2.0
(*Totino's* Microwave for One)	240	10.0	26.0	17.0	15	540	1.0
(*Totino's Pizza Party*), ½ pie	320	15.0	34.0	14.0	20	620	2.0
cheese, extra:							
(*Tombstone* Original 9"), ½ pie	420	20.0	42.0	19.0	30	730	3.0
(*Tombstone* Original 12"), ¼ pie	370	18.0	36.0	17.0	30	680	2.0
(*Tombstone For One*)	540	27.0	41.0	30.0	45	910	3.0
cheese, four:							
(*Celeste* for One Original)	480	22.0	41.0	26.0	45	920	4.0
(*Celeste* Rising Crust), ⅙ pie	340	16.0	46.0	10.0	20	770	4.0
(*Tombstone Special Order* 12"), ⅕ pie	400	20.0	37.0	19.0	40	760	2.0
(*Wolfgang Puck's*), ½ pie	360	17.0	40.0	15.0	25	530	5.0
zesty (*Celeste* for One)	470	21.0	44.0	24.0	40	970	4.0
"cheese," nondairy (*Amy's* Soy Cheeze), 4.33 oz.	280	12.0	37.0	11.0	0	490	2.0
cheese, three: Italian style (*Tombstone* ThinCrust), ¼ pie	380	20.0	25.0	22.0	45	730	2.0

Food and Measure	cal.	prot. (gms)	carbo. (gms)	fat (gms)	chol. (mgs)	sod. (mgs)	fiber (gms)
Pizza *(cont.)*							
chicken, spicy (*Wolfgang Puck's*), ½ pie	360	19.0	36.0	16.0	45	620	5.0
combination:							
(*Jeno's Crisp 'n Tasty*)	520	17.0	50.0	28.0	25	1130	3.0
(*Totino's* Family Size), pie	310	11.0	29.0	17.0	20	720	2.0
(*Totino's* Microwave for One)	310	10.0	26.0	18.0	15	720	1.0
(*Totino's Pizza Party*), ½ pie	390	14.0	35.0	21.0	15	910	2.0
(*Weight Watchers* Deluxe), 6.6 oz.	380	21.0	52.0	11.0	40	550	6.0
deluxe:							
(*Celeste* Large), ¼ pie	350	14.0	35.0	18.0	20	880	4.0
(*Celeste* Large Premium), ¼ pie . . .	390	16.0	34.0	21.0	35	840	2.0
(*Celeste* for One) . . .	470	18.0	46.0	25.0	25	1140	5.0
(*Tombstone* Original 9″), ⅓ pie	320	15.0	28.0	16.0	30	620	2.0
(*Tombstone* Original 12″), ⅕ pie	320	15.0	29.0	16.0	30	640	2.0
ham and shrimp, Hawaiian style (*Contessa*), ½ pie	340	16.0	46.0	11.0	35	750	2.0
hamburger:							
(*Jeno's Crisp 'n Tasty*)	500	17.0	50.0	25.0	25	1080	3.0
(*Tombstone* Original 9″), ⅓ pie	310	14.0	28.0	16.0	30	620	2.0
(*Tombstone* Original 12″), ⅕ pie	320	15.0	29.0	16.0	30	660	2.0
(*Totino's Pizza Party*), ½ pie	380	15.0	34.0	20.0	15	850	2.0
meat, four:							
(*Tombstone Special Order 9″*), ⅓ pie	400	19.0	35.0	20.0	45	910	2.0
(*Tombstone Special Order 12″*), ⅙ pie	350	17.0	31.0	18.0	40	810	2.0

Food and Measure	cal.	prot. (gms)	carbo. (gms)	fat (gms)	chol. (mgs)	sod. (mgs)	fiber (gms)
combo, Italian (*Tombstone* Thin Crust), 1/4 pie	410	20.0	25.0	25.0	50	940	2.0
meat, three:							
(*Celeste* Rising Crust), 1/6 pie	390	18.0	40.0	17.0	35	930	5.0
(*Jeno's Crisp 'n Tasty*)	500	17.0	50.0	26.0	25	1190	2.0
(*Totino's Pizza Party*), 1/2 pie	360	14.0	34.0	19.0	15	920	2.0
Mexican, supreme taco (*Tombstone* ThinCrust), 1/4 pie	380	16.0	26.0	23.0	50	850	2.0
mushroom spinach (*Wolfgang Puck's*), 1/2 pie	270	14.0	36.0	8.0	10	380	5.0
pepperoni:							
(*Celeste* Large), 1/4 pie	350	13.0	33.0	20.0	20	990	3.0
(*Celeste* Large Premium), 1/4 pie . . .	390	15.0	34.0	23.0	35	870	2.0
(*Celeste* for One) . . .	470	16.0	41.0	27.0	20	1100	4.0
(*Celeste* Rising Crust), 1/6 pie	380	17.0	43.0	16.0	30	950	6.0
(*Jeno's Crisp 'n Tasty*)	510	16.0	50.0	27.0	25	1170	2.0
(*Tombstone* Original 9"), 1/3 pie	340	15.0	28.0	19.0	30	740	2.0
(*Tombstone* Original 12"), 1/5 pie	340	15.0	29.0	18.0	35	750	2.0
(*Tombstone* For One)	580	25.0	41.0	35.0	50	1170	3.0
(*Tombstone* For One 1/2 Less Fat)	400	26.0	45.0	13.0	35	1040	4.0
(*Tombstone* Special Order 9"), 1/3 pie	400	19.0	35.0	21.0	45	880	2.0
(*Tombstone* Special Order 12"), 1/6 pie	360	16.0	31.0	19.0	40	790	2.0
(*Totino's* Family Size), 1/3 pie	410	14.0	38.0	22.0	20	990	2.0

Food and Measure	cal.	prot. (gms)	carbo. (gms)	fat (gms)	chol. (mgs)	sod. (mgs)	fiber (gms)
Pizza, pepperoni *(cont.)*							
(*Totino's* Microwave for One)	290	10.0	26.0	16.0	15	700	1.0
(*Totino's* Pizza Party), ½ pie	380	13.0	34.0	21.0	20	910	2.0
(*Weight Watchers*), 5.5 oz.	390	20.0	50.0	12.0	40	650	4.0
(*Wolfgang Puck's*), ½ pie	390	21.0	43.0	15.0	45	690	3.0
w/double cheese (*Tombstone Double Top*), ⅙ pie	350	19.0	25.0	20.0	45	850	2.0
Italian style (*Tombstone ThinCrust*), ¼ pie	420	20.0	25.0	27.0	55	950	2.0
pesto, w/tomatoes and broccoli (*Amy's*), 4.5 oz.	300	12.0	39.0	11.0	10	480	2.0
sausage:							
(*Celeste* for One) ...	530	23.0	52.0	27.0	25	1400	5.0
(*Jeno's Crisp 'n Tasty*)	520	16.0	50.0	28.0	20	1080	3.0
(*Tombstone* Original 9″), ⅓ pie	310	14.0	28.0	16.0	30	610	2.0
(*Tombstone* Original 12″), ⅕ pie	320	15.0	29.0	16.0	30	650	2.0
(*Tombstone* Special Order 9″), ⅓ pie	390	19.0	35.0	19.0	40	830	2.0
(*Totino's* Family Size), ⅓ pie	300	11.0	29.0	16.0	10	730	2.0
(*Totino's* Microwave for One)	290	9.0	26.0	17.0	10	650	1.0
(*Totino's* Pizza Party), ½ pie	380	14.0	35.0	20.0	15	880	2.0
w/double cheese (*Tombstone Double Top*), ⅙ pie	350	20.0	25.0	19.0	40	740	2.0
herb (*Wolfgang Puck's*), ½ pie ...	380	19.0	36.0	18.0	45	650	7.0

Food and Measure	cal.	prot. (gms)	carbo. (gms)	fat (gms)	chol. (mgs)	sod. (mgs)	fiber (gms)
Italian (*Tombstone For One*)	560	25.0	40.0	33.0	55	1130	3.0
Italian style (*Tombstone* ThinCrust), ¼ pie	400	19.0	25.0	24.0	50	880	2.0
three (*Tombstone Special Order* 12″), ⅙ pie	340	16.0	31.0	17.0	35	740	2.0
sausage and mushroom:							
(*Tombstone* Original 12″), ⅕ pie	320	15.0	29.0	16.0	30	630	2.0
(*Totino's Pizza Party*), ½ pie	360	14.0	34.0	19.0	20	850	2.0
sausage and pepperoni:							
(*Celeste* Large Premium), ¼ pie . . .	380	16.0	33.0	22.0	35	840	2.0
(*Tombstone* Original 9″), ⅓ pie	360	16.0	28.0	21.0	35	820	2.0
(*Tombstone* Original 12″), ⅕ pie	340	16.0	29.0	18.0	35	740	2.0
(*Tombstone For One*)	590	25.0	40.0	37.0	55	1200	3.0
w/double cheese (*Tombstone Double Top*), ⅙ pie	360	20.0	25.0	20.0	45	800	2.0
shrimp/pesto, ½ pie:							
basil (*Contessa*) . . .	300	14.0	40.0	11.0	35	510	2.0
roasted red (*Contessa*)	330	14.0	42.0	13.0	30	490	3.0
spinach (*Amy's*), 14 oz.	320	13.0	40	11.0	15	490	2.0
supreme:							
(*Celeste* Rising Crust), ⅙ pie	380	17.0	40.0	17.0	30	900	6.0
(*Celeste* Suprema Large), ⅕ pie	290	13.0	27.0	16.0	15	770	3.0
(*Celeste* Suprema for One)	500	22.0	49.0	27.0	25	1290	6.0

Food and Measure	cal.	prot. (gms)	carbo. (gms)	fat (gms)	chol. (mgs)	sod. (mgs)	fiber (gms)
Pizza, supreme *(cont.)*							
(*Jeno's Crisp 'n Tasty*)	520	17.0	50.0	28.0	25	1120	3.0
(*Tombstone* Original 12″), ⅕ pie	330	15.0	29.0	17.0	35	720	2.0
(*Tombstone For One*)	570	24.0	41.0	34.0	50	1130	3.0
(*Tombstone For One* ½ Less Fat)	400	27.0	45.0	13.0	35	1090	4.0
(*Tombstone Light*), ⅕ pie	270	25.0	30.0	9.0	20	710	2.0
(*Totino's* Microwave for One)	300	10.0	26.0	17.0	15	680	1.0
(*Totino's* Pizza Party), ½ pie	390	14.0	35.0	21.0	15	900	2.0
Italian style (*Tombstone* ThinCrust), ¼ pie	400	18.0	26.0	24.0	45	880	2.0
super (*Tombstone Special Order* 9″), ⅓ pie	400	19.0	36.0	21.0	45	900	2.0
super (*Tombstone Special Order* 12″), ⅙ pie	350	17.0	31.0	18.0	40	800	2.0
vegetable:							
(*Celeste* for One) ...	420	17.0	46.0	21.0	5	1120	5.0
(*Tombstone For One* ½ Less Fat)	360	22.0	46.0	10.0	15	730	5.0
(*Tombstone Light*), ⅕ pie	240	25.0	31.0	7.0	10	500	3.0
grilled, cheeseless (*Wolfgang Puck's* Fat Free), ½ pie	200	6.0	42.0	0	0	430	2.0
roasted (*Amy's*), 4 oz.	270	6.0	43.0	8.0	0	470	3.0
Pizza, croissant, frozen, 1 pc.:							
cheese (*Pepperidge Farm*)	390	12.0	39.0	20.0	90	770	6.0
deluxe (*Pepperidge Farm*)	450	14.0	40.0	27.0	85	910	7.0

Food and Measure	cal.	prot. (gms)	carbo. (gms)	fat (gms)	chol. (mgs)	sod. (mgs)	fiber (gms)
pepperoni (*Pepperidge Farm*)	420	15.0	39.0	23.0	90	810	5.0
Pizza, French bread, frozen, 1 pc.:							
cheese:							
(*Healthy Choice*) . . .	340	22.0	51.0	5.0	15	480	7.0
(*Lean Cuisine*)	320	15.0	48.0	7.0	15	480	4.0
(*Stouffer's*)	370	14.0	43.0	16.0	15	880	3.0
extra (*Stouffer's*)	400	16.0	49.0	16.0	25	950	4.0
five (*Stouffer's*)	420	17.0	48.0	18.0	25	850	3.0
deluxe:							
(*Lean Cuisine*)	300	16.0	46.0	6.0	25	590	4.0
(*Stouffer's*)	430	17.0	44.0	21.0	20	990	3.0
garlic, creamy (*Lean Cuisine*)	310	15.0	47.0	7.0	15	570	2.0
meat, three (*Stouffer's*)	460	20.0	48.0	21.0	35	1200	4.0
pepperoni:							
(*Healthy Choice*) . . .	340	24.0	49.0	5.0	20	580	5.0
(*Lean Cuisine*)	310	15.0	46.0	7.0	20	590	3.0
(*Stouffer's*)	430	16.0	46.0	20.0	15	990	3.0
pepperoni and mushroom (*Stouffer's*)	440	15.0	49.0	20.0	30	910	5.0
sausage:							
(*Healthy Choice*) . . .	320	21.0	48.0	5.0	25	580	5.0
(*Stouffer's*)	420	17.0	48.0	18.0	20	1260	3.0
sausage and pepperoni (*Stouffer's*)	470	18.0	47.0	23.0	25	1340	3.0
sun-dried tomatoes (*Lean Cuisine*)	340	19.0	48.0	8.0	20	580	3.0
supreme (*Healthy Choice*)	330	21.0	51.0	5.0	20	580	5.0
vegetable:							
(*Healthy Choice*) . . .	280	17.0	45.0	4.0	10	480	5.0
grilled (*Stouffer's*)	350	12.0	48.0	12.0	10	500	3.0
white (*Stouffer's*)	460	18.0	45.0	23.0	20	700	5.0
Pizza, stuffed (see also "Pizza Pocket"), frozen, 1/6 pkg., except as noted:							
(*Testa Rossa* Pueblo)	330	15.0	38.0	13.0	20	610	1.0

Food and Measure	cal.	prot. (gms)	carbo. (gms)	fat (gms)	chol. (mgs)	sod. (mgs)	fiber (gms)
Pizza, stuffed *(cont.)*							
cheese, five (*San Francisco Gourmet Foods*), ¼ pkg. . . .	410	18.0	52.0	15.0	30	880	1.0
Greek (*Testa Rossa*)	360	17.0	40.0	14.0	25	770	2.0
meat combo (*San Francisco Gourmet Foods*), ¼ pkg. . . .	410	18.0	49.0	17.0	30	940	1.0
pepperoni (*San Francisco Gourmet Foods*), ¼ pkg. . . .	420	19.0	49.0	17.0	35	970	1.0
pesto (*Testa Rossa*)	370	18.0	41.0	15.0	25	650	3.0
vegetable, roasted (*Testa Rossa*)	330	15.0	43.0	11.0	20	650	2.0
Pizza burrito, see "Burrito"							
Pizza crust:							
refrigerated (*Pillsbury All Ready*), ⅕ crust	150	5.0	27.0	2.0	0	380	<1.0
mix, dry:							
(*Betty Crocker*), ¼ crust	160	4.0	33.0	2.0	0	340	1.0
(*Martha White*), ¼ pkg.	160	5.0	32.0	1.0	0	250	1.0
(*Ragú Pizza Quick*), ⅓ cup	130	5.0	24.0	1.0	0	270	1.0
deep pan (*Martha White*), ⅕ pkg.	140	5.0	28.0	1.0	0	280	<1.0
Italian herb (*Betty Crocker*), ¼ crust	160	4.0	32.0	2.0	0	350	1.0
Pizza crust mix, ⅛ pkg.:							
deep dish (*Watkins*)	180	6.0	36.0	1.0	0	60	2.0
whole wheat (*Watkins*)	90	1.0	9.0	.5	0	40	0
Pizza crust seasoning, ⅛ pkg.:							
garden (*Watkins*)	10	0	2.0	0	0	120	0
Italian (*Watkins*)	10	0	2.0	0	0	100	0
Pizza entree, frozen, 1 pkg.:							
w/cheese (*Kid Cuisine Pirate*), 8 oz.	430	12.0	71.0	11.0	30	480	5.0

Food and Measure	cal.	prot. (gms)	carbo. (gms)	fat (gms)	chol. (mgs)	sod. (mgs)	fiber (gms)
hamburger (*Kid Cuisine* Big League), 8.3 oz.	400	14.0	61.0	11.0	25	530	6.0
Pizza entree, packaged, wedges, 1 cup:							
cheese, three (*Kid's Kitchen*)	270	10.0	44.0	7.0	25	1060	1.0
cheeseburger (*Kid's Kitchen*)	250	10.0	41.0	5.0	25	890	3.0
pepperoni (*Kid's Kitchen*)	260	10.0	38.0	8.0	25	1080	3.0
Pizza Hut, 1 slice of medium pie, except as noted:							
Edge, medium:							
chicken/veggie	120	6.0	16.0	3.0	10	310	1.0
meaty	150	7.0	15.0	7.0	15	430	1.0
veggies	110	4.0	16.0	2.5	5	250	1.0
works	140	6.0	16.0	5.0	10	360	1.0
Edge, large:							
chicken/veggie	160	8.0	21.0	4.0	10	430	2.0
meaty	200	9.0	19.0	10.0	25	580	1.0
veggies	140	6.0	21.0	3.5	5	340	2.0
works	180	8.0	21.0	7.0	15	470	2.0
hand-tossed:							
beef	280	15.0	32.0	10.0	20	860	2.0
cheese	280	16.0	32.0	10.0	25	770	2.0
chicken supreme	240	14.0	31.0	6.0	25	660	3.0
ham	230	13.0	30.0	6.0	25	710	2.0
Meat Lover's	290	15.0	32.0	11.0	35	820	3.0
pepperoni	260	12.0	31.0	9.0	30	750	3.0
Pepperoni Lover's	320	17.0	31.0	13.0	35	910	4.0
pork topping	290	14.0	22.0	13.0	25	780	2.0
sausage, Italian	300	15.0	32.0	12.0	30	780	3.0
super supreme	290	15.0	34.0	10.0	35	830	4.0
supreme	250	13.0	24.0	11.0	20	710	3.0
Veggie Lover's	240	11.0	34.0	7.0	20	650	3.0
pan pizza:							
beef	310	14.0	31.0	14.0	20	720	2.0
cheese	300	15.0	30.0	14.0	25	610	2.0

Food and Measure	cal.	prot. (gms)	carbo. (gms)	fat (gms)	chol. (mgs)	sod. (mgs)	fiber (gms)
Pizza Hut, pan pizza _(cont.)_							
chicken supreme	280	14.0	32.0	11.0	25	570	3.0
ham	250	12.0	31.0	9.0	10	590	2.0
Meat Lover's	360	17.0	30.0	19.0	40	870	3.0
pepperoni	280	12.0	31.0	12.0	20	640	3.0
Pepperoni Lover's	350	17.0	32.0	17.0	20	800	2.0
pork topping	300	14.0	31.0	13.0	30	720	3.0
sausage, Italian	350	16.0	31.0	18.0	40	740	3.0
super supreme	340	15.0	33.0	16.0	30	790	4.0
supreme	300	13.0	32.0	13.0	25	670	3.0
Veggie Lover's	240	10.0	31.0	9.0	10	480	3.0
Pizzeria Stuffed Crust:							
beef	410	20.0	49.0	14.0	30	1270	4.0
cheese	380	21.0	49.0	11.0	25	1160	4.0
chicken supreme	390	21.0	46.0	13.0	40	1130	4.0
ham	380	22.0	43.0	14.0	45	1250	4.0
Meat Lover's	500	25.0	47.0	23.0	60	1510	5.0
pepperoni	410	20.0	46.0	17.0	40	1250	4.0
Pepperoni Lover's	480	24.0	47.0	22.0	60	1440	4.0
pork topping	420	22.0	46.0	16.0	30	1290	4.0
sausage, Italian	430	20.0	46.0	19.0	35	1200	4.0
super supreme	470	24.0	49.0	20.0	50	1440	5.0
supreme	440	23.0	51.0	16.0	40	1380	4.0
Veggie Lover's	390	18.0	48.0	14.0	25	1140	5.0
Sicilian:							
beef	320	13.0	31.0	15.0	20	930	3.0
cheese	290	12.0	31.0	13.0	10	740	2.0
chicken supreme	270	13.0	32.0	10.0	15	730	3.0
ham	260	11.0	31.0	10.0	15	750	2.0
Meat Lover's	350	15.0	32.0	18.0	30	990	3.0
pepperoni	290	11.0	31.0	13.0	20	760	2.0
Pepperoni Lover's	330	14.0	31.0	17.0	30	910	2.0
pork topping	320	13.0	31.0	16.0	20	890	3.0
sausage, Italian	330	14.0	32.0	16.0	25	850	2.0
super supreme	320	14.0	32.0	16.0	25	930	3.0
supreme	310	13.0	32.0	15.0	20	860	3.0
Veggie Lover's	270	10.0	32.0	11.0	5	670	3.0
Thin 'N Crispy :							
beef	240	13.0	22.0	11.0	20	790	2.0
cheese	210	12.0	21.0	9.0	20	530	2.0
chicken supreme	220	14.0	26.0	11.0	25	550	2.0

Food and Measure	cal.	prot. (gms)	carbo. (gms)	fat (gms)	chol. (mgs)	sod. (mgs)	fiber (gms)
ham	190	10.0	23.0	6.0	15	560	1.0
Meat Lover's	310	16.0	25.0	16.0	35	900	3.0
pepperoni	220	10.0	22.0	9.0	20	610	2.0
Pepperoni Lover's	270	15.0	26.0	12.0	25	780	2.0
pork topping	270	14.0	22.0	13.0	25	780	2.0
sausage, Italian	300	15.0	24.0	16.0	35	740	3.0
super supreme	280	15.0	26.0	13.0	30	810	4.0
supreme	250	13.0	24.0	11.0	20	710	3.0
Veggie Lover's	170	7.0	23.0	6.0	10	460	3.0
starters/sides:							
Buffalo wings:							
hot, 4 pcs.	210	22.0	4.0	12.0	130	900	<1.0
mild, 5 pcs.	200	23.0	<1.0	12.0	150	510	0
garlic bread, 1 slice	150	3.0	16.0	8.0	0	240	1.0
breadstick, 1 pc.	130	3.0	20.0	4.0	0	170	1.0
breadstick dipping							
sauce, 1 serving	30	<1.0	5.0	.5	0	170	<1.0
Pizza pepper							
(*Lawry's*), ¼ tsp.	0	0	0	0	0	0	0
Pizza pocket (see also							
"Pizza, stuffed"),							
frozen, 1 pc.:							
(*Ken & Robert's Veg-*							
gie Pockets)	270	9.0	41.0	8.0	0	490	4.0
cheese:							
(*Amy's*)	290	14.0	38.0	9.0	20	390	3.0
double (*Hot Pockets*							
Pizza Minis)	240	7.0	32.0	9.0	15	430	3.0
double (*Hot Pockets*							
Toaster Breaks)	190	5.0	22.0	9.0	10	240	1.0
pepperoni:							
(*Big Stuffs*)	440	17.0	50.0	19.0	60	900	4.0
(*Croissant Pockets*)	360	14.0	41.0	12.0	40	800	3.0
(*Deli Stuffs*)	350	14.0	41.0	14.0	35	660	3.0
(*Hot Pockets*)	350	13.0	41.0	15.0	40	640	4.0
(*Hot Pockets* Pizza							
Minis)	250	7.0	31.0	11.0	15	500	3.0
(*Hot Pockets*							
Toaster Breaks)	200	5.0	21.0	10.0	10	350	2.0
deluxe (*Lean Pock-*							
ets)	270	15.0	37.0	7.0	35	580	3.0

Food and Measure	cal.	prot. (gms)	carbo. (gms)	fat (gms)	chol. (mgs)	sod. (mgs)	fiber (gms)
Pizza pocket *(cont.)*							
pepperoni and sausage:							
(*Hot Pockets*)	330	13.0	33.0	14.0	35	510	4.0
(*Hot Pockets* Pizza Minis)	230	8.0	31.0	9.0	15	460	4.0
sausage:							
(*Hot Pockets*)	340	14.0	37.0	15.0	35	550	3.0
(*Hot Pockets* Pizza Minis)	230	8.0	31.0	8.0	15	490	4.0
sausage and pepperoni (*Hot Pockets Toaster Breaks*)	180	5.0	22.0	8.0	10	350	1.0
supreme (*Croissant Pockets*)	390	13.0	40.0	20.0	40	790	3.0
vegetarian (*Amy's*) . . .	240	10.0	35.0	6.0	10	360	3.0
Pizza sauce, 1/4 cup:							
(*Hunt's*)	25	1.0	5.0	<1.0	0	190	2.0
(*Muir Glen*)	40	1.0	6.0	1.0	0	230	2.0
(*Pastorelli Italian Chef*)	40	2.0	6.0	1.0	0	310	2.0
(*Prince* Traditional Arabic)	20	1.0	4.0	0	0	330	1.0
(*Progresso*)	20	<1.0	4.0	0	0	170	1.0
(*Ragú Pizza Quick* 100% Natural)	30	1.0	4.0	1.0	0	270	1.0
(*Ragú Pizza Quick* Traditional)	40	1.0	5.0	0	340	1.0	
garlic and basil (*Ragú Pizza Quick*)	40	1.0	6.0	1.5	0	340	1.0
mushroom, chunky (*Ragú Pizza Quick*)	40	1.0	6.0	1.5	0	340	1.0
pepperoni flavor (*Ragú Pizza Quick*)	60	1.0	5.0	2.0	5	420	1.0
tomato, chunky (*Ragú Pizza Quick*)	50	1.0	7.0	1.5	0	300	1.0
Pizza seasoning (see also "Pizza crust seasoning"):							
(*Tone's/Presti's*), 3/4 tsp.	10	0	1.0	1.0	0	5	0

Food and Measure	cal.	prot. (gms)	carbo. (gms)	fat (gms)	chol. (mgs)	sod. (mgs)	fiber (gms)
and pasta, herbal or hot and sweet (*Chef Paul Prudhomme's Magic Seasoning Blends*), 1/4 tsp. . . .	0	0	0	0	0	95	0
Pizza snack (see also "Nacho snack"), frozen, 6 pcs.:							
cheese:							
(*Amy's*)	180	9.0	22.0	6.0	10	290	2.0
(*Totino's Pizza Rolls*)	210	9.0	25.0	8.0	10	420	1.0
combination (*Totino's Pizza Rolls*)	230	8.0	23.0	12.0	15	480	1.0
meat, three (*Totino's Pizza Rolls*)	220	8.0	24.0	10.0	15	460	1.0
pepperoni (*Totino's Pizza Rolls*)	240	8.0	24.0	12.0	15	550	1.0
sausage (*Totino's Pizza Rolls*)	230	8.0	24.0	11.0	10	390	1.0
supreme (*Totino's Pizza Rolls*)	220	7.0	25.0	10.0	10	380	1.0
Plantain:							
raw:							
(*Frieda's*), 3 oz. . . .	100	1.0	27.0	0	0	0	2.0
1 medium, 9.7 oz.	218	2.3	57.1	.7	0	7	4.1
sliced, 1/2 cup	91	1.0	23.6	.3	0	3	1.7
cooked, sliced, 1/2 cup	89	.6	24.0	.1	0	4	1.8
Plantain, frozen, fried (*Goya Tostones*), 3 medium pcs.	170	1.0	37.0	2.0	0	0	2.0
Plum, fresh:							
Japanese or hybrid, 2 1/8" fruit	36	.5	8.6	.4	0	tr.	<1.0
sliced, 1/2 cup	46	.7	10.7	.5	0	1	1.2
Plum, canned:							
in juice:							
1/2 cup	73	.7	19.1	<.1	0	2	1.3
3 plums and 2 tbsp. liquid	55	.5	14.4	<.1	0	1	1.0
in light syrup:							
1/2 cup	79	.5	20.5	.1	0	25	1.3

Food and Measure	cal.	prot. (gms)	carbo. (gms)	fat (gms)	chol. (mgs)	sod. (mgs)	fiber (gms)
Plum, canned, in light syrup *(cont.)*							
3 plums and 2¾ tbsp. liquid	83	.5	21.7	.1	0	26	1.3
in heavy syrup:							
½ cup	115	.5	30.0	.1	0	25	1.3
purple (*Oregon*), ½ cup	100	19.0	25.0	0	0	15	2.0
whole, purple (*Comstock/Wilderness*), ½ cup	110	1.0	26.0	0	0	35	2.0
Plum sauce:							
(*Ka•Me*), 2 tbsp.	70	0	16.0	0	0	360	0
(*La Choy*), 1 tbsp. . . .	25	0	6.0	0	0	5	0
dipping (*Trader Vic's*), 2 tbsp.	70	0	16.0	0	0	220	0
Pocket sandwich, see specific listings							
Poi, ½ cup	134	.5	32.7	.2	0	14	.5
Poke greens, canned (*Allens*), ½ cup	35	2.0	5.0	1.0	0	5	3.0
Pokeberry shoots:							
raw, ½ cup	18	2.1	3.0	.3	0	n.a.	1.4
boiled, drained, ½ cup	16	1.9	2.5	.3	0	n.a.	1.2
Polenta, refrigerated, 2 slices, ½", except as noted:							
plain:							
(*Frieda's*), 4 oz. . . .	100	3.0	21.0	0	0	440	3.0
(*San Gennaro*)	70	2.0	15.0	0	0	310	1.0
basil and garlic (*San Gennaro*)	71	2.0	15.0	0	0	310	1.0
sun-dried tomato (*San Gennaro*)	74	2.0	16.0	0	0	310	1.0
Polenta dishes, mix, dry, 1.8-oz. cont., except as noted:							
(*Fantastic Foods International Fantastica*), ⅜ cup	260	8.0	46.0	5.0	5	550	4.0
cheese, three (*Fantastic Foods* Cup)	210	7.0	37.0	3.0	10	590	3.0

Food and Measure	cal.	prot. (gms)	carbo. (gms)	fat (gms)	chol. (mgs)	sod. (mgs)	fiber (gms)
Mediterranean (*Fantastic Foods* Cup)	200	7.0	36.0	3.0	5	560	3.0
Mexicana, spicy (*Fantastic Foods* Cup)	210	6.0	39.0	3.0	10	560	4.0
Santa Fe (*Fantastic Foods* Cup)	220	7.0	40.0	3.0	10	590	4.0
Polenta dishes, packaged, ½ pkg.:							
green chili and cilantro, w/black bean sauce (*San Gennaro*)	140	6.0	25.0	2.0	0	530	2.0
mushroom and onion, w/chicken sausage sauce (*San Gennaro*)	130	6.0	21.0	2.0	13	650	1.0
spinach and cheese, w/marinara sauce (*San Gennaro*)	120	4.0	22.0	2.0	3	664	2.0
Polenta mix (see also "Cornmeal"):							
(*Contadina*), 3 tbsp.	110	2.0	26.0	.5	0	0	0
(*Fantastica*), 1 cup*	260	8.0	46.0	5.0	5	550	4.0
Polish sausage (see also "Kielbasa"), 3-oz. link:							
(*Ball Park*)	240	11.0	3.0	20.0	60	950	0
beef (*Hebrew National*)	240	12.0	1.0	22.0	50	680	0
hot (*Ball Park*)	240	11.0	3.0	20	60	950	0
Pollock, meat only:							
Atlantic, 4 oz.:							
raw	104	22.1	0	1.1	80	98	0
baked, broiled, or microwaved	134	28.3	0	1.4	103	125	0
walleye, 4 oz.:							
raw	91	19.5	0	.9	81	112	0
baked, broiled, or microwaved	128	26.7	0	1.3	109	132	0
Pomegranate:							
(*Frieda's*), 5 oz.	100	1.0	24.0	0	0	0	1.0
w/peel, 9.7-oz. fruit	104	1.5	26.4	.5	0	5	.9

Food and Measure	cal.	prot. (gms)	carbo. (gms)	fat (gms)	chol. (mgs)	sod. (mgs)	fiber (gms)
Pomegranate juice							
(*R.W. Knudsen Organic*), 8 fl. oz.	150	0	37.0	0	0	10	0
Pomegranate syrup, see "Grenadine syrup"							
Pompano, Florida, meat only:							
raw, 4 oz.	186	21.0	0	10.7	57	74	0
baked, broiled, or microwaved, 4 oz. . . .	239	26.4	0	13.8	73	86	0
Popcorn:							
(*Arrowhead Mills*), ¼ cup	180	6.0	36.0	2.5	0	0	6.0
(*Orville Redenbacher's Smartpop*), 1.1 oz.	90	3.0	20.0	2.0	0	320	5.0
(*Pop•Secret* Homestyle), 3 tbsp.	170	2.0	16.0	12.0	0	450	3.0
butter/butter flavor:							
(*America's Best*), 5 cups*	90	4.0	23.0	2.0	0	210	9.0
(*Jolly Time Blast O Butter*), 3½ cups*	150	3.0	19.0	11.0	0	340	9.0
(*Jolly Time Blast O Butter* Light), 4 cups*	130	3.0	21.0	6.0	0	340	6.0
(*Jolly Time Butter 'Licious*), 4 cups*	140	3.0	18.0	9.0	0	320	6.0
(*Jolly Time Butter 'Licious* Light), 4 cups*	120	3.0	21.0	6.0	0	290	7.0
(*Jolly Time Healthy Pop*), 5 cups* . . .	90	4.0	23.0	2.0	0	210	9.0
(*Orville Redenbacher's*), 1.1 oz.	135	2.0	14.0	10.0	0	345	3.5
(*Orville Redenbacher's* Light), 1.1 oz.	110	2.5	18.0	5.0	0	325	4.0
(*Pop•Secret*), 4 cups*	150	3.0	16.0	10.0	0	210	3.0

Food and Measure	cal.	prot. (gms)	carbo. (gms)	fat (gms)	chol. (mgs)	sod. (mgs)	fiber (gms)
(*Pop•Secret* Light), 6 cups*	120	3.0	20.0	5.0	0	260	4.0
(*Pop•Secret* Light Snack Size), 1/4 cup	160	4.0	26.0	7.0	0	440	5.0
(*Pop•Secret* Light *Movie Theater*), 6 cups*	130	3.0	20.0	5.0	0	250	3.0
(*Pop•Secret* 99% Fat Free), 6 cups*	110	4.0	23.0	2.0	0	230	4.0
(*Pop•Secret* Snack Size), 1/4 cup	230	4.0	24.0	16.0	0	400	6.0
(*Pop•Secret Jumbo Pop*), 3 tbsp.	170	2.0	18.0	11.0	0	320	3.0
(*Pop•Secret Land O Lakes*), 3 tbsp.	180	3.0	17.0	12.0	0	330	3.0
(*Pop•Secret Movie Theater*), 3 tbsp.	180	2.0	17.0	13.0	0	300	3.0
(*Rudenbudder's* Movie Theater), 1.1 oz.	145	2.0	14.0	10.0	0	310	3.5
(*Rudenbudder's* Movie Theater Light), 1.1 oz.	105	2.5	18.0	4.5	0	310	4.5
zesty (*Rudenbudder's*), 1.1 oz.	145	2.0	13.5	10.5	0	360	3.0
caramel (*Orville Redenbacher's*), 1.1 oz.	140	1.0	18.0	8.0	0	40	1.5
cheddar:							
(*Jolly Time* Microwave), 3 cups*	160	3.0	17.0	10.0	0	350	4.0
(*Pop•Secret*), 5 cups*	150	3.0	16.0	10.0	0	230	3.0
white/golden (*Orville Redenbacher's*), 1.1 oz.	150	2.0	13.0	12.0	0	335	3.0
natural flavor:							
(*Jolly Time* Micro), 4 cups*	150	3.0	16.0	10.0	0	410	6.0

Food and Measure	cal.	prot. (gms)	carbo. (gms)	fat (gms)	chol. (mgs)	sod. (mgs)	fiber (gms)
Popcorn, natural flavor *(cont.)*							
(*Jolly Time* Micro Light), 4 cups*	120	3.0	20.0	5.0	0	320	7.0
(*Orville Redenbacher's*), 1.1 oz.	135	2.0	15.0	9.0	0	425	3.5
(*Orville Redenbacher's Light*), 1.1 oz.	110	2.5	18.0	5.0	0	360	4.0
(*Pop•Secret*), 4 cups*	150	3.0	16.0	10.0	0	280	3.0
(*Pop•Secret* Light), 6 cups*	130	3.0	20.0	5.0	0	260	3.0
(*Pop•Secret* 99% Fat Free), 6 cups*	110	4.0	23.0	2.0	0	230	4.0
white/yellow (*Jolly Time*), 5 cups air- popped	100	4.0	24.0	.5	0	0	6.0
Popcorn, popped:							
(*Bachman* Lite), 5 cups, 1.1 oz.	120	4.0	23.0	1.5	0	115	4.0
(*Frieda's*), 2 cups	120	4.0	23.0	1.5	0	0	5.0
(*Northern Lites* 50% Less Fat), 4 cups	130	3.0	22.0	3.5	0	210	4.0
(*Wise* Baby White Lowfat), 2½ cups	140	3.0	18.0	6.0	0	80	2.0
butter/butter flavor:							
(*Chester's*), 3 cups	160	2.0	15.0	12.0	0	330	3.0
(*Chester's* Micro- wave), 5 cups . . .	200	3.0	22.0	12.0	0	300	4.0
(*Old Dutch* Gourmet White), 2¾ cups	160	2.0	17.0	9.0	0	200	2.0
(*Smartfood*), 3 cups	150	2.0	15.0	9.0	5	240	1.0
(*Smartfood* Re- duced Fat), 3 cups	130	3.0	21.0	4.0	0	410	4.0
(*Weight Watchers*), .7 oz.	90	2.0	14.0	2.5	0	100	3.0
(*Wise*), 1-oz. bag	150	2.0	14.0	10.0	0	320	2.0
(*Wise* Lite), 4 cups	140	3.0	22.0	5.0	0	160	3.0
caramel:							
(*Chester's*), ¾ cup	130	1.0	27.0	2.0	0	220	1.0

Food and Measure	cal.	prot. (gms)	carbo. (gms)	fat (gms)	chol. (mgs)	sod. (mgs)	fiber (gms)
(*Weight Watchers*), .9 oz.	100	1.0	22.0	1.0	0	45	1.0
(*Wise* Choice Fat Free), ¾ cup	110	<1.0	26.0	0	0	95	<1.0
caramel w/peanuts:							
(*Cracker Jack*), ½ cup	120	2.0	23.0	2.0	0	70	1.0
(*Cracker Jack* Fat Free), ¾-cup	110	<1.0	26.0	0	0	70	1.0
(*Moore's*), ¾ cup	110	0	26.0	1.0	0	90	1.0
cheddar (*Wise* Buttery), 2 cups	160	2.0	13.0	11.0	10	270	2.0
cheddar, white:							
(*Chester's*), 3 cups	190	3.0	17.0	13.0	<5	300	3.0
(*Old Dutch* Premium), 2 cups	160	3.0	15.0	10.0	<5	380	2.0
(*Smartfood*), 2 cups	190	3.0	17.0	12.0	5	310	2.0
(*Smartfood* Reduced Fat), 3 cups	140	4.0	19.0	6.0	<5	280	3.0
(*Weight Watchers*), .7 oz.	90	2.0	12.0	4.0	0	125	2.0
(*Wise*), 2 cups	160	3.0	13.0	11.0	5	400	2.0
cheddar, yellow (*Old Dutch*), 2½ cups	160	3.0	16.0	9.0	5	400	2.0
cheese flavored:							
(*Moore's*), 2 cups	160	2.0	15.0	10.0	<5	250	2.0
hot (*Wise/Moore's*), 2 cups	150	2.0	15.0	9.0	5	300	2.0
toffee:							
butter (*Cracker Jack* Fat Free), ¾ cup	110	1.0	26.0	0	0	85	1.0
butter (*Wise* Fat Free), ¾ cup	110	<1.0	26.0	0	0	95	<1.0
crunch (*Smartfood* Lowfat), ¾ cup	110	1.0	25.0	1.0	0	220	1.0
Popcorn cake, 1 cake, except as noted:							
caramel:							
(*Orville Redenbacher's*), ½ oz.	60	1.5	14.0	0	0	20	1.0

Food and Measure	cal.	prot. (gms)	carbo. (gms)	fat (gms)	chol. (mgs)	sod. (mgs)	fiber (gms)
Popcorn cake, caramel *(cont.)*							
apple (*Quaker*)	55	1.0	12.0	1.0	0	50	0
chocolate chip (*Quaker*)	60	1.0	13.0	1.0	0	20	0
barbecue (*Orville Redenbacher's* Mini), ½ oz.	60	2.0	11.0	1.0	0	80	1.0
butter (*Orville Redenbacher's*), ½ oz.	55	1.5	12.0	1.0	0	60	2.0
butterscotch (*Orville Redenbacher's* Clusters), 1.1 oz.	115	.5	28.0	0	0	135	2.0
cheddar, white: (*Orville Redenbacher's*), ½ oz. ....,	55	2.0	11.5	1.0	0	75	1.5
mild (*Quaker* Grain)	45	1.0	8.0	1.0	0	130	0
nacho cheese (*Orville Redenbacher's* Mini), 8 pcs., ½ oz.	55	2.0	12.0	1.0	0	90	1.5
w/nuts (*Orville Redenbacher's* Clusters), 1.1 oz.	120	1.5	25.0	4.5	0	130	2.0
w/rice: (*Lundberg* Mini), 5 cakes	70	1.0	12.0	1.0	0	100	2.0
(*Lundberg* Organic Unsalted)	60	1.0	14.0	0	0	0	2.0
Popcorn seasoning (*Tone's*), ¼ tsp. ...	0	0	0	0	0	630	0
Poppy seed, 1 tsp.	15	.5	.7	1.3	0	1	.8
Poppy seed filling, see "Pastry filling"							
Porgy, see "Scup"							
Pork (see also "Pork, refrigerated"), meat only, 4 oz., except as noted:							
leg, see "Ham"							
loin, whole:							
braised, lean w/fat	417	30.8	0	31.6	116	74	0

Food and Measure	cal.	prot. (gms)	carbo. (gms)	fat (gms)	chol. (mgs)	sod. (mgs)	fiber (gms)
braised, lean only	310	37.4	0	16.6	119	85	0
broiled, lean w/fat	392	26.7	0	30.9	107	75	0
broiled, lean only	291	31.6	0	17.3	108	85	0
roasted, lean w/fat	362	26.6	0	27.5	102	71	0
roasted, lean only	272	30.5	0	15.8	102	78	0
loin, blade:							
braised, lean w/fat	465	27.2	0	38.7	122	78	0
braised, lean only	355	33.7	0	23.3	128	92	0
broiled, lean w/fat	446	23.4	0	38.4	111	76	0
broiled, lean only	340	28.2	0	24.3	113	87	0
roasted, lean w/fat	413	23.9	0	34.5	102	69	0
roasted, lean only	316	28.0	0	21.9	101	77	0
loin, center:							
braised, lean w/fat	401	33.3	0	28.7	121	58	0
braised, lean only	308	39.4	0	15.5	126	62	0
broiled, lean w/fat	358	31.1	0	25.1	110	79	0
broiled, lean w/fat, 3.1 oz. (3.7 oz. raw chop w/bone)	275	23.9	0	19.2	84	61	0
broiled, lean only.	262	36.3	0	11.9	111	88	0
broiled, lean only, 2.5 oz. (3.7 oz. raw chop w/bone, fat)	166	23.0	0	7.5	71	56	0
roasted, lean w/fat	346	28.8	0	24.7	103	73	0
roasted, lean only	272	32.3	0	14.8	103	78	0
loin, center rib:							
braised, lean w/fat	416	32.4	0	30.8	108	54	0
braised, lean only	314	39.1	0	16.4	110	59	0
broiled, lean w/fat	389	27.9	0	29.9	106	69	0
broiled, lean only	293	32.7	0	16.9	107	76	0
roasted, lean w/fat	361	28.1	0	26.8	92	50	0
roasted, lean only	278	32.0	0	15.6	86	52	0
loin, top:							
braised, lean w/fat	432	31.4	0	33.1	108	53	0
braised, lean only	314	39.1	0	16.4	110	59	0
broiled, lean w/fat	408	26.9	0	32.5	105	67	0
broiled, lean only	293	32.7	0	16.9	107	76	0
roasted, lean only	278	32.0	0	15.6	90	52	0
shoulder, whole:							
roasted, lean w/fat	370	25.0	0	29.1	109	77	0

Food and Measure	cal.	prot. (gms)	carbo. (gms)	fat (gms)	chol. (mgs)	sod. (mgs)	fiber (gms)
Pork, shoulder, whole *(cont.)*							
roasted, lean only	277	28.8	0	17.0	110	86	0
shoulder, arm (picnic),							
roasted, lean w/fat	375	25.3	0	29.6	107	79	0
roasted, lean w/fat,							
diced, 1 cup.....	463	31.3	0	36.5	132	97	0
roasted, lean only	259	30.3	0	14.3	108	91	0
roasted, lean only,							
diced, 1 cup.....	319	37.4	0	17.7	133	112	0
shoulder, Boston							
blade:							
braised, lean w/fat	421	29.9	0	32.5	126	76	0
braised, lean only	333	35.3	0	19.9	132	85	0
broiled, lean w/fat	397	24.8	0	32.3	117	85	0
broiled, lean only	311	28.5	0	20.9	119	95	0
roasted, lean only	290	27.6	0	19.1	111	83	0
sirloin:							
braised, lean w/fat	399	31.7	0	29.2	120	61	0
braised, lean only	296	38.0	0	14.8	125	67	0
broiled, lean w/fat	375	27.4	0	28.6	110	62	0
broiled, lean w/fat,							
3 oz. (3.7 oz. raw							
chop w/bone) ...	278	20.3	0	21.2	81	46	0
broiled, lean only	276	32.1	0	15.4	111	68	0
broiled, lean only,							
2.4 oz. (3.7 oz.							
raw chop w/bone,							
fat)	165	19.2	0	9.2	67	41	0
roasted, lean w/fat	330	28.4	0	23.1	103	67	0
roasted, lean only	268	31.2	0	14.9	102	70	0
spareribs, lean w/fat,							
braised, 6.3 oz.							
(1 lb. raw w/bone)	703	51.4	0	53.6	214	165	0
tenderloin, lean only,							
roasted	188	32.6	0	5.5	105	76	0
Pork, cured (see also							
"Ham"), 4 oz.:							
arm (picnic), roasted:							
lean w/fat	318	23.2	0	24.2	66	1216	0
lean only	193	28.3	0	8.0	54	1396	0

Food and Measure	cal.	prot. (gms)	carbo. (gms)	fat (gms)	chol. (mgs)	sod. (mgs)	fiber (gms)
blade roll, lean w/fat, roasted	325	19.6	.4	26.6	76	1103	0
Pork, pickled (see also "Pig's feet"), 2 oz.:							
hocks (*Hormel*)	110	9.0	0	8.0	45	530	0
tidbits (*Hormel*)	100	8.0	0	8.0	45	530	0
Pork, refrigerated, 4 oz., except as noted:							
barbecue sauce, w/shredded pork (*Lloyd's*), ¼ cup ...	90	8.0	9.0	2.5	15	340	1.0
blade steak (*Hormel Always Tender*)	260	17.0	0	21.0	65	470	0
boneless roast (*Hormel Always Tender Chef's Prime*)	160	21.0	0	9.0	60	470	0
chops:							
center cut (*Hormel Always Tender*)	190	20.0	0	12.0	65	460	0
loin (*Hormel Always Tender*)	190	20.0	0	12.0	65	470	0
loin, center cut, boneless (*Hormel Always Tender*)	160	21.0	0	9.0	60	470	0
loin filet and roast:							
(*Hormel Always Tender Original*)	130	21.0	0	4.5	50	330	0
(*Mosey's Time for Dinner*), 5 oz. ...	190	31.0	3.0	6.0	130	520	0
honey mustard (*Hormel Always Tender*)	140	20.0	4.0	5.0	55	390	0
lemon garlic (*Hormel Always Tender*)	130	20.0	1.0	5.0	50	690	0
mesquite barbecue (*Hormel Always Tender*)	130	20.0	2.0	5.0	50	710	0

Food and Measure	cal.	prot. (gms)	carbo. (gms)	fat (gms)	chol. (mgs)	sod. (mgs)	fiber (gms)
Pork, refrigerated, loin filet and roast *(cont.)*							
salsa (*Hormel Always Tender*)	140	20.0	2.0	5.0	55	590	0
shoulder roast:							
(*Hormel Always Tender* Country Roast)	200	15.0	1.0	15.0	60	520	0
onion garlic (*Hormel Always Tender*)	200	15.0	2.0	1.0	60	570	0
spareribs:							
(*Hormel Always Tender*)	280	17.0	0	23.0	80	470	0
(*Hormel Always Tender* Country-style Ribs)	260	17.0	0	21.0	65	470	0
(*Hormel Always Tender* Ribs)	240	18.0	0	18.0	80	470	0
(*Hormel Always Tender* Special Trim Ribs)	280	17.0	0	23.0	80	470	0
(*Lloyd's*), 3 ribs w/sauce, 5 oz.	380	20.0	15.0	27.0	65	920	1.0
tenderloin:							
peppercorn (*Hormel Always Tender*)	130	19.0	2.0	4.5	60	670	0
teriyaki (*Hormel Always Tender*)	140	21.0	4.0	4.0	65	540	0
Pork batter, frying (*House of Tsang*), 4 tbsp.	140	3.0	32.0	.5	0	1300	0
Pork belly, raw, 1 oz.	147	2.7	0	15.1	20	9	0
Pork dinner, frozen, 1 pkg.:							
boneless, rib-shape:							
(*Swanson*), 10½ oz.	470	16.0	58.0	19.0	30	900	5.0
(*Swanson Hungry Man*), 14.1 oz.	750	29.0	74.0	37.0	85	1440	9.0
riblet (*Banquet Extra Helping*), 15¼ oz.	720	27.0	62.0	40.0	80	1590	7.0

Food and Measure	cal.	prot. (gms)	carbo. (gms)	fat (gms)	chol. (mgs)	sod. (mgs)	fiber (gms)
chop, country fried (*Marie Callender's*), 15 oz.	550	26.0	50.0	27.0	65	2240	9.0
Pork entree, canned, chow mein (*Chun King* Bi-Pack), 1 cup	80	7.0	9.0	1.0	10	1185	1.5
Pork entree, freeze-dried, sweet and sour, w/rice (*Mountain House*), 1 cup	270	10.0	40.0	8.0	25	760	2.0
Pork entree, frozen (see also "Pork, refrigerated"), 1 pkg.:							
cutlet: (*Banquet*), 10¼ oz.	420	11.0	38.0	25.0	35	1060	4.0
breaded (*Stouffer's* Homestyle), 10 oz.	420	26.0	27.0	18.0	70	1230	7.0
honey roasted (*Lean Cuisine Cafe Classics*), 9½ oz.	250	17.0	32.0	6.0	45	590	3.0
patty, grilled, glazed (*Healthy Choice*), 9.6 oz.	300	16.0	44.0	6.0	45	380	4.0
riblet, boneless (*Banquet*), 10 oz.	400	17.0	40.0	19.0	45	1070	4.0
and roasted potato (*Stouffer's Hearty Portions*), 15 oz.	540	28.0	68.0	17.0	70	1480	8.0
sandwich, see "Pork sandwich"							
Pork fat, roasted, 1 oz.	167	2.2	0	17.5	24	177	0
Pork gravy, in jars (*Franco-American Golden*), ¼ cup	45	1.0	3.0	4.0	5	340	1.0
Pork gravy mix, ¼ cup*:							
(*Durkee*)	10	.5	3.0	0	0	240	0
(*French's*)	10	0	3.0	.5	0	250	0
roasted (*Knorr*)	25	1.0	4.0	.5	0	350	0

Food and Measure	cal.	prot. (gms)	carbo. (gms)	fat (gms)	chol. (mgs)	sod. (mgs)	fiber (gms)
Pork lunch meat (see also "Ham"), 2 oz.:							
(*Hormel Deli Pork Roast*)	70	12.0	1.0	1.5	30	570	0
seasoned (*Boar's Head*)	80	14.0	0	3.0	35	310	0
Pork rind snack, ½ oz.:							
(*Baken-ets*)	80	8.0	<1.0	5.0	20	330	<1.0
(*Baken-ets* Cracklins)	80	7.0	<1.0	6.0	15	550	<1.0
(*Herr's*)	80	9.0	0	5.0	20	270	0
(*Old Dutch Bac'n Puffs*)	80	8.0	0	5.0	15	340	0
hot and spicy:							
(*Baken-ets*)	80	8.0	<1.0	5.0	20	440	<1.0
(*Baken-ets* Cracklins)	80	7.0	<1.0	5.0	20	320	<1.0
Pork sandwich, frozen, barbecued, 1 pc.:							
(*Hormel Quick Meal*)	360	15.0	38.0	16.0	45	560	1.0
rib shaped (*Hormel Quick Meal*)	430	14.0	40.0	24.0	50	660	1.0
Pork seasoning mix:							
(*Durkee/French's* Roasting Bag), ⅙ pkg.	25	.5	5.0	0	0	320	0
(*Shake'n Bake* Original Recipe), ⅛ pkg. . . .	40	1.0	9.0	0	0	320	0
barbecue glaze (*Shake 'n Bake*), ⅛ pkg. . . .	35	0	8.0	0	0	250	0
extra crispy (*Oven Fry*), ⅛ pkg.	60	2.0	11.0	1.5	0	340	0
hot and spicy (*Shake'n Bake*), ⅛ pkg.	45	1.0	8.0	.5	0	220	0
sparerib (*Durkee* Roasting Bag), ⅐ pkg.	25	0	5.0	0	0	430	0
Pork and beans, see "Baked beans" and specific bean listings							

Food and Measure	cal.	prot. (gms)	carbo. (gms)	fat (gms)	chol. (mgs)	sod. (mgs)	fiber (gms)
Pork and veal seasoning (*Chef Paul Prudhomme's Magic Seasoning Blends*), ¼ tsp.	0	0	0	0	0	130	0
Posole, see "Corn, dried"							
Pot pie, see specific entree listings							
Pot roast, see "Beef dinner, frozen" and "Beef entree, frozen"							
Pot roast seasoning mix, see "Sauerbraten seasoning mix"							
Potato:							
raw:							
all varieties (*Frieda's*), ½ cup, 3 oz.	70	2.0	15.0	0	0	5	1.0
unpeeled, 1 lb.	269	7.1	61.2	.3	0	21	5.4
peeled, 2½" potato	88	2.3	20.1	.1	0	7	1.8
peeled, diced, ½ cup	59	1.6	13.5	.1	0	5	1.2
baked:							
in skin, 4¾" x 2⅓"	220	4.7	51.0	.2	0	16	4.8
w/out skin, 4 oz.	105	2.2	24.4	.1	0	6	1.7
w/out skin, ½ cup	57	1.2	13.2	.1	0	3	.9
boiled in skin, baby (*Frieda's*), 4 oz. ...	86	2.4	19.4	.1	0	3	n.a.
boiled in skin, peeled:							
2½" potato	119	2.5	27.4	.1	0	6	2.4
½ cup	68	1.5	15.7	.1	0	3	1.4
boiled w/out skin:							
2½" potato	116	2.3	27.0	.1	0	7	2.4
½ cup	67	1.3	15.6	.1	0	4	1.4
microwaved in skin:							
4¾" x 2⅓" potato	212	4.9	48.7	.2	0	16	<5.0
peeled, ½ cup	78	1.6	18.2	.1	0	5	1.2
skin only, 2 oz.	75	2.5	16.8	.1	0	9	n.a.

Food and Measure	cal.	prot. (gms)	carbo. (gms)	fat (gms)	chol. (mgs)	sod. (mgs)	fiber (gms)
Potato *(cont.)*							
mashed, w/whole milk:							
½ cup	81	2.0	18.4	.6	2	318	2.1
w/butter, ½ cup . . .	111	2.0	17.5	4.4	13	309	2.1
w/margarine, ½ cup	111	2.0	17.5	4.4	2	309	2.1
Potato, canned:							
w/liquid, 4 oz.	45	1.5	9.8	.2	0	341	1.8
drained, 1.2-oz. potato	21	.5	4.8	.1	0	n.a.	<1.0
whole:							
(*Butterfield/Sunshine*), 2½ pcs., 5.6 oz.	90	2.0	20.0	0	0	330	2.0
(*Seneca*), cup	80	2.0	17.0	0	0	300	2.0
(*Seneca* No Salt), cup	80	2.0	17.0	0	0	30	2.0
new (*Del Monte*), 2 pcs. w/liquid . . .	60	1.0	13.0	0	0	360	2.0
sliced:							
(*Butterfield*), ½ cup	100	2.0	22.0	0	0	390	4.0
(*Del Monte*), ⅔ cup	60	1.0	13.0	0	0	360	2.0
diced (*Butterfield*), ⅔ cup	100	2.0	22.0	0	0	350	3.0
Potato, frozen (see also "Potato dishes, frozen"), 3 oz., except as noted:							
whole (*Birds Eye*), 3 pcs.	50	1.0	13.0	0	0	25	1.0
au gratin (*Cascadian Farm*), cup	110	5.0	15.0	4.0	10	290	1.0
fried or french-fried:							
(*Cascadian Farm* Oven French Fries)	130	2.0	24.0	4.0	0	10	2.0
(*Ore-Ida* Crinkle Cuts)	160	2.0	23.0	7.0	0	15	2.0
(*Ore-Ida* Oven Chips)	180	2.0	25.0	8.0	0	360	1.0
(*Ore-Ida* Shoestrings)	150	2.0	22.0	6.0	0	20	2.0
(*Ore-Ida* Steak Fries)	110	2.0	19.0	3.0	0	20	1.0

Food and Measure	cal.	prot. (gms)	carbo. (gms)	fat (gms)	chol. (mgs)	sod. (mgs)	fiber (gms)
(*Ore-Ida* Wedges)	110	2.0	18.0	3.0	0	20	2.0
(*Ore-Ida* Crispers!)	220	2.0	23.0	13.0	0	420	2.0
(*Ore-Ida* Fast Food Fries)	160	2.0	22.0	7.0	0	270	2.0
(*Ore-Ida* Golden Crinkles)	120	2.0	19.0	3.5	0	15	2.0
(*Ore-Ida* Golden Twirls)	160	2.0	22.0	7.0	0	260	2.0
(*Ore-Ida* Pixie Crinkles)	130	2.0	21.0	4.5	0	25	2.0
(*Ore-Ida* Snackin' Fries), 5-oz. pkg.	310	3.0	40.0	15.0	0	300	3.0
(*Ore-Ida* Waffle Fries)	150	2.0	21.0	7.0	0	270	2.0
(*Ore-Ida* Zesties) . . .	160	2.0	20.0	7.0	0	360	1.0
hash brown:							
(*Cascadian Farm*), 1 cup	70	2.0	15.0	0	0	20	2.0
(*Ore-Ida* Patties), 3-oz. pc.	70	2.0	16.0	0	0	30	1.0
(*Ore-Ida* Toaster), 2 pcs., 3.6 oz. . . .	210	2.0	25.0	11.0	0	500	2.0
(*Ore-Ida* Golden Patties), 2.4-oz. pc.	150	2.0	16.0	8.0	0	170	2.0
mashed (*Ore-Ida*), ²/₃ cup*	70	3.0	10.0	2.5	8	150	1.0
O'Brien (*Ore-Ida*), ³/₄ cup	60	1.0	14.0	0	0	25	2.0
w/peppers and onions (*Cascadian Farm* Country Style), ³/₄ cup	80	2.0	19.0	0	0	5	1.0
puffs:							
(*Cascadian Farm* Spud Puppies)	150	2.0	19.0	8.0	0	320	2.0
(*Hot Tots*)	160	2.0	20.0	7.0	0	370	2.0
(*Tater Tots*), 9 pcs., 3 oz.	150	2.0	20.0	8.0	0	290	2.0
mini (*Ore-Ida*), 10 pcs., 3 oz. . . .	180	2.0	21.0	10.0	0	300	2.0

Food and Measure	cal.	prot. (gms)	carbo. (gms)	fat (gms)	chol. (mgs)	sod. (mgs)	fiber (gms)
Potato, frozen, puffs *(cont.)*							
onion (*Tater Tots*),							
9 pcs., 3 oz.	150	2.0	21.0	7.0	0	390	2.0
Potato, mix, see "Potato dishes, mix"							
Potato, refrigerated, mashed (*Diner's Choice*), ⅔ cup	110	3.0	19.0	2.0	0	210	1.0
Potato, stuffed, see "Potato dishes, frozen"							
Potato, sweet, see "Sweet potato"							
Potato chips and crisps, 1 oz., except as noted:							
(*Barbara's* No Salt) . . .	150	2.0	15.0	10.0	0	20	1.0
(*Barbara's* Regular/ Ripple)	150	2.0	16.0	10.0	0	180	1.0
(*Herr's/Herr's* Ripple)	140	2.0	16.0	8.0	0	180	1.0
(*Kettle* Chips)	130	2.0	18.0	6.0	0	140	2.0
(*Lay's*)	150	2.0	15.0	10.0	0	180	1.0
(*Lay's* Adobadas)	170	2.0	18.0	10.0	0	240	1.0
(*Lay's* Baked)	110	2.0	23.0	1.5	0	150	2.0
(*Lay's* Deli Style)	150	1.0	160	10.0	0	180	1.0
(*Lay's* Wavy)	160	2.0	15.0	10.0	0	210	1.0
(*Lay's* WOW)	75	2.0	18.0	0	0	200	1.0
(*Munchos*)	150	1.0	18.0	10.0	0	270	1.0
(*No Fries* Original) . . .	110	2.0	24.0	0	0	230	1.0
(*Old Dutch*)	150	2.0	16.0	8.0	0	130	1.0
(*Old Dutch Ripl*)	150	2.0	17.0	8.0	0	140	<1.0
(*Pringles* Original) . . .	160	1.0	15.0	11.0	0	170	1.0
(*Pringles* Original Fat Free)	70	1.0	15.0	0	0	160	1.0
(*Pringles* Ridges)	150	1.0	15.0	10.0	0	150	1.0
(*Pringles Right Crisp* Original)	140	2.0	19.0	7.0	0	135	1.0
(*Ruffles*)	150	2.0	14.0	10.0	0	180	1.0
(*Ruffles* Baked)	110	2.0	23.0	1.5	0	180	2.0
(*Ruffles* Reduced Fat)	130	2.0	18.0	6.7	0	160	1.0
(*Ruffles* WOW)	75	2.0	17.0	0	0	200	1.0

Food and Measure	cal.	prot. (gms)	carbo. (gms)	fat (gms)	chol. (mgs)	sod. (mgs)	fiber (gms)
(*Sun Chips*)	140	2.0	19.0	6.0	0	115	2.0
(*Terra Yukon Gold*) . . .	130	2.0	19.0	5.0	0	80	0
(*Wise* Cottage Fries No Salt)	150	2.0	14.0	10.0	0	0	1.0
(*Wise* Lightly Salted)	150	2.0	14.0	10.0	0	85	1.0
(*Wise* New York Deli Style)	150	2.0	14.0	10.0	0	170	1.0
(*Wise* Ridged Cut/Cottage Fries)	150	2.0	14.0	10.0	0	190	1.0
barbecue:							
(*Lay's* Red Pepper Grill)	150	2.0	16.0	10.0	0	220	1.0
(*Lay's KC Masterpiece*)	150	2.0	15.0	10.0	0	200	1.0
(*Lay's KC Masterpiece Baked*)	120	2.0	22.0	3.0	0	210	2.0
(*Munchos*)	160	1.0	15.0	10.0	0	250	1.0
(*No Fries*)	110	2.0	24.0	0	0	140	1.0
(*Old Dutch*)	150	2.0	15.0	9.0	0	300	1.0
(*Old Dutch* Ripples)	150	2.0	16.0	9.0	0	180	<1.0
(*Pringles*)	150	2.0	15.0	10.0	0	200	1.0
(*Pringles* Fat Free)	70	1.0	15.0	0	0	220	1.0
(*Pringles Right Crisps*)	140	2.0	18.0	7.0	0	160	1.0
(*Terra Yukon Gold*)	130	3.0	19.0	5.0	0	90	2.0
(*Wise*)	160	2.0	15.0	10.0	0	210	1.0
barbecue, mesquite:							
(*Kettle* Chips)	130	2.0	19.0	6.0	0	230	2.0
(*Lay's WOW*)	75	2.0	170	0	0	250	1.0
(*Pringles* Ridges)	150	1.0	15.0	10.0	0	220	1.0
(*Ruffles KC Masterpiece*)	150	1.0	15.0	10.0	0	190	1.0
(*Wise Krunchers!*)	140	2.0	16.0	8.0	0	200	1.0
blue (*Terra Blues*)	140	3.0	17.0	6.0	0	115	1.0
cheddar:							
(*Andy Capp Cheddar Fries*)	140	2.0	17.0	7.0	0	340	0
(*Health Valley* Puffs)	110	2.0	21.0	3.0	<5	260	1.0
(*Lay's* Deli Style) . . .	150	2.0	16.0	10.0	0	190	1.0
(*Sun Chips* Harvest)	140	2.0	19.0	6.0	0	115	2.0

Food and Measure	cal.	prot. (gms)	carbo. (gms)	fat (gms)	chol. (mgs)	sod. (mgs)	fiber (gms)
Potato chips and crisps *(cont.)*							
cheddar/sour cream:							
(*Old Dutch*)	160	2.0	16.0	9.0	0	190	1.0
(*Old Dutch* Ripples)	150	2.0	15.0	9.0	0	190	1.0
(*Pringles* Ridges)	150	1.0	15.0	10.0	0	200	1.0
(*Ruffles*)	160	2.0	14.0	10.0	0	190	1.0
(*Ruffles* Baked)	120	2.0	21.0	3.0	0	270	2.0
(*Wise*)	160	2.0	15.0	10.0	0	220	1.0
cheese:							
(*Pringles* Cheez							
Ums)	150	1.0	15.0	10.0	0	10	1.0
au gratin (*Lay's*							
Wavy)	150	2.0	140	10.0	<5	200	1.0
chili (*Lay's* Deli Style)	150	1.0	16.0	10.0	0	210	1.0
Dijon, golden (*Ruffles*)	150	1.0	16.0	9.0	0	190	1.0
dill (*Wise*)	150	2.0	14.0	10.0	0	220	1.0
hot:							
(*Andy Capp Hot*							
Fries)	140	2.0	18.0	7.0	0	220	0
(*Lay's* Flamin')	150	2.0	16.0	10.0	0	180	1.0
(*Wise*)	150	1.0	14.0	10.0	0	260	1.0
jalapeño:							
(*Wise Krunchers!*)	140	2.0	16.0	8.0	0	210	1.0
cheddar (*Kettle*							
Chips)	130	2.0	17.0	6.0	0	190	1.0
jack (*Wise*)	150	2.0	14.0	10.0	0	220	1.0
onion, French:							
(*Old Dutch* Ripples)	150	2.0	15.0	10.0	0	180	1.0
(*Ruffles*)	150	2.0	15.0	10.0	0	190	1.0
(*Sun Chips*)	140	2.0	18.0	7.0	0	115	2.0
onion and garlic:							
(*Lay's*)	150	2.0	16.0	9.0	0	200	1.0
(*Old Dutch*)	140	2.0	16.0	8.0	0	210	1.0
(*Terra Yukon Gold*)	130	2.0	19.0	50	0	65	1.0
(*Wise*)	150	2.0	14.0	10.0	0	310	1.0
pizza (*Pringles* Pizza-							
Licious)	160	1.0	14.0	11.0	0	200	1.0
puffs, 1½ cups:							
cheddar or garlic							
w/cheese (*Health*							
Valley Low Fat)	110	2.0	21.0	3.0	5	260	1.0

Food and Measure	cal.	prot. (gms)	carbo. (gms)	fat (gms)	chol. (mgs)	sod. (mgs)	fiber (gms)
zesty ranch (*Health Valley* Low Fat)	110	2.0	21.0	2.5	0	260	1.0
ranch:							
(*Lay's Hidden Valley* Wavy)	160	2.0	14.0	11.0	0	150	1.0
(*Pringles*)	150	2.0	15.0	10.0	0	130	1.0
(*Pringles Right Crisps*)	140	2.0	18.0	7.0	0	160	1.0
(*Ruffles*)	150	2.0	15.0	9.0	0	280	1.0
puffs (*Health Valley*)	110	2.0	21.0	2.5	0	260	1.0
salsa (*Andy Capp Salsa Fries*)	130	2.0	18.0	6.0	0	170	0
salt and pepper (*Terra Yukon Gold*)	130	3.0	19.0	5.0	0	120	1.0
salt and vinegar:							
(*Kettle* Chips)	130	1.0	18.0	6.0	0	360	1.0
(*Lay's*)	150	2.0	15.0	10.0	0	300	1.0
(*Pringles*)	160	1.0	15.0	11.0	0	200	1.0
(*Terra Yukon Gold*)	130	2.0	20.0	5.0	0	110	2.0
(*Wise*)	150	2.0	14.0	10.0	0	290	1.0
sour cream/onion:							
(*Lay's*)	160	2.0	12.0	11.0	0	200	1.0
(*Lay's* Baked)	120	2.0	21.0	3.0	0	210	2.0
(*Pringles*)	160	2.0	15.0	10.0	0	135	1.0
(*Pringles* Fat Free)	70	1.0	15.0	0	0	190	1.0
(*Pringles Right Crisps*)	140	2.0	18.0	7.0	0	140	1.0
(*Ruffles* Reduced Fat)	130	3.0	18.0	6.0	0	200	1.0
(*Wise*)	150	2.0	16.0	9.0	0	220	1.0
sticks:							
(*French's*), ¾-oz. bag	120	1.0	11.0	8.0	0	135	<1.0
hot (*Chester's* Fries Flamin')	140	2.0	17.0	7.0	0	240	<1.0
sweet potato, see "Sweet potato chips"							
yogurt–green onion:							
(*Barbara's*)	150	2.0	15.0	9.0	0	240	1.0

Food and Measure	cal.	prot. (gms)	carbo. (gms)	fat (gms)	chol. (mgs)	sod. (mgs)	fiber (gms)
Potato chips and crisps, yogurt–green onion *(cont.)*							
(*Terra Yukon Gold*)	130	2.0	19.0	5.0	0	75	1.0
Potato dishes, canned or packaged, scalloped, w/ham:							
(*Hormel Microwave*), 1 cup	240	7.0	20.0	14.0	35	920	2.0
(*Nalley*), 7½-oz. can	210	8.0	27.0	7.0	15	800	3.0
Potato dishes, frozen:							
au gratin:							
(*Stouffer's* Side Dish), ½ cup	150	6.0	20.0	5.0	15	510	3.0
ham and broccoli (*Banquet* Family), ⅔ cup	210	7.0	16.0	13.0	30	970	2.0
baked, twice, butter flavor (*Ore-Ida*), 1 pc.	160	3.0	24.0	6.0	0	330	3.0
broccoli and cheese baked (*Smart Ones*), 10 oz.	250	11.0	39.0	6.0	20	570	6.0
casserole, garden (*Healthy Choice*), 9¼ oz.	210	11.0	30.0	5.0	10	520	6.0
cheddar:							
(*Lean Cuisine* Deluxe), 10 oz.	270	12.0	40.0	7.0	20	590	6.0
broccoli (*Healthy Choice*), 10½ oz.	330	13.0	53.0	7.0	25	550	6.0
cheddared:							
(*The Budget Gourmet* Side Dish), 5½ oz.	250	7.0	22.0	15.0	35	690	3.0
and broccoli (*The Budget Gourmet* Side Dish), 5 oz.	160	6.0	16.0	8.0	25	460	2.0
mozzarella, w/chicken (*The Budget Gourmet*), 8½ oz.	300	8.0	33.0	16.0	30	650	4.0
puffs, 5 pcs.:							
(*Cohen's Famous*)	340	5.0	36.0	20.0	0	380	2.0

Food and Measure	cal.	prot. (gms)	carbo. (gms)	fat (gms)	chol. (mgs)	sod. (mgs)	fiber (gms)
spinach (*Cohen's Famous*)	320	4.0	30.0	20.0	0	330	2.0
roasted, w/broccoli and cheddar sauce (*Lean Cuisine*), 10¼ oz.	260	12.0	39.0	6.0	15	590	7.0
scalloped:							
(*Stouffer's* Entree 40 oz.), ½ cup . . .	140	4.0	19.0	5.0	3	560	2.0
(*Stouffer's* Side Dish 11½ oz.), ½ cup	140	4.0	17.0	6.0	<5	450	2.0
w/smoked turkey ham (*Lean Cuisine American Favorites*), 10 oz.	250	10.0	38.0	6.0	25	590	6.0
soufflé, kugel (*Melrose*), ½ cup	200	4.0	23.0	10.0	25	400	3.0
stuffed, 1 pc., except as noted:							
bacon and cheese (*Larry's*)	200	5.0	24.0	10.0	5	570	1.0
broccoli and cheese (*Ore-Ida* Topped Baked), ½ baker	160	6.0	25.0	4.0	10	480	2.0
cheddar cheese (*Oh Boy!*)	130	3.0	22.0	4.0	<5	270	2.0
cheese (*Larry's*) . . .	200	4.0	24.0	9.0	5	550	1.0
onion, sour cream, chives (*Oh Boy!*)	110	2.0	22.0	2.0	<5	260	2.0
wedges, cheese, broccoli, and bacon (*Marie Callender's*), 13 oz.	420	20.0	50.0	15.0	55	1480	7.0
wedges, Swiss cheese, 13 oz.:							
and chicken (*Marie Callender's*)	390	26.0	42.0	13.0	50	1070	5.0
ham and broccoli (*Marie Callender's*)	380	20.0	45.0	13.0	45	1230	5.0

Food and Measure	cal.	prot. (gms)	carbo. (gms)	fat (gms)	chol. (mgs)	sod. (mgs)	fiber (gms)
Potato dishes, mix:							
(*Betty Crocker Potato Shakers* Original):							
²/₃ cup*	140	3.0	23.0	4.0	<5	560	2.0
lower fat, ²/₃ cup*	120	3.0	23.0	1.5	<5	560	2.0
au gratin:							
(*Betty Crocker*):							
½ cup*	150	3.0	22.0	6.0	5	600	1.0
low fat, ½ cup*	110	3.0	22.0	1.0	<5	560	1.0
(*Betty Crocker 9 oz.*):							
½ cup*	150	3.0	23.0	6.0	<5	630	1.0
low fat, ½ cup*	110	3.0	23.0	1.0	<5	590	1.0
(*Hungry Jack*), ½ cup*	150	3.0	26.0	4.5	10	620	1.0
bacon and cheese (*Knorr Skillet Potatoes*), ½ cup	110	3.0	18.0	2.0	10	590	2.0
broccoli au gratin (*Betty Crocker*):							
½ cup*	140	3.0	21.0	6.0	<5	530	2.0
low fat, ½ cup*	110	3.0	21.0	2.5	0	500	2.0
cheddar (*Betty Crocker*):							
½ cup*	120	3.0	21.0	2.5	<5	600	1.0
stove-top, ½ cup*	140	3.0	21.0	4.5	5	580	1.0
cheddar/bacon:							
(*Betty Crocker*):							
½ cup*	150	3.0	21.0	6.0	<5	650	1.0
low fat, ½ cup*	120	3.0	21.0	3.0	0	620	1.0
(*Hungry Jack*), ½ cup*	150	4.0	24.0	4.5	10	540	2.0
twice baked (*Betty Crocker*):							
²/₃ cup*	210	6.0	22.0	11.0	85	580	1.0
low fat, ²/₃ cup*	130	6.0	22.0	2.0	<5	530	1.0
cheddar, cheesy (*Knorr Skillet Potatoes*), ½ cup	130	4.0	19.0	4.0	10	850	2.0

Food and Measure	cal.	prot. (gms)	carbo. (gms)	fat (gms)	chol. (mgs)	sod. (mgs)	fiber (gms)
cheddar/sour cream (*Betty Crocker*), ½ cup*	130	3.0	25.0	3.0	5	580	1.0
cheese, three (*Betty Crocker*), ½ cup*	150	3.0	23.0	6.0	<5	600	1.0
chicken/vegetable (*Betty Crocker*):							
⅔ cup*	140	4.0	23.0	4.0	<5	520	2.0
low fat, ⅔ cup*	120	4.0	23.0	2.5	<5	510	2.0
garlic, roasted (*Knorr Skillet Potatoes*), ⅔ cup	120	3.0	23.0	1.0	0	570	3.0
hash browns (*Betty Crocker*), ½ cup*	190	3.0	30.0	8.0	0	550	3.0
hash browns, onion (*Knorr Skillet Potatoes*), ⅓ cup	100	2.0	20.0	.5	0	620	2.0
julienne (*Betty Crocker*), ½ cup*	150	3.0	21.0	6.0	<5	630	1.0
mashed:							
(*Betty Crocker Potato Buds*):							
⅔ cup*	160	3.0	19.0	8.0	<5	460	1.0
low fat, ⅔ cup*	120	3.0	19.0	4.0	0	420	1.0
(*Hungry Jack Flakes*), ½ cup*	160	3.0	20.0	7.0	<5	240	1.0
(*Hungry Jack Idaho*):							
flakes, ½ cup*	150	3.0	20.0	6.0	<5	240	1.0
granules, ½ cup*	160	3.0	22.0	7.0	<5	300	2.0
butter flavor (*Hungry Jack*):							
½ cup*	150	3.0	19.0	7.0	<5	350	1.0
parsley, ½ cup*	150	3.0	19.0	7.0	<5	380	1.0
butter and herb (*Betty Crocker*):							
½ cup*	160	3.0	20.0	8.0	5	470	1.0
lower fat, ½ cup*	130	3.0	20.0	4.5	<5	450	1.0
cheese, four (*Betty Crocker*):							
½ cup*	150	3.0	20.0	7.0	<5	570	2.0

Food and Measure	cal.	prot. (gms)	carbo. (gms)	fat (gms)	chol. (mgs)	sod. (mgs)	fiber (gms)
Potato dishes, mix, mashed, cheese, four *(cont.)*							
lower fat, ½ cup*	120	3.0	20.0	4.0	0	540	2.0
chicken and herb (*Betty Crocker*):							
½ cup*	150	3.0	21.0	7.0	<5	520	1.0
lower fat, ½ cup*	120	3.0	21.0	3.5	0	490	1.0
garlic, roasted (*Betty Crocker*):							
½ cup*	150	3.0	19.0	8.0	<5	400	2.0
lower fat, ½ cup*	130	3.0	19.0	4.5	0	380	2.0
garlic flavor (*Hungry Jack*), ½ cup* ...	150	3.0	19.0	7.0	<5	360	1.0
sour cream/chive:							
(*Betty Crocker*):							
½ cup*	150	3.0	21.0	7.0	5	440	1.0
lower fat, ½ cup*	120	3.0	21.0	3.5	<5	420	1.0
(*Hungry Jack*), ½ cup*	150	3.0	19.0	7.0	<5	380	1.0
mashed, stuffed, 1 pkg., except as noted:							
broccoli cheddar:							
(*Fantastic Foods*), ¼ cup	100	4.0	20.0	1.5	5	320	2.0
(*Fantastic Foods Cup*)	190	8.0	35.0	3.0	10	480	3.0
butter, creamery (*Fantastic Foods Cup*)	200	7.0	36.0	3.0	10	480	3.0
cheddar:							
(*Fantastic Foods*), ¼ cup	100	4.0	21.0	1.5	5	320	2.0
(*Fantastic Foods Cup*)	180	7.0	35.0	3.0	10	480	3.0
garlic and herbs:							
(*Fantastic Foods*), ¼ cup	100	3.0	22.0	1.5	0	250	2.0
(*Fantastic Foods Cup*)	180	6.0	37.0	2.0	5	480	3.0

Food and Measure	cal.	prot. (gms)	carbo. (gms)	fat (gms)	chol. (mgs)	sod. (mgs)	fiber (gms)
jalapeño jack cheese (*Fantastic Foods* Cup)	200	7.0	36.0	3.0	10	480	3.0
sour cream and chive:							
(*Fantastic Foods*), ¼ cup	100	3.0	21.0	1.5	5	280	2.0
(*Fantastic Foods* Cup)	180	6.0	37.0	2.5	5	480	3.0
pancake, see "Potato pancake mix"							
ranch (*Betty Crocker*), ½ cup*	160	3.0	25.0	6.0	<5	610	2.0
scalloped.							
(*Betty Crocker*):							
½ cup*	160	3.0	23.0	6.0	<5	610	1.0
low fat, ⅔ cup*	110	3.0	23.0	1.0	0	570	1.0
(*Betty Crocker* 8¼ oz.*):							
½ cup*	150	3.0	23.0	6.0	<5	620	1.0
low fat, ⅔ cup*	110	3.0	23.0	1.0	0	580	1.0
scalloped, cheesy:							
(*Betty Crocker*):							
½ cup*	140	3.0	21.0	6.0	<5	540	3.0
low fat, ½ cup*	110	3.0	21.0	3.0	<5	510	3.0
(*Hungry Jack*), ½ cup*	150	3.0	24.0	5.0	10	570	1.0
scalloped, cheese and bacon (*Knorr Skillet Potatoes*), ½ cup	110	3.0	18.0	2.0	10	590	2.0
scalloped, creamy (*Hungry Jack*), ½ cup*	150	3.0	24.0	5.0	10	460	2.0
sour cream/chive:							
(*Betty Crocker*), ½ cup*	160	3.0	22.0	7.0	5	600	2.0
(*Hungry Jack*), ½ cup*	160	3.0	23.0	6.0	15	510	1.0
Southwestern (*Knorr Skillet Potatoes*), ½ cup	140	3.0	25.0	2.5	0	750	3.0

Food and Measure	cal.	prot. (gms)	carbo. (gms)	fat (gms)	chol. (mgs)	sod. (mgs)	fiber (gms)
Potato entree, frozen, see "Potato dishes, frozen"							
Potato entree, packaged, w/curried garbanzos and rice (*Tamarind Tree* Alu Chole), 1 pkg.	350	12.0	63.0	6.0	0	620	9.0
Potato flour, 1 cup . . .	628	14.3	143.0	1.4	0	61	10.9
Potato pancake, frozen:							
(*Empire Kosher*), 2-oz. cake	80	1.0	15.0	2.0	0	200	8.0
(*Golden*), 1 -oz. cake	70	2.0	10.0	3.0	4	187	1.0
mini (*Empire Kosher*), 2 cakes, 2 oz.	90	1.0	16.0	2.5	0	160	6.0
Potato pancake mix:							
(*Hungry Jack*), 2 tbsp.	70	2.0	16.0	0	0	360	1.0
(*Hungry Jack*), 3 cakes*, 3"	90	3.0	16.0	1.5	50	380	1.0
(*Knorr*), 2 tbsp.	80	2.0	18.0	0	0	420	2.0
(*Manischewitz*), 3 tbsp., 3 cakes* . . .	80	2.0	18.0	1.0	0	500	2.0
(*Manischewitz Latka*), 2 tbsp., 3 cakes* . . .	80	2.0	18.0	1.0	0	600	2.0
(*Streit's*), 2½ tbsp.	90	2.0	18.0	1.0	0	360	2.0
Potato salad, refrigerated (*Shally Sherman Foods*), ⅔ cup	180	2.0	28.0	7.0	5	970	3.0
Potato salad seasoning (*Tone's*), 1 tsp.	5	.2	.3	.2	0	1498	.1
Potato seasoning:							
cheddar, crispy (*Shake 'n Bake*), ⅙ pkt. . . .	30	2.0	2.0	2.0	5	380	0
cheddar, savory (*Lipton Recipe Secrets*), 1 tbsp.	60	1.0	1.0	5.0	5	420	0
garlic herb (*Lipton Recipe Secrets*), 1 tbsp.	50	0	2.0	5.0	5	290	0

Food and Measure	cal.	prot. (gms)	carbo. (gms)	fat (gms)	chol. (mgs)	sod. (mgs)	fiber (gms)
herb and garlic (*Shake 'n Bake*), ⅙ pkt.	20	0	5.0	0	0	370	0
onion, California (*Lipton Recipe Secrets*), 1 tbsp.	60	0	2.0	5.0	5	340	0
Potato sticks, see "Potato chips and crisps"							
Potato topping, in jars, 2 tbsp.:							
asparagus dill (*Sam Fulton's Tater Toppins*)	20	0	1.0	1.0	5	50	0
bean, five (*Sam Fulton's Tater Toppins Fiesta*)	15	1.0	3.0	0	0	60	<1.0
garlic Parmesan (*Sam Fulton's Tater Toppins*)	30	1.0	2.0	1.0	5	50	0
mushroom (*Sam Fulton's Tater Toppins Medley*)	10	0	2.0	0	0	60	0
Potato-cheddar pocket, frozen (*Ken & Robert's Veggie Pockets*), 4½-oz. pc.	260	6.0	42.0	8.0	0	370	2.0
Poultry, see specific listings							
Poultry seasoning:							
(*Chef Paul Prudhomme's Magic Seasoning Blends*), ¼ tsp. ...	0	0	0	0	0	105	0
1 tsp.	5	.1	1.0	.1	0	tr.	.2
Pout, ocean, meat only:							
raw, 4 oz.	90	18.9	0	1.0	59	69	0
baked, broiled, or microwaved, 4 oz. ...	116	24.2	0	1.3	76	88	0

Food and Measure	cal.	prot. (gms)	carbo. (gms)	fat (gms)	chol. (mgs)	sod. (mgs)	fiber (gms)
Preserves, see "Jam and preserves"							
Pretzel, 1 oz., except as noted:							
(*Bachman* Petite Unsalted), 1.1 oz.	120	3.0	25.0	1.0	0	50	1.0
(*Goldfish*), 1.1 oz. . . .	120	3.0	22.0	2.5	0	430	<1.0
bagel shaped (*Manischewitz*)	110	3.0	22.0	0	0	260	1.0
beer (*Quinlan*)	110	2.0	21.0	2.0	0	420	1.0
cheddar:							
(*Combos*)	130	3.0	18.0	5.0	0	310	0
(*Combos*), 1.8-oz. bag	240	5.0	33.0	9.0	5	560	1.0
(*Rold Gold*)	110	3.0	23.0	0	0	440	1.0
cheese:							
(*Handi-Snacks*), 1.1-oz. pc.	110	4.0	11.0	6.0	15	420	<1.0
(*Sargento MooTown Snackers*), .9-oz. pc.	90	3.0	12.0	3.0	10	320	0
cheddar (*Combos*)	130	3.0	19.0	5.0	0	310	1.0
cheddar (*Combos*), 1.8-oz. bag	240	5.0	34.0	9.0	5	560	1.0
cheddar (*Combos*), 1.4-oz. bag	180	4.0	26.0	7.0	5	430	1.0
nacho (*Combos*) . . .	130	3.0	19.0	4.5	0	320	1.0
nacho (*Combos*), 1.8-oz. bag	230	5.0	34.0	8.0	0	580	1.0
Dutch (*Mister Salty*), 2 pcs., 1.1 oz.	120	3.0	25.0	1.0	0	580	1.0
hard:							
(*Bachman*)	110	3.0	22.0	1.0	0	420	1.0
(*Bachman* Unsalted)	110	3.0	22.0	1.0	0	30	1.0
plain	108	2.6	22.5	1.0	0	486	.8
mini:							
(*Quinlan* Fat Free)	100	2.0	23.0	0	0	590	1.0
(*Quinlan* Fat Free No Salt)	100	2.0	24.0	0	0	10	1.0
mustard:							
(*Combos*)	130	2.0	19.0	4.0	0	270	1.0

Food and Measure	cal.	prot. (gms)	carbo. (gms)	fat (gms)	chol. (mgs)	sod. (mgs)	fiber (gms)
(*Combos*), 1.8-oz. bag	230	4.0	35.0	8.0	0	500	1.0
honey (*Rold Gold*)	110	3.0	23.0	0	0	380	1.0
nacho:							
(*Combos*)	130	3.0	19.0	5.0	0	320	1.0
(*Combos*), 1.8-oz. bag	230	5.0	34.0	8.0	0	580	1.0
9-grain (*Barbara's*) ...	100	4.0	21.0	1.5	0	180	3.0
nuggets (*Quinlan*) ...	110	2.0	22.0	2.0	0	280	<1.0
oat bran (*Weight Watchers*), 1½ oz.	170	4.0	33.0	2.5	0	250	3.0
pizza flavor:							
(*Combos* Pizzeria)	130	3.0	19.0	4.5	0	290	1.0
(*Combos* Pizzeria), 1.8-oz. bag	230	5.0	35.0	8.0	0	510	1.0
(*Combos* Pizzeria), 1.4-oz. bag	180	3.0	27.0	6.0	0	390	1.0
pepperoni (*Combos*)	140	2.0	17.0	7.0	5	280	0
pepperoni (*Combos*), 1.7-oz. bag	240	4.0	30.0	11.0	5	470	1.0
rods:							
(*Bachman*), 1.1 oz.	110	3.0	24.0	.5	0	260	1.0
(*Old Dutch*), 1.2 oz.	130	4.0	26.0	1.5	0	440	<1.0
(*Quinlan* Rods/ Logs)	110	2.0	22.0	1.5	0	310	1.0
(*Rold Gold*)	110	3.0	22.0	1.0	0	610	1.0
sourdough:							
(*Quinlan* Low Fat), .9-oz. pc.	90	2.0	18.0	1.0	0	470	<1.0
Bavarian or twists (*Barbara's*), 1.1 oz.	110	3.0	24.0	0	0	260	1.0
hard (*Rold Gold* Nuggets)	110	2.0	24.0	0	0	330	1.0
nuggets (*Quinlan* San Francisco)	110	2.0	22.0	1.5	0	430	1.0
sticks:							
(*Bachman Stix*)	100	2.0	20.0	1.0	0	1460	1.0
(*Old Dutch*)	110	3.0	22.0	1.5	0	280	<1.0
(*Quinlan*) ...,.....	110	3.0	22.0	1.0	0	570	<1.0
(*Quinlan* Fat Free)	100	3.0	22.0	0	0	570	<1.0

Food and Measure	cal.	prot. (gms)	carbo. (gms)	fat (gms)	chol. (mgs)	sod. (mgs)	fiber (gms)
Pretzel, sticks *(cont.)*							
(*Rold Gold* Fat Free)	110	3.0	23.0	0	0	530	1.0
sticks, sesame (*Barbara's*), 1.1 oz.	110	5.0	21.0	2.5	0	420	4.0
thins:							
(*Bachman* Thin 'n Right), 1.1 oz.	120	3.0	23.0	1.0	0	650	1.0
(*Old Dutch* Fat Free), 1.1 oz.	110	3.0	24.0	0	0	280	<1.0
(*Quinlan*)	110	2.0	22.0	1.0	0	760	<1.0
(*Quinlan* Fat Free)	100	3.0	22.0	0	0	630	<1.0
(*Quinlan* Party)	110	2.0	22.0	2.0	0	550	1.0
(*Quinlan* Ultra-Thin Fat Free)	100	2.0	22.0	0	0	750	1.0
(*Rold Gold* Crispy's)	110	3.0	22.0	1.5	0	670	1.0
(*Rold Gold* Fat Free)	110	2.0	24.0	0	0	520	1.0
twists:							
(*Bachman*)	100	3.0	22.0	1.0	0	650	1.0
(*Old Dutch*)	110	3.0	22.0	1.5	0	260	<1.0
(*Planters*)	100	3.0	23.0	.5	0	420	1.0
tiny (*Rold Gold* Fat Free)	100	3.0	23.0	0	0	420	1.0
Pretzel, soft:							
(*Superpretzel*), 2¼-oz. pc.	180	6.0	36.0	1.0	0	140	2.0
(*Superpretzel* Added Salt), 2¼-oz. pc.	180	6.0	36.0	1.0	0	930	2.0
bites (*Superpretzel*), 5 pcs., 1.9 oz.	140	3.0	32.0	.5	0	115	1.0
bites (*Superpretzel* Added Salt) 4 pcs., 1.9 oz.	140	3.0	32.0	.5	0	900	1.0
cheese-filled, cheddar (*Superpretzel* Softstix), 2 pcs., 1.8 oz.	140	5.0	24.0	2.5	10	250	1.0
Pretzel dip (*Nance's* Sweet & Sassy), 2 tbsp.	90	1.0	18.0	2.0	0	600	0
Prickly pear:							
(*Frieda's* Cactus Pear), 5 oz.	60	1.0	13.0	.5	0	5	5.0

Food and Measure	cal.	prot. (gms)	carbo. (gms)	fat (gms)	chol. (mgs)	sod. (mgs)	fiber (gms)
1 medium, 4.8 oz. ...	42	.8	9.9	.5	0	6	3.7
Profiterole, frozen							
(*Manzoni*), 3.5 oz.	320	3.0	41.0	16.0	45	90	2.0
Prosciutto:							
(*Boar's Head*), 1 oz.	60	8.0	0	3.0	15	770	0
(*Primissimo Pros-*							
cuitti), 2 oz.	120	15.0	0	7.0	50	1080	0
Prune, canned, in							
heavy syrup:							
(*Sonoma Organic*),							
3–4 pcs., 1.4 oz.	110	1.0	26.0	0	0	5	2.0
pitted, 4 oz.	119	1.0	31.5	.2	0	3	4.3
½ cup.............	123	1.0	32.5	.2	0	3	4.4
5 pcs., 2 tbsp. liquid	90	.8	23.9	.2	0	2	3.3
Prune, dried:							
(*Del Monte*), ¼ cup	120	1.0	29.0	0	0	5	3.0
(*Dole*), 2 oz.	140	1.0	36.0	1.0	0	<10	n.a.
(*Sunsweet* Breakfast),							
1½ oz., about							
8 pcs.	110	1.0	27.0	0	0	5	3.0
dehydrated, ½ cup ...	224	2.4	58.8	.5	0	4	n.a.
extra large (*Sonoma*							
Organic), ½ cup,							
1.4 oz. edible	120	1.0	29.0	0	0	5	3.0
w/pits, ½ cup	193	2.1	50.5	.4	0	3	5.7
pitted (*Sonoma* Or-							
ganic), ¼ cup,							
1.4 oz.	120	1.0	29.0	0	0	5	3.0
pitted, 10 prunes	201	2.2	52.7	.4	0	3	6.0
stewed, w/pits, un-							
sweetened, ½ cup	113	1.2	29.8	.2	0	2	7.0
Prune juice, 8 fl. oz.:							
(*Del Monte*)	170	1.0	43.0	0	0	20	1.0
(*R.W. Knudsen*)	170	1.0	45.0	0	0	20	0
Prune-plum pastry							
filling, see "Pastry							
filling"							
Pudding, ready-to-eat:							
banana:							
(*Comstock/Thank*							
You), ½ cup	200	3.0	36.0	4.0	0	280	0

Food and Measure	cal.	prot. (gms)	carbo. (gms)	fat (gms)	chol. (mgs)	sod. (mgs)	fiber (gms)
Pudding, banana *(cont.)*							
(*Hunt's Snack Pack*), 3½ oz. . . .	120	1.5	18.0	4.5	0	155	0
(*Imagine*), 3.7 oz.	140	1.0	28.0	3.0	0	40	0
(*Jell-O*), 4 oz.	170	3.0	25.0	7.0	0	170	0
(*Kozy Shack*), 4 oz.	130	3.0	22.0	3.0	10	150	0
cream (*Swiss Miss*), 3½ oz.	140	2.0	20.0	5.5	<5	155	0
butterscotch:							
(*Comstock/Thank You*), ½ cup	160	2.0	27.0	5.0	0	250	0
(*Hunt's Snack Pack*), 3½ oz. . . .	130	1.5	21.0	4.5	0	165	0
(*Imagine*), 3.7 oz.	140	1.0	28.0	3.0	0	55	<1.0
(*Swiss Miss*), 3½ oz.	155	3.0	23.0	6.0	<5	180	0
caramel apple (*Hunt's Snack Pack Puddin' Pie*), 4 oz.	180	2.0	26.0	8.0	0	165	0
chocolate:							
(*Comstock/Thank You*), ½ cup	190	3.0	33.0	5.0	0	180	0
(*Hunt's Snack Pack*), 3½ oz. . . .	145	2.0	22.0	5.0	0	140	0
(*Hunt's Snack Pack Fat Free*), 3½ oz.	85	2.0	19.0	0	0	135	0
(*Imagine*), 3.7 oz.	160	1.0	34.0	3.0	0	85	<1.0
(*Jell-O*), 4 oz.	160	2.0	28.0	5.0	0	190	0
(*Jell-O Free*), 4 oz.	100	3.0	23.0	0	0	190	0
(*Kozy Shack*), 4 oz.	140	3.0	24.0	3.5	5	150	1.0
(*Swiss Miss*), 3½ oz.	165	3.0	26.0	6.0	<5	175	0
(*Swiss Miss* Fat Free), 3½ oz. . . .	100	2.0	22.0	0	0	135	0
almond (*Healthy Choice*), ½ cup	110	2.5	21.0	1.5	0	110	0
cream (*Swiss Miss*), 3½ oz.	150	3.0	21.0	6.0	<5	150	0
fudge (*Comstock/ Thank You*), ½ cup	180	3.0	32.0	5.0	0	150	0

Food and Measure	cal.	prot. (gms)	carbo. (gms)	fat (gms)	chol. (mgs)	sod. (mgs)	fiber (gms)
fudge (*Hunt's Snack Pack*), 3½ oz.	145	2.0	23.0	5.0	<5	150	0
fudge (*Swiss Miss Fat Free*), 4 oz.	100	2.0	22.0	0	0	145	0
fudge, double (*Healthy Choice*), ½ cup	100	2.5	20.0	1.0	0	115	0
light (*Kozy Shack*), 4 oz.	110	4.0	22.0	1.0	5	150	1.0
marshmallow (*Hunt's Snack Pack*), 3½ oz. . . .	135	2.0	21.0	5.0	<5	120	0
milk (*Hunt's Snack Pack*), 3½ oz. . . .	145	2.0	23.0	5.0	0	150	0
milk (*Swiss Miss*), 4 oz.	165	2.0	27.0	6.0	<5	60	0
raspberry (*Healthy Choice*), ½ cup	100	2.5	19.0	2.0	0	110	0
chocolate-caramel swirl:							
(*Hunt's Snack Pack*), 3½ oz. . . .	145	2.0	23.0	5.0	0	145	0
(*Jell-O*), 4 oz.	160	3.0	27.0	5.0	0	180	0
(*Swiss Miss*), 4 oz.	170	2.0	26.0	6.0	0	180	0
chocolate–peanut butter swirl (*Hunt's Snack Pack*), 3½ oz.	145	2.5	21.0	6.0	<5	160	0
chocolate-vanilla parfait (*Swiss Miss Fat Free*), 3½ oz.	80	2.0	18.0	0	0	180	0
chocolate-vanilla swirl:							
(*Jell-O*), 4 oz.	160	3.0	27.0	5.0	0	180	0
(*Jell-O Free*), 4 oz.	100	3.0	23.0	0	0	210	0
(*Swiss Miss* Variety), 3½ oz.	160	2.0	25.0	6.0	<5	160	0
chocolate-vanilla-chocolate swirl (*Swiss Miss*), 4 oz.	170	3.0	26.0	6.0	<5	160	0
coconut cream (*Swiss Miss*), 3½ oz.	150	2.0	21.0	6.5	<5	150	0

Food and Measure	cal.	prot. (gms)	carbo. (gms)	fat (gms)	chol. (mgs)	sod. (mgs)	fiber (gms)
Pudding *(cont.)*							
flan/creme caramel							
(*Kozy Shack*), 4 oz.	150	4.0	25.0	3.5	40	90	0
lemon:							
(*Comstock/Thank You*), ½ cup	170	0	38.0	2.0	0	180	0
(*Hunt's Snack Pack*), 3½ oz. ...	125	0	24.0	3.0	0	50	0
(*Imagine*), 3.7 oz.	150	1.0	31.0	3.0	0	35	<1.0
mocha cream (*Swiss Miss*), 3½ oz.	150	3.0	21.0	6.0	0	150	0
mud pie (*Hunt's Snack Pack Puddin' Pie*), 4 oz.	200	2.0	30.0	8.0	0	165	0
rice, see "Rice pudding"							
tapioca:							
(*Comstock/Thank You*), ½ cup	160	2.0	27.0	4.0	0	180	0
(*Healthy Choice*), ½ cup	100	2.0	21.0	1.0	0	115	0
(*Hunt's Snack Pack*), 3½ oz. ...	125	1.5	21.0	4.0	0	145	0
(*Hunt's Snack Pack* Fat Free), 3½ oz.	80	2.0	18.0	0	0	140	0
(*Jell-O*), 4 oz.	140	0	26.0	4.0	0	160	0
(*Kozy Shack*), 4 oz.	140	3.0	25.0	3.0	5	160	0
(*Swiss Miss*), 4 oz.	140	2.0	24.0	3.5	<5	180	0
(*Swiss Miss* Fat Free), 3½ oz. ...	80	1.0	18.0	0	0	140	0
vanilla:							
(*Comstock/Thank You*), ½ cup	160	2.0	28.0	5.0	0	190	0
(*Hunt's Snack Pack*), 3½ oz. ...	135	2.0	21.0	5.0	0	150	0
(*Hunt's Snack Pack* Fat Free), 3½ oz.	80	2.0	18.0	0	0	145	0
(*Jell-O*), 4 oz.	160	3.0	25.0	5.0	0	170	0
(*Jell-O Free*), 4 oz.	100	2.0	23.0	0	0	240	0
(*Kozy Shack*), 4 oz.	130	3.0	22.0	3.0	10	150	0

Food and Measure	cal.	prot. (gms)	carbo. (gms)	fat (gms)	chol. (mgs)	sod. (mgs)	fiber (gms)
(*Swiss Miss*), 3½ oz.	160	2.5	24.0	6.0	<5	180	0
(*Swiss Miss* Fat Free), 3½ oz. ...	75	2.0	17.0	0	0	160	0
French (*Healthy Choice*), ½ cup	100	2.0	20.0	1.0	0	120	0
vanilla-chocolate parfait (*Swiss Miss*), 4 oz.	165	3.0	25.0	6.0	<5	200	0
vanilla-chocolate swirl (*Jell-O*), 4 oz.	160	3.0	26.0	5.0	0	180	0
Pudding and pie filling mix, ½ cup*, except as noted:							
banana:							
(*Jell-O* Sugar/Fat Free)	70	4.0	12.0	0	0	410	0
(*Watkins*), 1 tbsp. ..	35	0	9.0	0	0	160	0
banana cream:							
(*Jell-O*)	140	4.0	26.0	2.5	10	240	0
(*Jell-O* Instant)	150	4.0	29.0	2.5	10	410	0
butter pecan (*Jell-O* Instant)	160	4.0	29.0	3.0	10	410	0
butterscotch:							
(*Jell-O*)	160	4.0	30.0	2.5	10	190	0
(*Jell-O* Instant)	150	4.0	29.0	2.5	10	450	0
(*Jell-O* Sugar/Fat Free)	70	4.0	12.0	0	0	400	0
(*Watkins*), 1 tbsp. ..	35	0	9.0	0	0	240	0
chocolate:							
(*D-Zerta*)	60	5.0	11.0	0	0	65	<1.0
(*Jell-O*)	150	5.0	28.0	2.5	10	170	<1.0
(*Jell-O* Instant)	160	4.0	31.0	2.5	10	470	<1.0
(*Jell-O* Sugar Free)	90	5.0	12.0	2.5	10	170	<1.0
(*Jell-O* Sugar/Fat Free)	80	5.0	14.0	0	0	390	<1.0
(*My*T*Fine*)	90	0	22.0	0	0	140	<1.0
(*Watkins*), 1 tbsp. ..	30	0	7.0	0	0	115	0
milk (*Jell-O*)	150	4.0	28.0	2.5	10	170	<1.0
milk (*Jell-O* Instant)	160	5.0	31.0	3.0	10	460	<1.0

Food and Measure	cal.	prot. (gms)	carbo. (gms)	fat (gms)	chol. (mgs)	sod. (mgs)	fiber (gms)
Pudding and pie filling mix *(cont.)*							
chocolate fudge:							
(*Jell-O*)	150	5.0	28.0	2.5	10	170	1.0
(*Jell-O* Instant)	160	5.0	31.0	3.0	10	440	<1.0
(*Jell-O* Sugar/Fat							
Free)	80	5.0	14.0	0	0	390	<1.0
chocolate mousse, see							
"Mousse mix"							
coconut (*Watkins*),							
1 tbsp.	40	0	7.0	1.0	0	105	0
coconut cream:							
(*Jell-O*)	150	4.0	24.0	2.5	10	210	<1.0
(*Jell-O* Instant)	160	4.0	27.0	4.5	10	320	<1.0
custard:							
(*Jello-O Americana*)	140	5.0	25.0	2.5	10	190	0
Spanish style (*Goya*							
Flan), 1/4 oz. dry	60	0	13.0	.5	0	110	<1.0
flan:							
(*Alsa* Creme Cara-							
mel), 1 1/3 tbsp.							
mix, 1 tbsp. cara-							
mel	110	0	27.0	0	5	15	0
(*Jell-O*)	140	4.0	26.0	2.5	10	65	0
lemon:							
(*Jell-O*)	140	1.0	29.0	2.0	75	75	0
(*Jell-O* Instant)	150	4.0	29.0	2.5	10	360	0
(*Watkins*), 1 tbsp.	40	0	9.0	0	0	95	0
pistachio:							
(*Jell-O* Instant)	160	4.0	29.0	3.0	10	410	0
(*Jell-O* Sugar/Fat							
Free)	70	4.0	12.0	0	0	380	0
rice, see "Rice pud-							
ding mix"							
tapioca:							
(*Jell-O Americana*)	140	4.0	26.0	2.5	10	170	0
(*Watkins*), 1 tbsp.	35	0	9.0	0	0	160	0
vanilla:							
(*Jell-O*)	140	4.0	26.0	2.5	10	200	0
(*Jell-O* Instant)	150	4.0	29.0	2.5	10	410	0
(*Jell-O* Sugar Free)	80	4.0	11.0	2.5	10	170	0

Food and Measure	cal.	prot. (gms)	carbo. (gms)	fat (gms)	chol. (mgs)	sod. (mgs)	fiber (gms)
(*Jell-O* Sugar/Fat Free)	70	4.0	12.0	0	0	400	0
(*Watkins*), 1 tbsp.	35	0	9.0	0	0	140	0
French (*Jell-O* Instant)	150	4.0	29.0	2.5	10	410	0
Pudding, plum (*Crosse & Blackwell*), 1/3 pkg.	410	4.0	91.0	4.0	10	290	4.0
Pudding bar, all flavors, 1 pc.:							
(*Eskimo Pie*)	90	3.0	16.0	1.5	5	45	0
(*Eskimo Pie* Variety Pack)	80	3.0	15.0	1.5	5	65	<1.0
Pummelo:							
(*Frieda's*), 3.5 oz. . . .	38	.8	9.6	<.1	0	1	n.a.
1 medium, 5½"	228	4.6	58.6	.2	0	7	6.1
sections, ½ cup	36	.7	9.1	<.1	0	1	1.0
Pumpkin, ½ cup:							
fresh, pulp:							
raw, 1" cubes	15	.6	3.8	.1	0	1	1.0
boiled, drained, mashed	24	.9	6.0	.1	0	2	1.0
canned:							
(*Comstock* Pure)	50	1.0	10.0	0	0	0	4.0
(*Libby's* Solid Pack)	40	2.0	9.0	.5	0	5	5.0
(*Stokely*)	50	1.0	10.0	0	0	0	4.0
pie mix, see "Pie filling"							
w/or w/out winter squash	41	1.3	9.9	.3	0	6	3.4
Pumpkin butter (*Smucker's*), 1 tbsp.	45	0	11.0	0	0	25	0
Pumpkin flower:							
raw, ½ cup	3	.2	.5	<.1	0	1	<1.0
boiled, drained, ½ cup	10	.7	2.2	.1	0	4	.6
Pumpkin leaf:							
raw, ½ cup	4	.6	.5	.1	0	2	<1.0
boiled, drained, ½ cup	7	1.0	1.2	.1	0	3	.9
Pumpkin pie spice, 1 tsp.	6	.1	1.2	.2	0	1	.3

Food and Measure	cal.	prot. (gms)	carbo. (gms)	fat (gms)	chol. (mgs)	sod. (mgs)	fiber (gms)
Pumpkin seed:							
roasted, in shell:							
1 oz. or 85 seeds	127	5.3	15.3	5.5	0	5	n.a.
1 cup	285	11.9	34.4	12.4	0	12	n.a.
salted, 1 oz.	127	5.3	15.3	5.5	0	163	n.a.
roasted, shelled:							
1 oz.	148	9.4	3.8	12.0	0	5	1.8
salted, 1 oz.	148	9.4	3.8	12.0	0	163	1.8
dried, shelled, 1 oz. or							
142 kernels	154	7.0	5.1	13.0	0	5	n.a.
tamari-roasted, spicy							
(*Eden*), 1 oz.	170	11.0	5.0	11.0	0	80	3.0
Punch, see "Fruit							
drink blends," "Fruit							
juice blends," and							
specific fruit listings							
Purslane, ½ cup:							
raw	4	.3	.7	<.1	0	10	<1.0
boiled, drained	10	.9	2.1	.1	0	26	<1.0

Q

Food and Measure	cal.	prot. (gms)	carbo. (gms)	fat (gms)	chol. (mgs)	sod. (mgs)	fiber (gms)
Quail, raw:							
meat w/skin:							
quail, 3.8 oz.							
(4.3 oz. w/bone)	210	21.4	0	13.1	n.a.	58	0
1 oz.	54	5.6	0	3.4	n.a.	15	0
meat only:							
1 quail, 3.2 oz.							
(4.3 oz. w/bone							
and skin)	123	20.0	0	4.2	n.a.	47	0
1 oz.	38	6.2	0	1.3	n.a.	14	0
breast meat only:							
1 breast, 2 oz.	69	12.7	0	1.8	n.a.	31	0
1 oz.	35	6.4	0	.8	n.a.	16	0
Quesadilla dip,							
w/chicken (*Tos-*							
titos), 4 tbsp.	50	4.0	6.0	6.0	10	600	<2.0
Quiche, frozen, Flor-							
entine (*Nancy's*),							
6 oz.	440	18.0	35.0	26.0	180	620	1.0
Quince:							
(*Frieda's*), 5 oz.	80	1.0	21.0	0	0	5	3.0
1 medium, 5.3 oz. . . .	53	.4	14.1	.1	0	4	1.7
peeled, seeded, 1 oz.	16	.1	4.3	<.1	0	1	.5
Quinoa, dry:							
(*Eden*), 1/4 cup	170	7.0	31.0	2.5	0	0	3.0
(*Frieda's*), 1/3 cup	170	6.0	31.0	2.5	0	10	3.0
Quinoa seeds (*Arrow-*							
head Mills), 1/4 cup	140	5.0	25.0	2.0	0	0	4.0

R

Food and Measure	cal.	prot. (gms)	carbo. (gms)	fat (gms)	chol. (mgs)	sod. (mgs)	fiber (gms)
Rabbit, meat only:							
domesticated:							
roasted, 4 oz.	223	33.0	0	9.1	93	53	0
stewed, 4 oz.	234	34.5	0	9.5	98	42	0
stewed, diced, 1 cup	288	42.5	0	11.8	120	52	0
wild, stewed:							
4 oz.	196	37.4	0	4.0	139	51	0
diced, 1 cup	242	46.2	0	4.9	172	63	0
Radiatore pasta							
dishes, mix, dry:							
red beans, Barcelona							
(*Bean Cuisine* Pasta							
& Beans), 1.5 oz.	150	7.0	29.0	1.0	0	15	4.0
spicy tomato sauce							
(*DeBoles*), 2 oz. . . .	240	7.0	42.0	.5	0	500	2.0
w/sun-dried tomato-							
basil sauce (*An-*							
nie's), ²/₃ cup	260	10.0	49.0	2.5	5	390	2.0
Radicchio, fresh:							
(*Frieda's*), 2 cups,							
3 oz.	20	1.0	4.0	0	0	20	0
trimmed, 1 oz.	7	.4	1.3	.1	0	6	0
medium leaf, .3 oz.	2	.1	.4	<.1	0	2	0
shredded, ¹/₂ cup	5	.3	.9	.1	0	4	0
Radish:							
10 medium, ³/₄″–1″	7	.3	1.6	.2	0	11	.7
sliced, ¹/₂ cup	10	.4	2.1	.3	0	14	.9
Radish, black:							
(*Frieda's*), ³/₄ cup,							
3 oz.	15	1.0	3.0	0	0	20	1.0
1 oz.	5	.3	1.0	<.1	0	5	n.a.

Food and Measure	cal.	prot. (gms)	carbo. (gms)	fat (gms)	chol. (mgs)	sod. (mgs)	fiber (gms)
Radish, Chinese							
(*Frieda's* Lo Bok),							
⅔ cup, 3 oz.	25	1.0	5.0	0	0	55	2.0
Radish, Oriental:							
(*Frieda's* Daikon),							
⅔ cup, 3 oz.	15	1.0	3.0	0	0	20	1.0
raw, 1 medium, 7″ . . .	62	2.0	13.9	.3	0	71	5.4
raw, sliced, ½ cup . . .	8	.3	1.8	<.1	0	9	.7
boiled, drained, sliced,							
½ cup	13	.5	2.5	.2	0	10	1.2
dried, 1 oz.	77	2.2	18.0	.2	0	79	2.4
Radish, white-icicle:							
1 medium, .6 oz.	2	.2	.5	<.1	0	3	n.a.
sliced, ½ cup	7	.6	1.3	.1	0	8	n.a.
Raisin, ¼ cup, except							
as noted:							
(*Sun•Maid* Baking)	120	1.0	28.0	0	0	5	2.0
seeded, not packed	107	.9	28.5	.2	0	11	2.5
seedless:							
(*Sun•Maid* Snack							
Box), 1½ oz.	130	1.0	33.0	0	0	10	2.0
regular or golden							
(*Sun•Maid*)	130	1.0	31.0	0	0	10	2.0
golden, not packed	110	1.3	28.9	.2	0	5	1.5
Monukka/Thompson							
(*Sonoma* Organic)	130	1.0	31.0	0	0	10	2.0
not packed	109	1.2	28.7	.2	0	5	1.5
chocolate coated, see							
"Candy"							
Raisin, baking, semi-							
sweet chocolate							
coated (*Nestlé*),							
1⅓ tbsp.	70	<1.0	11.0	3.0	0	0	<1.0
Raisin sauce (*Reese*),							
¼ cup	150	0	36.0	0	0	55	n.a.
Ranch dip, 2 tbsp:							
(*Heluva* Good)	60	1.0	2.0	5.0	20	170	0
(*Heluva* Good Fat Free)	25	1.0	3.0	0	0	230	0
(*Kraft*)	60	1.0	3.0	4.0	0	210	0
(*Marie's* Homestyle)	130	1.0	2.0	13.0	15	280	0

Food and Measure	cal.	prot. (gms)	carbo. (gms)	fat (gms)	chol. (mgs)	sod. (mgs)	fiber (gms)
Ranch dip *(cont.)*							
(*T. Marzetti's* Veggie Dip)	140	1.0	1.0	14.0	25	200	0
(*T. Marzetti's* Veggie Dip Fat Free)	35	1.0	6.0	0	0	320	0
(*Nalley*)	110	1.0	2.0	11.0	10	240	0
(*Ruffles*)	70	1.0	4.0	6.0	0	240	1.0
(*Ruffles* Lowfat)	40	2.0	6.0	1.0	0	230	<1.0
bacon (*T. Marzetti's* Veggie Dip)	120	1.0	2.0	12.0	25	150	0
Southwestern:							
(*T. Marzetti's* Veggie Dip)	140	1.0	2.0	14.0	25	170	0
(*T. Marzetti's* Veggie Dip Fat Free)	30	1.0	6.0	0	0	380	0
Ranch dip mix, 2 tbsp.*, except as noted:							
(*Hidden Valley* Fiesta)	70	<1.0	2.0	6.0	15	260	0
(*Hidden Valley* Original)	70	<1.0	2.0	6.0	15	230	0
(*Hidden Valley* Original Reduced Calorie)	40	<1.0	2.0	3.0	10	240	0
pepper (*Watkins*), 1 tsp.	10	0	3.0	0	0	120	0
pepper, cracked (*Knorr*), ½ tsp. ...	5	0	<1.0	0	0	100	0
Rapini, see "Broccoli rabe"							
Raspberry, fresh, ½ cup	31	.6	7.1	.3	0	<1	4.2
Raspberry, canned, in heavy syrup, ½ cup:							
(*Comstock/Wilderness*)	100	1.0	23.0	0	0	35	3.0
(*Oregon*)	120	1.0	30.0	0	0	10	5.0
Raspberry, frozen:							
(*Birds Eye*), ½ cup ...	90	<1.0	22.0	0	0	5	5.0
(*Cascadian Farm*), 1 cup	60	1.0	15.0	1.0	0	0	7.0
sweetened, ½ cup ...	129	.9	32.7	.2	0	1	5.5

Food and Measure	cal.	prot. (gms)	carbo. (gms)	fat (gms)	chol. (mgs)	sod. (mgs)	fiber (gms)
Raspberry drink, 8 fl. oz.:							
hibiscus (*R.W. Knudsen*)	90	0	23.0	0	0	40	0
lemon (*Dole* Splash)	120	0	31.0	0	0	20	0
Raspberry drink, mix*, 8 fl. oz.:							
(*Kool-Aid*)	100	0	25.0	0	0	35	0
(*Kool-Aid* Presweetened)	60	0	17.0	0	0	0	0
Raspberry juice blends, 8 fl. oz.: except as noted:							
(*Dole* Country)	140	1.0	34.0	0	0	30	0
cranberry (*Apple & Eve*)	120	1.0	30.0	0	0	20	0
lemon (*Santa Cruz* Organic)	120	0	29.0	0	0	35	0
peach (*R.W. Knudsen*)	120	0	31.0	0	0	25	0
Raspberry nectar, 8 fl. oz.:							
(*R.W. Knudsen*)	120	0	30.0	0	0	25	0
(*Santa Cruz* Organic)	100	0	26.0	0	0	35	0
Raspberry pastry filling, see "Pastry filling" and "Pie filling"							
Raspberry syrup, ¼ cup:							
(*Maple Grove Farms*)	240	0	60.0	0	0	0	1.0
red (*Smucker's*)	210	0	52.0	0	0	0	0
Raspberry-tamarind dipping sauce (*Helen's Tropical Exotics*), 2 tbsp.	50	0	11.0	1.0	0	0	1.0
Rattlesnake beans, dried (*Frieda's*), ½ cup	120	7.0	22.0	0	0	0	9.0

Food and Measure	cal.	prot. (gms)	carbo. (gms)	fat (gms)	chol. (mgs)	sod. (mgs)	fiber (gms)
Ravioli, frozen or refrigerated (see also "Ravioli entree"), 1 cup, except as noted:							
beef and garlic (*Contadina*)	330	17.0	46.0	9.0	60	470	3.0
cheese:							
four (*Contadina*) ...	290	14.0	38.0	9.0	70	340	3.0
four (*Contadina* Light)	230	12.0	37.0	4.0	35	390	2.0
four (*Wolfgang Puck's*), 1 pkg.	330	18.0	16.0	20.0	55	610	2.0
and garlic (*Di Giorno Light Varieties*)	270	17.0	45.0	2.0	5	580	1.0
Italian herb (*Di Giorno*)	350	15.0	44.0	13.0	45	610	2.0
w/Italian sausage (*Di Giorno*), ¾ cup	340	16.0	41.0	12.0	50	630	2.0
chicken:							
and herb (*Contadina*), 1¼ cups	370	14.0	47.0	14.0	70	400	2.0
smoked (*Contadina*)	240	11.0	34.0	7.0	40	370	2.0
Gorgonzola (*Contadina*), 1¼ cups ...	360	15.0	47.0	12.0	60	400	3.0
mushroom spinach (*Wolfgang Puck's*), 1 pkg.	260	7.0	15.0	18.0	45	1280	3.0
tomato and cheese (*Di Giorno Light Varieties*)	280	14.0	49.0	3.0	10	490	2.0
vegetable, garden (*Contadina*)	250	11.0	39.0	5.0	40	500	2.0
Ravioli entree, canned or packaged, 1 cup, except as noted:							
(*Chef Boyardee Junior Micro*)...........	210	8.0	37.0	4.0	15	800	4.0

Food and Measure	cal.	prot. (gms)	carbo. (gms)	fat (gms)	chol. (mgs)	sod. (mgs)	fiber (gms)
(*Hormel Health Selections*)	190	8.0	32.0	2.5	10	510	3.0
beef:							
(*Chef Boyardee*) ...	230	7.0	35.0	7.0	15	1140	3.0
(*Chef Boyardee*), 7-oz. can	170	7.0	27.0	4.0	15	960	2.0
(*Chef Boyardee Micro Cup*), 7½ oz.	190	6.0	29.0	5.0	15	980	2.0
(*Chef Boyardee Mini*)	240	8.0	37.0	7.0	20	1180	3.0
(*Chef Boyardee 99% Fat Free*)	190	7.0	38.0	1.0	15	1150	2.0
(*Chef Boyardee Overstuffed*)	280	12.0	48.0	4.5	20	1190	4.0
(*Dinty Moore American Classics*), 1 bowl	300	20.0	34.0	9.0	55	810	3.0
(*Franco-American Superiore*)	280	11.0	38.0	9.0	20	1160	2.0
(*Nalley*), 7½-oz. can	240	11.0	26.0	10.0	35	930	5.0
(*Progresso*)	260	9.0	45.0	5.0	5	940	4.0
mini (*Kid's Kitchen*)	240	10.0	35.0	7.0	20	980	1.0
w/pasta in tomato and cheese (*Franco-American*)	230	7.0	42.0	3.5	10	1020	2.0
in sauce (*Nalley*), 7½-oz. can	230	9.0	33.0	7.0	15	1030	6.0
in tomato sauce (*Nalley*)	280	11.0	40.0	9.0	15	1240	7.0
cheese:							
(*Chef Boyardee 99% Fat Free*)	240	7.0	41.0	2.5	5	970	2.0
(*Progresso*)	220	7.0	43.0	2.0	<5	930	4.0
sausage, Italian (*Chef Boyardee Overstuffed*)	290	10.0	53.0	4.0	15	1230	4.0
w/tomato sauce (*Hormel Microwave*) ...	220	8.0	35.0	6.0	10	890	2.0

Food and Measure	cal.	prot. (gms)	carbo. (gms)	fat (gms)	chol. (mgs)	sod. (mgs)	fiber (gms)
Ravioli entree, frozen, 1 pkg., except as noted:							
(*Radical Ravioli* California Grill), 10.7 oz.	340	15.0	49.0	9.0	45	850	1.0
black bean (*Radical Ravioli* Santa Fe), 10.7 oz.	390	17.0	54.0	12.0	50	670	4.0
cheese:							
(*Kid Cuisine* Raptor), 9.82 oz. ...	310	7.0	59.0	5.0	15	730	5.0
(*Lean Cuisine*), 8½ oz.	270	11.0	40.0	7.0	45	580	5.0
(*Stouffer's*), 10⅝ oz.	380	15.0	51.0	13.0	100	700	6.0
marinara, w/spirals, garlic bread (*Marie Callender's*), 1 cup, 2 oz. garlic bread	470	16.0	57.0	20.0	20	670	8.0
parmigiana (*Healthy Choice*), 9 oz. ...	260	11.0	44.0	5.0	20	290	6.0
chicken:							
w/sauce (*Radical Ravioli*), 10.7 oz.	360	18.0	46.0	11.0	75	770	2.0
sausage, spicy (*Radical Ravioli*), 10.7 oz.	400	18.0	49.0	15.0	45	910	2.0
teriyaki (*Radical Ravioli*), 10.7 oz.	420	16.0	69.0	8.0	60	1070	2.0
Thai style (*Radical Ravioli*), 10.7 oz.	440	19.0	58.0	15.0	50	910	3.0
Florentine (*Smart Ones*), 8½ oz.	220	9.0	43.0	2.0	5	490	4.0
ricotta, w/sauce (*Amy's*), 9½ oz. ...	340	15.0	44.0	12.0	20	580	6.0
Red beans (see also "Kidney beans" and "Mexican beans"), canned, ½ cup:							
(*Allens*)	160	6.0	19.0	.5	0	310	9.0

Food and Measure	cal.	prot. (gms)	carbo. (gms)	fat (gms)	chol. (mgs)	sod. (mgs)	fiber (gms)
(*Bush's Best*)	110	6.0	19.0	.5	0	460	6.0
(*Green Giant/Joan of Arc*)	100	6.0	19.0	.5	0	350	6.0
small:							
(*Eden* Organic)	100	6.0	17.0	.5	0	65	5.0
(*Goya*)	90	7.0	18.0	.5	0	360	6.0
Red beans, mix, and fusilli, dry (*Marrakesh Express* Terrazza Florentine), ⅓ cup	220	10.0	43.0	1.0	<5	350	2.0
Red snapper, see "Snapper"							
Redfish, see "Ocean perch"							
Redfish seasoning, blackened (*Chef Paul Prudhomme's Magic Seasoning Blends*), ¼ tsp. . . .	0	0	0	0	0	95	0
Refried beans, canned, ½ cup:							
(*Allens*)	150	7.0	24.0	2.5	0	360	11.0
(*Chi-Chi's*)	150	7.0	23.0	3.0	0	530	5.0
(*Chi-Chi's* Fat Free) . . .	120	7.0	23.0	0	0	530	5.0
(*Gebhardt* No Fat)	85	7.0	16.0	0	0	510	4.0
(*Old El Paso*)	100	6.0	17.0	.5	0	570	6.0
(*Old El Paso* Fat Free)	100	6.0	18.0	0	0	480	6.0
(*Ortega*)	130	8.0	25.0	2.5	0	570	9.0
(*Rosarita* Authentic)	140	4.0	15.0	8.0	<5	500	3.0
(*Rosarita* No Fat)	90	n.a.	28.0	0	0	570	6.0
(*Rosarita* Traditional)	100	6.0	17.5	2.0	0	505	5.0
black beans:							
(*Old El Paso*)	110	6.0	18.0	2.0	0	340	6.0
(*Rosarita* Low Fat)	95	7.0	19.0	<1.0	0	525	7.5
w/cheese (*Old El Paso*)	130	7.0	18.0	3.5	5	500	6.0
w/green chilies:							
(*Old El Paso*)	100	6.0	17.0	.5	<5	720	6.0
(*Rosarita*)	90	5.0	17.0	2.0	0	500	5.0
jalapeño (*Gebhardt*)	95	5.0	18.0	1.5	0	410	6.0

Food and Measure	cal.	prot. (gms)	carbo. (gms)	fat (gms)	chol. (mgs)	sod. (mgs)	fiber (gms)
Refried beans, canned *(cont.)*							
w/salsa, zesty							
(*Rosarita* No Fat)	90	6.5	18.0	0	0	660	5.0
w/sausage (*Old El*							
Paso)	200	7.0	14.0	13.0	10	360	4.0
spicy:							
(*Old El Paso* Fat							
Free)	100	6.0	18.0	0	0	720	6.0
(*Rosarita*)	95	6.0	16.0	2.0	0	610	5.0
vegetarian:							
(*Gebhardt*)	95	6.0	15.0	2.0	0	515	3.5
(*Old El Paso*)	100	6.0	17.0	1.0	0	490	6.0
(*Rosarita*)	105	6.0	18.0	2.0	0	540	5.0
Refried beans, dried,							
w/cheese (*Al-*							
pineAire), 2¼ oz.	240	15.0	27.0	8.0	10	450	11.0
Refried beans, mix,							
dry, instant (*Fantas-*							
tic Foods), ⅓ cup	160	9.0	29.0	1.0	0	610	11.0
Relish, see "Pickle							
relish" and specific							
listings							
Remoulade sauce							
(*Zararain's*), ¼ cup	80	2.0	9.0	8.0	0	780	1.0
Rennet (*Junket*),							
1 tablet	1	0	0	0	0	165	0
Rhubarb, fresh:							
(*Frieda's*), ⅔ cup,							
3 oz.	20	1.0	4.0	0	0	0	2.0
diced, ½ cup	13	.6	2.8	.1	0	2	1.1
Rhubarb, canned, in							
extra-heavy syrup							
(*Oregon*), ½ cup . . .	180	<1.0	44.0	0	0	15	3.0
Rhubarb, frozen,							
cooked, sweetened,							
½ cup	139	.5	37.4	.1	0	2	2.4
Rice, dry, ¼ cup, ex-							
cept as noted:							
Arborio:							
(*Fantastic Foods*)	210	4.0	45.0	0	0	0	1.0

Food and Measure	cal.	prot. (gms)	carbo. (gms)	fat (gms)	chol. (mgs)	sod. (mgs)	fiber (gms)
brown (*Lundberg Nutra-Farmed*)	160	5.0	33.0	1.5	0	0	3.0
white (*Lundberg Nutra-Farmed*)	160	4.0	35.0	1.0	0	0	4.0
basmati, brown:							
(*Arrowhead Mills*)	150	3.0	33.0	1.0	0	0	2.0
(*Fantastic Foods*)	170	3.0	36.0	2.0	0	0	1.0
(*Lundberg* Organic)	160	4.0	34.0	1.5	0	0	2.0
(*Lundberg Nutra-Farmed* Royal) . . .	170	4.0	38.0	2.0	0	0	2.0
basmati, white:							
(*Casbah*)	158	3.0	36.0	0	0	0	1.0
(*Fantastic Foods*)	180	3.0	38.0	0	0	0	1.0
(*Lundberg* Organic)	180	4.0	38.0	.5	0	0	1.0
(*Lundberg Nutra-Farmed*)	180	4.0	41.0	.5	0	0	0
long grain (*Arrowhead Mills*)	150	4.0	34.0	0	0	0	1.0
blends:							
(*Lundberg Black Japonica*)	170	5.0	38.0	2.0	0	0	3.0
(*Lundberg Countrywild*)	150	3.0	35.0	1.5	0	0	3.0
(*Lundberg Jubilee*)	170	4.0	39.0	1.5	0	0	3.0
(*Lundberg Wild Blend*)	150	4.0	35.0	1.5	0	0	3.0
(*Watkins* Harvest Treasures Heartland Medley)	160	5.0	35.0	0	0	10	4.0
(*Watkins* Harvest Treasures Minnesota Medley)	160	5.0	34.0	.5	0	10	2.0
brown and wild (*Watkins* Harvest Treasures Medley)	160	4.0	34.0	0	0	10	3.0
jasmine (*Watkins* Harvest Treasures)	180	4.0	37.0	1.5	0	0	1.0
white and wild (*Watkins* Harvest Treasures Medley) . . .	160	4.0	34.0	0	0	5	1.0

Food and Measure	cal.	prot. (gms)	carbo. (gms)	fat (gms)	chol. (mgs)	sod. (mgs)	fiber (gms)
Rice *(cont.)*							
brown:							
(*Carolina/Mahatma/]River*)	150	3.0	32.0	1.0	0	0	1.0
(*Lundberg Wehani*)	170	3.0	38.0	1.5	0	0	3.0
(*Success*), ½ cup	150	4.0	33.0	1.0	0	5	2.0
precooked (*Lundberg*)	150	3.0	32.0	1.5	0	0	2.0
whole grain (*Minute* Instant), ½ cup	170	4.0	34.0	1.5	0	0	2.0
brown, long grain:							
(*Arrowhead Mills*)	150	3.0	33.0	1.0	0	0	2.0
(*Lundberg* Organic)	170	4.0	38.0	1.5	0	0	3.0
(*Lundberg Nutra-Farmed*)	170	3.0	37.0	2.0	0	0	3.0
(*Uncle Ben's* Instant), ½ cup	190	4.0	42.0	1.5	0	20	2.0
brown, quick (*Lundberg*)	150	3.0	32.0	1.5	0	0	2.0
brown, short grain:							
(*Arrowhead Mills*)	170	4.0	36.0	1.0	0	0	2.0
(*Lundberg Nutra-Farmed*/Organic)	170	3.0	40.0	1.5	0	0	3.0
glutinous or sweet . . .	171	3.2	37.8	.3	0	3	1.3
jasmine (*Fantastic Foods*)	170	3.0	38.0	0	0	0	1.0
sushi (*Lundberg* Organic)	160	3.0	36.0	0	0	0	1.0
white, long grain:							
(*Carolina*)	150	3.0	35.0	1.0	0	0	1.0
(*Mahatma*)	150	3.0	35.0	0	0	0	0
(*River/Water Maid*)	160	3.0	37.0	0	0	0	<1.0
(*Success*), ½ cup	190	4.0	44.0	0	0	5	<1.0
instant (*Carolina*)	160	4.0	36.0	0	0	0	1.0
instant (*Mahatma*)	160	4.0	36.0	0	0	5	1.0
instant (*Minute* Original), ½ cup	170	4.0	37.0	0	0	5	0
instant (*Minute* Boil-in-Bag), ½ cup	190	4.0	42.0	0	0	10	0
instant (*Minute* Premium), ½ cup . . .	170	3.0	36.0	0	0	5	0

Food and Measure	cal.	prot. (gms)	carbo. (gms)	fat (gms)	chol. (mgs)	sod. (mgs)	fiber (gms)
parboiled (*Uncle Ben's Converted*)	170	4.0	38.0	0	0	0	0
Rice, wild, see "Wild rice"							
Rice and beans, see "Rice dishes, frozen" and "Rice dishes, mix"							
Rice beverage, see " 'Milk,' nondairy"							
Rice bran, crude, 1 cup	262	11.1	41.2	17.3	0	4	18.0
Rice cake (see also "Popcorn cake"), 1 cake, except as noted:							
plain:							
(*Quaker/Mother's*)	35	1.0	7.0	0	0	15	0
(*Quaker/Mother's* Unsalted)	35	1.0	7.0	0	0	0	0
all varieties:							
(*Lundberg*), .6 oz.	60	1.0	14.0	0	0	120	2.0
(*Lundberg* Unsalted), .6 oz. . . .	60	1.0	14.0	0	0	0	2.0
bars (*Health Valley* Crisp Fat Free) . . .	110	1.0	26.0	0	0	5	1.0
apple cinnamon (*Crispy Cakes*)	35	1.0	7.0	<1.0	0	60	n.a.
banana nut (*Quaker*)	50	1.0	11.0	0	0	45	0
brown							
(*Lundberg* Mini), 5 cakes	60	1.0	14.0	0	0	115	2.0
toasted (*Crispy Cakes*)	30	1.0	7.0	<1.0	0	15	n.a.
cheese:							
cheddar (*Crispy Cakes*)	35	1.0	7.0	<1.0	0	50	n.a.
nacho (*Lundberg* Mini), 5 cakes . . .	60	1.0	13.0	.5	0	115	2.0
chocolate crunch (*Quaker*)	60	1.0	12.0	1.0	0	35	0

Food and Measure	cal.	prot. (gms)	carbo. (gms)	fat (gms)	chol. (mgs)	sod. (mgs)	fiber (gms)
Rice cake *(cont.)*							
cinnamon streusel							
(*Quaker*)	60	1.0	12.0	1.0	0	20	0
dill, creamy (*Lundberg*							
Mini), 5 cakes	60	1.0	13.0	1.0	0	55	2.0
peanut butter (*Quaker*)	60	1.0	12.0	1.0	0	60	0
pizza or ranch (*Crispy*							
Cakes)	30	1.0	7.0	<1.0	0	50	n.a.
w/popcorn, see "Pop-							
corn cake"							
vegetable, garden							
(*Crispy Cakes*)	35	1.0	7.0	<1.0	0	45	n.a.
Rice chips, brown							
(*Eden*), 1.1 oz.	150	2.0	19.0	7.0	0	100	0
Rice dishes, canned,							
1 cup, except as							
noted:							
fried (*La Choy*)	295	7.0	64.0	2.0	0	1295	3.5
Spanish:							
(*Old El Paso*)	130	3.0	28.0	1.0	0	1340	2.0
(*Van Camp's*),							
½ cup	90	30.0	19.0	1.5	0	645	1.5
Rice dishes, frozen,							
1 pkg., except as							
noted:							
and beans (*Smart*							
*One*santa Fe Style),							
10 oz.	300	12.0	49.0	8.0	20	620	6.0
beef, spicy, and broc-							
coli (*Uncle Ben's*							
Rice Bowl), 12 oz.	380	22.0	58.0	7.0	35	1660	5.0
and broccoli:							
(*Green Giant*)	320	8.0	15.0	12.0	5	1000	2.0
au gratin (*Freezer*							
Queen), 1 cup . . .	190	5.0	38.0	2.0	<5	560	3.0
in cheese sauce							
(*Birds Eye Side*							
Orders), 10 oz.	290	8.0	44.0	9.0	15	1110	2.0
chicken and vegeta-							
bles (*Uncle Ben's*							
Rice Bowl), 12 oz.	340	19.0	56.0	5.0	50	590	3.0

Food and Measure	cal.	prot. (gms)	carbo. (gms)	fat (gms)	chol. (mgs)	sod. (mgs)	fiber (gms)
pilaf, w/green beans (*The Budget Gourmet* Side Dish), 5 oz.	220	4.0	28.0	10.0	10	530	2.0
risotto, w/cheese and mushrooms (*Smart Ones*), 10 oz.	290	11.0	47.0	7.0	20	540	4.0
w/vegetables:							
(*Green Giant* Medley)	240	6.0	15.0	3.0	5	880	3.0
Caribbean (*Cascadian Farm Veggie Bowl*), 9 oz.	280	7.0	52.0	5.0	0	580	3.0
fiesta (*Cascadian Farm Veggie Bowl*), 9 oz.	340	12.0	52.0	11.0	15	330	7.0
Hunan style (*Smart Ones*), 10 1/3 oz.	280	7.0	45.0	8.0	0	630	5.0
Madras curry (*Cascadian Farm Veggie Bowl*), 9 oz.	270	7.0	49.0	5.0	0	650	3.0
Oriental (*The Budget Gourmet* Side Dish), 5.2 oz. . . .	200	4.0	23.0	11.0	5	500	2.0
pilaf (*Green Giant*)	230	6.0	15.0	3.0	5	1020	3.0
stir-fry (*The Budget Gourmet Value Classics*), 8 oz.	350	7.0	44.0	16.0	25	670	3.0
Szechuan (*Cascadian Farm Veggie Bowl*), 9 oz.	210	7.0	45.0	1.5	0	630	3.0
Szechuan style, spicy (*The Budget Gourmet Value Classics*), 8 oz.	290	10.0	41.0	9.0	15	890	3.0
teriyaki (*Cascadian Farm Veggie Bowl*), 9 oz.	270	9.0	44.0	7.0	0	630	2.0
teriyaki, stir-fry (*Uncle Ben's* Rice Bowl), 12 oz. . . .	340	8.0	70.0	3.0	0	1290	7.0

Food and Measure	cal.	prot. (gms)	carbo. (gms)	fat (gms)	chol. (mgs)	sod. (mgs)	fiber (gms)
Rice dishes, frozen, w/vegetables *(cont.)*							
white and wild (*Birds Eye Side Orders*), 1 cup . . .	180	4.0	31.0	4.0	10	480	2.0
white and wild (*Green Giant*) . . .	250	6.0	45.0	5.0	0	1000	3.0
wild rice pilaf (*The Budget Gourmet Value Classics*), 8 oz.	340	6.0	50.0	13.0	10	740	2.0
Rice dishes, mix, 2 oz. dry[1], except as noted:							
Alfredo broccoli (*Lipton* Rice & Sauce), 1 cup*	320	9.0	46.0	12.0	15	990	1.0
and beans:							
black (*Goya*), ¼ cup	160	5.0	34.0	0	0	570	3.0
black (*Mahatma*) . . .	200	7.0	39.0	1.5	0	930	5.0
black, Jamaican (*Fantastic Foods Healthy Complements*), ⅓ cup . . .	140	5.0	30.0	1.5	0	300	5.0
black, Mediterranean, pilaf (*Near East*)	270	7.0	52.0	5.0	0	990	5.0
black, savory (*Good Harvest*), ⅓ cup	160	6.0	31.0	2.0	0	320	4.0
black, spicy Jamaican (*Fantastic Foods* Cup), 2.4 oz.	250	10.0	52.0	1.5	0	530	6.0
black or red (*Watkins*), 1.4 oz., ⅙ pkg.	140	4.0	30.0	0	0	0	2.0
Cajun (*Rice-A-Roni*), 1 cup* . . .	280	8.0	52.0	5.0	0	1220	3.0
curry, Bombay, w/lentils (*Fantastic Foods* Cup), 2.4 oz.	250	9.0	53.0	1.5	0	590	5.0

[1] *Yield is approximately 1 cup prepared.*

Food and Measure	cal.	prot. (gms)	carbo. (gms)	fat (gms)	chol. (mgs)	sod. (mgs)	fiber (gms)
pinto (*Mahatma*) . . .	190	6.0	41.0	1.0	0	810	4.0
pinto, Tex-Mex (*Fantastic Foods* Cup), 2.3 oz.	240	8.0	48.0	2.5	0	590	6.0
red (*Goya*), ¼ cup	160	5.0	35.0	0	0	610	3.0
red (*Mahatma*)	190	7.0	40.0	1.0	0	790	6.0
red (*Rice-A-Roni*), 1 cup*	280	8.0	51.0	7.0	0	1200	5.0
red, Cajun (*Fantastic Foods* Cup), 2.3 oz.	230	10.0	46.0	3.0	0	480	8.0
red, New Orleans (*Fantastic Foods Healthy Complements*), ⅓ cup . . .	130	7.0	28.0	1.5	0	340	6.0
red, pilaf (*Near East*)	220	7.0	41.0	3.5	0	730	4.0
red, spicy (*Good Harvest*), ⅓ cup	160	5.0	32.0	1.0	0	280	3.0
tomato herb, pilaf (*Near East*)	270	7.0	52.0	5.0	0	945	5.0
vegetables, garden, pilaf (*Near East*)	270	7.0	52.0	5.0	0	1120	5.0
beef/beef flavor:							
(*Lipton* Rice & Sauce), 1 cup*	270	6.0	47.0	7.7	0	1010	1.0
(*Rice-A-Roni*), 1 cup*	320	7.0	51.0	9.5	0	1170	2.0
(*Rice-A-Roni* ⅓ Less Salt), 1 cup*	280	7.0	53.0	5.0	0	750	2.0
(*Success*)	190	5.0	43.0	.5	0	920	2.0
and mushroom (*Rice-A-Roni*), 1 cup*	290	7.0	51.0	7.0	0	1210	3.0
pilaf (*Near East*) . . .	220	5.0	42.0	4.5	0	850	1.0
broccoli:							
(*Rice-A-Roni*), 1 cup*	280	5.0	41.0	10.0	5	880	1.0
au gratin (*Rice-A-Roni*), 1 cup* . . .	370	8.0	47.0	17.0	5	890	2.0

Food and Measure	cal.	prot. (gms)	carbo. (gms)	fat (gms)	chol. (mgs)	sod. (mgs)	fiber (gms)
Rice dishes, mix, broccoli *(cont.)*							
au gratin (*Rice-A-Roni* ⅓ Less Salt), 1 cup*	320	8.0	49.0	11.0	5	590	2.0
au gratin (*Savory Classics*), 1 cup*	390	9.0	47.0	5.0	10	840	2.0
cheese (*Mahatma*)	200	5.0	41.0	1.5	5	620	2.0
cheese (*Success*)	210	5.0	40.0	4.5	5	840	1.0
brown:							
(*Arrowhead Mills Quick Original*), ⅓ cup	150	3.0	32.0	1.0	0	0	2.0
(*Arrowhead Mills Quick*), ⅓ cup	150	3.0	32.0	1.0	0	0	2.0
vegetable herb (*Arrowhead Mills Quick*), ¼ pkg.	150	4.0	30.0	1.0	0	160	3.0
brown and wild:							
(*Arrowhead Mills Quick*), ¼ pkg.	140	4.0	28.0	1.0	0	220	3.0
(*Success*)	190	6.0	40.0	1.0	0	830	3.0
Cajun style:							
(*Lipton* Rice & Sauce), 1 cup*	270	7.0	46.0	7.0	0	910	1.0
w/beans (*Lipton* Rice & Sauce), 1 cup*	310	10.0	52.0	7.5	0	530	7.0
cheddar, white, and herbs (*Rice-A-Roni*), 1 cup*	340	7.0	49.0	14.0	5	980	1.0
cheddar broccoli (*Lipton* Rice & Sauce), 1 cup*	280	7.0	46.0	9.0	5	1010	1.0
chicken/chicken flavor:							
(*Lipton* Rice & Sauce), 1 cup*	280	7.0	45.0	8.5	5	960	1.0
(*Mahatma*)	190	5.0	41.0	.5	0	970	1.0
(*Rice-A-Roni*), 1 cup*	310	7.0	52.0	9.0	0	1080	2.0
(*Rice-A-Roni* Low Fat), 1 cup*	210	5.0	41.0	3.0	0	820	1.0

Food and Measure	cal.	prot. (gms)	carbo. (gms)	fat (gms)	chol. (mgs)	sod. (mgs)	fiber (gms)
(*Rice-A-Roni* 1/3 Less Salt), 1 cup*	280	7.0	53.0	5.0	0	690	1.0
(*Savory Classics*), 1 cup*	300	8.0	52.0	8.0	5	1400	2.0
(*Success* Classic)	150	4.0	32.0	1.0	0	720	1.0
creamy (*Lipton* Rice & Sauce), 1 cup*	290	6.0	45.0	11.0	0	830	1.0
pilaf (*Eastern Traditions*)	200	6.0	41.0	1.0	0	690	1.0
pilaf (*Knorr*), 1/3 cup	210	5.0	45.0	1.0	0	1000	1.0
pilaf (*Lundberg* Quick Country)	220	5.0	47.0	3.0	0	370	4.0
pilaf (*Near East*) ...	220	5.0	42.0	4.5	0	940	1.0
pilaf, w/wild rice, Mediterranean (*Near East*)	220	5.0	43.0	4.0	0	910	1.0
roasted (*Lipton* Rice & Sauce), 1 cup*	260	5.0	46.0	7.5	0	880	1.0
Southwestern (*Lipton* Rice & Sauce), 1 cup*	260	5.0	47.0	7.5	0	840	1.0
chicken and broccoli: (*Lipton* Rice & Sauce), 1 cup*	280	7.0	46.0	8.5	0	910	2.0
(*Rice-A-Roni*), 1 cup*	290	7.0	51.0	7.0	0	1410	2.0
chicken and garlic (*Rice-A-Roni*), 1 cup*	260	5.0	42.0	9.0	0	840	1.0
chicken and herbs (*Near East*), 2 1/2 oz.	240	8.0	50.0	2.0	0	765	6.0
chicken and mushroom (*Rice-A-Roni*), 1 cup*	360	8.0	52.0	14.0	0	1480	2.0
chicken and vegetables: (*Rice-A-Roni*), 1 cup*	290	6.0	52.0	7.0	0	1470	2.0
savory (*Rice-A-Roni* Low Fat), 1 cup*	210	6.0	41.0	3.0	0	950	2.0

Food and Measure	cal.	prot. (gms)	carbo. (gms)	fat (gms)	chol. (mgs)	sod. (mgs)	fiber (gms)
Rice dishes, mix *(cont.)*							
chicken and wild rice, almond (*Savory Classics*), 1 cup*	310	7.0	53.0	9.0	0	1320	2.0
chili (*Lundberg One Step*)	180	6.0	42.0	1.0	0	420	5.0
curry:							
(*Lundberg One Step*)	160	5.0	38.0	1.5	0	400	5.0
basmati w/lentils (*Fantastic Foods Healthy Complements*), ¼ cup . . .	140	5.0	30.0	1.0	0	470	4.0
dolmas stuffing (*Casbah*), 1 oz.	130	3.0	24.0	1.0	0	270	2.0
fried:							
(*Chun King*), ½ cup	125	4.0	29.0	0	0	690	1.0
(*Rice-A-Roni*), 1 cup*	320	6.0	51.0	11.0	0	1590	2.0
(*Rice-A-Roni ⅓ Less Salt*), 1 cup*	260	6.0	52.0	3.5	0	930	2.0
garlic, roasted (*Near East*)	190	6.0	40.0	2.0	0	560	5.0
garlic basil (*Lundberg One Step*)	160	6.0	37.0	1.0	0	480	5.0
garlic herb (*Lundberg Quick*)	210	5.0	47.0	2.5	0	510	4.0
gumbo (*Mahatma*) . . .	160	3.0	31.0	2.5	0	720	1.0
herb and butter:							
(*Lipton* Rice & Sauce), 1 cup*	280	6.0	43.0	10.5	10	880	<1.0
(*Rice-A-Roni*), 1 cup*	310	6.0	53.0	9.0	5	1160	1.0
jambalaya (*Mahatma*)	190	4.0	43.0	1.0	0	700	<1.0
long grain and wild:							
(*Lipton* Rice & Sauce Original), 1 cup*	280	7.0	48.0	1.0	0	890	2.0
(*Mahatma*)	190	5.0	41.0	.5	0	710	2.0
(*Minute*), ⅓ box . . .	230	6.0	50.0	.5	0	950	1.0
(*Near East*)	190	5.0	43.0	.5	0	780	2.0

Food and Measure	cal.	prot. (gms)	carbo. (gms)	fat (gms)	chol. (mgs)	sod. (mgs)	fiber (gms)
(*Rice-A-Roni* Original), 1 cup*	240	5.0	43.0	6.0	0	1170	1.0
(*Success*)	190	5.0	42.0	0	0	890	1.0
chicken w/almonds (*Rice-A-Roni*), 1 cup*	290	7.0	51.0	9.0	0	1240	3.0
pilaf (*Rice-A-Roni*), 1 cup*	240	5.0	51.0	6.0	0	920	1.0
medley (*Lipton* Rice & Sauce), 1 cup*	270	7.0	44.0	8.5	5	870	2.0
Mexican:							
(*Goya*), 1/4 cup	160	3.0	37.0	0	0	520	0
(*Savory Classics* Fiesta), 1 cup*	310	8.0	55.0	7.0	0	1640	3.0
w/cheese (*AlpineAire*)	240	8.0	39.0	5.0	10	530	2.0
cheesy (*Old El Paso*), 2.5 oz.	250	4.0	55.0	2.0	<5	780	2.0
mushroom:							
(*Lipton* Rice & Sauce), 1 cup*	270	6.0	45.0	7.5	0	960	1.0
and herb (*Lipton* Rice & Sauce), 1 cup*	290	6.0	49.0	8.0	0	620	1.0
savory, pilaf (*Lundberg* Quick), 1 cup	190	4.0	41.0	2.5	0	590	3.0
Oriental:							
(*Rice-A-Roni*), 1 cup*	290	6.0	54.0	6.0	0	1220	2.0
(*Savory Classics*), 1 cup*	290	5.0	43.0	12.0	0	870	2.0
stir-fry (*Lipton* Rice & Sauce), 1 cup*	270	5.0	47.0	7.5	0	860	1.0
Parmesan, creamy (*Near East*), 2 1/2 oz.	240	8.0	48.0	3.0	10	775	3.0
pecan, roasted, and garlic (*Near East*)	215	6.0	37.0	5.0	0	525	4.0
pilaf (see also specific listings):							
(*Casbah*), 3/4 cup	210	6.0	38.0	.5	0	390	.5
(*Eastern Traditions*)	190	5.0	43.0	0	0	760	0

Food and Measure	cal.	prot. (gms)	carbo. (gms)	fat (gms)	chol. (mgs)	sod. (mgs)	fiber (gms)
Rice dishes, mix, pilaf *(cont.)*							
(*Eastern Traditions* Harvest)	190	6.0	40.0	1.0	0	770	2.0
(*Knorr* Original), ⅓ cup	210	5.0	46.0	.5	0	900	<1.0
(*Lipton* Rice & Sauce), 1 cup*	260	6.0	44.0	7.5	0	930	1.0
(*Mahatma*)	190	5.0	43.0	0	0	810	1.0
(*Rice-A-Roni*), 1 cup*	310	6.0	53.0	9.0	0	1100	1.0
(*Success*)	200	5.0	44.0	0	0	630	2.0
brown rice (*Near East*)	220	6.0	41.0	5.0	0	710	2.0
garden (*Savory Classics*), 1 cup*	240	6.0	41.0	6.0	0	1230	2.0
lemon herb (*Knorr*), ⅓ cup	260	6.0	55.0	2.0	0	790	<1.0
Mediterranean (*Good Harvest*), ⅓ cup	160	4.0	32.0	2.0	0	330	2.0
nutted (*Casbah*), ¾ cup	190	5.0	35.0	2.0	0	500	1.0
primavera (*Goya*), ¼ cup	160	5.0	35.0	0	0	570	1.0
risotto:							
(*Fantastic Foods Healthy Complements* Classico), ¼ cup	140	4.0	31.0	.5	0	410	<1.0
cheese, 3 (*Marrakesh Express*), ¼ cup	200	5.0	44.0	1.5	5	410	0
chicken and Parmesan (*Lipton* Rice & Sauce), 1 cup*	270	6.0	43.0	8.5	0	830	<1.0
garlic primavera (*Lundberg*), ¼ cup	140	4.0	29.0	1.0	0	520	1.0
Italian herb (*Lundberg*), ¼ cup	140	4.0	28.0	1.0	0	530	1.0

Food and Measure	cal.	prot. (gms)	carbo. (gms)	fat (gms)	chol. (mgs)	sod. (mgs)	fiber (gms)
Milanese (*Contadina*), ⅓ pkg.	220	5.0	45.0	3.0	0	700	<1.0
Milanese (*Knorr* Italian), ⅓ cup	260	4.0	59.0	1.0	0	880	1.0
Milanese, w/saffron (*Marrakesh Express*), ¼ cup . . .	210	4.0	48.0	0	0	70	0
mushroom (*Knorr* Italian), ⅓ cup . . .	280	6.0	62.0	1.0	0	1280	<1.0
mushroom, porcini (*Contadina*), ⅓ pkg.	220	5.0	44.0	2.5	0	800	<1.0
mushroom, wild (*Marrakesh Express*), ¼ cup . . .	200	5.0	44.0	.5	0	50	2.0
onion herb (*Knorr* Italian), ⅓ cup . . .	300	6.0	66.0	1.5	0	1390	1.0
Parmesan, creamy (*Lundberg*), ¼ cup	140	5.0	27.0	1.5	0	490	1.0
primavera (*Knorr* Italian), ⅓ cup . . .	280	6.0	61.0	1.0	<5	1250	1.0
primavera (*Marrakesh Express*), ¼ cup	200	5.0	44.0	.5	0	85	1.0
rosemary and potato (*Contadina*), ⅓ pkg.	190	4.0	42.0	1.5	0	490	1.0
tomato basil (*Lundberg*), ¼ cup	140	4.0	30.0	1.0	0	630	1.0
tomato–wild mushroom (*Good Harvest*), ⅓ cup	160	3.0	31.0	.5	0	340	1.0
sun-dried tomatoes and peas (*Marrakesh Express*), ¼ cup	200	5.0	45.0	.5	0	75	1.0
vegetable, garden (*Contadina*), ⅓ pkg.	190	4.0	40.0	2.0	0	800	2.0

Food and Measure	cal.	prot. (gms)	carbo. (gms)	fat (gms)	chol. (mgs)	sod. (mgs)	fiber (gms)
Rice dishes, mix *(cont.)*							
saffroned jasmine							
(*Casbah*), ¾ cup ...	200	6.0	38.0	.5	0	390	.5
salsa style (*Lipton*							
Rice & Sauce),							
1 cup*	220	4.0	37.0	7.0	0	540	2.0
scampi style (*Lipton*							
Rice & Sauce),							
1 cup*	270	6.0	44.0	8.5	5	900	1.0
Spanish:							
(*Fantastic Foods*							
Healthy Comple-							
ments Hacienda),							
⅜ cup	160	4.0	36.0	1.0	0	480	2.0
(*Good Harvest*),							
⅓ cup	160	5.0	32.0	1.0	0	390	4.0
(*Lipton* Rice &							
Sauce), 1 cup*	270	6.0	47.0	7.5	0	900	2.0
(*Mahatma*)	180	4.0	42.0	.5	0	760	2.0
(*Old El Paso*),							
2½ oz.	250	5.0	55.0	1.0	0	830	2.0
(*Rice-A-Roni*),							
1 cup*	270	6.0	46.0	8.0	0	1210	3.0
(*Success*)	190	5.0	43.0	.5	0	780	1.0
pilaf (*Casbah*),							
¾ cup	200	4.0	40.0	.5	0	430	1.0
pilaf (*Knorr*), ⅓ cup	230	5.0	50.0	1.0	0	1120	1.0
pilaf, brown (*Lund-*							
berg Quick Fiesta)	190	5.0	43.0	2.0	0	750	3.0
Stroganoff (*Rice-A-*							
Roni), 1 cup*	360	8.0	50.0	14.0	5	1040	1.0
teriyaki (*Lipton* Rice &							
Sauce), 1 cup*	270	5.0	45.0	8.0	0	910	1.0
wild, and bean (*Good*							
Harvest), ⅓ cup ...	160	5.0	31.0	1.5	0	310	3.0
yellow:							
(*Goya*)	180	4.0	40.0	.5	0	560	n.a.
(*Mahatma*)	190	4.0	43.0	0	0	970	<1.0
(*Vigo*)	190	5.0	43.0	0	0	730	.5
Spanish style							
(*Goya*), ¼ cup ...	170	4.0	37.0	0	0	640	1.0

Food and Measure	cal.	prot. (gms)	carbo. (gms)	fat (gms)	chol. (mgs)	sod. (mgs)	fiber (gms)
Rice entree, dried, 1 serving:							
black beans and (*AlpineAire* Santa Fe)	330	10.0	69.0	1.5	0	720	8.0
mushroom pilaf, w/vegetables (*AlpineAire*)	340	13.0	65.0	2.5	0	670	3.0
wild rice pilaf (*AlpineAire*)	330	11.0	58.0	7.0	0	830	7.0
Rice entree, frozen, see "Rice dishes, frozen"							
Rice flour:							
brown:							
(*Arrowhead Mills*), ¼ cup	120	3.0	27.0	1.0	0	0	2.0
1 cup	574	11.4	120.8	4.4	0	12	7.3
white:							
(*Arrowhead Mills*), ¼ cup	130	2.0	28.0	.5	0	0	1.0
1 cup	578	9.4	126.6	2.2	0	1	3.9
Rice pudding, ready-to-eat, ½ cup:							
(*Comstock/Thank You*)	160	3.0	32.0	3.0	0	280	1.0
(*Kozy Shack*)	130	4.0	23.0	3.0	17	140	1.0
Rice pudding mix:							
(*Jell-O Americana*), ½ cup*	160	5.0	30.0	2.5	10	160	0
(*Watkins*), 2 tbsp. . . .	50	1.0	11.0	0	0	170	0
cinnamon and raisin (*Uncle Ben's*), 1.5 oz.	160	2.0	37.0	1.0	0	180	0
cinnamon raisin (*Lundberg* Elegant), ½ cup	70	0	16.0	0	0	0	1.0
coconut (*Lundberg* Elegant), ½ cup	70	0	13.0	2.0	0	0	1.0
honey almond (*Lundberg* Elegant), ½ cup	70	2.0	15.0	.5	0	0	1.0

Food and Measure	cal.	prot. (gms)	carbo. (gms)	fat (gms)	chol. (mgs)	sod. (mgs)	fiber (gms)
Rice puffs (*Eden Arare*), 1.1 oz.	110	3.0	24.0	0	0	160	2.0
Rice seasoning mix:							
beef w/mushroom (*Knorr Rice Mates*), 1⅓ tbsp.	35	2.0	4.0	1.0	0	720	0
black bean, Santa Fe (*Knorr Rice Mates*), 1½ tbsp.	45	3.0	7.0	.5	0	860	2.0
broccoli au gratin (*Knorr Rice Mates*), 1½ tbsp.	50	2.0	4.0	3.0	5	650	0
chicken w/mushroom (*Knorr Rice Mates*), 1⅓ tbsp.	30	2.0	3.0	1.0	<5	840	0
Mexican (*Lawry's*), 1½ tbsp.	40	<1.0	9.0	0	0	840	0
Spanish (*Knorr Rice Mates*), 1½ tbsp.	35	2.0	6.0	.5	0	510	1.0
Rice syrup, brown (*Lundberg Nu- traFarmed Sweet Dreams*), ¼ cup ...	170	0	42.0	0	0	5	0
Rigatoni dishes, mix, white cheddar and broccoli sauce (*Pasta Roni*), 1 cup*	400	12.0	48.0	19.0	10	1010	3.0
Rigatoni entree, fro- zen, 1 pkg., except as noted:							
in cream sauce w/broccoli, chicken (*The Budget Gour- met Value Classics Low Fat*), 8 oz.	260	10.0	37.0	6.0	20	530	1.0
creamy, w/broccoli, chicken (*Smart Ones*), 9 oz.	240	16.0	39.0	3.5	25	780	4.0
jumbo, w/meatballs (*Lean Cuisine Hearty Portions*), 15⅜ oz.	440	25.0	64.0	9.0	35	820	7.0

Food and Measure	cal.	prot. (gms)	carbo. (gms)	fat (gms)	chol. (mgs)	sod. (mgs)	fiber (gms)
w/meat sauce (*Freezer Queen* Family), 1 cup	250	11.0	38.0	7.0	15	1450	5.0
Risotto, see "Rice dishes, mix"							
Rock candy syrup (*Trader Vic's*), 1 fl. oz.	90	0	23.0	0	0	15	0
Rockfish, meat only:							
raw, 4 oz.	107	21.3	0	1.8	39	68	0
baked, broiled, or microwaved, 4 oz. ...	137	27.3	0	2.3	50	87	0
Roe (see also "Caviar"):							
raw, 1 oz.	40	6.3	.4	1.8	106	n.a.	0
raw, 1 tbsp.	22	3.6	.2	1.0	60	n.a.	0
baked, broiled, or microwaved, 4 oz. ...	231	32.5	2.2	9.3	543	n.a.	0
Roll (see also "Biscuit" and "Bun, sweet"), 1 roll, except as noted:							
brown and serve: (*Pepperidge Farm* Hearth 12), 3 rolls	150	5.0	28.0	2.0	0	300	2.0
(*Roman Meal*), 2 rolls	140	5.0	26.0	2.0	0	290	2.0
(*Wonder*)	80	2.0	13.0	2.0	0	150	0
club (*Pepperidge Farm* 6)	120	5.0	22.0	1.5	0	240	2.0
French (*Pepperidge Farm* 2), ½ roll	180	8.0	34.0	2.0	0	400	2.0
French (*Pepperidge Farm* 3)	240	10.0	45.0	2.5	0	490	3.0
sourdough (*Wonder*)	70	2.0	13.0	1.5	0	130	0
wheat (*Wonder*) ...	80	2.0	13.0	1.5	0	140	0
club, grain (*Hearth Ridge*)	120	4.0	23.0	1.5	0	210	1.0
crescent, butter (*Pepperidge Farm* Heat & Serve)	110	3.0	13.0	5.0	15	160	1.0

Food and Measure	cal.	prot. (gms)	carbo. (gms)	fat (gms)	chol. (mgs)	sod. (mgs)	fiber (gms)
Roll *(cont.)*							
croissant, see "Croissant"							
dill-onion (*Awrey's* Deli Rounds)	150	4.0	30.0	1.5	10	280	2.0
dinner:							
(*Arnold* 12 Pack) . . .	110	4.0	19.0	2.5	0	140	1.0
(*Pepperidge Farm* Country), 3 rolls	150	9.0	22.0	3.0	0	230	1.0
(*Roman Meal*), 2 rolls	150	6.0	27.0	2.5	0	285	2.0
all varieties (*Awrey's*), 2 rolls, 1.6 oz.	110	3.0	19.0	2.0	0	210	<1.0
finger, poppy or sesame (*Pepperidge Farm*), 3 rolls	150	7.0	20.0	4.5	5	230	1.0
honey rich (*Wonder*), 2 rolls	100	3.0	17.0	1.5	0	240	0
parker house (*Pepperidge Farm*), 3 rolls	150	7.0	20.0	4.5	5	230	1.0
potato, hearty (*Pepperidge Farm* Deli Classic)	80	3.0	12.0	2.5	5	110	1.0
wheat (*Wonder*), 2 rolls	140	3.0	24.0	3.0	0	240	1.0
white (*Wonder*), 2 rolls	130	4.0	25.0	2.0	0	210	1.0
egg, twist (*Arnold Levy* Old Country)	170	5.0	30.0	4.0	5	240	1.0
French:							
(*Pepperidge Farm*)	100	4.0	19.0	1.0	0	230	1.0
club (*Hearth Ridge*)	120	4.0	23.0	1.5	0	230	0
7 grain (*Pepperidge Farm* 9)	80	4.0	19.0	2.0	0	270	2.0
sourdough (*Pepperidge Farm*)	100	4.0	18.0	1.0	0	240	1.0
garlic-dill or garlic-pepper (*Awrey's* Deli Rounds)	150	4.0	30.0	1.5	10	310	1.0

Food and Measure	cal.	prot. (gms)	carbo. (gms)	fat (gms)	chol. (mgs)	sod. (mgs)	fiber (gms)
golden twist (*Pepperidge Farm* Heat & Serve)	110	2.0	13.0	4.0	<5	160	1.0
hamburger:							
(*Arnold*)	140	5.0	25.0	2.0	0	280	1.0
(*Pepperidge Farm*)	130	5.0	22.0	2.5	0	230	1.0
(*Roman Meal*)	120	5.0	22.0	2.0	0	230	2.0
hoagie:							
(*Awrey's*)	230	6.0	46.0	1.0	0	470	2.0
(*Pepperidge Farm* Deli Classic)	200	7.0	32.0	4.5	0	340	2.0
French (*Hearth Ridge*)	220	7.0	41.0	2.5	0	410	1.0
grain (*Hearth Ridge*)	220	7.0	41.0	3.0	0	370	2.0
multi-grain (*Pepperidge Farm*)	200	7.0	32.0	4.5	0	340	2.0
sourdough (*Hearth Ridge*)	220	8.0	41.0	2.5	0	410	1.0
hot dog/frankfurter:							
(*Arnold*)	120	4.0	21.0	2.0	0	240	<1.0
(*Pepperidge Farm*)	140	5.0	24.0	2.5	0	270	<1.0
(*Roman Meal*)	110	4.0	20.0	2.0	0	215	2.0
Dijon (*Pepperidge Farm*)	140	6.0	23.0	3.0	0	240	2.0
potato (*Arnold*)	130	5.0	24.0	1.5	0	200	<1.0
Italian (*Bread du Jour*)	90	3.0	16.0	.5	0	190	0
kaiser:							
(*Arnold Levy* Old Country)	170	5.0	34.0	2.0	0	270	1.0
(*Awrey's*)	190	5.0	37.0	2.0	0	340	1.0
(*Hearth Ridge*)	220	7.0	41.0	2.5	0	410	1.0
(*Wonder* Bun)	180	5.0	33.0	3.0	0	270	1.0
multigrain (*Wonder* Bun)	140	4.0	25.0	2.0	0	210	1.0
onion (*Arnold Levy* Old Country)	160	5.0	31.0	3.0	5	210	3.0
party (*Pepperidge Farm* 20), 5 rolls . . .	170	7.0	26.0	4.5	10	240	2.0
potato (*Wonder* Bun)	110	4.0	22.0	1.0	0	220	1.0
sandwich roll/bun:							
(*Pepperidge Farm* Hearty)	230	8.0	39.0	5.0	0	360	2.0

Food and Measure	cal.	prot. (gms)	carbo. (gms)	fat (gms)	chol. (mgs)	sod. (mgs)	fiber (gms)
Roll, sandwich roll/bun *(cont.)*							
(*Roman Meal*)	185	7.0	35.0	3.0	0	390	3.0
multigrain (*Pepperidge Farm*)	150	6.0	24.0	3.0	0	230	3.0
onion (*Pepperidge Farm*)	150	5.0	26.0	3.0	0	270	1.0
potato (*Arnold*)	160	6.0	29.0	2.0	0	250	1.0
potato (*Pepperidge Farm*)	160	4.0	28.0	4.0	0	260	<1.0
potato, sesame (*Arnold*)	170	7.0	29.0	3.0	0	250	1.0
sesame (*Arnold*) ...	140	5.0	23.0	3.0	0	230	1.0
sesame (*Pepperidge Farm*)	140	5.0	23.0	3.0	0	240	1.0
sourdough (*Pepperidge Farm*)	170	6.0	28.0	3.5	0	290	1.0
sourdough:							
(*Bread du Jour*) ...	90	5.0	26.0	1.0	0	310	1.0
club (*Harvest Ridge*)	120	4.0	23.0	1.5	0	230	0
steak (*Wonder* Bun)	190	6.0	36.0	2.5	0	360	1.0
wheat:							
(*Wonder* Bun), 1½ oz.	120	4.0	21.0	2.0	0	210	1.0
(*Wonder* Bun), 1.9 oz.	140	5.0	24.0	2.0	0	280	2.0
(*Wonder* Bun), 2½ oz.	180	7.0	32.0	2.5	0	370	2.0
cracked (*Bread du Jour*)	100	3.0	17.0	1.0	0	290	1.0
white:							
(*Wonder* Bun), 1½ oz.	110	3.0	21.0	1.5	0	220	0
(*Wonder* Bun), 2 oz.	150	4.0	28.0	2.0	0	290	1.0
(*Wonder* Bun), 3 oz.	220	7.0	42.0	3.0	0	430	1.0
yellow (*Wonder*)	160	4.0	29.0	2.5	0	300	0
Roll, frozen or refrigerated, 1 pc.:							
crescent, 1 oz.:							
(*Pillsbury*)	110	2.0	11.0	6.0	0	220	0
(*Pillsbury* Reduced Fat)	100	2.0	12.0	4.5	0	230	0

Food and Measure	cal.	prot. (gms)	carbo. (gms)	fat (gms)	chol. (mgs)	sod. (mgs)	fiber (gms)
dinner, 1.4 oz.:							
wheat (*Pillsbury*)	110	4.0	18.0	2.0	0	270	1.0
white (*Pillsbury*) . . .	110	4.0	18.0	2.0	0	270	<1.0
garlic:							
(*New York*), 2 oz.	200	4.0	27.0	9.0	0	400	1.0
and cheese (*Pepper- idge Farm*),							
1.4 oz.	130	6.0	16.0	5.0	15	280	2.0
Roll, sweet, see "Bun, sweet"							
Roseapple, 1 oz.	7	.2	1.6	.1	0	<1	<1.0
Roselle, 1 oz., ½ cup	14	.3	3.2	.2	0	2	<1.0
Rosemary, dried,							
1 tsp.	4	.1	.8	.2	0	1	.2
Rotini dishes, mix, 1 cup*, except as noted:							
w/cheese, broccoli (*Kraft Velveeta*)	400	18.0	46.0	16.0	45	1240	2.0
mushroom sauce (*Knorr*), ⅔ cup	260	10.0	50.0	1.5	0	710	1.0
primavera (*Lipton Pasta & Sauce*)	320	10.0	45.0	11.5	15	980	2.0
three cheese (*Lipton Pasta & Sauce*)	320	11.0	44.0	12.0	15	970	<1.0
Roughy, orange, meat only:							
raw, 4 oz.	143	16.7	0	8.0	23	72	0
baked, broiled, or mi- crowaved, 4 oz. . . .	101	21.4	0	1.0	29	92	0
Rum runner mixer, frozen* (*Bacardi*),							
8 fl. oz.	140	0	35.0	0	0	10	0
Rutabaga, ½ cup:							
fresh, cubed:							
raw	25	.8	5.7	.1	0	14	1.8
boiled, drained	33	1.1	7.4	.2	0	17	1.5
fresh, boiled, drained, mashed	47	1.6	10.5	.3	0	25	2.2
canned (*Sunshine*) . . .	30	<1.0	7.0	0	0	220	3.0

Food and Measure	cal.	prot. (gms)	carbo. (gms)	fat (gms)	chol. (mgs)	sod. (mgs)	fiber (gms)
Rye, whole-grain:							
(*Arrowhead Mills*),							
¼ cup	160	6.0	34.0	1.0	0	0	6.0
1 cup	567	25.0	117.9	4.2	0	10	24.7
Rye flakes, rolled (*Arrowhead Mills*),							
⅓ cup	110	4.0	24.0	.5	0	0	4.0
Rye flour:							
(*Arrowhead Mills*),							
¼ cup	100	5.0	20.0	1.0	0	0	4.0
dark, 1 cup	415	18.0	88.0	3.4	0	2	n.a.
light, 1 cup	374	8.6	81.8	1.4	0	2	14.9
medium (*Pillsbury*),							
¼ cup	100	3.0	22.0	0	0	0	2.0
medium, 1 cup	361	9.9	79.0	1.8	0	3	14.9
Rye malt syrup (*Eden Organic*), 1 tbsp.	50	1.0	13.0	0	0	30	0
Rye-wheat flour (*Pillsbury's* Bohemian Style), ¼ cup	100	3.0	22.0	0	0	0	2.0

S

Food and Measure	cal.	prot. (gms)	carbo. (gms)	fat (gms)	chol. (mgs)	sod. (mgs)	fiber (gms)
Sablefish, meat only:							
raw, 4 oz.	222	15.2	0	17.4	56	64	0
baked, broiled, or microwaved,							
4 oz.	284	19.5	0	22.2	71	82	0
smoked, 4 oz.	291	20.0	0	22.8	73	836	0
Safflower kernels, dried, 1 oz.	147	4.6	9.7	10.9	0	<1	1.0
Safflower meal, partially defatted, 1 oz.	97	10.1	13.8	.7	0	n.a.	<3.0
Saffron, 1 tsp.	2	.1	.5	<.1	0	1	0
Sage, ground, 1 tsp.	2	.1	.4	.1	0	<1	0
Salad dressing, 2 tbsp.:							
bacon and tomato:							
(*Kraft*)	140	<1.0	2.0	14.0	<5	260	0
(*Kraft Deliciously Right* Lowfat) . . .	60	<1.0	3.0	5.0	<5	300	0
balsamic vinaigrette:							
(*Cardini's*)	150	0	2.0	16.0	0	210	0
(*Marzetti*)	100	0	4.0	9.0	0	330	0
(*Marzetti* Light)	50	0	4.0	4.0	0	340	0
(*Wish-Bone*)	60	0	3.0	5.0	0	280	0
berry vinaigrette (*Knott's Berry Farm*)	40	0	7.0	1.5	0	120	0
blue cheese:							
(*Bernstein's* Dressing/Dip)	180	2.0	0	20.0	10	210	0
(*Bernstein's* Lite)	80	1.0	1.0	8.0	20	220	0
(*Hidden Valley* Free)	20	0	4.0	0	0	270	0
(*Kraft* Free)	50	<1.0	12.0	0	0	340	1.0
(*Kraft Roka*)	90	1.0	5.0	7.0	10	470	0

Food and Measure	cal.	prot. (gms)	carbo. (gms)	fat (gms)	chol. (mgs)	sod. (mgs)	fiber (gms)
Salad dressing, blue cheese *(cont.)*							
(*Marie's*)	180	1.0	3.0	19.0	15	170	1.0
(*Marie's* Free)	30	<1.0	6.0	0	0	250	1.0
(*T. Marzetti's* Dip/ Dressing)	150	1.0	1.0	16.0	20	310	0
chunky (*Marzetti* 15 oz.)	150	1.0	1.0	16.0	20	310	0
chunky (*Marzetti* Light)	90	1.0	5.0	8.0	15	340	1.0
chunky (*Seven Seas*)	90	1.0	5.0	7.0	10	470	0
chunky (*Wish-Bone*)	170	1.0	3.0	17.0	0	290	0
chunky (*Wish-Bone* Free)	35	0	7.0	0	0	290	<1.0
creamy (*Bernstein's*)	110	1.0	2.0	13.0	5	180	0
creamy (*Bernstein's* Restaurant Bleu)	120	1.0	2.0	13.0	5	180	0
honey French (*Marzetti*)	160	1.0	11.0	13.0	0	270	0
sour cream (*T. Marzetti's* Dip/ Dressing)	170	1.0	1.0	18.0	25	190	0
Caesar:							
(*Bernstein's*)	100	1.0	1.0	10.0	15	190	0
(*Bernstein's* Extra Rich)	110	1.0	2.0	11.0	10	340	0
(*Cardini's* Free)	40	0	9.0	0	0	500	0
(*Cardini's* Lowfat)	45	1.0	7.0	1.5	20	250	0
(*Cardini's* "The Orig- inal Caesar Dress- ing")	160	1.0	1.0	17.0	35	240	0
(*Kraft*)	130	<1.0	2.0	13.0	<5	370	0
(*Kraft Deliciously Right* Lowfat) . . .	60	<1.0	2.0	5.0	<5	560	0
(*Marzetti*)	120	1.0	1.0	13.0	0	360	0
(*Marzetti* Free)	40	0	9.0	0	0	500	0
(*Marzetti* House) . . .	150	1.0	1.0	15.0	10	370	0
(*Marzetti* Lite)	70	1.0	2.0	6.0	3	640	0
(*Seven Seas Viva*)	120	<1.0	2.0	12.0	0	500	0
(*Weight Watchers*)	10	0	1.0	0	0	390	0

Food and Measure	cal.	prot. (gms)	carbo. (gms)	fat (gms)	chol. (mgs)	sod. (mgs)	fiber (gms)
(*Wish-Bone*)	110	1.0	2.0	10.0	5	300	0
(*Wish-Bone* Classic)	110	1.0	2.0	10.0	0	390	0
(*Wish-Bone* Free)	25	1.0	5.0	0	0	320	0
creamy (*Marzetti*)	160	1.0	1.0	17.0	35	240	0
creamy (*Seven Seas*)	140	<1.0	1.0	15.0	10	300	0
creamy (*Wish-Bone*)	180	1.0	1.0	18.0	10	290	0
garlic, roasted (*Knott's Berry Farm*)	140	<1.0	2.0	15.0	15	260	0
ranch (*Kraft*)	140	<1.0	1.0	15.0	10	300	0
carrot ginger (*Cary Randall's*)	5	0	1.0	0	0	130	1.0
chicken salad, Oriental (*Knott's Berry Farm*)	130	<1.0	4.0	12.0	0	220	0
citrus vinaigrette (*Knott's Berry Farm*)	40	0	8.0	1.0	0	120	0
coleslaw, see "slaw," below							
Dijon, creamy (*Bernstein's Light Fantastic*)	50	0	9.0	1.0	0	310	0
dill, creamy:							
(*Bernstein's Light Fantastic*)	45	1.0	6.0	2.0	0	320	0
(*Nasoya Vegi-Dressing*)	60	0	3.0	5.0	0	135	0
French:							
(*Hidden Valley Lowfat*)	35	0	7.0	1.0	0	210	0
(*Kraft*)	120	0	4.0	12.0	0	260	0
(*Kraft* Free)	50	0	12.0	0	0	300	<1.0
(*Kraft Catalina*)	140	0	8.0	11.0	0	390	0
(*Kraft Catalina* Free)	45	0	11.0	0	0	360	<1.0
(*Kraft Deliciously Right* Lowfat) . . .	50	0	6.0	3.0	0	260	0
(*Kraft Deliciously Right Catalina* Lowfat)	80	0	9.0	4.0	0	400	0

Food and Measure	cal.	prot. (gms)	carbo. (gms)	fat (gms)	chol. (mgs)	sod. (mgs)	fiber (gms)
Salad dressing, French *(cont.)*							
(*Marzetti* California)	160	0	11.0	12.0	0	250	0
(*Marzetti* Country)	160	0	7.0	15.0	10	180	0
(*Trader Vic's*)	130	0	0	14.0	0	200	0
(*Wish-Bone* Deluxe)	120	0	5.0	11.0	0	170	0
(*Wish-Bone* Lite)	50	0	8.0	2.0	5	240	0
creamy (*Nalley*) ...	110	0	6.0	9.0	0	240	0
herbal, creamy (*Bernstein's*)	130	0	8.0	11.0	0	260	0
honey (*Kraft Catalina*)	140	0	8.0	12.0	0	310	0
honey (*Marzetti* Light)	80	0	11.0	4.0	0	260	0
honey (*T. Marzetti's*)	170	0	10.0	14.0	0	240	0
style (*Marzetti* California Free)	40	0	10.0	0	0	290	0
style (*Weight Watchers*)	40	0	9.0	0	0	200	0
style (*Wish-Bone* Deluxe Free)	30	0	7.0	0	0	230	<1.0
sweet 'n spicy (*Wish-Bone*)	130	0	6.0	12.0	0	330	0
sweet 'n spicy (*Wish-Bone* Free)	30	0	7.0	0	0	220	0
tangy (*Marie's*)	130	0	8.0	11.0	0	260	0
fruit salad (*Knott's Berry Farm*)	70	0	8.0	4.0	0	125	0
fruit vinaigrette (*Knott's Berry Farm*)	45	0	9.0	1.0	0	120	0
garden, zesty (*Kraft Salsa*)	70	0	3.0	6.0	0	280	<1.0
garlic:							
creamy (*Kraft*)	110	0	2.0	11.0	0	350	0
creamy (*Wish-Bone* Free)	40	0	9.0	0	0	280	0
roasted (*Cardini's*)	130	0	1.0	14.0	4	310	0
roasted, creamy (*Wish-Bone*)	110	1.0	3.0	10.0	0	240	0
roasted, vinaigrette (*Cary Randall's*)	5	0	1.0	0	0	55	0

Food and Measure	cal.	prot. (gms)	carbo. (gms)	fat (gms)	chol. (mgs)	sod. (mgs)	fiber (gms)
roasted, vinaigrette							
(*JMarzetti*)	130	0	8.0	10.0	0	340	0
garlic cilantro							
(*Marie's*)	90	1.0	6.0	7.0	10	250	<1.0
green goddess							
(*Seven Seas*)	120	0	1.0	13.0	0	260	0
herb:							
garden (*Nasoya*							
Vegi-Dressing)	60	0	3.0	5.0	0	135	0
poppyseed							
(*Cardini's*)	35	0	7.0	1.0	0	300	0
and spices (*Seven*							
Seas)	120	0	1.0	12.0	0	320	0
honey Dijon:							
(*Hidden Valley* Free)	35	1.0	7.0	0	0	270	0
(*Kraft*) . . . . . , . . .	150	0	4.0	15.0	0	200	0
(*Kraft* Free)	50	<1.0	11.0	0	0	330	1.0
(*Marzetti*)	140	0	6.0	12.0	15	180	0
(*Marzetti* Free)	50	0	12.0	0	0	290	0
(*Weight Watchers*)	45	0	11.0	0	0	150	0
(*Wish-Bone* Free)	45	1.0	10.0	0	0	270	0
honey mustard:							
(*Bernstein's* Dress-							
ing/Dip)	130	0	7.0	12.0	5	100	0
(*Cardini's* Summer)	140	0	5.0	13.0	0	210	1.0
(*Cary Randall's*) . . .	35	1.0	8.0	0	0	95	<1.0
(*Knott's Berry Farm*)	130	0	4.0	13.0	<5	100	0
(*T. Marzetti's* Dip/							
Dressing)	130	0	6.0	12.0	15	170	0
(*Nalley* Restaurant							
Style)	130	0	7.0	12.0	5	100	0
spicy (*Cary Ran-*							
dall's Chile Out)	30	1.0	7.0	0	0	130	0
Italian:							
(*Bernstein's*)	140	0	1.0	16.0	0	230	0
(*Bernstein's* Re-							
duced Cal)	25	0	3.0	1.5	0	310	0
(*Bernstein's* Restau-							
rant Recipe)	80	1.0	12.0	4.0	0	390	0
(*Bernstein's* Wine							
Country)	110	0	2.0	11.0	0	250	0

Food and Measure	cal.	prot. (gms)	carbo. (gms)	fat (gms)	chol. (mgs)	sod. (mgs)	fiber (gms)
Salad dressing, Italian *(cont.)*							
(*Cardini's* Dressing/ Marinade)	120	0	1.0	13.0	0	220	0
(*Kraft* Free)	10	0	2.0	0	0	290	0
(*Kraft* Fat/Oil Free)	5	0	2.0	0	0	450	0
(*Kraft* House)	120	0	3.0	12.0	<5	240	0
(*Kraft* Presto)	140	0	2.0	15.0	0	290	0
(*Kraft* Zesty)	110	0	2.0	11.0	0	530	0
(*Kraft Deliciously Right* Lowfat) . . .	70	0	3.0	7.0	0	240	0
(*Marzetti*)	100	0	3.0	10.0	0	580	0
(*Marzetti* Free)	20	0	4.0	0	0	290	0
(*Marzetti* Zesty) . . .	100	0	3.0	10.0	0	590	0
(*Seven Seas* Free)	10	0	2.0	0	0	480	0
(*Seven Seas* Viva)	110	0	2.0	11.0	0	580	0
(*Seven Seas* Viva Reduced Cal)	45	0	2.0	4.0	0	390	0
(*Trader Vic's*)	80	0	<1.0	9.0	0	490	0
(*Weight Watchers*)	10	0	2.0	0	0	360	0
(*Wish-Bone*)	80	0	3.0	8.0	0	490	0
(*Wish-Bone* Classic House)	140	0	2.0	14.0	5	360	0
(*Wish-Bone* Free)	10	0	2.0	0	0	280	0
(*Wish-Bone* Lite)	15	0	2.0	.5	0	500	0
(*Wish-Bone Rubusto*)	90	0	4.0	8.0	0	550	0
w/blue cheese (*Marzetti*)	100	1.0	3.0	10.0	0	500	0
w/cheese (*Bern-stein's* Reduced Cal)	25	1.0	1.0	2.0	5	540	0
cheese, two (*Seven Seas*)	70	0	3.0	7.0	0	240	0
cheese and garlic (*Bernstein's*)	110	1.0	2.0	11.0	0	340	0
creamy (*Kraft*)	110	0	3.0	11.0	0	230	0
creamy (*Kraft Deliciously Right* Lowfat)	50	0	3.0	5.0	0	250	0
creamy (*Marzetti*)	160	0	1.0	17.0	15	240	0

Food and Measure	cal.	prot. (gms)	carbo. (gms)	fat (gms)	chol. (mgs)	sod. (mgs)	fiber (gms)
creamy (*Nasoya Vegi-Dressing*)	60	0	3.0	5.0	0	170	0
creamy (*Seven Seas*)	110	0	2.0	12.0	0	510	0
creamy (*Seven Seas Lowfat*)	60	0	2.0	5.0	0	490	0
creamy (*Weight Watchers*)	30	0	7.0	0	0	360	0
creamy (*Wish-Bone*)	110	1.0	4.0	10.0	0	240	0
creamy (*Wish-Bone Free*)	35	0	9.0	0	0	250	0
garlic (*Marie's*)	180	0	3.0	19.0	15	220	0
w/garlic, onion, and peppers (*Bernstein's* Classico)	40	0	6.0	1.5	0	300	0
herb garlic, creamy (*Bernstein's*)	130	1.0	3.0	13.0	5	280	0
olive oil (*Wish-Bone* Classic)	60	0	4.0	5.0	0	350	0
olive oil/oil blend (*Seven Seas* Lowfat)	50	0	2.0	5.0	0	450	0
Parmesan (*Hidden Valley* Free)	20	0	4.0	0	0	240	0
Romano (*Marzetti*)	150	0	1.0	16.0	0	420	0
sweet (*Marzetti*) . . .	150	0	7.0	14.0	0	250	0
Italian vinaigrette: garlic, roasted (*Marzetti* House)	120	0	2.0	13.0	0	520	0
garlic, roasted (*Marzetti* 16 oz.)	130	0	8.0	10.0	0	340	0
Javanese (*Trader Vic's*)	150	1.0	1.0	16.0	1	390	0
lemon herb (*Cardini's* Dressing/Marinade)	130	0	1.0	13.0	0	220	0
lemon vinaigrette (*Marzetti* Free)	35	0	9.0	0	0	270	0
lime dill (*Cardini's* Dressing/Marinade)	130	0	1.0	14.0	0	220	0
mayonnaise type, see "Mayonnaise"							

Food and Measure	cal.	prot. (gms)	carbo. (gms)	fat (gms)	chol. (mgs)	sod. (mgs)	fiber (gms)
Salad dressing *(cont.)*							
olive oil vinaigrette (*Wish-Bone*)	60	0	4.0	5.0	0	250	0
Oriental:							
(*Bernstein's Light Fantastic*)	60	0	11.0	1.0	0	310	0
(*Wish-Bone*)	70	0	5.0	5.0	0	440	0
Parmesan:							
creamy (*Hidden Valley* Free)	30	1.0	5.0	0	0	250	0
and onion (*Wish-Bone*)	110	1.0	5.0	10.0	5	260	0
and onion (*Wish-Bone* Free)	45	1.0	9.0	0	0	320	<1.0
pepper (*Marzetti* 15 oz.)	160	1.0	1.0	16.0	10	230	0
peppercorn (*Marzetti*)	160	0	1.0	17.0	10	260	0
Romano and provolone (*Bernstein's* Cheese Fantastico!)	110	1.0	2.0	11.0	5	410	0
Romano and provolone (*Bernstein's Light Fantastic* Cheese Fantastico!)	30	1.0	5.0	1.0	n.a.	360	0
pepper, roasted, vinaigrette (*Cary Randall's*)	10	0	2.0	0	0	60	0
peppercorn:							
cracked (*Marzetti*)	150	1.0	1.0	16.0	25	290	0
ground (*Knott's Berry Farm*)	160	<1.0	1.0	17.0	0	210	0
pesto:							
(*Cardini's* Pasta Dressing/Marinade)	140	0	1.0	14.0	0	250	0
hemp, vinaigrette (*Cary Randall's*)	130	0	1.0	14.0	0	35	0
poppyseed:							
(*Knott's Berry Farm*)	120	0	10.0	9.0	0	190	0

Food and Measure	cal.	prot. (gms)	carbo. (gms)	fat (gms)	chol. (mgs)	sod. (mgs)	fiber (gms)
(*Marzetti*)	160	0	11.0	13.0	15	310	0
(*Marzetti* 15 oz.) ...	140	0	10.0	11.0	10	230	0
(*Marzetti* Free)	60	0	14.0	0	0	190	0
ranch:							
(*Bernstein's* Dressing/Dip)	110	0	1.0	12.0	10	200	0
(*Bernstein's* Dressing/Dip Lite)	70	0	2.0	6.0	10	210	0
(*Bernstein's* Light Fantastic)	35	1.0	7.0	.5	5	240	0
(*Hidden Valley* Original Lowfat)	40	0	5.0	3.0	0	270	0
(*Hidden Valley* Original Reduced Cal)	80	0	2.0	7.0	0	270	0
(*Kraft*)	170	0	2.0	18.0	5	270	0
(*Kraft* Free)	50	<1.0	11.0	0	0	310	<1.0
(*Kraft Deliciously Right* Lowfat) ...	110	0	2.0	11.0	10	310	0
(*Kraft Salsa*)	130	0	1.0	13.0	10	320	0
(*Marzetti*)	150	1.0	1.0	16.0	10	210	0
(*Marzetti* Free)	25	0	7.0	0°	0	380	1.0
(*Nalley* Free)	40	1.0	8.0	0	0	470	0
(*Nalley* Homestyle)	100	0	6.0	8.0	10	250	0
(*Ott's* Buttermilk)	140	0	1.0	15.0	0	120	0
(*Seven Seas*)	150	0	2.0	16.0	5	250	0
(*Seven Seas* Free)	50	<1.0	12.0	0	0	330	1.0
(*Seven Seas* Lowfat)	100	0	5.0	9.0	0	320	0
(*Wish-Bone*)	160	0	1.0	17.0	10	200	0
(*Wish-Bone* Free)	40	0	9.0	0	0	280	<1.0
(*Wish-Bone* Lite)	100	0	5.0	8.0	5	300	0
and bacon (*Marzetti*)	160	1.0	1.0	17.0	10	250	0
buttermilk (*Kraft*)	150	0	2.0	16.0	<5	230	0
buttermilk (*Marzetti*)	160	0	1.0	17.0	10	240	0
Caesar (*Marzetti*)	180	1.0	2.0	19.0	5	300	0
creamy (*Marie's*)	190	<1.0	3.0	20.0	15	170	0
cucumber (*Kraft*)	150	0	2.0	15.0	0	220	0
cucumber (*Kraft Deliciously Right* Lowfat)	60	0	2.0	5.0	0	450	0
Dijon (*Grey Poupon* Reduced Fat/Cal)	50	1.0	4.0	3.5	<5	135	0

Food and Measure	cal.	prot. (gms)	carbo. (gms)	fat (gms)	chol. (mgs)	sod. (mgs)	fiber (gms)
Salad dressing, ranch *(cont.)*							
garden (*Marzetti*)	160	0	1.0	17.0	10	210	0
Italian (*Bernstein's*)	150	0	3.0	15.0	n.a.	25	0
Italian (*Hidden Valley* Reduced Cal)	50	0	2.0	5.0	0	240	0
Parmesan (*Cardini's*)	130	1.0	1.0	14.0	20	250	0
Parmesan (*Cardini's* Lowfat)	45	1.0	7.0	2.0	0	350	0
Parmesan (*Marie's*)	180	1.0	2.0	14.0	10	140	<1.0
Parmesan garlic (*Bernstein's*)	110	1.0	3.0	11.0	5	330	0
Parmesan garlic (*Bernstein's Light Fantastic*)	45	2.0	7.0	1.0	5	280	0
peppercorn (*Kraft*)	170	<1.0	1.0	18.0	10	340	0
peppercorn (*Kraft* Free)	50	<1.0	11.0	0	0	360	1.0
peppercorn (*Marzetti*)	180	1.0	2.0	19.0	10	230	0
peppercorn (*Marzetti* Free) . . .	35	0	8.0	0	0	380	1.0
sour cream and onion (*Kraft*)	170	0	1.0	18.0	10	240	0
zesty (*Marie's* Low Fat)	30	0	7.0	<1.0	0	310	0
raspberry vinaigrette:							
(*Knott's Berry Farm* Low Fat)	50	0	8.0	2.0	0	110	0
(*Marzetti*)	110	0	4.0	11.0	0	65	0
(*Marzetti* Free)	20	0	5.0	0	0	590	0
(*Marzetti* House) . . .	110	0	3.0	11.0	0	90	0
zesty (*Marie's* Free)	35	0	8.0	0	0	35	0
red wine vinaigrette:							
(*Marzetti* Light)	30	0	3.0	1.5	0	460	0
(*Wish-Bone*)	80	0	9.0	5.0	0	230	0
(*Wish-Bone* Free)	35	0	7.0	0	0	230	0
zesty (*Marie's* Free)	40	0	10.0	0	0	300	0
red wine vinegar:							
(*Kraft/Seven Seas* Free)	15	0	3.0	0	0	400	0

Food and Measure	cal.	prot. (gms)	carbo. (gms)	fat (gms)	chol. (mgs)	sod. (mgs)	fiber (gms)
(*Seven Seas* Lowfat)	60	0	2.0	5.0	0	310	0
and oil (*Cardini's*)	90	0	3.0	8.0	0	440	0
and oil (*Marzetti*)	90	0	3.0	8.0	0	440	0
and oil (*Seven Seas*)	110	0	2.0	11.0	0	510	0
Romano, see "Parmesan," above							
Roquefort (*Bernstein's Dressing/Dip*)	140	1.0	1.0	15.0	20	210	0
Russian:							
(*Kraft*)	130	0	10.0	10.0	0	280	0
(*Seven Seas Viva*)	150	0	3.0	16.0	0	230	0
(*Wish-Bone*)	110	0	15.0	6.0	0	350	0
salsa and sour cream (*Bernstein's* Dressing/Dip)	90	0	2.0	9.0	15	160	0
sesame w/soy (*Trader Vic's* South Pacific)	110	<1.0	3.0	11.0	0	200	0
sesame garlic (*Nasoya Vegi-Dressing*)	60	0	3.0	5.0	0	125	0
slaw:							
(*Hidden Valley* Free)	35	0	9.0	0	0	200	0
(*Kraft*)	150	0	8.0	12.0	25	420	0
(*Marzetti* 15 oz.) . . .	170	0	6.0	16.0	25	370	0
(*Marzetti* Free)	45	0	11.0	0	0	400	0
(*Marzetti* Light)	100	0	10.0	7.0	25	380	0
(*Marzetti* Light 15 oz.)	100	0	10.0	7.0	30	380	0
(*Marzetti* Low Fat)	60	0	11.0	1.5	20	370	0
(*Marzetti* Original)	170	0	6.0	16.0	25	390	0
spinach salad (*Marzetti*)	80	0	14.0	2.0	0	250	0
sweet and saucy (*Marzetti*)	140	0	9.0	12.0	0	300	0
sweet and sour:							
(*Marzetti*)	160	0	10.0	13.0	0	220	0
(*Marzetti* Free)	50	0	13.0	0	0	300	0
(*Old Dutch*)	50	0	13.0	0	0	480	0
Thousand Island: (*Bernstein's* Dressing/Dip)	120	0	4.0	11.0	15	180	0

Food and Measure	cal.	prot. (gms)	carbo. (gms)	fat (gms)	chol. (mgs)	sod. (mgs)	fiber (gms)
Salad dressing, Thousand Island *(cont.)*							
(*Hidden Valley* Lowfat)	35	0	6.0	1.0	0	240	0
(*Kraft*)	110	0	5.0	10.0	10	310	0
(*Kraft* Free)	45	0	11.0	0	0	300	1.0
(*Kraft Deliciously Right* Lowfat) . . .	70	0	8.0	4.0	5	320	0
(*Marzetti*)	140	0	4.0	14.0	15	240	0
(*Marzetti* 15 oz.)	150	0	5.0	15.0	25	230	0
(*Marzetti* Free)	45	0	11.0	0	0	370	0
(*Nalley*)	120	0	4.0	11.0	15	180	0
(*Nalley* Free)	30	0	8.0	0	0	210	0
(*Nasoya Vegi-Dressing*)	60	0	6.0	4.0	0	140	0
(*Wish-Bone*)	140	0	7.0	12.0	10	340	0
(*Wish-Bone* Free)	35	0	9.0	0	0	290	<1.0
w/bacon (*Kraft*) . . .	120	0	5.0	12.0	0	190	0
tomato, sun-dried:							
basil (*Cary Randall's*)	10	0	2.0	0	0	70	0
vinaigrette (*Knott's Berry Farm*)	100	<1.0	3.0	9.0	0	230	0
vinaigrette (*Marzetti*)	130	0	6.0	11.0	0	330	0
white wine vinaigrette:							
(*Wish-Bone*)	60	0	4.0	4.5	0	260	0
zesty (*Marie's* Free)	40	0	10.0	0	0	310	0
Salad dressing mix*, 2 tbsp.:							
bacon (*Hidden Valley*)	120	1.0	2.0	12.0	10	220	0
blue cheese (*Hidden Valley*)	120	<1.0	2.0	12.0	10	200	0
buttermilk:							
(*Good Seasons Farm*)	120	1.0	2.0	12.0	10	260	0
(*Hidden Valley* Original)	110	<1.0	1.0	11.0	10	240	0
Caesar, gourmet (*Good Seasons*) . . .	150	0	3.0	16.0	0	300	0
cheese garlic (*Good Seasons*)	140	0	1.0	16.0	0	330	0

Food and Measure	cal.	prot. (gms)	carbo. (gms)	fat (gms)	chol. (mgs)	sod. (mgs)	fiber (gms)
garlic and herbs (*Good Seasons*)	140	0	1.0	15.0	0	340	0
herb, zesty (*Good Seasons* Free)	10	0	2.0	0	0	260	0
honey mustard:							
(*Good Seasons*) . . .	150	0	3.0	15.0	0	240	0
(*Good Seasons* Free)	20	0	5.0	0	0	280	0
Dijon (*Hidden Valley*)	120	<1.0	4.0	12.0	10	210	0
Italian:							
(*Good Seasons*) . . .	140	0	1.0	15.0	0	320	0
(*Good Seasons* Free)	10	0	3.0	0	0	290	0
(*Good Seasons* Reduced Cal)	50	0	2.0	5.0	0	280	0
creamy (*Good Seasons* Free)	20	<1.0	3.0	0	0	280	0
mild (*Good Seasons*)	150	0	2.0	15.0	0	370	0
zesty (*Good Seasons*)	140	0	1.0	15.0	0	220	0
zesty (*Good Seasons* Reduced Cal)	50	0	2.0	5.0	0	260	0
Mexican spice (*Good Seasons*)	140	0	2.0	15.0	0	310	0
Oriental sesame (*Good Seasons*)	150	0	3.0	16.0	0	360	0
ranch:							
(*Good Seasons*) . . .	120	1.0	2.0	12.0	10	220	0
(*Good Seasons* Reduced Cal)	60	1.0	3.0	4.5	5	240	0
(*Hidden Valley* Original Lowfat)	30	1.0	4.0	1.0	0	240	0
(*Hidden Valley* Original Milk)	120	<1.0	2.0	12.0	10	210	0
(*Hidden Valley* Original Reduced Cal)	70	1.0	2.0	6.0	5	240	0
Italian (*Hidden Valley*)	140	<1.0	3.0	14.0	0	250	0

Food and Measure	cal.	prot. (gms)	carbo. (gms)	fat (gms)	chol. (mgs)	sod. (mgs)	fiber (gms)
Salad toppers (see also "Croutons"), 1 tbsp.:							
bacon cheddar or Caesar (*Pepperidge Farm*)	35	1.0	4.0	2.0	0	85	0
cinnamon raisin (*Pepperidge Farm*)	35	1.0	4.0	2.0	0	15	0
garlic Italian (*Pepperidge Farm*)	35	1.0	4.0	1.5	0	70	0
Salami, 2 oz., except as noted:							
beef:							
(*Boar's Head*)	120	10.0	0	9.0	25	470	0
(*Hansel 'n Gretel*)	170	7.0	4.0	14.0	35	660	0
(*Hebrew National*), 3 slices, 2 oz. . . .	150	8.0	0	13.0	35	420	0
(*Hebrew National* Chub)	170	8.0	0	14.0	40	420	0
(*Hebrew National* Reduced Fat)	110	8.0	0	8.0	30	380	0
(*Oscar Mayer* Machiach), 2 slices, 1.6 oz.	120	6.0	1.0	10.0	30	510	0
beer (*Oscar Mayer*), 2 slices, 1.6 oz. . . .	110	6.0	1.0	9.0	30	580	0
cooked:							
(*Boar's Head*)	130	8.0	0	11.0	40	550	0
(*Hansel 'n Gretel*)	160	7.0	4.0	12.0	40	770	0
(*Russer Light*)	90	8.0	4.0	5.0	40	400	0
cotto:							
(*Oscar Mayer*), 2 slices, 1.6 oz.	110	6.0	0	9.0	35	500	0
beef (*Oscar Mayer*), 1-oz. slice	60	4.0	1.0	4.5	20	360	0
dry or hard, 1 oz.:							
(*Boar's Head*)	110	6.0	<1.0	9.0	25	490	0
(*Hansel 'n Gretel*)	230	12.0	2.0	20.0	50	920	0
(*Homeland*)	110	5.0	0	10.0	35	450	0
(*Oscar Mayer* Hard), 3 slices, 1 oz. . . .	100	7.0	1.0	8.0	25	510	0

Food and Measure	cal.	prot. (gms)	carbo. (gms)	fat (gms)	chol. (mgs)	sod. (mgs)	fiber (gms)
Genoa:							
(*Boar's Head*)	180	12.0	1.0	14.0	55	970	0
(*Di Lusso*)	210	12.0	0	18.0	50	940	0
(*Hansel 'n Gretel*)	220	11.0	3.0	18.0	50	980	0
(*Hormel Pillow Pack*)	210	12.0	0	18.0	50	940	0
(*Oscar Mayer*), 3 slices, 1 oz.	100	5.0	0	9.0	25	490	0
(*San Remo Brand*), 1 oz.	120	6.0	0	9.0	30	470	0
"Salami," vegetarian, frozen (*Worthington*), 3 slices	130	12.0	2.0	8.0	0	800	2.0
Salisbury steak, see "Beef dinner" and "Beef entree"							
Salmon, fresh, meat only, 4 oz.:							
Atlantic, farmed:							
raw	207	22.6	0	12.3	67	66	0
baked, broiled, or microwaved	234	25.0	0	14.0	71	69	0
Atlantic, wild:							
raw	161	22.5	0	7.2	62	50	0
baked, broiled, or microwaved	206	28.8	0	9.2	81	64	0
Chinook:							
raw	204	22.8	0	11.9	75	53	0
baked, broiled, or microwaved	262	29.2	0	15.2	96	68	0
chum:							
raw	136	22.8	0	4.3	84	112	0
baked, broiled, or microwaved	175	29.3	0	5.5	108	73	0
coho, farmed:							
raw	182	24.1	0	8.7	58	53	0
baked, broiled, or microwaved	202	27.6	0	9.3	71	59	0
coho, wild:							
raw	165	25.0	0	6.7	51	53	0

Food and Measure	cal.	prot. (gms)	carbo. (gms)	fat (gms)	chol. (mgs)	sod. (mgs)	fiber (gms)
Salmon, , coho, wild *(cont.)*							
baked, broiled, or microwaved	158	26.6	0	4.9	62	66	0
boiled, poached, or steamed	209	31.0	0	8.5	65	60	0
pink:							
raw	132	22.6	0	3.9	59	76	0
baked, broiled, or microwaved	169	29.0	0	5.0	76	98	0
sockeye:							
raw	191	24.2	0	9.7	70	53	0
baked, broiled, or microwaved	245	31.0	0	12.4	99	75	0
Salmon, canned,							
¼ cup, except as noted:							
chum:							
(*Peter Pan*)	90	13.0	0	4.0	40	270	0
drained, 4 oz.	160	24.3	0	6.2	44	552	0
coho (*Peter Pan*)	90	12.0	0	5.0	40	270	0
king (*Peter Pan*)	140	12.0	0	10.0	40	270	0
Norwegian fillet (*Abelvaer*), 3 oz.	170	16.0	0	12.0	42	460	0
pink, skinless fillet:							
(*Bumble Bee*)	70	14.0	0	2.0	40	220	0
(*Chicken of the Sea*), 2 oz.	60	10.0	0	2.0	20	280	0
(*Peter Pan*)	90	12.0	0	5.0	40	270	0
red:							
(*Peter Pan*)	110	13.0	0	7.0	40	270	0
blueback (*Rubinstein's*)	110	13.0	0	7.0	40	270	0
sockeye (*Icy Point*)	110	13.0	0	7.0	40	270	0
Salmon, smoked:							
Atlantic, imported (*Nova*), 2 oz.	50	11.0	<1.0	1.0	20	650	0
Chinook:							
4 oz.	133	20.7	0	4.9	26	889	0
lox, 4 oz.	133	20.7	0	4.9	26	2268	0
lox:							
(*Vita*), 2 oz.	50	11.0	<1.0	1.0	20	800	0
(*Vita*), 3-oz. pkg.	80	16.0	1.0	1.5	35	1200	0

Food and Measure	cal.	prot. (gms)	carbo. (gms)	fat (gms)	chol. (mgs)	sod. (mgs)	fiber (gms)
Norwegian (*Frionor*), 2 oz.	93	12.0	0	5.0	39	484	0
Nova:							
(*Vita*), 2 oz.	50	11.0	<1.0	1.0	20	580	0
(*Vita*), 3-oz. pkg.	80	16.0	1.0	1.5	35	960	0
(*Vita* Premium), 2 oz.	50	11.0	<1.0	1.0	20	650	0
bits (*Vita*), 2 oz.	50	11.0	<1.0	1.0	20	650	0
w/color (*Vita*), 3-oz. pkg.	80	16.0	1.0	1.5	35	870	0
pastrami style (*Ducktrap River* Spruce Point), 2 oz.	130	11.0	0	9.0	10	690	0
roasted (*Ducktrap River*), 2 oz.	100	13.0	0	6.0	10	430	0
sockeye (*Lascco* Copper River), 2 oz.	70	15.0	0	1.0	30	400	0
Salmon, smoked, spread:							
(*Vita*), 1/4 cup	180	5.0	29.0	5.0	35	440	0
cream cheese (*Vita*), 2 tbsp.	100	2.0	1.0	9.0	25	80	0
Salmon burger, frozen, 1 pc.:							
(*Ocean Beauty*)	80	18.0	1.0	.5	35	380	1.0
(*Vita*)	90	14.0	5.0	2.0	30	290	<1.0
Salmon entree, frozen:							
cake, stuffed (*Five Star*), 1 pc.	190	9.0	17.0	10.0	75	420	<1.0
grilled, fillet, 1 pc.:							
creamy dill (*Mrs. Paul's/Van de Kamp's*)	90	16.0	1.0	2.5	30	200	0
honey mustard (*Mrs. Paul's/Van de Kamp's*)	90	16.0	3.0	2.0	30	380	0
nuggets (*Vita* Alaskan), 6 pcs., 4 1/4 oz.	240	16.0	24.0	9.0	40	430	0
Salmon oil, see "Oil"							
Salmon roll, see "Fish roll"							

Food and Measure	cal.	prot. (gms)	carbo. (gms)	fat (gms)	chol. (mgs)	sod. (mgs)	fiber (gms)
Salsa, 2 tbsp., except as noted:							
(*Christopher Ranch*)	15	0	2.0	1.0	0	120	0
(*Gracias* Chunky Original)	15	1.0	2.0	0	0	125	0
(*La Victoria* Brava), 1 tbsp.	0	0	0	0	0	35	0
(*La Victoria* Ranchera)	10	0	2.0	0	0	170	0
(*La Victoria* Victoria)	5	0	1.0	0	0	160	0
(*Old El Paso* Verde)	10	0	2.0	0	0	95	0
(*Watkins JR's* Thick & Chunky)	10	0	2.0	0	0	218	0
all styles:							
(*Chi-Chi's*)	10	0	2.0	0	0	150	0
(*Chi-Chi's* Verde)	15	0	3.0	0	0	180	0
(*Del Monte* Traditional/Thick & Chunky/Fire Roasted)	10	0	2.0	0	0	210	0
(*Heluva* Good/ *Heluva* Good Thick & Chunky)	10	0	2.0	0	0	180	0
(*Muir Glen* Fat Free)	10	<1.0	2.0	0	0	160	0
(*Old El Paso* Homestyle)	10	0	2.0	0	0	220	0
(*Old El Paso* Thick 'n Chunky)	10	0	2.0	0	0	230	0
(*Pace* Thick & Chunky)	10	0	3.0	0	0	220	0
(*Rosarita*)	10	0	2.0	0	0	210	0
(*Tostitos*), 4 tbsp.	30	2.0	6.0	0	0	520	2.0
(*Valley of Mexico* Fire Roasted)	10	0	2.0	0	0	125	0
(*Valley of Mexico* Fire Roasted Salsa Verde)	10	0	2.0	0	0	100	0
black bean and corn (*Muir Glen*)	10	<1.0	3.0	0	0	125	0
cheese, see "Cheese dip"							

Food and Measure	cal.	prot. (gms)	carbo. (gms)	fat (gms)	chol. (mgs)	sod. (mgs)	fiber (gms)
fajita:							
(*Gracias* Superba)	10	0	2.0	0	0	160	0
(*Nalley Superba*) . . .	10	0	2.0	0	0	160	0
fruit, tropical (*Watkins*)	60	0	13.0	0	0	430	0
garden (*Tostitos* Ultimate), 4 tbsp.	30	2.0	6.0	0	0	460	2.0
garden pepper medley (*Muir Glen*)	10	0	2.0	0	0	140	0
garlic:							
(*Del Monte*)	10	0	2.0	0	0	210	0
cilantro (*Muir Glen*)	10	0	2.0	0	0	165	<1.0
roasted (*Newman's Own*)	10	1.0	2.0	0	0	150	1.0
roasted, hot (*Muir Glen*)	10	0	3.0	0	0	140	<1.0
roasted, medium or mild (*Muir Glen*)	10	<1.0	3.0	0	0	165	<1.0
green chili:							
(*La Victoria*)	10	0	1.0	0	0	170	0
(*Old El Paso*)	10	0	2.0	0	0	110	<1.0
hot:							
(*Gold's* Extra Chunky), 1 tbsp.	5	0	1.0	0	0	90	0
(*Gracias*)	15	0	2.0	0	0	135	0
(*La Victoria* Thick N Chunky)	10	0	1.0	0	0	135	0
jalapeño:							
green (*La Victoria* Jalapena)	10	0	1.0	0	0	180	0
red (*La Victoria* Jalapena)	10	0	2.0	0	0	150	0
medium:							
(*Gracias* Superba)	10	0	2.0	0	0	140	0
(*Muir Glen* 11 oz.)	10	0	2.0	0	0	180	0
(*Muir Glen* 16 oz.)	10	0	2.0	0	0	220	<1.0
(*Nalley Salsa Superba*)	10	0	2.0	0	0	140	0
mild:							
(*Gracias* Superba)	10	0	2.0	0	0	150	0
(*Muir Glen*)	10	0	2.0	0	0	220	<1.0

Food and Measure	cal.	prot. (gms)	carbo. (gms)	fat (gms)	chol. (mgs)	sod. (mgs)	fiber (gms)
Salsa, mild *(cont.)*							
(*Nalley Salsa Suberba*)	10	0	2.0	0	0	150	0
mild or medium:							
(*La Victoria Suprema*)	10	0	2.0	0	0	180	0
(*La Victoria* Thick N Chunky)	10	0	1.0	0	0	160	0
(*Newman's Own*)	10	0	2.0	0	0	105	0
onion, roasted, and pepper (*Muir Glen*)	10	0	2.0	0	0	140	0
peach (*Newman's Own*)	25	0	6.0	0	0	90	1.0
picante (see also "Picante sauce"):							
(*La Victoria* Medium)	10	0	1.0	0	0	150	0
(*La Victoria* Mild)	10	0	1.0	0	0	180	0
pico de gallo (*Chi-Chi's*)	10	0	2.0	0	0	170	0
pineapple (*Newman's Own*)	15	0	3.0	0	0	90	1.0
sweet and zesty (*Tostitos*), 4 tbsp.	40	<2.0	6.0	0	0	460	2.0
taco, see "Taco sauce"							
Salsa seasoning (*Lawry's*), ½ tsp.	5	0	1.0	0	0	90	0
Salsa–sour cream dip mix, dry (*Watkins*), 1 tsp.	10	0	3.0	0	0	210	0
Salsify:							
raw:							
(*Frieda's*), ¾ cup, 3 oz.	70	3.0	16.0	0	0	15	3.0
untrimmed, 1 lb.	325	13.0	73.4	.8	0	79	13.0
sliced, ½ cup	55	2.2	12.5	.1	0	13	2.2
boiled, drained, sliced, ½ cup	46	1.9	10.5	.1	0	11	2.1
Salt (see also specific listings), ¼ tsp.:							
(*Morton Lite*)	0	0	0	0	0	290	0

Food and Measure	cal.	prot. (gms)	carbo. (gms)	fat (gms)	chol. (mgs)	sod. (mgs)	fiber (gms)
iodized/non-iodized							
(*Morton*)	0	0	0	0	0	590	0
kosher (*Morton*)	0	0	0	0	0	450	0
seasoned:							
(*House of Tsang*							
Hong King)	0	0	0	0	0	170	0
(*Lawry's*)	0	0	0	0	0	380	0
(*Morton*)	0	0	0	0	0	325	0
red pepper							
(*Lawry's*)	0	0	0	0	0	330	0
Salt, substitute:							
(*Morton*), 1/4 tsp.	0	0	0	0	0	610	0
seasoned:							
(*Lawry's* Salt Free),							
1/4 tsp.	0	0	0	0	0	0	0
(*Morton*), 1 tsp. . . .	2	0	.5	0	0	<1	0
Salt pork, raw, 1 oz.	212	1.4	0	22.8	25	404	0
Sandwich, see specific listings							
Sandwich sauce, 1/4 cup, except as noted:							
(*Durkee Famous*), 1 tbsp.	60	.5	2.0	6.0	15	330	0
(*Frank's RedHot* Buffalo), 1 tbsp.	5	0	1.0	0	0	470	0
(*Kraft*), 1 tbsp.	50	0	3.0	5.0	<5	100	0
Sloppy Joe:							
(*Del Monte* Original)	70	1.0	16.0	0	0	680	0
(*Green Giant*)	50	2.0	11.0	0	0	420	2.0
(*Green Giant* w/Meat)	200	14.0	11.0	11.0	45	470	2.0
(*Heinz*), 1/2 cup	70	3.0	14.0	.5	0	770	2.0
(*Hormel Not-So-Sloppy Joe* Sauce)	60	1.0	13.0	0	0	640	1.0
(*Libby's*), 1/3 cup . . .	45	1.0	10.0	0	0	430	1.0
(*Manwich* Bold) . . .	60	.5	13.0	1.0	0	800	1.0
(*Manwich* Original)	30	<1.0	7.0	0	0	335	1.0
(*Manwich* Thick & Chunky)	45	1.5	9.0	.5	0	735	1.0

Food and Measure	cal.	prot. (gms)	carbo. (gms)	fat (gms)	chol. (mgs)	sod. (mgs)	fiber (gms)
Sandwich sauce, Sloppy Joe *(cont.)*							
barbecue (*Manwich*)	60	1.0	14.0	0	0	890	1.0
hickory flavor (*Del Monte*)	70	1.0	18.0	0	0	700	0
Sandwich sauce mix							
(*Manwich*), ¼ oz.	20	0	5.0	0	0	355	0
Sandwich spread (see also "Meat spread," "Sandwich sauce," and specific listings):							
(*Hellmann's*), 1 tbsp.	50	0	3.0	5.0	<5	170	0
(*Kraft* Spread & Burger Sauce), 1 tbsp. . . .	50	0	3.0	5.0	<5	100	0
(*Loma Linda*), ¼ cup	80	4.0	7.0	4.5	0	260	3.0
Sapodilla:							
1 medium, 3″ x 2½″	140	.7	33.9	1.9	0	20	9.0
½ cup	100	.5	24.1	1.3	0	15	6.4
Sapote:							
(*Frieda's*), 5 oz.	190	3.0	47.0	1.0	0	15	4.0
1 medium, 11.2 oz.	301	4.8	76.0	1.4	0	21	5.9
trimmed, 1 oz.	38	.6	9.6	.2	0	3	.7
Sardine, fresh, see "Herring"							
Sardine, canned:							
Atlantic, in oil:							
drained, 2 oz.	118	14.8	0	6.5	81	286	0
2 medium, 3″ long	50	5.9	0	2.8	34	121	0
in hot sauce (*Chicken of the Sea*), 3¾-oz. can	220	16.0	2.0	16.0	145	560	1.0
lemon (*Goya*), ¼ cup	120	10.0	0	9.0	20	300	0
in mustard sauce (*Underwood*), 3¾-oz. can	180	17.0	2.0	12.0	105	820	1.0
in olive oil, drained:							
(*Goya*), ¼ cup	130	13.0	0	9.0	20	20	0
skinless, boneless (*Granadaisa*), ¼ cup	120	13.0	0	7.0	24	280	0

Food and Measure	cal.	prot. (gms)	carbo. (gms)	fat (gms)	chol. (mgs)	sod. (mgs)	fiber (gms)
in soy oil, drained:							
(*Underwood*), 3 oz.	220	18.0	1.0	16.0	100	310	0
skinless, boneless (*King Oscar*),							
3 pcs.	120	13.0	0	7.0	20.0	350	0
spiced (*Goya*), ¼ cup	120	12.0	0	9.0	20	280	0
in tomato sauce:							
(*Del Monte*), 2 oz., ½ fish, w/sauce	80	10.0	1.0	4.0	35	170	<1.0
(*Goya*), ¼ cup	130	12.0	1.0	9.0	20	300	0
(*Underwood*),							
3¾-oz. can	180	16.0	4.0	11.0	115	960	1.0
Pacific, 2 oz.	101	9.3	n.a.	6.8	35	235	<1.0
Sardine oil, see "Oil"							
Sauce, see specific listings							
Sauerbraten seasoning mix (*Knorr*),							
1 tbsp.	35	<1.0	6.0	1.0	0	440	0
Sauerkraut, 2 tbsp., except as noted:							
(*Boar's Head*)	5	0	1.0	0	0	180	<1.0
(*Claussen*), ¼ cup . . .	5	0	1.0	0	0	210	1.0
(*Comstock*)	10	0	2.0	0	0	130	0
(*Del Monte*)	0	0	<1.0	0	0	180	<1.0
(*Eden* Organic), ½ cup	25	2.0	4.0	0	0	580	3.0
(*Frank's/Snowfloss*)	5	<1.0	1.0	0	0	180	<1.0
(*Hebrew National*) . . .	5	0	1.0	0	0	180	1.0
(*Hebrew National*), ½ cup	25	0	4.0	0	0	800	0
(*Hebrew National/ Shorr's* New), ½ cup	50	1.0	11.0	1.0	0	550	0
(*Pickle Eater's* Kozmic Kraut)	0	0	1.0	0	0	180	0
(*Pickle Eater's* Reduced Sodium)	0	0	.6	0	0	134	0
(*Seneca*)	5	0	1.0	0	0	200	<1.0
(*Silver Floss*)	5	0	1.0	0	0	180	1.0
(*Silver Floss*), ½ cup	25	1.0	4.0	0	0	700	0
Bavarian style:							
(*Bush's Best*)	15	0	3.0	0	0	105	1.0

Food and Measure	cal.	prot. (gms)	carbo. (gms)	fat (gms)	chol. (mgs)	sod. (mgs)	fiber (gms)
Sauerkraut, Bavarian style *(cont.)*							
(*Del Monte*)	15	0	4.0	0	0	180	0
(*Frank's/Snowfloss*)	15	<1.0	3.0	0	0	170	<1.0
(*Seneca*)	10	0	3.0	0	0	190	<1.0
chopped or shredded							
(*Bush's Best*)	5	0	1.0	0	0	180	1.0
sweet and sour							
(*Stokely*)	20	0	5.0	0	0	210	1.0
Sauerkraut juice:							
(*Bush's Best*), 8 fl. oz.	15	2.0	1.0	0	0	1670	0
(*Stokely*), 8 fl. oz. . . .	20	1.0	4.0	0	0	1720	0
Sausage (see also specific listings), cooked, 2 links, except as noted:							
andouille (*Aidell's* Cajun Brand), 3½-oz. link	220	16.0	1.0	17.0	55	770	<1.0
beef:							
(*Jones Dairy Farm* Golden Brown)	170	7.0	1.0	15.0	40	410	0
hot, jalapeño (*Hebrew National*), 3-oz. link	260	10.0	1.0	24.0	55	670	0
smoked (*Healthy Choice*), 2 oz. . . .	70	8.0	6.0	1.5	20	480	0
smoked (*Oscar Mayer* Smokies), 1 link	120	5.0	1.0	5.0	30	420	0
brown and serve:							
(*Jones Golden Brown*), 1 patty	150	5.0	1.0	14.0	30	240	0
(*Little Sizzlers*), 3 links	230	8.0	1.0	22.0	45	670	0
(*Little Sizzlers*), 2 patties	190	7.0	1.0	18.0	40	560	0
beef, smoked (*Jones Dairy Farm*)	180	6.0	1.0	17.0	35	360	0
light (*Jones Dairy Farm*)	100	7.0	1.0	8.0	25	280	0

Food and Measure	cal.	prot. (gms)	carbo. (gms)	fat (gms)	chol. (mgs)	sod. (mgs)	fiber (gms)
pork (*Jones Dairy Farm*)	190	5.0	1.0	18.0	35	280	0
pork and bacon (*Jones Dairy Farm*)	180	6.0	1.0	17.0	35	420	0
cheese, smoked: (*Oscar Mayer* Little Smokies), 6 links	180	7.0	1.0	16.0	40	590	0
(*Oscar Mayer* Smokies), 1 link	130	6.0	1.0	12.0	30	450	0
chicken, 3½-oz. link, except as noted: and apple: fresh, raw (*Aidell's*), 2 oz.	100	8.0	1.0	7.0	40	300	<1.0
smoked (*Aidell's*)	210	16.0	1.0	16.0	90	730	<1.0
apricot w/rosemary (*Bilinski's*)	120	15.0	8.0	3.0	60	650	1.0
broccoli w/cheese (*Bilinski's*)	110	15.0	1.0	3.5	65	710	0
jalapeño (*Bilinski's*)	130	21.0	1.0	4.0	85	870	0
lemon, smoked (*Aidell's*)	210	15.0	1.0	16.0	90	700	<1.0
pesto (*Bilinski's*) ...	110	17.0	0	4.5	70	740	0
spinach w/garlic, fennel (*Bilinski's*)	100	15.0	2.0	3.0	60	640	1.0
sun-dried tomato w/basil (*Bilinski's*)	120	17.0	5.0	3.5	55	770	0
teriyaki, fresh, raw (*Aidell's*)	210	15.0	6.0	15.0	85	590	<1.0
chicken and turkey (see also "turkey and chicken," below), 3½-oz. link: curry, smoked (*Aidell's* Burmese)	220	18.0	3.0	15.0	95	730	<1.0
smoked (*Aidell's* New Mexico Brand)	210	15.0	2.0	16.0	80	600	<1.0
Thai, fresh, raw (*Aidell's*)	200	15.0	1.0	16.0	75	600	<1.0

Food and Measure	cal.	prot. (gms)	carbo. (gms)	fat (gms)	chol. (mgs)	sod. (mgs)	fiber (gms)
Sausage, chicken and turkey *(cont.)*							
Thai, smoked (*Aidell's*)	220	18.0	0	16.0	80	770	<1.0
chorizo:							
beef, raw (*Aidell's*), 3½-oz. link	400	13.0	3.0	37.0	70	550	<1.0
pork, spicy (*Battistoni*), 1 oz.	80	4.0	0	7.0	20	180	0
dinner, (*Jones Dairy Farm* All Natural), 1.4-oz. link	150	6.0	1.0	14.0	35	310	0
duck and turkey, smoked (*Aidell's*), 3½-oz. link	220	17.0	1.0	16.0	60	700	<1.0
Italian, 2-oz. link, mild or hot, except as noted:							
chicken, w/peppers, onions (*Bilinski's*), 3½-oz. link	120	19.0	1.0	4.0	80	800	0
pork, raw (*Aidell's*), 3½-oz. link	230	16.0	0	18.0	40	550	0
pork, raw (*Paisano*)	140	9.0	0	11.0	30	390	0
pork, w/peppers and onions (*Garden State*), 2½-oz. link	180	13.0	2.0	13.0	55	360	0
turkey (*Perdue*)	80	10.0	0	4.0	45	320	0
turkey, raw (*Aidell's*), 3½-oz. link	190	19.0	1.0	12.0	65	500	<1.0
turkey, raw (*Perdue*)	80	10.0	0	4.0	45	340	0
turkey, hot, raw (*Shady Brook Farms*)	100	12.0	0	5.0	40	460	0
turkey, sweet, raw (*Shady Brook Farms*)	100	12.0	1.0	5.0	40	420	0
lamb and beef, w/rosemary, fresh, raw (*Aidell's*), 3½-oz. link	220	16.0	2.0	16.0	65	600	<1.0

Food and Measure	cal.	prot. (gms)	carbo. (gms)	fat (gms)	chol. (mgs)	sod. (mgs)	fiber (gms)
pickled, smoked or hot (*Hormel*), 6 links . . .	140	8.0	1.0	11.0	40	380	0
pork:							
(*Johnsonville* Original Breakfast), 3 links	190	10.0	1.0	16.0	40	610	0
(*Jones Dairy Farm* All Natural Light)	130	8.0	1.0	11.0	20	420	0
(*Jones Dairy Farm* All Natural Little Links), 3 links . . .	190	8.0	1.0	17.0	45	420	0
(*Little Sizzlers*), 3 links or 2 patties	230	8.0	0	22.0	45	610	0
(*Oscar Mayer*)	180	9.0	1.0	16.0	45	450	0
(*Tobin's First Prize* Little Links)	190	8.0	1.0	18.0	40	340	0
(*Tobin's First Prize* Patties), 1 patty	170	6.0	0	16.0	30	310	1.0
fresh, ½ oz. (1 oz. raw link)	48	2.6	.1	4.1	11	168	0
light (*Jones Dairy Farm* Golden Brown)	100	7.0	1.0	8.0	30	230	0
maple (*Jones Dairy Farm* Golden Brown)	190	5.0	1.0	18.0	35	260	0
mild (*Jones Dairy Farm* Golden Brown)	190	6.0	1.0	18.0	35	300	0
spicy (*Jones Dairy Farm* Golden Brown)	190	6.0	1.0	18.0	35	300	0
pork, patty:							
(*Jones Dairy Farm* All Natural), 1 pc.	130	5.0	0	12.0	30	250	0
(*Jones Dairy Farm* Golden Brown), 1 pc.	150	5.0	1.0	14.0	30	240	0
(*Little Sizzlers*), 2 pcs.	210	10.0	0	23.0	50	680	0

Food and Measure	cal.	prot. (gms)	carbo. (gms)	fat (gms)	chol. (mgs)	sod. (mgs)	fiber (gms)
Sausage *(cont.)*							
pork, smoked:							
(*Ball Park*), 4-oz. link	240	11.0	3.0	20.0	60	970	0
(*Boar's Head*), 4½ oz.	400	17.0	2.0	36.0	75	1050	0
(*Light & Lean 97* Dinner), 1 link . . .	60	8.0	2.0	2.0	20	640	0
(*Oscar Mayer* Little Smokies), 6 links	170	7.0	1.0	16.0	40	580	0
(*Oscar Mayer* Smokie Links), 1 link	130	5.0	1.0	12.0	25	430	0
w/barbecue sauce (*Lloyd's* Little Smokies), 6 links w/sauce, 3 oz.	280	9.0	26.0	13.0	30	620	0
hot (*Boar's Head*), 3.2 oz.	280	12.0	1.0	25.0	55	740	0
hot or regular (*Hill-shire Farm*), 1 link	250	10.0	3.0	23.0	35	620	0
whiskey fennel (*Aidell's*), 3½-oz. link	200	7.0	1.0	17.0	60	520	<1.0
pork roll, original or hot (*Jones Dairy Farm* All Natural), 2 oz.	230	9.0	1.0	21.0	50	430	0
pork and turkey, breakfast (*Healthy Choice*), 2 links or patties	50	7.0	1.0	2.0	15	300	0
pork and veal, smoked, 3½-oz. link:							
bier (*Aidell's*)	240	17.0	0	19.0	35	720	0
hunter (*Aidell's*) . . .	240	17.0	0	19.0	35	720	0
smoked (*Healthy Choice*), 2 oz.	70	7.0	2.0	1.5	20	480	0
tomato-basil (*Healthy Choice*), 2 oz.	70	8.0	2.0	1.5	15	480	0

Food and Measure	cal.	prot. (gms)	carbo. (gms)	fat (gms)	chol. (mgs)	sod. (mgs)	fiber (gms)
turkey, raw, except as noted:							
(*Shady Brook Farms* Old World), 4 oz.	190	20.0	3.0	11.0	65	850	0
breakfast, (*Perdue*)	100	9.0	0	7.0	40	330	0
breakfast (*Shady Brook Farms*), 2 oz.	80	10.0	.5	4.0	35	480	0
breakfast (*Wampler*), 4 oz.	230	17.0	1.0	17.0	100	880	0
breakfast, cooked (*Perdue*)	100	9.0	0	7.0	45	350	0
cranberry, smoked (*Aidell's*), 3½-oz. link	210	16.0	1.0	16.0	85	730	<1.0
Italian, see "Italian," above							
w/scallions and herbs, fresh (*Aidell's*), 3½-oz. link	200	15.0	1.0	12.0	70	700	<1.0
turkey and chicken, 3½-oz. link:							
artichoke, smoked (*Aidell's*)	180	14.0	2.0	14.0	75	610	<1.0
pesto, smoked (*Aidell's*)	220	18.0	1.0	16.0	75	780	<1.0
w/sun-dried tomatoes and basil (*Aidell's*)	200	19.0	0	14.0	80	730	<1.0
w/sun-dried tomatoes and basil, fresh, raw (*Aidell's*)	200	15.0	1.0	15.0	85	550	<1.0
Sausage, canned:							
pickled, regular or hot (*Hormel*), 6 links, 2 oz.	140	8.0	1.0	11.0	40	380	0
Vienna:							
(*Goya*), 3 links	130	5.0	1.0	12.0	50	320	0
(*Hormel*), 2 oz. . . .	150	5.0	0	14.0	45	420	0

Food and Measure	cal.	prot. (gms)	carbo. (gms)	fat (gms)	chol. (mgs)	sod. (mgs)	fiber (gms)
Sausage, canned, Vienna *(cont.)*							
(*Libby's*), 3 links . . .	150	6.0	<1.0	14.0	45	460	0
chicken (*Hormel*), 2 oz.	110	6.0	1.0	9.0	55	400	0
chicken (*Libby's*), 3 links	100	6.0	0	8.0	50	450	0
"Sausage," vegetarian:							
.9-oz. link	64	4.6	2.5	4.5	0	222	.7
1.3-oz. patty	97	7.0	3.7	6.9	0	337	1.1
canned:							
(*Loma Linda* Linketts), 2 links	70	7.0	1.0	4.5	0	160	1.0
(*Loma Linda* Little Links), 2 links . . .	90	8.0	2.0	6.0	0	230	2.0
(*Worthington* Saucettes), 1 link	90	6.0	1.0	6.0	0	200	1.0
frozen:							
(*Green Giant* Breakfast), 3 links	110	12.0	5.0	5.0	0	340	4.0
(*Green Giant* Breakfast), 2 patties . . .	100	10.0	5.0	4.0	0	280	3.0
(*Morningstar Farms* Breakfast), 2 links	60	8.0	2.0	2.5	0	340	2.0
(*Morningstar Farms* Breakfast), 1 patty	70	8.0	2.0	3.0	0	270	2.0
(*Worthington* Prosage Links), 2 links	60	8.0	2.0	2.5	0	340	2.0
(*Worthington* Prosage Patties), 1 patty	80	9.0	3.0	3.0	0	300	2.0
bits (*Morningstar Farms* Sausage Style Crumbles), ²/₃ cup	90	11.0	5.0	3.0	0	370	3.0
roll (*Worthington* Prosage), ⁵/₈" slice	140	10.0	2.0	10.0	0	390	2.0
mix* (*Fantastic Nature's Sausage*), 2 links or 1 patty . . .	65	6.0	7.0	1.5	0	240	2.0

Food and Measure	cal.	prot. (gms)	carbo. (gms)	fat (gms)	chol. (mgs)	sod. (mgs)	fiber (gms)
refrigerated:							
(*Morningstar Farms* Breakfast), 2 patties	120	15.0	5.0	5.0	0	380	3.0
Sausage biscuit, see "Breakfast sandwich"							
Sausage hash, canned (*Mary Kitchen*), 1 cup	410	20.0	23.0	27.0	85	1020	2.0
Sausage seasoning, pork (*Tone's*), 1 tsp.	12	.4	2.7	.3	0	1	.7
Sausage stick, 1 pc., except as noted:							
(*Slim Jim Big Slim*)	70	1.0	1.0	6.0	10	190	0
beef/beef jerky:							
(*Boar's Head*), .6 oz.	100	3.0	2.0	9.0	20	240	0
(*Rustlers Roundup* Jerky), .22 oz.	30	2.0	1.0	2.0	10	140	<1.0
(*Slim Jim Big Jerk*)	25	2.0	1.0	1.5	<5	135	0
(*Slim Jim Super Jerk*)	35	3.0	1.0	2.0	<5	200	0
chopped (*Slim Jim Cannister*), 7 pcs.	130	11.0	1.0	8.0	10	710	1.0
chopped (*Slim Jim Giant*)	70	5.0	2.0	4.0	10	360	0
chopped (*Slim Jim Handipak*), 1 box	70	6.0	2.0	5.0	10	400	0
hot:							
(*Rustlers Roundup* Flamin' Hot), .3 oz.	40	2.0	1.0	3.0	10	140	<1.0
red pepper (*Pemmican Tender Jerky*), 1-oz. bag	80	11.0	6.0	2.0	35	470	1.0
mild or spicy:							
(*Slim Jim* Cannister), 3 pcs. . . .	150	6.0	2.0	14.0	15	410	1.0

Food and Measure	cal.	prot. (gms)	carbo. (gms)	fat (gms)	chol. (mgs)	sod. (mgs)	fiber (gms)
Sausage stick, mild or spicy *(cont.)*							
(*Slim Jim* Handipak), 1 box, 5 pcs.	210	9.0	2.0	19.0	25	570	1.0
smoked:							
(*Rustlers Roundup* Steak Strip), .8 oz.	60	8.0	1.0	2.0	20	580	0
hickory, and peppered (*Pemmican Tender Jerky*), 2-oz. bag	160	24.0	7.0	4.0	70	1450	1.0
hickory, and peppered (*Pemmican Tender Jerky*), 1-oz. bag	80	12.0	3.0	2.0	35	720	1.0
mild or spicy (*Slim Jim*), 1.4-oz. box	210	9.0	2.0	19.0	25	570	1.0
spicy:							
(*Rustlers Roundup*), .3 oz.	50	2.0	<1.0	4.0	10	140	<1.0
(*Rustlers Roundup*), ½ oz.	70	3.0	1.0	6.0	20	250	<1.0
(*Slim Jim* Caddy)	50	2.0	0	4.5	5	125	0
(*Slim Jim* Giant), 1-oz. pc.	150	6.0	2.0	14.0	15	410	1.0
(*Slim Jim* Super Slim)	100	4.0	1.0	9.0	10	260	0
(*Slim Jim* Super Slim Twin Pack), 1 pkg.	190	8.0	2.0	17.0	20	510	1.0
(*Slim Jim Tabasco* Super Slim)	100	3.0	2.0	8.0	5	290	0
teriyaki:							
(*Pemmican Tender Jerky*), 2-oz. bag	190	26.0	5.0	7.0	70	1470	1.0
(*Pemmican Tender Jerky*), 1-oz. bag	90	13.0	3.0	3.0	35	730	1.0
turkey, peppered (*Pemmican Snacks*), 1 oz.	60	10.0	4.0	.5	20	670	0

Food and Measure	cal.	prot. (gms)	carbo. (gms)	fat (gms)	chol. (mgs)	sod. (mgs)	fiber (gms)
Savory, ground:							
1 tsp.	4	.1	1.0	.1	0	<1	<1.0
summer (*Tone's*), 1 tsp.	4	.1	1.0	.1	0	1	<1.0
Scallion, see "Onion, green"							
Scallop, meat only:							
raw, 4 oz.	100	19.0	2.7	.9	38	183	0
raw, 2 large or 5 small, 1.1 oz.	26	5.0	.7	.2	10	48	0
"Scallop," imitation:							
from surimi, 4 oz. . . .	112	14.5	12.1	.5	25	902	0
frozen, bay style (*Louis Kemp Scallop Delights*), ½ cup . . .	80	9.0	12.0	0	10	550	0
"Scallop," vegetarian, canned:							
(*Loma Linda Tender Bits*), 6 pcs.	110	11.0	7.0	4.5	0	440	3.0
(*Worthington Vegetable Skallops*), ½ cup	90	15	3.0	1.5	0	410	3.0
Scallop entree, frozen:							
fried (*Mrs. Paul's*), 5½-oz. pkg.	330	18.0	39.0	11.0	35	660	2.0
w/linguine (*Contessa Entrees for 2*), 2 cups	310	18.0	53.0	3.0	35	450	4.0
Scallop squash, ½ cup:							
raw, sliced	12	.8	2.5	.1	0	1	1.2
boiled, drained, sliced	14	.9	3.0	.2	0	1	1.1
boiled, drained, mashed.	19	1.2	4.0	.2	0	1	1.4
Scone, all fruit varieties (*Health Valley*), 1 pc.	180	4.0	43.0	0	0	190	5.0
Scorpion drink mixer (*Trader Vic's*), 4 oz.	80	0	21.0	0	0	20	0
Scrapple (*Jones Dairy Farm*), 2 oz.	120	5.0	7.0	8.0	30	280	0

Food and Measure	cal.	prot. (gms)	carbo. (gms)	fat (gms)	chol. (mgs)	sod. (mgs)	fiber (gms)
Scrod, fresh, see "Cod, Atlantic"							
Scup, meat only:							
raw, 4 oz.	119	21.4	0	3.1	n.a.	48	0
baked, broiled, or microwaved, 4 oz. . . .	153	27.5	0	4.0	n.a.	61	0
Sea bass, meat only:							
raw, 4 oz.	110	20.9	0	2.3	47	77	0
baked, broiled, or microwaved, 4 oz. . . .	141	26.8	0	2.9	60	99	0
Sea trout, meat only:							
raw, 4 oz.	118	19.0	0	4.1	94	66	0
baked, broiled, or microwaved, 4 oz. . . .	151	24.3	0	5.3	120	84	0
Seabreeze drink mixer (*Mr & Mrs T*), 4 fl. oz.	90	0	21.0	0	0	40	0
Seafood, see specific listings							
Seafood bites, frozen (*Matlaw's*), 2 pcs.	60	2.0	8.0	1.5	5	60	0
Seafood dip (see also specific listings), (*Heluva* Good), 2 tbsp.	60	1.0	3.0	4.5	20	250	0
Seafood sauce (see also specific listings), cocktail, ¼ cup:							
(*Crosse & Blackwell*)	100	1.0	23.0	0	0	710	0
(*Del Monte*)	100	1.0	24.0	0	0	910	0
(*Heinz*)	60	1.0	15.0	0	0	690	1.0
(*Heluva* Good)	40	0	10.0	0	0	410	0
(*Nalley*)	65	1.0	15.0	0	0	470	0
(*Sauceworks*)	60	1.0	13.0	.5	0	800	<1.0
hot and spicy (*Bookbinder's*)	70	1.0	15.0	1.5	0	1040	1.0

Food and Measure	cal.	prot. (gms)	carbo. (gms)	fat (gms)	chol. (mgs)	sod. (mgs)	fiber (gms)
Seafood seasoning (see also "Fish seasoning and coating mix"):							
(*Chef Paul Prudhomme's Magic Seasoning Blends*), ¼ tsp. . . .	0	0	0	0	0	115	0
(*Old Bay*), ½ tsp.	0	0	0	0	0	330	0
Seafood stuffing, frozen (*Massachusetts Bay Clam Co.*), 1 oz.	80	2.0	7.0	5.0	2	230	.5
Seasoning (see also specific listings):							
(*Ac'cent*), ⅛ tsp.	0	0	0	0	0	160	0
(*Maggi*), 1 tsp.	0 .	<1.0	0	0	0	410	0
(*Sa-son* con Culantro), ¼ tsp.	0	0	0	0	0	170	0
(*Sa-son Ac'cent*), ¼ tsp.	0	0	0	0	0	150	0
(*Sazon Goya* con Achiote), ¼ tsp.	0	0	0	0	0	160	0
(*Sazon Goya* con Azafran), ¼ tsp. . . .	0	0	0	0	0	150	0
Seasoning blend (*Watkins* All Purpose), ¼ tsp.	0	0	0	0	0	0	0
Seasoning and coating mix (see also specific listings), ⅛ pkt.:							
country (*Shake 'n Bake*)	35	0	5.0	2.0	0	240	0
glaze, honey mustard (*Shake 'n Bake*)	45	0	9.0	1.0	0	290	0
glaze, tangy honey (*Shake 'n Bake*)	45	0	10.0	1.0	0	280	0
Italian herb (*Shaken 'n Bake*)	40	1.0	7.0	.5	0	300	0

Food and Measure	cal.	prot. (gms)	carbo. (gms)	fat (gms)	chol. (mgs)	sod. (mgs)	fiber (gms)
Seaweed:							
agar:							
raw, 1 oz.	7	.2	1.9	tr.	0	3	.1
dried, 1 oz.	87	1.8	22.9	.1	0	29	2.2
flakes or bar (*Eden*),							
1 tbsp.	10	0	2.0	0	0	10	2.0
arame (*Eden*), ½ cup	30	1.0	7.0	0	0	120	7.0
hiziki (*Eden*), ½ cup	30	0	6.0	0	0	160	6.0
Irish moss, raw, 1 oz.	14	.4	3.5	<.1	0	19	.4
kelp, raw, 1 oz.	12	.5	2.7	.2	0	66	.4
kombu (*Eden*), ½ of							
7″ pc.	10	0	2.0	0	0	90	1.0
laver, raw, 1 oz.	10	1.6	1.4	.1	0	1	4.1
nori (*Eden*), 1 sheet	10	1.0	1.0	0	0	5	1.0
spirulina, 1 oz.:							
raw	8	1.7	.7	.1	0	28	n.a.
dried	82	16.3	6.8	2.2	0	297	1.0
wakame:							
(*Eden*), ½ cup	25	2.0	4.0	0	0	660	4.0
raw, 1 oz.	13	.9	2.6	.2	0	247	.1
flakes (*Eden*), 1 tsp.	3	0	0	0	0	72	2.0
Semolina,							
wholegrain, 1 cup	602	21.2	121.6	1.8	0	2	6.5
Semolina flour, mix							
(*Arrowhead Mills*),							
½ cup	240	9.0	50.0	1.0	0	0	4.0
Sesame flour, 1 oz.:							
high fat	149	8.7	7.6	10.5	0	12	1.8
partially defatted	109	11.5	10.0	3.4	0	12	1.7
low fat	95	14.2	10.1	.5	0	11	1.4
Sesame meal, par-							
tially defatted, 1 oz.	161	4.8	7.4	13.6	0	11	1.1
Sesame oil, see "Oil"							
Sesame paste (see							
also "Tahini"), from							
whole seeds,							
1 tbsp.	95	2.9	4.1	8.1	0	2	.9
Sesame seasoning,							
½ tsp.:							
(*Eden* Shake)	10	0	0	.5	0	40	<1.0

Food and Measure	cal.	prot. (gms)	carbo. (gms)	fat (gms)	chol. (mgs)	sod. (mgs)	fiber (gms)
garlic or seaweed (*Eden* Shake)	10	0	0	.5	0	35	<1.0
Sesame seeds:							
whole:							
brown (*Arrowhead Mills*), ¼ cup	200	7.0	8.0	20.0	0	20	5.0
roasted, toasted, 1 oz.	161	4.8	7.3	13.6	0	3	4.0
kernels, decorticated:							
(*Arrowhead Mills*), ¼ cup	210	7.0	5.0	20.0	0	0	5.0
dried, 1 tsp.	16	.7	.3	1.5	0	1	<1.0
toasted, 1 oz.	161	4.8	7.4	13.6	0	11	4.8
Sesbania flower:							
raw, 1 cup	5	.3	1.4	<.1	0	3	n.a.
steamed, ½ cup	11	.6	2.7	<.1	0	6	n.a.
Shad, meat only:							
raw, 4 oz.	223	19.2	0	15.6	n.a.	58	0
baked, broiled, or microwaved, 4 oz. ...	286	24.6	0	20.0	n.a.	74	0
Shallot:							
fresh or stored:							
(*Frieda's*), 1 tbsp., 1 oz.	20	1.0	5.0	0	0	0	0
peeled, 1 oz.	20	.7	4.8	<.1	0	3	<1.0
chopped, 1 tbsp. ...	7	.3	1.7	<.1	0	1	<1.0
freeze-dried, 1 tbsp.	3	.1	.7	tr.	0	1	<1.0
Shark, meat only, raw, 4 oz.	148	23.8	0	5.1	58	90	0
Sheepshead, meat only:							
raw, 4 oz.	123	22.9	0	2.7	n.a.	81	0
baked, broiled, or microwaved, 4 oz. ...	143	29.5	0	1.8	n.a.	83	0
Shellie beans, canned w/liquid, ½ cup	37	2.1	7.6	.2	0	408	4.1
Shells, pasta, entree, frozen:							
and American cheese (*Stouffer's*), ½ of 12-oz. pkg.	260	11.0	31.0	10.0	20	1190	2.0

Food and Measure	cal.	prot. (gms)	carbo. (gms)	fat (gms)	chol. (mgs)	sod. (mgs)	fiber (gms)
Shells, pasta, entree *(cont.)*							
marinara (*Healthy Choice*), 12 oz. pkg.	390	25.0	55.0	8.0	40	390	5.0
Shells, pasta, mix:							
Alfredo, garlic (*Fantastic Foods Healthy Complements*), ⅔ cup	210	10.0	38.0	3.0	5	460	2.0
and cheddar, white (*Pasta Roni*), 1 cup*	390	12.0	48.0	17.0	10	1030	2.0
cheddar sauce, white (*DeBoles*), 2.7 oz.	260	11.0	50.0	4.0	10	750	3.0
w/cheese:							
(*Kraft Velveeta*), 1 cup*	360	16.0	44.0	13.0	40	1030	1.0
bacon (*Kraft Velveeta*), 1 cup*	360	17.0	43.0	14.0	40	1140	1.0
salsa (*Kraft Velveeta*), 1 cup*	380	17.0	47.0	14.0	40	1180	2.0
Sherbet (see also "Ice" and "Sorbet"), ½ cup:							
berry rainbow (*Edy's/ Dreyer's*)	130	1.0	29.0	1.0	5	35	0
orange:							
(*Breyers*)	120	n.a.	26.0	1.0	5	25	0
(*Breyers* Fat Free)	110	n.a.	27.0	0	0	25	0
Swiss (*Edy's/ Dreyer's*)	160	1.0	31.0	3.0	5	40	0
vanilla swirl (*Edy's/ Dreyer's*)	120	2.0	23.0	2.0	10	40	0
rainbow:							
(*Breyers*)	120	n.a.	27.0	1.5	5	15	0
(*Breyers* Fat Free)	110	n.a.	28.0	0	0	25	0
raspberry:							
(*Breyers*)	120	n.a.	28.0	1.5	5	15	0
(*Breyers* Fat Free)	120	n.a.	28.0	0	0	20	0
strawberry kiwi (*Edy's/Dreyer's*)	120	1.0	27.0	1.0	5	30	0
tropical:							
(*Breyers*)	120	n.a.	27.0	1.0	5	15	0

Food and Measure	cal.	prot. (gms)	carbo. (gms)	fat (gms)	chol. (mgs)	sod. (mgs)	fiber (gms)
(*Breyers* Fat Free)	110	n.a.	27.0	0	0	25	0
Sherbet bar, lemon (*Good Humor Smile!*), 1 bar	110	n.a.	24.0	1.0	<5	15	0
Sherbet cup, orange:							
(*Carnation*), 3 fl. oz.	90	1.0	19.0	1.0	5	20	0
(*Carnation*), 5 fl. oz.	150	1.0	32.0	1.5	5	30	0
Shortening, 1 tbsp.:							
(*Jewel/Swiftning*)	110	0	0	12.0	1	10	0
(*Wesson*)	110	0	0	12.0	0	0	0
lard or vegetable oil	115	0	0	12.8	n.a.	0	0
vegetable:							
(*Snowdrift*)	110	0	0	12.0	1	0	0
regular/butter flavor (*Crisco*)	110	0	0	12.0	0	0	0
Shrimp, meat only:							
raw, 4 oz.	120	23.0	1.0	2.0	173	168	0
raw, 4 large, 1 oz. . . .	30	5.7	.3	.5	43	42	0
boiled or steamed:							
4 oz.	112	23.7	n.a.	1.2	221	254	0
4 large	22	4.6	n.a.	.2	43	49	0
Shrimp, canned, drained, 1 cup	154	29.6	1.3	2.5	222	216	0
Shrimp, freeze-dried, whole (*AlpineAire*), 1 oz.	110	23.0	2.0	1.0	0	170	0
"Shrimp," imitation:							
from surimi, 4 oz. . . .	115	14.1	10.4	1.7	41	800	0
frozen, jumbo (*Captain Jac*), 3 pcs., 3 oz.	90	9.0	11.0	1.0	10	510	.0
Shrimp cocktail:							
(*Vita*), ½ cup	100	8.0	16.0	.5	75	820	1.0
(*Vita*), 4-oz. jar	100	7.0	18.0	.5	65	810	1.0
Shrimp entree, canned, chow mein (*La Choy* Bi-Pack), 1 cup	65	6.0	9.0	1.0	20	1015	1.5
Shrimp entree, freeze-dried, 1 serving:							
Alfredo (*AlpineAire*)	300	17.0	40.0	8.0	25	700	0

Food and Measure	cal.	prot. (gms)	carbo. (gms)	fat (gms)	chol. (mgs)	sod. (mgs)	fiber (gms)
Shrimp entree, freeze-dried *(cont.)*							
Newburg (*AlpineAire*)	310	15.0	48.0	6.0	15	520	3.0
Shrimp entree, frozen:							
and angel hair pasta (*Lean Cuisine Cafe Classics*), 10 oz.	290	16.0	42.0	6.0	55	590	1.0
breaded:							
butterfly (*Van de Kamp's*), 7 pcs.	300	11.0	32.0	14.0	80	570	2.0
popcorn (*Van de Kamp's*), 20 pcs.	270	11.0	31.0	11.0	70	760	1.0
popcorn, garlic-herb (*Gorton's*), 3.6 oz.	270	11.0	24.0	14.0	90	600	n.a.
whole (*Van de Kamp's*), 7 pcs.	240	13.0	26.0	10.0	50	520	2.0
fajitas (*Contessa* Entrees for 2), 2½ pcs.	260	13.0	42.0	4.5	55	960	5.0
and linguine (*Contessa* Entrees for 2), 2 cups	310	18.0	53.0	3.0	35	450	4.0
marinara:							
(*Healthy Choice*), 10½ oz.	250	10.0	44.0	4.0	55	360	5.0
(*Smart Ones*), 9 oz.	180	9.0	31.0	2.0	40	570	4.0
stir-fry (*Contessa* Entrees for 2), 2¼ cups	170	9.0	38.0	0	70	490	3.0
and vegetables (*Healthy Choice* Maria), 12½ oz.	290	15.0	46.0	5.0	40	540	5.0
Shrimp sauce (*Crosse & Blackwell*), ¼ cup	110	1.0	25.0	0	0	790	0
Shrimp spice (*Tone's* Craboil), 1 tsp.	10	.3	1.2	.6	1	1	.3
Sloppy Joe sauce, see "Sandwich sauce"							

Food and Measure	cal.	prot. (gms)	carbo. (gms)	fat (gms)	chol. (mgs)	sod. (mgs)	fiber (gms)
Smelt, rainbow, meat only:							
raw, 4 oz.	110	20.0	0	2.8	80	68	0
baked, broiled, or microwaved, 4 oz. . . .	141	25.6	0	3.5	102	87	0
Snack bar (see also "Cookie" and "Granola and cereal bar"), 1 bar:							
blueberry, raspberry, or strawberry (*Sweet Rewards* Fat Free)	120	1.0	29.0	0	0	80	<1.0
brownie (*Sweet Rewards* Low Fat)	120	2.0	24.0	2.0	0	105	<1.0
chocolate chip (*Sweet Rewards* Low Fat)	110	2.0	23.0	2.0	0	115	0
chocolate chunk:							
(*Golden Grahams Treats* S'Mores)	90	1.0	17.0	2.5	0	100	0
(*Golden Grahams Treats* S'Mores King Size)	190	1.0	34.0	5.0	0	210	1.0
fudge, double (*Sweet Rewards* Fat Free Supreme)	100	2.0	25.0	0	0	980	1.0
marshmallow (*Golden Grahams Treats*) . . .	90	1.0	17.0	2.0	0	110	0
Snack chips and crisps (see also "Snack mix" and specific listings), 1 oz., except as noted:							
(*Chex* Mix Bold Party Blend), ½ cup, 1.1 oz.	140	3.0	20.0	6.0	0	440	1.0
(*Chex* Mix Traditional), ⅔ cup, 1.1 oz.	130	3.0	21.0	4.0	0	410	1.0

Food and Measure	cal.	prot. (gms)	carbo. (gms)	fat (gms)	chol. (mgs)	sod. (mgs)	fiber (gms)
Snack chips and crisps (*cont.*)							
apple cinnamon (*Crunchwells Crumpet Chips*)	110	4.0	21.0	1.0	0	230	n.a.
cheddar (*Chex* Mix), ½ cup, 1.1 oz.	130	3.0	20.0	5.0	0	330	1.0
cheese (*Pub Stix* Baked)	110	3.0	21.0	2.0	0	350	1.0
hot and spicy (*Chex Mix*), cup, 1.1 oz.	130	3.0	21.0	4.5	0	420	2.0
multigrain chips: (*Barbara's* Pinta) . . .	130	2.0	19.0	6.0	0	70	2.0
salsa (*Barbara's* Pinta)	130	2.0	19.0	6.0	0	210	2.0
onion: (*Funyons*)	140	2.0	18.0	7.0	0	250	<1.0
rings (*Wise*)	140	0	20.0	6.0	0	420	0
Parmesan garlic (*Crunchwells Crumpet Chips*)	100	4.0	20.0	1.0	0	310	n.a.
pizza (*Pub Stix* Baked)	110	3.0	21.0	2.0	0	360	1.0
raspberry (*Crunchwells Crumpet Chips*)	110	4.0	21.0	1.0	0	210	n.a.
spicy barbecue (*Crunchwells Crumpet Chips*)	100	4.0	20.0	1.0	0	560	n.a.
Snack mix, ½ cup, except as noted:							
(*Blue Diamond* Beach House), 1 oz.	110	3.0	7.0	8.0	0	20	1.0
(*Blue Diamond* Hot House), 1 oz.	150	4.0	13.0	9.0	0	320	1.0
(*Blue Diamond* Smoke House), 1 oz.	140	4.0	14.0	8.0	0	370	2.0
(*Cheez-It* Party Mix)	140	4.0	19.0	5.0	0	270	1.0
(*Chex Mix*), ⅔ cup . . .	130	3.0	22.0	3.5	0	280	1.0
(*Chex Mix* Bold n' Zesty)	150	3.0	17.0	7.0	0	390	5.0
(*Goldfish* Original) . . .	5.0	5.0	21.0	8.0	5	360	2.0

Food and Measure	cal.	prot. (gms)	carbo. (gms)	fat (gms)	chol. (mgs)	sod. (mgs)	fiber (gms)
cheddar (*Goldfish* Zesty)	180	1.0	19.0	10.0	<5	390	1.0
honey mustard and onion (*Pepperidge Farm*)	180	4.0	19.0	10.0	<5	390	1.0
lightly seasoned (*Pepperidge Farm*)	170	4.0	22.0	8.0	<5	400	1.0
mini (*Ritz*)	150	2.0	21.0	7.0	0	430	1.0
nacho cheese (*Cheez-It Party Mix*)	130	3.0	20.0	4.5	0	330	1.0
nutty, extra (*Pepperidge Farm*)	180	5.0	20.0	9.0	25	330	2.0
Snail, sea, see "Whelk"							
Snapper, meat only:							
raw, 4 oz.	113	23.3	0	1.5	42	73	0
baked, broiled, or microwaved, 4 oz. . . .	145	3.0	0	2.0	53	65	0
Snow peas, see "Peas, edible-podded"							
Snow pea sprouts (*Jonathan's*), 1 cup	40	3.0	8.0	0	0	0	3.0
Soft drinks, carbonated, 8 fl. oz., except as noted:							
apple:							
(*R.W. Knudsen Spritzer*), 12 fl. oz.	160	0	40.0	0	0	25	0
green (*Nehi* Lockjaw)	120	0	32.0	0	0	35	0
spiced (*Natural Brew*), 12 fl. oz.	170	0	42.0	0	0	18	0
apple raspberry (*Fruitworks*), 12 fl. oz.	160	0	42.0	0	0	110	0
berry (*After the Fall Spritzer* Berrymeister), 12 fl. oz.	170	<1.0	42.0	0	0	25	0

Food and Measure	cal.	prot. (gms)	carbo. (gms)	fat (gms)	chol. (mgs)	sod. (mgs)	fiber (gms)
Soft drinks *(cont.)*							
birch beer:							
brown (*Canada Dry*)	110	0	27.0	0	0	40	0
clear (*Canada Dry*)	100	0	27.0	0	0	25	0
blueberry (*Minute Maid*)	110	0	29.0	0	0	9	0
boysenberry (*R.W. Knudsen Spritzer*), 12 fl. oz.	160	0	40.0	0	0	25	0
cactus cooler (*Canada Dry*)	100	0	27.0	0	0	25	0
cafe mocha (*Natural Brew*), 12 fl. oz. . . .	150	0	34.0	0	0	0	0
cherry:							
(*Cott's* Natural Red)	120	0	32.0	0	0	30	0
(*Crush*)	120	0	34.0	0	0	30	0
(*Snapple* French)	120	0	29.0	0	0	0	0
(*Sunkist*)	130	0	35.0	0	0	25	0
black (*After the Fall Spritzer*), 12 fl. oz.	180	<1.0	45.0	0	0	20	0
black (*Canada Dry*)	120	0	33.0	0	0	25	0
black (*IBC*)	120	0	32.0	0	0	40	0
black (*Minute Maid*)	110	0	29.0	0	0	11	0
black (*R.W. Knudsen Spritzer*), 12 fl. oz.	170	0	42.0	0	0	20	0
lemon (*Sundrop*)	120	0	31.0	0	0	15	0
lime (*Slice*), 12 fl. oz.	160	0	43.0	0	0	50	0
lime (*Snapple* Rickey)	110	0	27.0	0	0	0	0
spice (*Slice*), 12 fl. oz.	150	0	40.0	0	0	35	0
red (*Nehi* Lockjaw)	120	0	32.0	0	0	35	0
wild (*Canada Dry*)	100	0	28.0	0	0	25	0
cherry Amaretto (*Natural Brew*), 12 fl. oz.	160	0	40.0	0	0	20	0
chocolate (*Arizona* Lite Fudge)	60	0	15.0	0	0	15	0
citrus (*Citra*)	90	0	25.0	0	0	40	0

Food and Measure	cal.	prot. (gms)	carbo. (gms)	fat (gms)	chol. (mgs)	sod. (mgs)	fiber (gms)
club soda:							
(*Canada Dry*)	0	0	0	0	0	60	0
(*Schweppes*)	0	0	0	0	0	45	0
cola:							
(*Coca-Cola* Classic/ Caffeine Free) ...	97	0	27.0	0	0	9	0
(*Cotts*)	100	0	27.0	0	0	10	0
(*Pepsi/Pepsi* Caffeine Free), 12 fl. oz.	150	0	41.0	0	0	35	0
(*RC/RC* Caffeine Free)	110	0	29.0	0	0	35	0
(*Santa Cruz Organic* Gold), 12 fl. oz.	140	0	36.0	0	0	0	0
(*Slice*), 12 fl. oz. ...	160	0	43.0	0	0	35	0
cherry (*Coca-Cola*)	104	0	28.0	0	0	4	0
cherry (*IBC*)	110	0	29.0	0	0	25	0
cherry (*RC*)	110	0	29.0	0	0	35	0
cherry (*R.W. Knudsen Spritzer*), 12 fl. oz.	170	0	42.0	0	0	20	0
cherry, wild (*Pepsi*), 12 fl. oz.	160	0	43.0	0	0	35	0
draft (*RC*)	120	0	33.0	0	0	35	0
ginseng (*Natural Brew*), 12 fl. oz.	170	0	42.0	0	0	18	0
Jamaica (*Canada Dry*)	100	0	27.0	0	0	10	0
Collins mixer:							
(*Canada Dry*)	90	0	21.0	0	0	15	0
(*Schweppes*)	90	0	21.0	0	0	15	0
cranberry (*R.W. Knudsen Spritzer*), 12 fl. oz.	190	1.0	45.0	0	0	65	0
cream/creme:							
(*A&W*)	110	0	28.0	0	0	30	0
(*Barq's* Red)	115	0	31.0	0	0	19	0
(*Cotts*)	100	0	29.0	0	0	35	0
(*Hires*)	120	0	32.0	0	0	30	0
(*IBC*)	120	0	32.0	0	0	45	0
(*Mug*), 12 fl. oz. ...	170	0	48.0	0	0	65	0

Food and Measure	cal.	prot. (gms)	carbo. (gms)	fat (gms)	chol. (mgs)	sod. (mgs)	fiber (gms)
Soft drinks, cream/creme *(cont.)*							
(*Snapple* Creme D' Vanilla)	130	0	33.0	0	0	0	0
blue (*Nehi*)	130	0	32.0	0	0	35	0
vanilla (*After the Fall Spritzer* Creamie), 12 fl. oz	170	1.0	42.0	0	0	25	0
vanilla (*Canada Dry*)	110	0	30.0	0	0	30	0
vanilla (*Natural Brew*), 12 fl. oz.	170	0	42.0	0	0	18	0
vanilla (*R.W. Knudsen Spritzer*), 12 fl. oz.	160	0	35.0	0	0	20	0
vanilla, French (*Barq's*)	112	0	30.0	0	0	20	0
(*Delaware Punch*)	123	0	33.0	0	0	26	0
(*Dr Pepper*)	100	0	27.0	0	0	35	0
(*Dr. Slice*), 12 fl. oz	140	0	39.0	0	0	35	0
(*Fresca*)	3	0	<1.0	0	0	1	0
fruit punch/blend:							
(*Cotts*)	110	0	30.0	0	0	25	0
(*Crush* Fruity Red)	120	0	32.0	0	0	25	0
(*Crush* Tropical Punch)	120	0	33.0	0	0	30	0
(*Minute Maid*)	113	0	32.0	0	0	19	0
(*Nehi*)	130	0	34.0	0	0	35	0
(*Old Colony*)	130	0	37.0	0	0	30	0
(*Slice*), 12 fl. oz. . . .	190	0	50.0	0	0	55	0
(*Sunkist*)	120	0	33.0	0	0	25	0
(*Sunkist* Citrus) . . .	90	0	25.0	0	0	25	0
(*Welch's* Tropical Punch)	130	0	34.0	0	0	30	0
Tahitian treat (*Canada Dry*)	110	0	30.0	0	0	25	0
(*Fruitworks* Pink Lemonade), 12 fl. oz.	170	0	46.0	0	0	80	0
ginger ale:							
(*After the Fall Spritzer* Nantucket), 12 fl. oz.	160	1.0	40.0	0	0	25	0
(*Canada Dry*)	80	0	22.0	0	0	25	0

Food and Measure	cal.	prot. (gms)	carbo. (gms)	fat (gms)	chol. (mgs)	sod. (mgs)	fiber (gms)
(*Canada Dry* Golden)	90	0	24.0	0	0	10	0
(*Cotts*)	70	0	20.0	0	0	20	0
(*Natural Brew* Outrageous), 12 fl. oz.	170	0	42.0	0	0	18	0
(*Nehi*)	100	0	24.0	0	0	35	0
(*R.W. Knudsen* Spritzer), 12 fl. oz.	160	1.0	40.0	0	0	25	0
(*Santa Cruz* Organic), 12 fl. oz.	150	1.0	38.0	0	0	70	0
(*Schweppes*)	80	0	22.0	0	0	25	0
cherry (*Canada Dry*)	100	0	27.0	0	0	25	0
cranberry (*Canada Dry*)	90	0	25.0	0	0	15	0
grape, dry (*Schweppes*)	90	0	26.0	0	0	25	0
lemon (*Canada Dry*)	90	0	25.0	0	0	15	0
mint (*Cotts*)	110	0	27.0	0	0	20	0
raspberry (*After the Fall Spritzer*), 12 fl. oz.	140	0	35.0	0	0	15	0
raspberry (*Schweppes*)	90	0	26.0	0	0	25	0
strawberry (*After the Fall Spritzer*), 12 fl. oz.	150	0	37.0	0	0	15	0
ginger beer (*Schweppes*)	90	0	25.0	0	0	50	0
grape:							
(*Cotts*)	110	0	30.0	0	0	25	0
(*Crush*)	130	0	35.0	0	0	30	0
(*Fanta*)	117	0	31.0	0	0	9	0
(*Minute Maid*)	113	0	30.0	0	0	9	0
(*Nehi*)	120	0	32.0	0	0	35	0
(*Old Colony*)	150	0	38.0	0	0	30	0
(*R.W. Knudsen* Spritzer), 12 fl. oz.	170	1.0	41.0	0	0	30	0
(*Schweppes*)	120	0	33.0	0	0	30	0
(*Slice*), 12 fl. oz. ...	190	0	51.0	0	0	70	0

Food and Measure	cal.	prot. (gms)	carbo. (gms)	fat (gms)	chol. (mgs)	sod. (mgs)	fiber (gms)
Soft drinks, grape *(cont.)*							
(Sunkist)	130	0	36.0	0	0	25	0
Concord *(Canada Dry)*	110	0	29.0	0	0	30	0
Concord *(After the Fall Spritzer)*, 12 fl. oz.	180	<1.0	48.0	0	0	30	0
grapefruit:							
(Schweppes)	100	0	27.0	0	0	50	0
(Squirt)	100	0	27.0	0	0	15	0
lemon *(Canada Dry Half & Half)*	100	0	27.0	0	0	25	0
lemon *(Cotts* Half & Half)	100	0	26.0	0	0	25	0
ruby red *(Squirt)* ...	120	0	31.0	0	0	15	0
guava *(Santa Cruz* Organic)	150	1.0	38.0	0	0	70	0
guava berry *(Fruitworks)*, 12 fl. oz.	170	0	46.0	0	0	80	0
(Hi-Spot)	100	0	28.0	0	0	40	0
(Josta), 12 fl. oz.	160	0	44.0	0	0	40	0
kiwi-lime *(R.W. Knudsen Spritzer)*, 12 fl. oz.	160	1.0	40.0	0	0	25	0
kiwi-strawberry:							
(After the Fall Spritzer), 12 fl. oz.	150	0	38.0	15	0		
(Nehi)	120	0	32.0	0	0	35	0
lemon:							
(Cott's Lemon-Up)	100	0	28.0	0	0	40	0
(Nehi Lockjaw)	120	0	32.0	0	0	35	0
bitter *(Canada Dry)*	100	0	26.0	0	0	10	0
bitter *(Schweppes)*	110	0	28.0	0	0	20	0
sour *(Canada Dry)*	90	0	21.0	0	0	15	0
sour *(Schweppes)*	100	0	26.0	0	0	25	0
lemonade (see also "Lemonade"):							
(Nehi)	90	0	35.0	0	0	35	0
(Santa Cruz Organic), 12 fl. oz.	150	1.0	38.0	0	0	70	0

Food and Measure	cal.	prot. (gms)	carbo. (gms)	fat (gms)	chol. (mgs)	sod. (mgs)	fiber (gms)
Jamaican (*R.W. Knudsen Spritzer*), 12 fl. oz.	170	0	41.0	0	0	25	0
raspberry (*Santa Cruz* Organic), 12 fl. oz.	150	1.0	38.0	0	0	70	0
lemon-lime:							
(*R.W. Knudsen Spritzer*), 12 fl. oz.	170	1.0	42.0	0	0	25	0
(*Santa Cruz* Organic), 12 fl. oz.	150	1.0	38.0	0	0	70	0
(*Schweppes*)	90	0	25.0	0	0	50	0
(*Slice*), 12 fl. oz.	150	0	40.0	0	0	55	0
lime:							
(*Canada Dry* Island)	120	0	33.0	0	0	15	0
Caribbean (*After the Fall Spritzer*), 12 fl. oz.	170	<1.0	41.0	0	0	20	0
mandarin lime (*R.W. Knudsen Spritzer*), 12 fl. oz.	170	1.0	42.0	0	0	25	0
mango, 12 fl. oz.:							
(*After the Fall Spritzer*)	190	<1.0	45.0	0	0	30	0
(*R.W. Knudsen Fandango Spritzer*)	190	1.0	45.0	0	0	30	0
ginger (*After the Fall Spritzer*)	150	0	36.0	0	0	10	0
(*Mello Yello*)	118	0	32.0	0	0	9	0
(*Mountain Dew* Regular/Caffeine Free), 12 fl. oz.	170	0	46.0	0	0	70	0
(*Mr. Pibb*)	97	0	26.0	0	0	7	0
(*Nehi* Wild Red)	120	0	32.0	0	0	35	0
orange:							
(*Canada Dry* Sunripe)	110	0	290	0	0	25	0
(*Cotts*)	120	0	33.0	0	0	25	0
(*Crush*)	120	0	34.0	0	0	30	0

Food and Measure	cal.	prot. (gms)	carbo. (gms)	fat (gms)	chol. (mgs)	sod. (mgs)	fiber (gms)
Soft drinks, orange *(cont.)*							
(*Fanta*)	118	0	32.0	0	0	9	0
(*Fruitworks*)	110	0	26.0	0	0	10	0
(*Minute Maid*)	118	0	32.0	0	0	0	0
(*Nehi*)	120	0	35.0	0	0	35	0
(*Orangina*),							
10 fl. oz.	120	<1.0	28.0	0	0	115	0
(*Slice*)	170	0	46.0	0	0	55	0
(*Sunkist*)	130	0	35.0	0	0	30	0
(*Welch's*)	120	0	34.0	0	0	30	0
creme (*Natural*							
Brew), 12 fl. oz.	160	0	40.0	0	0	20	0
mango (*Santa Cruz*							
Organic), 12 fl.							
oz.	150	1.0	38.0	0	0	70	0
mimosa (*After the*							
Fall Spritzer),							
12 fl. oz.	170	1.0	39.0	0	0	35	0
passion							
(*Fruitworks*),							
12 fl. oz.	160	0	43.0	0	0	110	0
passion fruit (*R.W.*							
Knudsen							
Spritzer),							
12 fl. oz.	160	0	40.0	0	0	25	0
peach:							
(*Canada Dry*)	110	0	30.0	0	0	25	0
(*Crush*)	120	0	33.0	0	0	25	0
(*Nehi*)	120	0	34.0	0	0	35	0
(*R.W. Knudsen*							
Spritzer),							
12 fl. oz.	160	2.0	37.0	0	0	35	0
(*Sunkist*)	110	0	30.0	0	0	25	0
(*Welch's*)	130	0	37.0	0	0	20	0
Georgia (*After the*							
Fall Spritzer),							
12 fl. oz.	150	<1.0	37.0	0	0	35	0
papaya (*Fruitworks*),							
12 fl. oz.	170	0	46.0	0	0	110	0
piña colada (*Nehi*) . . .	110	0	31.0	0	0	35	0

Food and Measure	cal.	prot. (gms)	carbo. (gms)	fat (gms)	chol. (mgs)	sod. (mgs)	fiber (gms)
pineapple:							
(*Canada Dry*)	100	0	26.0	0	0	25	0
(*Cotts*)	120	0	31.0	0	0	25	0
(*Crush*)	120	0	34.0	0	0	30	0
(*Minute Maid*)	109	0	30.0	0	0	9	0
(*Nehi*)	130	0	36.0	0	0	35	0
(*Old Colony*)	150	0	38.0	0	0	30	0
(*Slice*), 12 fl. oz. . . .	190	0	51.0	0	0	70	0
(*Sunkist*)	120	0	32.0	0	0	25	0
(*Welch's*)	130	0	35.0	0	0	45	0
mandarin (*After the Fall Spritzer*), 12 fl. oz.	160	<1.0	38.0	0	0	20	0
raspberry:							
(*After the Fall Spritzer*), 12 fl. oz.	170	<1.0	42.0	0	0	35	0
(*Nehi* Lockjaw)	120	0	32.0	0	0	35	0
red (*R.W. Knudsen* Spritzer), 12 fl. oz.	170	0	38.0	0	0	25	0
(*RC Dr. Nehi*)	120	0	26.0	0	0	35	0
(*RC Kick*)	120	0	33.0	0	0	50	0
(*RC Upper 10*)	110	0	29.0	0	00	0	0
(*Red Rattler*)	111	0	30.0	0	0	20	0
root beer:							
(*A&W*)	120	0	31.0	0	0	30	0
(*Barq's/Barq's* Caffeine Free)	111	0	30.0	0	0	24	0
(*Barrelhead*)	100	0	27.0	0	0	30	0
(*Cotts*)	100	0	27.0	0	0	20	0
(*Hires*)	120	0	31.0	0	0	45	0
(*IBC*)	110	0	29.0	0	0	40	0
(*Mug*), 12 fl. oz. . . .	160	0	43.0	0	0	65	0
(*Natural Brew* Draft), 12 fl. oz.	180	0	44.0	0	0	0	0
(*Nehi*)	130	0	32.0	0	0	35	0
(*Snapple* Tru)	110	0	29.0	0	0	0	0
seltzer:							
plain (*Canada Dry*)	0	0	0	0	0	0	0

Food and Measure	cal.	prot. (gms)	carbo. (gms)	fat (gms)	chol. (mgs)	sod. (mgs)	fiber (gms)
Soft drinks, seltzer *(cont.)*							
plain or flavored							
(*Schweppes*)	0	0	0	0	0	10	0
all flavors (*Canada Dry*)	0	0	0	0	0	10	0
all flavors (*Snapple*)	0	0	0	0	0	0	0
(*7Up*)	100	0	26.0	0	0	50	0
(*Slice* Red), 12 fl. oz.	190	0	51.0	0	0	55	0
sour mixer (*Canada Dry*)	80	0	22.0	0	0	30	0
(*Sprite*)	96	0	26.0	0	0	23	0
strawberry:							
(*Crush*)	110	0	30.0	0	0	30	0
(*Minute Maid*)	113	0	31.0	0	0	0	0
(*Nehi*)	110	0	31.0	0	0	35	0
(*R.W. Knudsen Spritzer*), 12 fl. oz.	170	0	42.0	0	0	25	0
(*Slice*), 12 fl. oz. . . .	170	0	47.0	0	0	55	0
(*Sunkist*)	120	0	33.0	0	0	25	0
(*Welch's*)	120	0	34.0	0	0	30	0
California (*Canada Dry*)	100	0	27.0	0	0	30	0
melon (*Fruitworks*), 12 fl. oz.	160	0	44.0	0	0	110	0
(*Sundrop*)	120	0	34.0	0	0	20	0
(*Surge*)	116	0	31.0	0	0	3	0
(*Tab*)	1	0	<1.0	0	0	4	0
tangerine, 12 fl. oz.:							
(*After the Fall Spritzer*)	180	<1.0	44.0	0	0	35	0
(*R.W. Knudsen Spritzer*)	170	2.0	40.0	0	0	35	0
citrus (*Fruitworks*)	150	0	42.0	0	0	80	0
tonic water:							
(*Canada Dry*)	90	0	24.0	0	0	15	0
(*Cotts*)	80	0	23.0	0	0	10	0
(*Schweppes*)	80	0	23.0	0	0	20	0
cranberry (*Schweppes*)	80	0	21.0	0	0	20	0
lime (*Canada Dry*)	90	0	24.0	0	0	20	0

Food and Measure	cal.	prot. (gms)	carbo. (gms)	fat (gms)	chol. (mgs)	sod. (mgs)	fiber (gms)
tropical passion (*After the Fall Spritzer*), 12 fl. oz.	170	<1.0	42.0	0	0	20	0
(*Vernor's*)	100	0	26.0	0	0	15	0
watermelon (*Nehi*) ...	120	0	34.0	0	0	35	0
(*Wink II*)	110	0	29.0	0	0	25	0
Sole:							
fresh, see "Flatfish"							
frozen (*Van de Kamp's*), 4-oz. fillet	110	23.0	0	1.5	50	125	0
Sole entree, frozen:							
au gratin (*Oven Poppers*), 5-oz. pc. ...	220	24.0	5.0	11.0	75	450	<1.0
breaded, fillet (*Mrs. Paul's*), 1 pc.	160	8.0	15.0	8.0	25	360	1.0
stuffed, 5-oz. pc., except as noted:							
w/broccoli, cheese (*Oven Poppers*)	150	20.0	4.0	6.0	55	330	1.0
w/crab (*Oven Poppers*)	250	17.0	15.0	13.0	70	400	1.0
w/crab, miniatures (*Oven Poppers*), 2-oz. pc.	120	6.0	8.0	7.0	25	140	0
w/garlic, shrimp, almonds (*Oven Poppers*)	250	19.0	15.0	13.0	80	430	2.0
w/shrimp, lobster (*Oven Poppers*)	150	20.0	7.0	5.0	80	430	1.0
w/spinach, cheese (*Oven Poppers*)	210	15.0	13.0	10	70	270	0
Sopressata, mini (*Cinghiale*), 1 oz.	100	8.0	<1.0	8.0	15	540	0
Sorbet (see also "Ice" and "Sherbet"), ½ cup:							
banana strawberry (*Häagen-Dazs*)	140	<1.0	34.0	0	0	5	<1.0
(*Ben & Jerry's Doonesbury*)	140	0	33.0	0	0	15	0

Food and Measure	cal.	prot. (gms)	carbo. (gms)	fat (gms)	chol. (mgs)	sod. (mgs)	fiber (gms)
Sorbet *(cont.)*							
berries, wild (*Real Fruit* Chunky)	110	0	27.0	0	0	5	0
cherry cordial (*Edy's/ Dreyer's*)	160	1.0	38.0	0	0	65	0
chocolate:							
(*Columbo* Cha Cha)	100	0	25.	0	0	70	1.0
(*Häagen-Dazs*)	120	2.0	28.0	0	0	70	2.0
devil's food (*Ben & Jerry's*)	170	2.0	36.0	2.5	0	60	2.0
and ice cream:							
orange (*Häagen-Dazs*)	190	2.0	24.0	9.0	60	45	0
raspberry (*Häagen-Dazs*)	190	3.0	23.0	9.0	60	45	<1.0
lemon:							
(*Columbo* Twist) . . .	100	0	24.0	0	0	15	0
(*Edy's/Dreyer's*) . . .	140	0	34.0	0	0	25	0
(*Häagen-Dazs* Zesty)	120	0	31.0	0	0	0	<1.0
peel (*Real Fruit* Chunky)	100	0	25.0	0	0	5	0
swirl (*Ben & Jerry's*)	120	0	30.0	0	0	15	0
mango:							
(*Häagen-Dazs*)	120	0	31.0	0	0	0	<1.0
lime (*Ben & Jerry's*)	130	0	33.0	0	0	10	0
orange (*Edy's/ Dreyer's*)	120	1.0	30.0	0	0	15	0
Margarita (*Häagen-Dazs*)	130	0	31.0	0	0	25	0
passion fruit (*Ben & Jerry's Purple Passion Fruit*)	140	0	22.0	0	0	25	0
peach:							
(*Columbo* Retreat)	100	0	24.0	0	0	15	0
(*Edy's/Dreyer's*) . . .	120	0	31.0	0	0	5	0
(*Häagen-Dazs* Orchard)	140	<1.0	35.0	0	0	0	<1.0
(*Real Fruit* Chunky Georgia)	110	0	28.0	0	0	5	0

Food and Measure	cal.	prot. (gms)	carbo. (gms)	fat (gms)	chol. (mgs)	sod. (mgs)	fiber (gms)
raspberry:							
(*Columbo* Jazz)	100	0	24.0	0	0	15	0
(*Häagen-Dazs*)	120	0	30.0	0	0	0	2.0
kiwi (*Edy's/Dreyer's*)	130	0	31.0	0	0	10	0
lemonade (*Häagen-Dazs*)	120	0	30.0	0	0	5	<1.0
red (*Real Fruit* Chunky)	110	0	27.0	0	0	5	0
strawberry:							
(*Columbo* Swing)	100	0	24.0	0	0	15	0
(*Edy's/Dreyer's*) . . .	120	0	31.0	0	0	10	0
(*Häagen-Dazs*)	130	0	32.0	0	0	0	<1.0
(*Real Fruit* Chunky)	100	0	26.0	0	0	5	0
kiwi (*Ben & Jerry's*)	140	1.0	34.0	0	0	15	0
tropical blend (*Real Fruit* Chunky)	120	1.0	29.0	0	0	5	0
Sorbet bar, 1 bar:							
berry, wild (*Häagen-Dazs*)	90	0	22.0	0	0	5	<1.0
chocolate (*Häagen-Dazs*)	80	1.0	20.0	0	0	50	1.0
Sorghum, whole grain, 1 cup	650	21.7	143.3	6.3	0	n.a.	n.a.
Sorghum syrup:							
(*Arrowhead Mills*), 1 tbsp.	60	0	16.0	0	0	0	0
½ cup	479	0	123.7	0	0	13	0
1 tbsp.	61	0	15.7	0	0	2	0
Sorrel, see "Dock"							
Soup, canned, ready-to-serve, 1 cup, except as noted:							
bean:							
4 (*Arrowhead Mills*)	130	6.0	23.0	2.0	0	770	5.0
black (*Goya*)	210	12.0	34.0	2.5	0	1400	10.0
black (*Green's Farm*), 7½ oz. . . .	160	10.0	32.0	1.5	0	510	9.0
black (*Health Valley*)	110	8.0	28.0	0	0	290	10.0
black (*Progresso* Hearty)	170	8.0	30.0	1.5	<5	730	10.0

Food and Measure	cal.	prot. (gms)	carbo. (gms)	fat (gms)	chol. (mgs)	sod. (mgs)	fiber (gms)
Soup, canned, ready-to-serve, bean *(cont.)*							
smoky (*Arrowhead Mills*)	140	8.0	25.0	1.0	0	880	7.0
bean w/bacon (*Grandma Brown's*)	190	9.0	31.0	3.5	0	700	10.0
bean and ham:							
(*Campbell's Chunky*)	190	14.0	29.0	2.0	10	880	10.0
(*Campbell's Home Cookin'*)	180	9.0	32.0	2.0	10	710	8.0
(*Progresso*)	160	10.0	25.0	2.0	10	870	8.0
bean and vegetable:							
(*Health Valley*)	140	10.0	32.0	0	0	250	13.0
black bean (*Health Valley*)	110	11.0	24.0	0	0	280	12.0
beef:							
barley (*Progresso*)	130	10.0	13.0	4.0	25	780	3.0
barley (*Progresso* 99% Fat Free) . . .	140	11.0	20.0	2.0	20	470	3.0
chowder, chunky (*Nalley*), 7½ oz.	110	4.0	17.0	3.0	5	970	2.0
noodle (*Progresso*)	140	13.0	15.0	3.5	30	950	1.0
pasta (*Campbell's Chunky*)	140	11.0	18.0	3.0	20	970	2.0
and potato (*Healthy Choice*)	115	11.0	16.0	1.0	5	450	<1.0
beef broth:							
(*College Inn* No Fat)	20	4.0	0	0	0	620	0
(*Health Valley*)	20	5.0	0	0	0	160	0
(*Swanson* Clear) . . .	20	2.0	1.0	1.0	<5	820	0
beef vegetable:							
(*Progresso* 99% Fat Free)	160	11.0	24.0	2.0	10	870	3.0
country (*Campbell's Chunky*)	150	10.0	14.0	4.0	25	900	1.0
country (*Campbell's Chunky*), 10¾ oz.	190	13.0	22.0	5.0	30	1130	3.0
and rotini (*Progresso*)	130	13.0	14.0	2.5	25	780	4.0
borscht:							
(*Gold's*)	70	1.0	16.0	0	0	780	1.0

Food and Measure	cal.	prot. (gms)	carbo. (gms)	fat (gms)	chol. (mgs)	sod. (mgs)	fiber (gms)
(*Manischewitz*)....	80	<1.0	21.0	0	0	680	2.0
(*Manischewitz* Low Cal)	25	<1.0	6.0	0	0	530	3.0
(*Manischewitz* Reduced Sodium)	80	<1.0	21.0	0	0	350	0
w/shredded beets (*Manischewitz*)	90	1.0	21.0	0	0	540	3.0
chicken:							
(*Progresso* Chickarina)	130	8.0	12.0	5.0	20	1010	<1.0
hearty (*Healthy Choice*)	120	8.0	20.0	2.0	<5	480	2.0
rotisserie seasoned (*Progresso*).....	100	7.0	15.0	1.5	15	920	2.0
chicken barley (*Progresso*)	110	8.0	16.0	1.5	15	850	3.0
chicken broccoli, cheese and potato:							
(*Campbell's Chunky*)	200	9.0	14.0	12.0	25	1120	1.0
(*Campbell's Chunky*), 10¾ oz.	250	11.0	17.0	15.0	30	1400	1.0
chicken broth:							
(*Arrowhead Mills*)	60	0	12.0	1.0	0	740	0
(*Campbell's Healthy Request*)	20	3.0	1.0	0	0	450	0
(*Campbell's Healthy Request* Low Sodium), 10½ oz.	40	4.0	2.0	2.0	5	140	0
(*College Inn*)	25	1.0	1.0	1.5	<5	1050	0
(*College Inn* Low Salt)	25	1.0	1.0	2.0	5	640	0
(*College Inn* No Fat)	10	1.0	1.0	0	0	640	0
(*Health Valley*)	45	7.0	0	1.5	25	250	0
(*Progresso*)	20	2.0	1.0	1.5	0	920	0
(*Swanson*)	20	2.0	1.0	.5	0	980	0
(*Swanson Fat Free Natural Goodness*)	15	0	1.0	0	0	620	1.0

Food and Measure	cal.	prot. (gms)	carbo. (gms)	fat (gms)	chol. (mgs)	sod. (mgs)	fiber (gms)
Soup, canned, ready-to-serve, chicken broth *(cont.)*							
w/Italian herbs or roasted garlic (*Swanson*)	20	1.0	3.0	.5	<5	950	0
w/onion (*Swanson*)	25	0	5.0	.5	<5	980	0
chicken chowder, w/noodles (*Nalley*), 7½ oz.	120	8.0	15.0	3.5	25	1060	1.0
chicken corn chowder:							
(*Campbell's Chunky*)	250	10.0	18.0	15.0	25	870	3.0
(*Campbell's Chunky*), 10¾ oz.	310	12.0	22.0	19.0	30	1080	4.0
(*Campbell's Healthy Request* Hearty)	150	7.0	24.0	3.0	15	480	2.0
chicken and mush-room chowder (*Campbell's Chunky*)	210	8.0	18.0	12.0	20	1030	1.0
chicken noodle:							
(*Campbell's Chunky Classic*)	130	9.0	16.0	3.0	20	1050	2.0
(*Campbell's Chunky Classic*), 10¾ oz.	160	12.0	20.0	4.0	25	1310	3.0
(*Campbell's Healthy Request*)	100	5.0	14.0	3.0	15	480	1.0
(*Campbell's Healthy Request* Low So-dium), 10¾ oz.	170	11.0	18.0	5.0	50	120	2.0
(*Campbell's Simply Home*)	80	5.0	12.0	1.0	10	810	1.0
(*Progresso*)	90	9.0	9.0	2.0	25	950	<1.0
(*Progresso* 99% Fat Free)	90	7.0	13.0	1.5	20	950	1.0
egg (*Campbell's Home Cookin'*)	90	16.0	13.0	2.0	15	940	1.0
egg (*Campbell's Home Cookin'*), 10¾ oz.	110	8.0	16.0	2.0	20	1150	1.0

Food and Measure	cal.	prot. (gms)	carbo. (gms)	fat (gms)	chol. (mgs)	sod. (mgs)	fiber (gms)
chicken pasta:							
(*Campbell's Simply Home*)	90	6.0	14.0	1.0	5	850	1.0
(*Healthy Choice*) . . .	110	7.0	17.0	2.0	<5	480	2.0
Alfredo (*Healthy Choice*)	120	9.0	18.0	2.0	10	480	<1.0
and mushroom (*Campbell's Chunky*)	120	8.0	16.0	4.0	15	930	1.0
w/roasted garlic (*Campbell's Home Cookin'*)	120	6.0	17.0	3.0	5	850	1.0
chicken and penne, spicy (*Progresso*)	110	9.0	14.0	1.5	15	950	1.0
chicken rice:							
(*Campbell's Healthy Request* Hearty)	110	5.0	16.0	2.5	15	480	1.0
(*Campbell's Home Cookin'*)	100	4.0	19.0	1.0	10	900	2.0
(*Campbell's Home Cookin'*), 10¾ oz.	140	8.0	22.0	2.0	20	1080	2.0
(*Healthy Choice*) . . .	110	7.0	16.0	2.0	<5	480	1.0
w/vegetables (*Progresso*)	90	6.0	13.0	2.0	10	890	1.0
w/vegetables (*Progresso* 99% Fat Free)	110	7.0	16.0	2.0	10	780	1.0
white/wild (*Campbell's Simply Home*)	100	5.0	19.0	1.0	5	810	1.0
white/wild (*Progresso*)	100	7.0	15.0	1.5	15	850	1.0
white/wild, savory (*Campbell's Chunky*)	140	9.0	18.0	3.0	25	840	2.0
chicken and rotini (*Progresso* Hearty)	90	8.0	12.0	1.5	15	970	<1.0
chicken vegetable: (*Arrowhead Mills*)	100	9.0	10.0	3.0	20	1230	2.0

Food and Measure	cal.	prot. (gms)	carbo. (gms)	fat (gms)	chol. (mgs)	sod. (mgs)	fiber (gms)
Soup, canned, ready-to-serve, chicken vegetable *(cont.)*							
(*Campbell's Chunky* Hearty)	90	6.0	12.0	2.0	10	800	2.0
(*Campbell's Healthy Request*)	110	6.0	18.0	2.0	10	480	2.0
(*Campbell's Home Cookin'*)	120	5.0	18.0	2.5	10	720	2.0
(*Progresso*)	90	7.0	13.0	1.5	15	820	2.0
(*Progresso* Home-style)	90	7.0	11.0	1.5	15	900	<1.0
Italian style (*Campbell's Home Cookin'*)	130	8.0	20.0	1.5	15	880	3.0
spicy (*Campbell's Chunky*)	90	7.0	13.0	1.0	10	870	3.0
chili beef, w/beans (*Campbell's Chunky*), 11 oz. . . .	300	21.0	38.0	7.0	20	1080	9.0
clam chowder:							
(*Healthy Choice*) . . .	120	6.0	23.0	1.5	10	480	5.0
(*Nalley* Puget Sound), 7½ oz.	140	6.0	14.0	6.0	5	650	3.0
clam chowder, Manhattan:							
(*Campbell's Chunky*)	130	6.0	20.0	4.0	5	900	3.0
(*Campbell's Chunky*), 10¾ oz.	170	7.0	25.0	4.0	5	1120	4.0
(*Progresso*)	110	12.0	11.0	2.0	10	710	3.0
clam chowder, New England:							
(*Campbell's Chunky*)	240	7.0	21.0	15.0	10	980	2.0
(*Campbell's Chunky*), 10¾ oz.	300	9.0	26.0	18.0	15	1210	3.0
(*Campbell's Healthy Request*)	120	5.0	17.0	3.0	15	480	1.0
(*Campbell's Home Cookin'*)	190	5.0	14.0	13.0	10	960	1.0

Food and Measure	cal.	prot. (gms)	carbo. (gms)	fat (gms)	chol. (mgs)	sod. (mgs)	fiber (gms)
(*Campbell's Home Cookin'*), 10¾ oz.	240	7.0	17.0	16.0	15	1200	1.0
(*Campbell's Home Cookin'* 98% Fat Free)	110	4.0	17.0	3.0	10	780	2.0
(*Progresso*)	190	6.0	20.0	10.0	15	920	1.0
(*Progresso* 99% Fat Free)	130	5.0	22.0	2.0	5	700	1.0
clam and rotini chowder (*Progresso*) . . .	190	7.0	21.0	9.0	10	800	0
corn and vegetable (*Health Valley*)	70	5.0	17.0	0	0	135	7.0
corn chowder, chicken (*Healthy Choice*) . . .	160	8.0	26.0	2.5	5	470	4.0
crab, red, vegetable (*Chincoteague*)	90	7.0	10.0	2.5	20	600	2.0
egg flower (*Rice Road*)	90	2.0	15.0	2.5	15	1000	1.0
escarole, in chicken broth (*Progresso*)	25	1.0	3.0	1.0	<5	930	1.0
gazpacho	57	8.7	.8	2.2	0	1183	<2.0
gumbo, w/chicken, sausage (*Healthy Choice* Zesty)	90	7.0	13.0	1.5	10	480	2.0
hot and sour (*Rice Road*)	90	3.0	15.0	3.0	0	1340	2.0
Italian, carotene (*Health Valley*)	80	7.0	19.0	0	0	240	6.0
lentil: (*Health Valley*)	90	9.0	20.0	0	0	240	9.0
(*Progresso*)	140	9.0	22.0	2.0	0	750	7.0
(*Progresso* 99% Fat Free)	130	8.0	20.0	1.5	0	440	6.0
and carrots (*Health Valley*)	90	10.0	25.0	0	0	220	14.0
red (*Arrowhead Mills*)	100	6.0	17.0	1.5	0	320	3.0
savory (*Campbell's Home Cookin'*)	130	8.0	23.0	1.0	0	770	4.0
macaroni and bean (*Progresso*)	160	7.0	23.0	4.0	<5	800	6.0

Food and Measure	cal.	prot. (gms)	carbo. (gms)	fat (gms)	chol. (mgs)	sod. (mgs)	fiber (gms)
Soup, canned, ready-to-serve *(cont.)*							
meatballs and pasta							
pearls (*Progresso*)	140	7.0	13.0	7.0	15	700	0
minestrone: (*Arrow-*							
head Mills)	110	5.0	19.0	2.0	0	637	4.0
(*Campbell's Healthy*							
Request Hearty)	120	5.0	22.0	2.0	<5	480	3.0
(*Campbell's Home*							
Cookin' Old							
World)	120	0	25.0	1.0	0	870	3.0
(*Campbell's Simply*							
Home)	110	5.0	21.0	1.5	5	840	4.0
(*Health Valley*)	90	8.0	23.0	0	0	190	10.0
(*Progresso*)	120	5.0	21.0	2.0	0	960	5.0
(*Progresso* 99% Fat							
Free)	130	7.0	23.0	1.5	0	710	4.0
beef (*Progresso*) . . .	140	10.0	18.0	3.0	10	970	3.0
chicken (*Progresso*)	110	9.0	15.0	1.5	15	890	2.0
Italian (*Health Val-*							
ley)	80	8.0	21.0	0	0	210	11.0
Parmesan							
(*Progresso*)	100	3.0	16.0	2.5	0	700	3.0
shells, Italian herb							
(*Progresso* Pasta							
Soup)	120	5.0	22.0	1.5	0	1050	4.0
Tuscany (*Campbell's*							
Home Cookin')	190	5.0	21.0	9.0	5	870	5.0
mushroom:							
broth (*Arrowhead*							
Mills)	10	0	1.0	0	0	520	0
cream of (*Camp-*							
bell's Healthy Re-							
quest Low So-							
dium), 10½ oz.	200	3.0	18.0	14.0	20	65	3.0
cream of (*Camp-*							
bell's Home							
Cookin' 98% Fat							
Free)	80	1.0	15.0	2.0	5	810	1.0
mushroom barley:							
(*Arrowhead Mills*)	70	2.0	13.0	1.0	0	730	2.0
(*Health Valley*)	60	5.0	15.0	0	0	220	8.0

Food and Measure	cal.	prot. (gms)	carbo. (gms)	fat (gms)	chol. (mgs)	sod. (mgs)	fiber (gms)
mushroom chicken, creamy (*Progresso* 99% Fat Free)	90	7.0	12.0	2.0	10	840	1.0
mushroom rice, country (*Campbell's Home Cookin'*)	90	6.0	16.0	.5	0	820	2.0
noodles, Oriental, w/vegetables (*Campbell's Home Cookin'*)	100	4.0	18.0	1.0	10	890	3.0
onion, creamy (*Arrowhead Mills*)	100	2.0	21.0	1.5	0	662	2.0
Oriental broth (*Swanson*)	15	1.0	3.0	0	0	1070	0
pasta:							
Bolognese (*Health Valley* Pasta Soup)	100	4.0	20.0	0	0	290	4.0
cacciatore (*Health Valley* Pasta Soup)	100	4.0	20.0	0	0	290	4.0
Chinese (*Rice Road*)	70	1.0	12.0	2.0	0	1260	1.0
fagioli (*Health Valley* Pasta Soup)	120	6.0	25.0	0	0	290	4.0
primavera (*Health Valley* Pasta Soup)	110	3.0	23.0	0	0	290	3.0
roasted garlic, lentil (*Progresso*)	120	7.0	20.0	1.5	0	960	5.0
Romano (*Health Valley* Pasta Soup)	100	4.0	20.0	0	0	290	4.0
pea, split: (*Campbell's Healthy Request* Low Sodium), 10¾ oz.	240	12.0	38.0	4.0	5	50	5.0
(*Health Valley*)	110	10.0	23.0	0	0	160	8.0
(*Progresso* 99% Fat Free)	170	10.0	29.0	1.5	0	620	5.0
w/bacon (*Grandma Brown's*)	210	12.0	31.0	4.0	0	520	6.0

Food and Measure	cal.	prot. (gms)	carbo. (gms)	fat (gms)	chol. (mgs)	sod. (mgs)	fiber (gms)
Soup, canned, ready-to-serve, pea, split *(cont.)*							
and carrots (*Health Valley*)	110	8.0	17.0	0	0	230	4.0
green (*Progresso*)	170	10.0	25.0	3.0	5	870	5.0
pea, split, w/ham:							
(*Campbell's Chunky*)	190	14.0	27.0	3.0	20	1120	3.0
(*Campbell's Healthy Request*)	170	10.0	29.0	1.5	10	480	4.0
(*Campbell's Home Cookin'*)	170	10.0	30.0	1.5	10	860	6.0
(*Progresso*)	150	9.0	20.0	4.0	15	830	5.0
penne:							
in chicken broth (*Progresso Hearty*)	80	4.0	14.0	1.0	0	1020	<1.0
oregano, Italian-style vegetable (*Proggresso Pasta Soups*)	90	3.0	15.0	2.0	0	960	1.0
peppercorn vegetable (*Progresso Pasta Soups*)	100	3.0	20.0	1.0	0	920	2.0
pepper steak (*Campbell's Chunky*)	130	9.0	18.0	3.0	20	830	3.0
potato, baked:							
(*Healthy Choice*) . . .	130	4.0	27.0	2.0	<5	480	5.0
w/bacon bits, chives (*Campbell's Chunky*)	170	7.0	20.0	7.0	10	890	2.0
w/cheddar, bacon bits (*Campbell's Chunky*)	180	5.0	23.0	8.0	10	840	2.0
w/steak, cheese (*Campbell's Chunky*)	200	8.0	21.0	9.0	20	970	2.0
potato, broccoli and cheese (*Progresso*)	160	5.0	21.0	6.0	<5	960	1.0
potato, creamy, w/roasted garlic:							
(*Campbell's Healthy Request*)	110	2.0	22.0	2.5	<5	480	3.0

Food and Measure	cal.	prot. (gms)	carbo. (gms)	fat (gms)	chol. (mgs)	sod. (mgs)	fiber (gms)
(*Campbell's Home Cookin'*)	180	3.0	21.0	9.0	5	800	2.0
potato, ham and cheese (*Progresso*)	170	6.0	21.0	7.0	10	860	1.0
potato, white cheddar (*Progresso* 99% Fat Free)	140	4.0	26.0	2.5	5	930	2.0
potato ham chowder (*Campbell's Chunky* Old Fashioned)	220	6.0	16.0	14.0	20	840	3.0
potato leek (*Health Valley*)	70	4.0	15.0	0	0	230	3.0
rotini:							
herb, vegetable (*Progresso*).....	120	5.0	21.0	1.5	0	990	4.0
tomato-basil (*Progresso*).....	120	5.0	22.0	1.5	<5	890	2.0
and vegetable (*Health Valley* Pasta)	100	4.0	20.0	0	0	290	4.0
sirloin burger w/vegetable:							
(*Campbell's Chunky*)	210	13.0	18.0	9.0	25	1010	4.0
(*Campbell's Chunky*), 10¾ oz.	250	16.0	22.0	11.0	30	1250	5.0
steak and potato:							
(*Campbell's Chunky*)	150	9.0	19.0	4.0	20	890	3.0
(*Campbell's Chunky*), 10¾ oz.	190	12.0	24.0	5.0	30	1110	4.0
tomato:							
(*Campbell's*)	100	2.0	22.0	.5	<5	760	1.0
(*Health Valley*)	90	4.0	22.0	0	0	250	4.0
(*Muir Glen*)	60	3.0	12.0	0	0	660	3.0
(*Progresso*)	100	2.0	19.0	2.0	0	790	1.0
(*Progresso* Hearty)	100	2.0	19.0	2.0	0	800	1.0
basil (*Progresso*)	100	2.0	19.0	2.0	0	790	1.0
black bean (*Muir Glen*)	100	6.0	20.0	.5	0	490	4.0
creamy (*Campbell's*)	130	3.0	26.0	1.5	5	760	2.0

Food and Measure	cal.	prot. (gms)	carbo. (gms)	fat (gms)	chol. (mgs)	sod. (mgs)	fiber (gms)
Soup, canned, ready-to-serve, tomato *(cont.)*							
garden (*Campbell's Home Cookin'*)	100	4.0	22.0	.5	5	720	3.0
minestrone (*Muir Glen*) . . . . :	80	3.0	18.0	1.0	0	490	3.0
rice (*Muir Glen*) . . .	80	3.0	18.0	1.0	0	490	2.0
w/tomato pieces (*Campbell's Healthy Request Low Sodium*), 10½ oz.	170	4.0	28.0	6.0	10	60	2.0
tomato vegetable:							
(*Arrowhead Mills*)	90	2.0	17.0	2.0	0	820	2.0
(*Progresso*)	90	3.0	15.0	2.0	0	990	4.0
garden (*Progresso 99% Fat Free*) . . .	100	3.0	19.0	1.5	0	660	2.0
ravioli (*Campbell's Chunky*)	150	5.0	26.0	3.0	10	1000	3.0
ravioli (*Campbell's Healthy Request Hearty*)	140	4.0	26.0	1.0	5	480	3.0
tortellini:							
cheese, w/chicken, vegetables (*Campbell's Chunky*)	110	5.0	18.0	2.0	15	860	2.0
cheese and herb, tomato (*Progresso Pasta Soups*)	140	4.0	23.0	3.0	<5	700	2.0
in chicken broth (*Progresso*)	70	3.0	10.0	2.0	10	970	2.0
turkey noodle (*Progresso*)	90	7.0	11.0	1.5	20	1080	<1.0
turkey rice:							
w/vegetables (*Progresso*)	110	7.0	18.0	1.0	15	1040	1.0
wild rice (*Healthy Choice*)	70	10.0	8.5	1.0	<5	410	3.0
vegetable:							
(*Campbell's Chunky*)	130	3.0	22.0	4.0	0	870	4.0

Food and Measure	cal.	prot. (gms)	carbo. (gms)	fat (gms)	chol. (mgs)	sod. (mgs)	fiber (gms)
(*Campbell's Chunky*), 10¾ oz.	160	4.0	28.0	5.0	0	1090	5.0
(*Campbell's Healthy Request* Hearty)	100	3.0	20.0	1.0	0	470	2.0
(*Campbell's Home Cookin'* Fiesta)	140	3.0	24.0	3.0	0	740	4.0
(*Health Valley*)	80	5.0	18.0	0	0	230	6.0
(*Progresso*)	90	3.0	15.0	2.0	<5	810	2.0
(*Progresso* 99% Fat Free)	70	2.0	13.0	1.0	0	870	2.0
carotene (*Health Valley*)	70	5.0	17.0	0	0	240	6.0
country (*Campbell's Home Cookin'*)	110	3.0	21.0	1.5	10	750	2.0
country (*Campbell's Home Cookin'*), 10¾ oz.	140	4.0	27.0	1.5	10	940	2.0
garden (*Campbell's Simply Home*) ...	110	4.0	21.0	.5	5	720	2.0
garden (*Health Valley*)	80	6.0	17.0	0	0	250	4.0
w/pasta (*Campbell's Chunky* Hearty)	140	4.0	24.0	3.0	<5	920	3.0
Southwestern, w/black beans (*Campbell's Healthy Request*)	140	5.0	28.0	1.0	0	480	5.0
vegetable barley (*Health Valley*)	90	6.0	19.0	0	0	210	4.0
vegetable beef: (*Campbell's Chunky* Old Fashioned)	150	10.0	17.0	5.0	15	870	3.0
(*Campbell's Chunky* Old Fashioned), 10¾ oz.	180	13.0	20.0	6.0	20	1090	4.0
(*Campbell's Healthy Request* Hearty)	140	9.0	20.0	2.5	20	480	3.0
(*Campbell's Home Cookin'*)	110	9.0	15.0	1.5	20	930	3.0

Food and Measure	cal.	prot. (gms)	carbo. (gms)	fat (gms)	chol. (mgs)	sod. (mgs)	fiber (gms)
Soup, canned, ready-to-serve, vegetable beef *(cont.)*							
chunky (*Campbell's Healthy Request Low Sodium*), 10¾ oz.	160	13.0	11.0	4.5	80	95	4.0
w/pasta (*Campbell's Simply Home*) . . .	120	6.0	19.0	1.5	10	790	2.0
vegetable broth:							
(*Arrowhead Mills*)	15	0	3.0	0	0	590	0
(*College Inn*)	20	0	5.0	0	0	780	0
(*Swanson* Clear) . . .	20	0	3.0	1.0	0	1000	0
Soup, canned, condensed, undiluted, ½ cup:							
asparagus, cream of (*Campbell's*)	90	3.0	11.0	3.5	5	860	1.0
barley and mushroom (*Manischewitz*)	100	3.0	16.0	2.5	0	1040	4.0
bean:							
w/bacon (*Campbell's*)	180	8.0	25.0	5.0	<5	890	7.0
black (*Campbell's*)	110	5.0	19.0	2.0	0	1000	5.0
and ham, w/bacon (*Campbell's Healthy Request*)	150	7.0	26.0	2.0	5	480	7.0
beef:							
broth, double rich (*Campbell's*)	15	3.0	1.0	0	<5	900	0
consommé (*Campbell's*)	25	4.0	2.0	0	<5	820	0
noodle (*Campbell's*)	70	5.0	8.0	2.5	15	920	1.0
w/vegetables, barley (*Campbell's*)	80	5.0	11.0	2.0	15	920	2.0
broccoli:							
cream of (*Campbell's*)	100	2.0	9.0	6.0	<5	770	1.0
cream of (*Campbell's* 98% Fat Free)	80	2.0	12.0	3.0	<5	720	1.0

Food and Measure	cal.	prot. (gms)	carbo. (gms)	fat (gms)	chol. (mgs)	sod. (mgs)	fiber (gms)
cream of (*Campbell's Healthy Request*)	70	2.0	9.0	2.0	5	480	1.0
broccoli cheese:							
(*Campbell's*)	110	3.0	9.0	7.0	10	860	2.0
cheddar and onion (*Healthy Choice*)	90	3.0	15.0	2.0	5	560	2.0
cream of (*Campbell's 98% Fat Free*)	80	3.0	11.0	3.0	10	850	1.0
celery, cream of:							
(*Campbell's*)	110	2.0	9.0	7.0	<5	900	1.0
(*Campbell's 98% Fat Free*)	80	2.0	11.0	3.5	5	900	1.0
(*Campbell's Healthy Request*)	70	2.0	11.0	2.0	5	480	1.0
(*Healthy Choice*) ...	75	1.0	14.0	2.0	<5	365	3.0
cheese:							
cheddar (*Campbell's*)	90	4.0	10.0	4.0	15	950	1.0
nacho (*Campbell's Fiesta*)	140	5.0	11.0	8.0	15	810	2.0
chicken:							
alphabet, w/vegetables (*Campbell's*)	80	4.0	11.0	2.0	10	880	1.0
broth (*Campbell's*)	30	2.0	2.0	2.0	<5	770	0
broth (*Manischewitz*)	15	<1.0	2.0	.5	0	740	2.0
cream of (*Campbell's*)	130	3.0	11.0	8.0	10	890	1.0
cream of (*Campbell's 98% Fat Free*)	80	3.0	9.0	3.0	10	910	0
cream of (*Campbell's Healthy Request*)	70	2.0	12.0	2.0	15	480	0
cream of, and broccoli (*Campbell's*)	120	4.0	9.0	8.0	15	860	1.0

Food and Measure	cal.	prot. (gms)	carbo. (gms)	fat (gms)	chol. (mgs)	sod. (mgs)	fiber (gms)
Soup, canned, condensed, chicken *(cont.)*							
cream of, and broccoli (*Campbell's Healthy Request*)	80	3.0	10.0	2.5	5	480	1.0
cream of, w/herbs (*Campbell's*)	80	3.0	9.0	4.0	10	920	1.0
cream of, roasted (*Healthy Choice*)	80	2.0	13.0	3.0	<5	350	3.0
dumplings (*Campbell's*)	80	4.0	10.0	3.0	25	1050	2.0
gumbo (*Campbell's*)	60	2.0	9.0	1.5	10	990	1.0
w/kreplach (*Manischewitz*)	35	2.0	5.0	1.0	0	880	3.0
w/matzo balls (*Manischewitz*)	80	3.0	9.0	4.0	25	880	2.0
mushroom, cream of (*Campbell's*)	130	3.0	9.0	9.0	15	1000	1.0
noodle (*Campbell's*)	70	3.0	9.0	2.0	15	980	1.0
noodle (*Campbell's Homestyle*)	70	4.0	9.0	2.5	20	970	1.0
noodle (*Campbell's Healthy Request*)	70	3.0	9.0	2.0	15	480	0
noodle (*Campbell's Noodle O's*)	80	4.0	10.0	3.0	15	980	1.0
noodle (*Manischewitz*)	35	2.0	6.0	.5	0	830	1.0
noodle, creamy (*Campbell's*)	130	5.0	12.0	7.0	15	880	2.0
noodle, curly (*Campbell's*)	80	3.0	12.0	2.5	15	840	1.0
rice (*Campbell's*)	70	3.0	9.0	2.5	<5	940	0
w/rice (*Campbell's Healthy Request*)	60	2.0	10.0	2.5	15	480	<1.0
and stars (*Campbell's*)	70	3.0	9.0	2.0	<5	1010	1.0
vegetable (*Campbell's*)	80	3.0	12.0	2.0	10	940	2.0
vegetable (*Campbell's Healthy Request*)	80	3.0	12.0	2.0	5	480	1.0

Food and Measure	cal.	prot. (gms)	carbo. (gms)	fat (gms)	chol. (mgs)	sod. (mgs)	fiber (gms)
vegetable, Southwestern (Campbell's)	110	7.0	18.0	1.5	10	900	4.0
w/white and wild rice (Campbell's)	70	3.0	9.0	2.0	10	900	1.0
chili beef, w/beans (Campbell's Fiesta)	170	7.0	24.0	5.0	15	910	4.0
clam chowder, Manhattan:							
(Campbell's)	60	2.0	12.0	.5	<5	910	2.0
(Chincoteague)	100	8.0	13.0	2.0	15	990	1.0
clam chowder, New England:							
(Campbell's)	90	4.0	13.0	2.5	5	980	1.0
(Cape Cod Premium 99% Fat Free) ...	60	2.0	10.0	1.0	5	650	0
(Chincoteague)	80	5.0	10.0	2.5	10	590	<1.0
corn chowder (Chincoteague)	100	2.0	16.0	3.5	0	890	1.0
crab, cream of (Chincoteague)	200	11.0	23.0	6.0	35	830	0
garlic, cream of roasted (Healthy Choice)	60	<1.0	13.0	1.0	<5	490	3.0
lentil (Manischewitz)	140	7.0	24.0	2.0	0	1310	4.0
lobster bisque (Chincoteague)	90	4.0	10.0	4.0	15	650	0
minestrone:							
(Campbell's)	90	4.0	15.0	1.5	5	910	4.0
(Campbell's Healthy Request)	90	4.0	17.0	1.0	0	480	2.0
Manischewitz)	90	3.0	16.0	1.50		760	2.0
mushroom:							
beefy (Campbell's)	70	5.0	6.0	3.0	10	1000	1.0
cream of (Campbell's)	110	2.0	9.0	7.0	<5	870	1.0
cream of (Campbell's 98% Fat Free)	70	1.0	9.0	3.0	<5	830	0

Food and Measure	cal.	prot. (gms)	carbo. (gms)	fat (gms)	chol. (mgs)	sod. (mgs)	fiber (gms)
Soup, canned, condensed, mushroom *(cont.)*							
cream of (*Campbell's Healthy Request*)	70	1.0	10.0	2.5	10	480	0
cream of (*Healthy Choice*)	55	1.0	13.0	1.0	<5	480	3.0
cream of, w/roasted garlic (*Campbell's*)	70	2.0	10.0	2.5	<5	790	<1.0
golden (*Campbell's*)	80	2.0	10.0	3.0	<5	930	1.0
noodle (see also "chicken," above):							
double, in chicken broth (*Campbell's*)	100	4.0	15.0	2.5	15	810	2.0
and ground beef (*Campbell's*)	100	5.0	11.0	4.02	5	900	2.0
stars, super (*Campbell's*)	50	2.0	7.0	1.5	<5	950	<1.0
onion:							
cream of (*Campbell's*)	110	2.0	13.0	6.0	20	910	1.0
French (*Campbell's*)	70	2.0	10.0	2.5	<5	980	1.0
oyster stew (*Campbell's*)	90	2.0	6.0	6.0	20	940	0
pasta, *Rugrats*, w/chicken in broth (*Campbell's*)	60	2.0	9.0	1.5	<5	920	1.0
pea:							
green (*Campbell's*)	180	9.0	29.0	3.0	<5	890	5.0
split, w/ham (*Campbell's*)	180	10.0	28.0	3.5	<5	860	5.0
pepperpot (*Campbell's*)	100	4.0	9.0	5.0	15	1020	1.0
potato, cream of (*Campbell's*)	90	2.0	14.0	3.0	10	890	1.0
Scotch broth (*Campbell's*)	80	4.0	9.0	3.0	5	900	1.0
shrimp, cream of (*Campbell's*)	100	2.0	8.0	7.0	20	890	1.0
tomato:							
(*Campbell's*)	80	2.0	19.0	0	0	760	1.0

Food and Measure	cal.	prot. (gms)	carbo. (gms)	fat (gms)	chol. (mgs)	sod. (mgs)	fiber (gms)
(*Campbell's Healthy Request*)	90	1.0	18.0	1.5	0	460	1.0
bisque (*Campbell's*)	130	2.0	24.0	3.0	<5	900	2.0
garden, w/herbs (*Healthy Choice*)	80	2.0	18.0	1.0	0	300	3.0
Italian, w/basil, oreggano (*Campbell's*)	100	2.0	23.0	.5	0	820	2.0
rice (*Campbell's* Old Fashioned)	120	2.0	23.0	2.0	<5	790	1.0
turkey:							
noodle (*Campbell's*)	80	4.0	10.0	2.5	15	970	1.0
vegetable (*Campbell's*)	80	3.0	11.0	2.5	10	840	2.0
vegetable:							
(*Campbell's*)	80	2.0	17.0	.5	<5	920	2.0
(*Campbell's* Old Fashioned)	70	2.0	10.0	2.5	<5	950	2.0
(*Campbell's Healthy Request*)	90	3.0	16.0	1.0	5	480	2.0
beef (*Campbell's*)	80	4.0	14.0	1.0	10	890	2.0
beef (*Campbell's Healthy Request*)	80	5.0	11.0	2.0	5	480	2.0
California style (*Campbell's*)	60	3.0	10.0	1.0	5	850	2.0
hearty, w/pasta (*Campbell's*)	90	2.0	18.0	1.0	0	830	2.0
hearty, w/pasta (*Campbell's Healthy Request*)	90	3.0	16.0	1.0	5	480	2.0
vegetarian (*Campbell's*)	90	3.0	18.0	1.0	0	770	2.0
won ton (*Campbell's*)	45	4.0	5.0	1.0	15	940	1.0
Soup, frozen:							
clam chowder (*Marie Callender's*), 13½-oz. bowl	590	24.0	87.0	16.0	25	1740	11.0
corn chowder (*Cascadian Farm Veggie Bowl*), 9-oz. pkg.	170	7.0	29.0	4.0	10	570	2.0

Food and Measure	cal.	prot. (gms)	carbo. (gms)	fat (gms)	chol. (mgs)	sod. (mgs)	fiber (gms)
Soup, frozen *(cont.)*							
mushroom and barley							
(*Ratner's*), 1 cup . . .	120	5.0	23.0	1.0	0	690	3.0
split pea (*Ratner's*),							
1 cup	110	5.0	18.0	2.0	30	470	7.0
vegetable (*Ratner's*),							
1 cup	120	5.0	21.0	1.0	0	650	4.0
Soup, packaged,							
readyto-serve,							
1 cup:							
broccoli, creamy							
(*Imagine*)	70	5.0	12.0	1.0	0	450	3.0
broth, no-chicken							
(*Imagine*)	45	2.0	5.0	2.0	0	500	0
butternut squash,							
creamy (*Imagine*)	90	3.0	19.0	2.0	0	430	3.0
chicken broth (*Swan-*							
son Clear)	10	1.0	<1.0	.5	<5	910	0
corn, sweet, creamy							
(*Imagine*)	90	2.0	18.0	3.0	0	480	5.0
gazpacho (*Imagine*)	60	<1.0	5.0	0	0	720	<1.0
mushroom (*Imagine*)	60	<1.0	5.0	0	0	720	<1.0
potato leek (*Imagine*)	90	<1.0	11.0	2.0	0	550	<1.0
tomato (*Imagine*)	90	1.0	10.0	1.5	0	620	2.0
vegetable broth (*Imag-*							
ine)	30	0	3.0	1.0	0	580	0
Soup, mix (see also							
"Soup base mix"),							
dry, 1 pkg., except							
as noted:							
asparagus, creamy:							
(*Fantastic*							
Foods Cup)	130	6.0	22.0	2.5	5	480	3.0
(*Maggi*), 1/4 pkg.	60	2.0	10.0	2.0	0	940	0
bean:							
black (*Bean-Cuisine*							
Island), 1 oz.	100	6.0	17.0	0	0	0	7.0
black (*Fantastic*							
Foods							
Jumpin' Cup) . . .	210	12.0	39.0	1.0	0	470	8.0
black (*Knorr* Cup)	190	9.0	10.0	1.0	0	660	10.0

Food and Measure	cal.	prot. (gms)	carbo. (gms)	fat (gms)	chol. (mgs)	sod. (mgs)	fiber (gms)
black (*Knorr* Taste Breaks)	190	9.0	36.0	1.0	0	660	10.0
black (*Manischewitz* Instant)	200	11.0	37.0	1.0	0	320	5.0
black (*Smart Soup*)	190	10.0	32.0	1.5	0	560	13.0
black, spicy, w/couscous (*Health Valley*), ⅓ cup	130	6.0	29.0	0	0	190	5.0
black, zesty, w/rice (*Health Valley*), cup	100	5.0	22.0	0	0	190	4.0
five (*Fantastic Foods* Hearty Cup)	230	12.0	43.0	1.0	0	480	10.0
four (*Manischewitz*), ⅕ pkg. ...	110	6.0	20.0	.5	0	900	6.0
lima w/barley (*Manischewitz*), ⅙ pkg.	08	4.0	19.0	.5	0	670	3.0
multi (*AlpineAire*), 1¾ oz.	170	9.0	28.0	3.0	0	570	8.0
navy (*Knorr* Cup)	130	6.0	25.0	.5	0	820	7.0
rice, see "rice and beans," below							
seven, and barley, all varieties (*Arrowhead Mills*), ¼ cup	170	12.0	35.0	0	0	330	7.0
thirteen, bouillabaisee (*Bean Cuisine*), 1 oz.	100	6.0	18.0	0	0	0	5.0
white (*Bean Cuisine* Provençal), 1 oz.	100	6.0	17.0	0	0	0	5.0
bean, w/bacon and ham (*Campbell's* Microwave)	180	8.0	26.0	6.0	10	750	7.0
bean and ham (*Hormel* Micro Cup)	190	9.0	29.0	4.0	15	680	7.0
bean and pasta (*Bean Cuisine* Ultima Pasta E Fagioli), 1 oz. ...	100	6.0	18.0	.5	0	0	4.0

Food and Measure	cal.	prot. (gms)	carbo. (gms)	fat (gms)	chol. (mgs)	sod. (mgs)	fiber (gms)
Soup, mix *(cont.)*							
beef noodle (*Maggi*),							
¼ pkg.	50	2.0	9.0	1.0	0	1110	0
beef vegetable (*Hormel* Micro Cup)	90	6.0	15.0	1.0	10	790	1.0
broccoli, cream of:							
(*AlpineAire*), 1.2 oz.	130	5.0	16.0	5.0	15	870	1.0
(*Knorr* Soup/Recipe), 3 tbsp.	70	2.0	10.0	2.5	0	730	1.0
broccoli cheese:							
(*Cup-a-Soup*)	70	2.0	9.0	3.0	5	550	<1.0
cheddar (*Fantastic Foods* Cup)	160	7.0	26.0	3.0	10	590	2.0
w/ham (*Hormel* Micro Cup)	170	4.0	10.0	13.0	40	710	1.0
and rice (*Uncle Ben's* Hearty) . . .	160	7.0	26.0	3.0	5	870	1.0
chicken:							
broth (*Cup-a-Soup*)	20	1.0	3.0	0	0	440	0
broth w/pasta (*Cup-a-Soup*)	45	2.0	8.0	0	0	450	0
country, w/pasta and herbs (*Lipton Soup Secrets Kettle Style*), 1 cup*	100	4.0	18.0	1.5	5	740	1.0
cream of (*Cup-a-Soup*)	70	1.0	12.0	2.0	0	640	<1.0
creamy (*Maggi*), ¼ pkg.	60	2.0	9.0	1.5	0	1070	0
noodle (*Campbell's* Microwave)	90	5.0	10.0	4.0	20	850	1.0
noodle (*Campbell's* Soup/Recipe), 3 tbsp.	90	4.0	15.0	1.5	10	660	0
noodle (*Cup-a-Soup*)	50	2.0	8.0	1.0	10	540	0
noodle (*Hormel* Micro Cup)	110	8.0	13.0	2.5	35	790	0
noodle (*Knorr* Taste Breaks)	120	4.0	20.0	2.0	20	910	1.0

Food and Measure	cal.	prot. (gms)	carbo. (gms)	fat (gms)	chol. (mgs)	sod. (mgs)	fiber (gms)
noodle (*Maggi*), ¼ pkg.	50	2.0	9.0	1.0	0	910	0
noodle (*Manischewitz* Instant)	140	3.0	26.0	2.0	15	840	0
noodle, double (*Campbell's* Soup/ Recipe)	170	7.0	32.0	2.0	30	740	1.0
noodle, hearty (*Cup-a-Soup*)	60	3.0	10.0	1.0	15	590	0
noodle, w/white chicken meat (*Lipton* Soup Mix), 3 tbsp.	80	3.0	11.0	2.0	15	690	0
'n onion (*Lipton Soup Secrets Kettle Style*), 1 cup*	120	4.0	24.0	1.5	5	740	1.0
w/pasta and beans (*Lipton Soup Secrets Kettle Style*), 1 cup* ...	110	5.0	19.0	1.5	5	700	3.0
rice (*Campbell's* Microwave)	120	5.0	20.0	2.5	10	1130	2.0
rice (*Hormel* Micro Cup)	110	5.0	17.0	3.0	15	950	1.0
rice (*Maggi*), ¼ pkg.	50	1.0	10.0	1.0	0	910	0
rice (*Manischewitz* Instant)	130	3.0	28.0	1.0	0	840	1.0
rice (*Mrs. Grass*), ¼ pkg.	80	2.0	15.0	1.0	0	1000	0
seashell (*Maggi*), ¼ pkg.	50	2.0	9.0	1.0	0	640	0
thyme (*Aunt Patsy's Pantry*), 2 tbsp.	100	4.0	20.0	.5	0	350	2.0
vegetable (*Knorr* Cup)	120	4.0	21.0	1.5	<5	860	1.0
vegetable (*Smart Soup*)	130	6.0	24.0	1.5	25	590	1.0
chili (*Fantastic ChaCha Hearty Cup*)	220	18.0	37.0	1.0	0	470	13.0

Food and Measure	cal.	prot. (gms)	carbo. (gms)	fat (gms)	chol. (mgs)	sod. (mgs)	fiber (gms)
Soup, mix *(cont.)*							
clam chowder, New England (*Hormel* Micro Cup)	130	5.0	17.0	5.0	25	820	1.0
corn chowder:							
(*AlpineAire* Kernel's), 2 oz.	200	13.0	35.0	1.5	0	151	1.0
(*Knorr* Cup)	140	3.0	26.0	3.0	10	700	2.0
(*Smart Soup*)	100	4.0	23.0	1.0	0	300	1.0
and potato, creamy (*Fantastic Foods* Cup)	170	6.0	34.0	2.0	5	440	3.0
w/tomatoes (*Health Valley*), ¼ cup ...	100	4.0	21.0	0	0	190	3.0
couscous:							
(*Casbah* Moroccan Stew Cup)	180	5.0	38.0	0	0	460	2.0
w/lentil (*Fantastic Foods* Cup)	230	12.0	44.0	1.0	0	480	7.0
garlic, roasted, herb (*Knorr* Soup/Recipe), 3 tbsp.	80	2.0	13.0	1.5	0	860	0
garlic mushroom, creamy (*Fantastic Foods* Cup)	160	7.0	28.0	3.0	10	480	2.0
herb:							
fiesta, w/red pepper (*Lipton Recipe Secrets*), 1 cup*	30	1.0	6.0	0	0	560	0
fine (*Knorr* Soup/ Recipe), 3 tbsp.	110	3.0	13.0	5.0	<5	910	0
golden, w/lemon (*Lipton Recipe Secrets*), 1 cup*	35	<1.0	7.0	.5	0	510	0
Italian, w/tomato (*Lipton Recipe Secrets*), 1 cup*	40	<1.0	9.0	.5	0	510	0
savory, w/garlic (*Lipton Recipe Secrets*), 1 cup*	30	1.0	6.0	0	0	480	0

Food and Measure	cal.	prot. (gms)	carbo. (gms)	fat (gms)	chol. (mgs)	sod. (mgs)	fiber (gms)
leek (*Knorr* Soup/Recipe), 2 tbsp.	70	2.0	9.0	2.5	<5	810	0
lentil:							
(*Fantastic Foods* Country Cup)	230	15.0	41.0	1.0	0	480	12.0
(*Smart Soup*)	190	9.0	35.0	1.0	0	490	5.0
hearty (*Knorr* Taste Breaks)	200	10.0	38.0	1.0	0	820	5.0
hearty (*Manischewitz*)	140	6.0	26.0	1.0	0	1090	2.0
homestyle, w/bow-tie pasta (*Lipton Soup Secrets Kettle Style*), 1 cup*	130	7.0	22.0	1.0	0	750	5.0
w/couscous (*Health Valley*), 1/3 cup	130	7.0	28.0	0	0	190	5.0
matzo ball (*Manischewitz* Instant)	40	1.0	9.0	1.5	14	800	1.0
minestrone: (*AlpineAire*), 1 3/4 oz.	170	7.0	33.0	1.0	0	440	6.0
(*Fantastic Foods* Cup)	150	6.0	29.0	1.0	0	480	4.0
(*Lipton Soup Secrets Kettle Style*), 1 cup* . . .	110	4.0	21.0	1.0	0	750	4.0
(*Manischewitz*), 1/4 pkg.	150	9.0	27.0	0	0	700	3.0
(*Manischewitz* Instant)	210	9.0	39.0	1.5	0	760	6.0
(*Smart Soup*)	120	4.0	24.0	.5	0	590	3.0
Mediterranean (*Knorr*), 3 tbsp.	100	2.0	18.0	2.0	0	810	3.0
mushroom:							
beefy (*Lipton Recipe Secrets*), 1 1/2 tbsp.	35	1.0	7.0	0	0	640	0
creamy (*Cup-a-Soup*)	60	1.0	10.0	2.0	0	610	0
noodle:							
chicken free (*Fantastic* Ramen Cup)	140	8.0	26.0	.5	0	540	4.0

Food and Measure	cal.	prot. (gms)	carbo. (gms)	fat (gms)	chol. (mgs)	sod. (mgs)	fiber (gms)
Soup, mix, noodle *(cont.)*							
onion and Oriental (*Sanwa* Ramen), ½ block	180	11.0	26.0	7.0	0	700	1.0
ring noodle (*Cup-a-Soup*)	50	2.0	9.0	1.0	10	560	0
noodle, beef:							
(*Campbell's* Baked Ramen), ½ block	140	4.0	30.0	1.0	0	830	1.0
(*Campbell's* Fried Ramen)	290	6.0	41.0	11.0	<5	1220	2.0
(*Campbell's* Low Fat Ramen)	210	6.0	44.0	1.0	0	980	2.0
(*Campbell's/Sanwa* Ramen), ½ block	170	3.0	26.0	6.0	0	750	1.0
(*Nissin Cup Noodles*)	300	6.0	38.0	14.0	0	100	2.0
(*Nissin Cup Noodles* Twin), 1.2 oz.	150	3.0	20.0	6.0	0	720	1.0
(*Nissin Top Ramen*)	190	4.0	28.0	7.0	0	700	<1.0
hot sauce (*Nissin Cup Noodles*)	290	6.0	35.0	14.0	0	1090	2.0
picante (*Nissin Top Ramen*)	180	4.0	26.0	7.0	0	830	1.0
noodle, chicken:							
(*Campbell's* Baked Ramen), ½ block	140	4.0	30.0	1.0	0	720	1.0
(*Campbell's* Low Fat Ramen)	210	6.0	43.0	1.0	0	1150	2.0
(*Knorr* Box), 2 tbsp.	90	3.0	17.0	1.0	15	800	0
(*Nissin Cup Noodles*)	300	6.0	36.0	14.0	<5	1170	2.0
(*Nissin Cup Noodles* Twin), 1.2 oz.	150	3.0	20.0	7.0	0	710	<1.0
(*Nissin Top Ramen*)	180	4.0	26.0	7.0	0	800	<1.0
broth (*Mrs. Grass*), ¼ pkg.	60	2.0	10.0	1.5	20	880	0
w/broth (*Lipton* Soup Mix), 2 tbsp.	60	2.0	9.0	2.0	15	720	0

Food and Measure	cal.	prot. (gms)	carbo. (gms)	fat (gms)	chol. (mgs)	sod. (mgs)	fiber (gms)
w/broth (*Lipton Ring O-Noodle* Soup Mix), 2 tbsp.	70	2.0	10.0	2.0	15	720	0
w/broth, extra noodle (*Lipton* Soup Mix), 3 tbsp.	90	3.0	15.0	1.5	25	680	<1.0
w/broth, giggle noodle (*Lipton* Soup Mix), 2 tbsp.	70	2.0	11.0	2.0	20	750 ·	0
w/broth, real (*Campbell's* Quality), 3 tbsp.	100	3.0	17.0	1.5	10	740	1.0
Cajun (*Nissin Cup Noodles*)	300	7.0	37.0	14.0	0	1240	2.0
Cajun (*Nissin Top Ramen*)	180	4.0	26.0	7.0	0	890	<1.0
creamy (*Nissin Cup Noodles*)	300	7.0	39.0	13.0	5	1240	2.0
creamy (*Nissin Top Ramen*)	190	5.0	26.0	7.0	<5	710	1.0
flavor, hearty (*Knorr* Cup)	120	4.0	20.0	2.0	20	910	1.0
flavor, savory (*Knorr*), 3 tbsp.	70	3.0	11.0	1.5	10	650	1.0
hot sauce (*Nissin Cup Noodles*)	300	6.0	37.0	13.0	<5	1130	2.0
mushroom (*Nissin Cup Noodles*)	300	5.0	38.0	14.0	0	1140	2.0
mushroom (*Nissin Top Ramen*)	190	4.0	27.0	7.0	0	720	1.0
sesame (*Nissin Top Ramen*)	190	4.0	27.0	7.0	0	900	1.0
spicy (*Campbell's Baked Ramen*), ½ block	140	4.0	30.0	1.0	0	780	1.0
spicy (*Campbell's/ Sanwa Ramen*), ½ block	170	3.0	26.0	6.0	0	740	1.0
spicy (*Nissin Cup Noodles*)	300	6.0	38.0	14.0	0	1120	3.0

Food and Measure	cal.	prot. (gms)	carbo. (gms)	fat (gms)	chol. (mgs)	sod. (mgs)	fiber (gms)
Soup, mix, noodle, chicken *(cont.)*							
teriyaki (*Nissin Cup Noodles*)	300	7.0	37.0	14.0	0	1030	2.0
teriyaki (*Nissin Top Ramen*)	190	4.0	28.0	7.0	0	600	1.0
vegetable (*Nissin Cup Noodles*)	300	7.0	37.0	14.0	0	1120	2.0
vegetable (*Nissin Cup Noodles Twin*), 1.2 oz. ...	160	3.0	21.0	7.0	0	720	<1.0
vegetable (*Nissin Top Ramen*)	190	4.0	27.0	7.0	0	790	1.0
w/vegetables (*Health Valley*), ⅓ cup	110	3.0	24.0	0	0	190	3.0
noodle, chili (*Nissin Top Ramen*)	190	4.0	26.0	8.0	0	690	<1.0
noodle, onion, French (*Nissin Cup Noodles*)	300	7.0	40.0	12.0	5	1170	2.0
noodle, Oriental (*Nissin Top Ramen*) ...	190	4.0	26.0	7.0	0	830	1.0
noodle, pork:							
(*Campbell's Ramen*), ½ block	170	4.0	26.0	6.0	0	850	1.0
(*Nissin Cup Noodles*)	300	6.0	36.0	14.0	0	1130	2.0
(*Nissin Top Ramen*)	180	4.0	26.0	7.0	0	760	<1.0
noodle, seafood (*Nissin Cup Noodles*)	300	7.0	36.0	14.0	0	1240	2.0
noodle, shrimp:							
(*Campbell's Fried Ramen*), ½ block	170	3.0	26.0	6.0	0	740	1.0
(*Nissin Cup Noodles*)	300	6.0	38.0	14.0	10	1070	2.0
(*Nissin Cup Noodles Twin*), 1.2 oz. ...	150	3.0	21.0	6.0	<5	730	<1.0
(*Nissin Top Ramen*)	190	4.0	27.0	7.0	0	800	1.0
hot sauce (*Nissin Cup Noodles*)	300	7.0	38.0	13.0	10	1210	2.0

Food and Measure	cal.	prot. (gms)	carbo. (gms)	fat (gms)	chol. (mgs)	sod. (mgs)	fiber (gms)
picante (*Nissin Cup Noodles*)	310	6.0	37.0	15.0	5	980	2.0
noodle, vegetable:							
curry (*Fantastic Foods* Ramen Cup)	140	6.0	28.0	1.0	0	490	3.0
miso (*Fantastic Foods* Ramen Cup)	130	5.0	25.0	1.0	0	540	2.0
tomato(*Fantastic Foods* Ramen Cup)	150	5.0	31.0	1.0	0	490	3.0
onion:							
(*Campbell's* Soup & Recipe), 1 tbsp.	20	0	5.0	0	0	530	0
(*Lipton Recipe Secrets*), 1 tbsp.	20	0	4.0	0	0	610	0
(*Mrs. Grass* Reduced Sodium), ¼ pkg.	3	51.0	7.0	0	0	490	0
(*Mrs. Grass* Soup/ Recipe), ¼ pkg.	35	1.0	6.0	.5	0	980	0
beefy (*Lipton Recipe Secrets*), 1 tbsp.	25	1.0	5.0	.5	0	610	0
French (*Knorr* Soup/ Recipe), 2 tbsp.	35	1.0	6.0	1.0	0	790	0
golden (*Lipton Recipe Secrets*), 1 tbsp.	50	1.0	9.0	1.0	0	700	0
onion mushroom:							
(*Lipton Recipe Secrets*), 1 tbsp.	30	1.0	5.0	.5	0	640	0
(*Mrs. Grass* Soup/ Recipe), ¼ pkg.	60	2.0	10.0	1.0	0	1080	0
orzo thyme (*Buckeye*), ¼ pkg.	210	7.0	41.0	1.0	0	270	2.0
oxtail, tomato beef flavor (*Knorr* Soup/ Recipe), 2 tbsp. . . .	60	2.0	9.0	2.0	<5	1030	0

Food and Measure	cal.	prot. (gms)	carbo. (gms)	fat (gms)	chol. (mgs)	sod. (mgs)	fiber (gms)
Soup, mix *(cont.)*							
pasta:							
Italiano (*Health Valley* Fat Free),							
½ cup	140	5.0	31.0	0	0	190	3.0
marinara,Parmesan, or Mediterranean (*Health Valley* Healthy Pasta),							
½ cup	100	5.0	20.0	0	0	190	1.0
spiral,w/chicken broth (*Lipton* Soup Mix),							
3 tbsp.	60	2.0	11.0	1.0	0	660	0
pasta and bean (*Casbah Pasta Fasul*) . . .	160	11.0	12.0	0	0	470	2.0
pea, green (*Cup-a-Soup*)	80	4.0	12.0	1.0	0	520	3.0
pea, split:							
(*AlpineAire* Souper), 1.2 oz.	200	14.0	34.0	1.5	0	380	9.0
(*Fantastic* Hearty Cup)	190	12.0	35.0	1.0	0	470	8.0
(*Knorr* Taste Breaks)	150	8.0	28.0	1.0	0	730	4.0
(*Smart Soup*)	150	8.0	28.0	.5	0	460	7.0
w/barley (*Manischewitz*), ⅕ pkg. . . .	110	7.0	21.0	0	0	780	3.0
garden, w/carrots (*Health Valley*),							
½ cup	130	8.0	22.0	0	0	190	2.0
potato, creamy:							
(*Maggi*), ¼ pkg.	70	2.0	11.0	2.0	0	820	0
w/broccoli (*Health Valley*), ⅓ cup . . .	70	4.0	17.0	0	0	190	3.0
w/cheddar (*AlpineAire*), 2 oz.	220	9.0	30.0	7.0	20	1020	1.0
potato cheese, w/ham (*Hormel* Micro Cup)	190	4.0	15.0	13.0	50	750	1.0
potato leek:							
(*Knorr* Cup)	130	4.0	22.0	2.5	10	920	1.0
(*Smart Soup*)	120	6.0	23.0	1.0	5	590	1.0

Food and Measure	cal.	prot. (gms)	carbo. (gms)	fat (gms)	chol. (mgs)	sod. (mgs)	fiber (gms)
creamy (*Fantastic Foods* Cup)	120	4.0	21.0	2.0	.5	590	2.0
rice (*Casbah Thai Yum*)	160	4.0	30.0	0	0	470	2.0
rice and beans:							
(*Casbah* La Fiesta)	170	6.0	34.0	1.0	0	400	4.0
Cajun (*Casbah* Jambalaya)	128	4.0	27.0	0	0	490	2.0
Mexican(*Campbell's* Soupsations)	210	2.0	41.0	1.5	<5	930	6.0
red (*Smart Soup*)	180	8.0	35.0	1.0	0	460	7.0
seafood, creamy (*Maggi*), ¼ pkg.	80	5.0	10.0	2.5	20	1130	<1.0
spicy (*Maggi* Thick n Spicy), ½ pkg.	110	4.0	18.0	2.0	0	1400	1.0
spinach, cream of (*Knorr* Soup/Recipe), 2 tbsp.	70	2.0	10.0	2.5	0	760	<1.0
tomato:							
(*Cup-a-Soup*)	100	2.0	20.0	1.0	5	510	<1.0
basil (*Knorr* Soup/ Recipe), 3 tbsp.	80	2.0	13.0	2.5	0	920	0
vegetable:							
(*Knorr* Soup/Recipe), 2 tbsp.	30	1.0	6.0	.5	0	730	1.0
(*Lipton Recipe Secrets*), 1⅔ tbsp.	30	<1.0	7.0	0	0	600	1.0
barley (*Fantastic Foods* Hearty Cup)	150	6.0	29.0	.5	0	470	6.0
beef (*Campbell's* Microwave)	90	5.0	13.0	2.0	10	780	2.0
chickenflavor (*Cup-a-Soup*)	50	1.0	10.0	1.0	10	520	0
chicken flavor (*Knorr*) ....:	120	4.0	21.0	1.5	<5	860	1.0
chicken flavor, creamy (*Cup-a-Soup*)	80	2.0	10.0	4.5	0	590	<1.0
cream of, savory (*Knorr*), 3 tbsp.	100	2.0	12.0	4.5	0	870	1.0

Food and Measure	cal.	prot. (gms)	carbo. (gms)	fat (gms)	chol. (mgs)	sod. (mgs)	fiber (gms)
Soup, mix, vegetable *(cont.)*							
w/mushrooms (*Manischewitz*),							
⅕ pkg.	120	7.0	22.0	0	0	700	3.0
spring (*Cup-a-Soup*)	45	2.0	8.0	1.0	10	500	<1.0
spring (*Knorr* Soup/ Recipe), 2 tbsp.	25	1.0	5.0	0	0	610	1.0
vegetarian (*Knorr* Cup)	160	6.0	32.0	1.0	0	870	3.0
Soup base mix,							
⅛ pkg., except as noted:							
beef:							
(*Watkins* Soup/ Gravy), 2 tsp. . . .	15	1.0	2.0	1.0	0	730	0
barley vegetable (*Wyler's Soup Starter*)	100	3.0	20.0	.5	0	960	0
ground, vegetable (*Wyler's Soup Starter*)	80	3.0	17.0	.5	0	990	2.0
stew, hearty (*Wyler's Stew Starter*)	60	1.0	15.0	0	0	660	2.0
vegetable (*Wyler's Soup Starter*) . . .	90	3.0	19.0	.5	0	990	2.0
cheese (*Watkins* Soup/ Gravy), 2½ tbsp.	90	2.0	12.0	3.0	5	490	0
chicken:							
(*Watkins* Soup/ Gravy), 2 tsp. . . .	15	1.0	2.0	1.0	0	560	0
noodle (*Watkins* Soup/Gravy), 1 tbsp.	25	1.0	5.0	0	5	470	0
noodle (*Wyler's Soup Starter*) . . .	80	2.0	17.0	.5	5	960	1.0
vegetable, hearty (*Wyler's Soup Starter*), ⅐ pkg.	70	2.0	16.0	0	0	850	2.0
w/white and wild rice (*Wyler's Soup Starter*)	70	2.0	15.0	0	0	790	1.0

Food and Measure	cal.	prot. (gms)	carbo. (gms)	fat (gms)	chol. (mgs)	sod. (mgs)	fiber (gms)
cream (*Watkins* Soup/ Gravy), 2½ tbsp.	90	2.0	4.0	10.0	15	1146	0
mushroom (*Watkins* Soup/Gravy), 2 tbsp.	60	2.0	9.0	2.0	0	490	0
onion (*Watkins* Soup/ Gravy), 2 tsp.	20	1.0	3.0	1.0	0	390	0
tomato (*Watkins* Soup/Gravy), 5 tsp.	45	1.0	10.0	0	0	420	1.0
vegetable, vegetarian (*Watkins* Soup/ Gravy), 2 tsp.	15	0	3.0	0	0	760	0
Sour cream, see "Cream, sour"							
Sour cream dip mix (*Durkee*), 2 tsp. . . .	25	1.0	4.0	.5	0	200	0
Soursop, ½ cup	75	1.1	18.9	.3	0	16	3.7
Soy bean, see "Soy- bean"							
Soy beverage, 8 fl. oz., except as noted:							
(*Edensoy/Edensoy* Ex- tra)	130	10.0	13.0	4.0	0	105	0
(*Edensoy/Edensoy* Ex- tra), 8.45 fl. oz. . . .	135	10.0	14.0	4.0	0	110	0
(*Soy Dream* Original)	140	8.0	14.0	5.0	0	140	0
(*Soy Moo* Fat Free) . . .	110	6.0	22.0	0	0	60	1.0
carob (*Soy Dream*) . . .	210	7.0	36.0	4.5	0	150	0
chocolate (*Soy Dream* Enriched)	210	7.0	35.0	4.5	0	150	0
vanilla:							
(*Edensoy/Edensoy* Extra)	150	6.0	23.0	3.0	0	90	0
(*Edensoy/Edensoy* Extra), 8.45 fl. oz.	150	6.0	24.0	3.0	0	95	0
(*Soy Dream*)	170	8.0	23.0	5.0	0	140	0
(*Soy Dream* En- riched)	160	8.0	21.0	5.0	0	160	0

Food and Measure	cal.	prot. (gms)	carbo. (gms)	fat (gms)	chol. (mgs)	sod. (mgs)	fiber (gms)
Soy beverage mix, dry, ¼ cup:							
all purpose (*Loma Linda Soyagen*)	130	6.0	12.0	6.0	0	150	3.0
carob (*Loma Linda Soyagen*)	130	6.0	13.0	6.0	0	170	2.0
Soy butter, mix, roasted (*Morningstar Farms/Natural Touch*), 2 tbsp.	170	6.0	10.0	11.0	0	170	1.0
Soy flour: (*Arrowhead Mills*), ½ cup	200	16.0	16.0	9.0	0	0	8.0
stirred, 1 cup:							
full fat, raw	371	29.4	29.9	17.6	0	11	8.2
full fat, roasted	375	29.6	28.6	18.6	0	11	n.a.
defatted	329	47.0	38.4	1.2	0	20	17.5
low fat	287	40.9	33.4	2.4	0	16	9.0
Soy meal, defatted, raw, 1 cup	414	54.8	49.0	2.9	0	3	14.0
Soy milk, see "Soy beverage"							
Soy protein, concentrate, 1 oz.:							
acid/water wash	94	16.5	8.8	.1	0	255	<2.0
w/alcohol	94	16.5	8.8	.1	0	1	<2.0
Soy sauce, 1 tbsp., except as noted:							
(*Chun King*)	10	1.0	1.5	0	0	1225	0
(*Chun King* Lite)	15	1.5	2.0	0	0	540	0
(*House of Tsang* Light)	5	0	0	0	0	930	0
(*House of Tsang* Low Sodium)	5	0	0	0	0	300	0
(*Kikkoman*)	10	2.0	0	0	0	920	0
(*Kikkoman* Lite)	10	1.0	1.0	0	0	605	0
(*La Choy*)	10	1.5	1.0	0	0	1225	0
(*La Choy* Lite)	15	1.5	2.0	0	0	530	0
dark (*House of Tsang*)	10	0	1.0	0	0	920	0
garlic, spicy (*Watkins*)	10	1.0	1.0	0	0	930	0
ginger flavor: (*House of Tsang*)	20	1.0	4.0	0	0	760	0

Food and Measure	cal.	prot. (gms)	carbo. (gms)	fat (gms)	chol. (mgs)	sod. (mgs)	fiber (gms)
(*House of Tsang* Low Sodium) ...	10	0	2.0	0	0	320	0
hot:							
(*Try Me Dragon Sauce*), 1 tsp. ...	5	<1.0	<1.0	0	0	260	0
honey (*Watkins*) ...	20	1.0	5.0	0	0	700	0
Polynesian (*Trader Vic's*)	10	<1.0	1.0	0	0	400	0
shoyu:							
(*Eden* Imported Organic)	15	2.0	2.0	0	0	1040	0
(*Eden* Imported Traditional)	15	2.0	2.0	0	0	1010	0
(*Eden* Reduced Sodium)	10	2.0	2.0	0	0	500	0
tamari:							
(*Eden* Domestic) ...	15	2.0	2.0	0	0	860	0
(*Eden* Imported) ...	10	2.0	2.0	0	0	990	0
Soybean, ½ cup, except as noted:							
green:							
raw, shelled	188	16.6	14.1	8.7	0	n.a.	5.4
boiled, drained	127	11.1	10.0	5.8	0	n.a.	3.8
dried:							
raw (*Arrowhead Mills*), ¼ cup	170	15.0	14.0	8.0	0	0	10.0
boiled	149	14.3	8.5	7.7	0	1	5.2
dry-roasted	387	34.0	28.1	18.6	0	2	7.0
roasted	405	30.3	28.9	21.8	0	140	7.0
Soybeans, canned, black (*Eden Organic*), ½ cup	90	9.0	9.0	1.5	0	0	5.0
Soybean cake or curd, see "Tofu"							
Soybean kernels, roasted, toasted:							
1 oz. or 95 kernels ...	129	10.5	8.7	6.8	0	1	1.0
whole, 1 cup	490	40.0	33.0	25.9	0	4	3.9
whole, salted, 1 cup	490	40.0	33.0	25.9	0	176	3.9

Food and Measure	cal.	prot. (gms)	carbo. (gms)	fat (gms)	chol. (mgs)	sod. (mgs)	fiber (gms)
Soybean sprouts (*Jonathan's*), 1 cup, 3 oz.	100	11.0	8.0	6.0	0	10	2.0
Spaetzel, see "Noodle, egg"							
Spaghetti, see "Pasta"							
Spaghetti dishes, mix:							
w/meat sauce (*Kraft* Dinner), 5.5 oz. . . .	330	12.0	46.0	11.0	15	830	3.0
mild (*Kraft* American Dinner), 2 oz.	200	8.0	40.0	1.5	<5	520	1.0
tangy (*Kraft* Italian Dinner), 2 oz.	200	9.0	38.0	2.0	<5	610	1.0
Spaghetti entree, canned or packaged, 1 cup, except as noted:							
(*Hormel Health Selections*)	180	10.0	30.0	2.0	20	580	3.0
w/franks:							
(*Franco-American SpaghettiO's*) . . .	250	10.0	32.0	11.0	25	1210	4.0
rings (*Kid's Kitchen*)	240	9.0	32.0	9.0	30	810	1.0
w/meat sauce (*Hormel* Microwave).	220	10.0	31.0	7.0	20	790	2.0
w/meatballs:							
(*Chef Boyardee*) . . .	270	8.0	29.0	12.0	30	1050	2.0
(*Chef Boyardee* Micro Cup), 7½ oz.	210	7.0	25.0	9.0	20	870	1.0
(*Chef Boyardee* 99% Fat Free)	220	10.0	40.0	2.0	10	1300	3.0
(*Dinty Moore American Classics*), 1 bowl	290	13.0	44.0	7.0	20	1020	3.0
(*Franco-American SpaghettiO's*) . . .	260	11.0	31.0	11.0	20	1150	5.0
(*Kid's Kitchen*)	220	11.0	28.0	7.0	25	950	1.0
rings (*Kid's Kitchen*)	230	11.0	31.0	7.0	25	1190	1.0

Food and Measure	cal.	prot. (gms)	carbo. (gms)	fat (gms)	chol. (mgs)	sod. (mgs)	fiber (gms)
in tomato sauce (*Franco-American Superiore*)	260	11.0	39.0	7.0	15	1090	5.0
in tomato-cheese sauce (*Franco-American Spaghettio's*)	190	5.0	36.0	2.0	5	990	2.0
in tomato-meat sauce (*Chef Boyardee*) . . .	220	10.0	40.0	2.0	10	1300	3.0
Spaghetti entree, dried, 1 serving:							
marinara w/mushrooms (*AlpineAire*)	290	13.0	52.0	2.5	0	210	2.0
w/meat, sauce (*Mountain House*)	200	12.0	27.0	5.0	15	910	3.0
Spaghetti entree, frozen, 1 pkg., except as noted:							
carbonara (*The Budget Gourmet*), 8 oz. . . .	340	12.0	43.0	13.0	35	670	2.0
marinara:							
(*The Budget Gourmet Value Classics* Low Fat), 8 oz.	260	8.0	43.0	6.0	5	690	3.0
(*Smart Ones*), 9 oz.	280	9.0	46.0	7.0	5	690	4.0
w/cheese garlic bread (*Marie Callender's*), 1 cup and 2 oz. bread	410	13.0	61.0	13.0	20	680	6.0
w/meat sauce:							
(*Lean Cuisine*), 11½ oz.	290	11.0	50.0	5.0	20	570	7.0
(*Smart Ones*), 11½ oz.	280	17.0	43.0	5.0	15	670	5.0
(*Stouffer's*), 10 oz.	350	15.0	46.0	12.0	35	570	5.0
and garlic bread (*Marie Callender's*), 1 cup and 2 oz. bread	360	16.0	51.0	13.0	10	700	5.0

Food and Measure	cal.	prot. (gms)	carbo. (gms)	fat (gms)	chol. (mgs)	sod. (mgs)	fiber (gms)
Spaghetti entree, frozen *(cont.)*							
w/meatballs:							
(*Lean Cuisine*),							
9½ oz.	280	16.0	40.0	6.0	20	570	4.0
(*Stouffer's*),							
12⅝ oz.	440	19.0	56.0	15.0	50	830	5.0
and sauce,							
w/seasoned beef							
(*Healthy Choice*),							
10 oz.	280	14.0	43.0	6.0	30	470	5.0
Spaghetti sauce, see							
"Pasta sauce"							
Spaghetti squash:							
fresh (*Frieda's*),							
¾ cup, 3 oz.	30	1.0	6.0	0	0	15	1.0
baked or boiled,							
drained, ½ cup	23	.5	5.0	.2	0	14	1.1
Spanakopita, see							
"Spinach-feta appe-							
tizer"							
Spareribs, see "Pork"							
Spelt:							
flakes, see "Cereal,							
ready-to-eat"							
flour (*Arrowhead*							
Mills), ¼ cup	100	4.0	24.0	.5	0	0	5.0
Spinach, fresh,							
½ cup:							
raw, chopped	6	.8	1.0	.1	0	22	.8
boiled, drained	21	2.7	3.4	.2	0	63	2.2
Spinach, canned,							
½ cup:							
(*Allens Popeye*)	45	2.0	7.0	1.0	0	310	4.0
(*Allens Popeye* Low							
Sodium)	35	2.0	4.0	1.0	0	35	3.0
(*Bush's Best*)	30	3.0	4.0	0	0	390	2.0
(*Del Monte*)	30	2.0	4.0	0	0	360	2.0
(*Del Monte* No Salt)	30	2.0	4.0	0	0	85	2.0
chopped (*Allens*							
Popeye/Sunshine)	40	2.0	6.0	1.0	0	310	4.0

Food and Measure	cal.	prot. (gms)	carbo. (gms)	fat (gms)	chol. (mgs)	sod. (mgs)	fiber (gms)
Spinach, frozen (see also "Spinach dishes"):							
(*Green Giant*), ¾ cup	25	3.0	3.0	0	0	65	3.0
(*Green Giant Harvest Fresh*), ½ cup	25	3.0	3.0	0	0	240	2.0
leaf:							
(*Birds Eye*), ⅓ cup	20	2.0	3.0	0	0	75	1.0
(*Seabrook*), 1 cup	20	2.0	2.0	0	0	110	2.0
whole or cut							
(*Freshlike*), 1 cup	20	2.0	2.0	0	0	110	2.0
chopped:							
(*Birds Eye*), ⅓ cup	20	3.0	3.0	0	0	80	2.0
(*Cascadian Farm*), ⅓ cup	20	2.0	3.0	0	0	65	3.0
(*Freshlike*), ⅓ cup	20	2.0	2.0	0	0	115	2.0
(*Seabrook*), ⅓ cup	20	2.0	2.0	0	0	115	2.0
in butter sauce, cut (*Green Giant*), ½ cup	40	2.0	5.0	1.5	<5	280	2.0
Spinach, New Zealand, chopped:							
raw, 1 oz. or ½ cup	4	.4	.7	.1	0	37	n.a.
boiled, drained, ½ cup	11	1.2	2.0	.2	0	97	n.a.
Spinach, water (*Frieda's* Ong Choy), 2 cups, 3 oz.	20	2.0	3.0	0	0	65	2.0
Spinach dip, 2 tbsp.:							
(*Marie's*)	140	2.0	3.0	14.0	10	200	0
(*T. Marzetti's* Veggie Dip)	140	1.0	1.0	14.0	25	240	0
Spinach dishes, frozen:							
au gratin (*The Budget Gourmet* Side Dish), 5 oz.	160	5.0	8.0	12.0	30	690	2.0
creamed:							
(*Birds Eye Side Dish*), ½ cup	100	3.0	7.0	7.0	35	630	1.0
(*Green Giant*), ½ cup	80	4.0	10.0	3.0	0	520	2.0

Food and Measure	cal.	prot. (gms)	carbo. (gms)	fat (gms)	chol. (mgs)	sod. (mgs)	fiber (gms)
Spinach dishes, creamed *(cont.)*							
(*Seabrook*), ½ cup	120	4.0	10.0	6.0	15	450	3.0
(*Stouffer's* Side Dish), ½ cup, 4½ oz.	160	4.0	8.0	12.0	15	380	2.0
(*Tabatchnick*), 7½ oz.	60	2.0	8.0	2.0	5	270	2.0
Indian (*Deep* Palak Paneer), 5 oz.	230	8.0	7.0	19.0	25	690	4.0
soufflé (*Stouffer's* Side Dish), ½ cup, 4 oz.	150	6.0	9.0	10.0	120	480	0
Spinach entree, packaged, w/rice, 1 pkg.:							
w/cheese (*Tamarind Tree* Palak Paneer)	380	14.0	46.0	15.0	35	640	6.0
w/garbanzos (*Tamarind Tree* Saag Chole)	370	14.0	55.0	10.0	0	800	13.0
Spinach Masala sauce, cooking (*Shahi* Indian Magic), ¼ cup	40	1.0	3.0	2.5	0	550	1.0
Spinach-artichoke dip (*Classy Delights*), 2 tbsp.	25	0	2.0	1.5	5	55	0
Spinach-feta appetizer, frozen:							
(*Cohen's*), 5 pcs., 3 oz.	220	7.0	24.0	11.0	35	400	1.0
(*The Fillo Factory*), 5 pcs., 5 oz.	360	11.0	38.0	19.0	65	610	2.0
Spinach-feta pocket, frozen (*Amy's*), 4½-oz. pc.	200	9.0	27.0	7.0	15	420	2.0
Spinach-feta snack (*Amy's*), 6 pcs.	160	6.0	21.0	6.0	15	390	2.0
Spiny lobster, meat only:							
raw, 4 oz.	127	23.4	2.8	1.7	80	201	0
boiled or steamed, 2-lb. lobster w/shell	233	43.1	5.1	3.2	146	370	0

Food and Measure	cal.	prot. (gms)	carbo. (gms)	fat (gms)	chol. (mgs)	sod. (mgs)	fiber (gms)
boiled or steamed, 4 oz.	138	29.9	3.5	2.2	102	257	0
Spirals, pasta, mix, 4 cheese (*Fantastic Foods Healthy Complements*), ⅔ cup	210	10.0	38.0	3.0	5	450	2.0
Split peas:							
boiled, ½ cup	116	8.2	20.7	.4	0	2	8.1
green, dry, ¼ cup:							
(*Arrowhead Mills*)	170	12.0	31.0	.5	0	20	7.0
(*Goya*)	110	11.0	27.0	0	0	25	11.0
yellow (*Goya*), ¼ cup	110	10.0	28.0	0	0	20	12.0
Sports drink, 8 fl. oz.:							
(*Arizona Total Sport*)	60	0	16.0	0	0	35	0
(*Powerade Jagged Ice/ Mountain Blast*)	73	0	19.0	0	0	28	0
(*Powerade Tidal Burst*)	72	0	19.0	0	0	28	0
all flavors:							
(*All Sport*)	70	0	20.0	0	0	55	0
(*Recharge*)	70	<1.0	18.0	0	0	25	0
berry or lime (*Recharge* Plus)	80	1.0	18.0	0	0	25	0
fruit punch or lemon-lime (*Powerade*)	72	0	19.0	0	0	28	0
lemon-lime (*Gatorade*)	55	0	15.0	0	0	110	0
orange-tangerine (*Powerade*)	71	0	19.0	0	0	28	0
Spot, meat only:							
raw, 4 oz.	140	21.0	0	5.6	n.a.	33	0
baked, broiled, or microwaved, 4 oz.	179	26.9	0	7.1	n.a.	42	0
Sprouts (see also specific listings), 1 cup:							
fresh:							
spicy (*Frieda's*)	10	1.0	1.0	0	0	0	1.0
stir-fry (*Frieda's*)	15	2.0	3.0	0	0	0	0
canned, bean:							
(*Chun King*)	10	1.0	1.0	0	0	0	1.0
(*La Choy*)	20	2.0	4.0	0	0	75	1.5
Squab, fresh, raw:							
meat w/skin, 4 oz.	333	20.9	0	27.0	n.a.	n.a.	0

Food and Measure	cal.	prot. (gms)	carbo. (gms)	fat (gms)	chol. (mgs)	sod. (mgs)	fiber (gms)
Squab *(cont.)*							
breast meat only,							
4 oz.	161	19.8	0	8.5	n.a.	n.a.	0
Squash (see also spe-							
cific squash list-							
ings):							
canned (*Stokely*),							
½ cup	50	1.0	10.0	0	0	0	4.0
frozen, ½ cup:							
(*Stilwell*)	15	<1.0	2.0	0	0	15	1.0
winter (*Birds Eye*)	50	1.0	12.0	0	0	0	4.0
winter (*Cascadian*							
Farm)	50	2.0	11.0	0	0	5	1.0
Squid, meat only, raw,							
4 oz.	104	17.7	3.5	1.6	265	50	0
St. Honore, frozen							
dessert (*Manzoni*),							
3½ oz.	290	3.0	38.0	14.0	50	75	1.0
Star fruit, see							
"Carambola"							
Steak, see "Beef"							
Steak sauce, 1 tbsp.,							
except as noted:							
(*A.1.*)	15	0	3.0	0	0	250	0
(*A.1.* Bold)	20	0	5.0	0	0	190	0
(*Crosse & Blackwell*)	30	0	7.0	0	0	95	0
(*Heinz 57*)	15	0	4.0	0	0	220	0
(*HP*)	15	0	3.0	0	0	150	0
(*Hunt's*)	10	0	2.0	0	0	250	0
(*Maull's*)	20	0	5.0	0	0	250	0
(*Peter Luger* Steak							
House)	30	0	7.0	0	0	125	0
(*Texas Best*)	15	0	4.0	0	0	220	0
(*Trappey's* Great							
American)	16	0	4.0	0	0	150	0
(*Watkins*)	20	0	4.0	0	0	220	0
and burger (*Try Me*							
Bullfighter)	15	0	4.0	0	0	220	0
Caribbean (*Tabasco*)	15	0	4.0	0	0	160	0
garlic peppercorn (*Lea*							
& Perrins)	25	0	6.0	0	0	110	0

Food and Measure	cal.	prot. (gms)	carbo. (gms)	fat (gms)	chol. (mgs)	sod. (mgs)	fiber (gms)
New Orleans style:							
(*Tabasco*)	15	0	4.0	0	0	270	0
(*Trappey's Chef-Magic*)	10	0	2.0	0	0	70	<1.0
peppercorn (*Lawry's Weekday Gourmet*), 2 tbsp.	40	<1.0	3.0	3.0	0	370	0
sweet:							
mild (*Maull's*)	20	0	4.0	0	0	190	0
spicy (*Lea & Perrins*)	25	0	6.0	0	0	140	0
Steak seasoning, blackened (*Chef Paul Prudhomme's Magic Seasoning Blends*), 1/4 tsp. ...	0	0	0	0	0	80	0
Stir-fry entree mix, see "Vegetable entree mix" and specific listings							
Stir-fry sauce (see also "Marinade" and specific listings), 1 tbsp., except as noted:							
(*House of Tsang* Classic)	25	0	4.0	1.0	0	570	0
(*House of Tsang Bangkok Padang*)	45	1.0	4.0	2.5	0	250	0
(*House of Tsang Saigon Sizzle*)	40	0	8.0	1.0	0	380	0
(*Ka•Me*)	10	1.0	1.0	0	0	570	0
(*Kikkoman*)	15	<1.0	3.0	0	0	530	0
(*Lawry's*)	25	<1.0	4.0	.5	0	330	0
(*Newman's Own*)	10	0	4.0	.5	0	85	0
garlic and ginger (*Rice Road*)	25	0	3.0	1.0	0	310	0
lemon (*Rice Road*) ...	15	0	4.0	0	0	310	0
and marinade (*Mary Rose Halu*)	25	0	6.0	0	0	340	0

Food and Measure	cal.	prot. (gms)	carbo. (gms)	fat (gms)	chol. (mgs)	sod. (mgs)	fiber (gms)
Stir-fry sauce *(cont.)*							
and rib, garlic (*Mi-Kee*)	30	0	10	0	0	550	0
spicy, Szechuan (*House of Tsang*)	20	0	4.0	.5	0	520	0
sweet and sour:							
(*House of Tsang*)	35	0	8.0	0	0	50	0
(*La Choy*), ½ cup	150	2.0	35.0	<1.0	0	840	1.0
teriyaki (*Rice Road*)	20	0	4.0	0	0	310	0
Stomach, pork, raw, 1 oz.	44	4.7	0	2.7	55	15	0
Strawberry, fresh:							
1 pint	97	2.0	22.5	1.2	0	4	7.4
½ cup	23	.5	5.2	.3	0	1	1.7
Strawberry, canned, ½ cup:							
in light syrup (*Oregon*)	100	1.0	23.0	0	0	5	2.0
in heavy syrup:							
½ cup	117	.7	29.9	.3	0	5	2.2
whole (*Comstock/ Wilderness*)	140	1.0	33.0	0	0	35	6.0
Strawberry, dried (*Frieda's*), ½ cup, 1.4 oz.	150	1.0	34.0	0	0	0	3.0
Strawberry, freeze-dried, whole (*AlpineAire*), ½ oz. ...	50	1.0	12.0	0	0	0	2.0
Strawberry, frozen:							
(*Big Valley*), ⅔ cup ...	50	<1.0	12.0	0	0	0	2.0
(*Cascadian Farm*), 1 cup	90	1.0	20.0	0	0	0	6.0
(*Stilwell*), ⅔ cup	50	<1.0	13.0	1.0	0	5	2.0
whole (*Birds Eye*), ½ cup	100	<1.0	25.0	0	0	0	1.0
halves, ½ cup:							
(*Birds Eye*)	120	<1.0	31.0	0	0	0	1.0
in light syrup (*Birds Eye*)	70	<1.0	17.0	0	0	0	1.0
unsweetened, ½ cup	26	.3	6.8	.1	0	1	1.6

Food and Measure	cal.	prot. (gms)	carbo. (gms)	fat (gms)	chol. (mgs)	sod. (mgs)	fiber (gms)
Strawberry drink:							
(*Capri Sun* Cooler),							
6.75 fl. oz.	100	0	26.0	0	0	20	0
(*Farmer's Market*),							
8 fl. oz.	120	0	30.0	0	0	0	0
(*Snapple* Squeeze),							
8 fl. oz.	120	0	30.0	0	0	10	0
nectar:							
(*Kern's*), 8 fl. oz.	150	0	36.0	0	0	5	0
(*Libby's/Kern's*),							
11.5 fl. oz.	210	0	52.0	0	0	10	0
Strawberry drink							
blends, 8 fl. oz., ex-							
cept as noted:							
(*Fruitopia Strawberry*							
Passion Awareness)	114	0	30.0	0	0	58	0
banana:							
(*Arizona* Colada) ...	140	0	34.0	.5	0	25	0
(*R.W. Knudsen*) ...	120	0	30.0	0	0	25	0
(*Veryfine*),							
11.5 fl. oz.	190	0	48.0	0	0	30	0
(*Wipper Snapple*),							
10 fl. oz.	160	0	40.0	0	0	60	0
cactus (*R.W. Knud-*							
sen)	120	0	29.0	0	0	10	0
guava:							
(*R.W. Knudsen*) ...	110	0	27.0	0	0	25	0
(*Santa Cruz Or-*							
ganic)	100	0	24.0	0	0	25	0
kiwi:							
(*R.W. Knudsen*) ...	120	0	30.0	0	0	25	0
(*Tropicana Twister*)	130	0	33.0	0	0	20	0
(*V8 Splash*)	110	0	28.0	0	0	40	0
melon:							
(*Veryfine* Chiller							
Shivering)	120	0	29.0	0	0	5	0
(*Veryfine* Chiller							
Shivering),							
11.5 fl. oz.	160	0	41.0	0	0	10	0
orange:							
(*Season's Best*) ...	130	1.0	31.0	0	0	25	0

Food and Measure	cal.	prot. (gms)	carbo. (gms)	fat (gms)	chol. (mgs)	sod. (mgs)	fiber (gms)
Strawberry drink blends, orange *(cont.)*							
(*Tropicana Bursters*)	130	1.0	30.0	0	0	15	0
raspberry (*Kool-Aid Bursts*), 6.75 fl. oz.	100	0	24.0	0	0	30	0
Strawberry drink mix*, 8 fl. oz.:							
(*Kool-Aid*)	100	0	25.0	0	0	25	0
(*Kool-Aid Presweetened*)	60	0	16.0	0	0	0	0
raspberry:							
(*Kool-Aid Incrediberry*)	100	0	25.0	0	0	10	0
(*Kool-Aid Incrediberry Presweetened*)	60	0	16.0	0	0	0	0
Strawberry filling, see "Pastry filling" and "Pie filling"							
Strawberry juice, 8 fl. oz.:							
(*Veryfine* Juice-Up)	140	0	36.0	0	0	15	0
nectar (*R.W. Knudsen*)	120	0	30.0	0	0	25	0
Strawberry milk (*Nestlé Quik*), 1 cup	230	7.0	33.0	8.0	30	100	1.0
Strawberry milk drink mix (*Nestlé Quik*), 3 tbsp.	100	0	24.0	0	0	0	0
Strawberry snack (*Weight Watchers*), ¹/₂ oz.	50	0	13.0	0	0	125	2.0
Strawberry syrup, ¹/₄ cup, except as noted:							
(*Hershey's*), 2 tbsp.	100	0	26.0	0	0	10	0
(*Knott's Berry Farm*), 2 tbsp.	120	0	30.0	0	0	0	0
(*Maple Grove Farms*)	230	0	57.0	0	0	0	0
(*R.W. Knudsen*)	150	0	38.0	0	0	0	0
(*Smucker's*)	210	0	52.0	0	0	0	0
(*Smucker's* Light) . . .	130	0	33.0	0	0	0	0

Food and Measure	cal.	prot. (gms)	carbo. (gms)	fat (gms)	chol. (mgs)	sod. (mgs)	fiber (gms)
(*Smucker's* Sundae), 2 tbsp.	110	0	27.0	0	0	70	0
Strawberry topping, 2 tbsp.:							
(*Kraft*)	110	0	29.0	0	0	15	0
(*Mrs. Richardson's Fat Free*)	70	0	18.0	0	0	15	<1.0
(*Smucker's*)	100	0	260	0	0	0	0
Strawberry-banana nectar (*Kern's*), 8 fl. oz.	150	0	36.0	0	0	5	0
Strawberry-peach-banana smoothie (*Del Monte Blenders*), 5.5 fl. oz.	150	<1.0	39.0	0	0	10	1.0
String beans, see "Green beans"							
Stroganoff gravy (*Pepperidge Farm*), ¼ cup	30	2.0	4.0	1.0	<5	240	0
Stroganoff mix, vegetarian (*Natural Touch*), 4 tbsp.	90	5.0	10.0	3.5	10	610	3.0
Stroganoff sauce, beef (*Lawry's*), 1 tbsp.	20	0	5.0	0	0	500	0
Stroganoff seasoning mix (*Durkee*), ⅛ pkg.	10	.5	3.0	0	0	350	0
Strudel, apple (*Entenmann's*), ¼ strudel	320	3.0	44.0	15.0	0	250	2.0
Stuffing (see also "Stuffing mix"):							
apple and raisin (*Pepperidge Farm*), ½ cup	140	4.0	27.0	1.5	0	520	2.0
Cajun rice (*Good Harvest*), ½ cup	130	3.0	24.0	2.0	0	390	1.0

Food and Measure	cal.	prot. (gms)	carbo. (gms)	fat (gms)	chol. (mgs)	sod. (mgs)	fiber (gms)
Stuffing *(cont.)*							
chicken, classic (*Pepperidge Farm*),							
½ cup	130	5.0	24.0	1.5	0	490	3.0
corn bread:							
(*Arnold*), 2 cups ...	250	9.0	49.0	4.0	0	800	2.0
(*Brownberry*),							
2 cups	250	8.0	51.0	3.50	800		2.0
(*Pepperidge Farm*),							
¾ cup	170	4.0	33.0	2.0	0	480	2.0
honey pecan (*Pepperidge Farm*),							
½ cup	140	3.0	23.0	5.0	0	400	<1.0
country style (*Pepperidge Farm*), ¾ cup	140	5.0	27.0	1.5	0	380	2.0
cube (*Pepperidge Farm*), ¾ cup	140	4.0	28.0	1.5	0	530	2.0
garden and herb, country (*Pepperidge Farm*), ½ cup	150	4.0	22.0	5.0	0	360	2.0
herb-seasoned:							
(*Arnold*), 2 cups ...	240	9.0	48.0	3.0	0	740	4.0
(*Brownberry*), 1 cup	200	7.0	41.0	2.5	0	630	3.0
(*Pepperidge Farm*),							
¾ cup	170	5.0	33.0	1.5	0	600	3.0
sage and onion:							
(*Arnold*), 2 cups ...	240	9.0	48.0	3.0	0	960	4.0
(*Pepperidge Farm* Box), ½ cup	150	5.0	28.0	1.5	0	520	2.0
Santa Fe (*Good Harvest*), ½ cup	110	3.0	21.0	1.5	0	330	.5
seasoned (*Arnold*), 2 cups...........	250	9.0	49.0	3.0	0	820	2.0
sourdough, San Francisco (*Good Harvest*), ½ cup	110	3.0	19.0	2.0	0	480	.5
vegetable, harvest, and almond (*Pepperidge Farm*), ½ cup	140	5.0	23.0	3.0	0	300	2.0

Food and Measure	cal.	prot. (gms)	carbo. (gms)	fat (gms)	chol. (mgs)	sod. (mgs)	fiber (gms)
wild rice and mush-room (*Pepperidge Farm*), ²/₃ cup	170	5.0	22.0	6.0	0	410	2.0
wild rice trio (*Good Harvest*), ½ cup ...	140	3.0	27.0	2.5	0	470	.5
Stuffing mix, ⅙ box dry, except as noted:							
(*Kellogg's Crouettes*), 1 cup	120	5.0	25.0	0	0	460	0
for beef (*Stove Top*)	110	4.0	22.0	1.0	0	520	1.0
chicken flavor:							
(*Stove Top*)	110	4.0	20.0	1.0	0	440	<1.0
(*Stove Top* Flexible Serving), ½ cup	120	3.0	19.0	3.0	0	460	<1.0
(*Stove Top* Lower Sodium)	110	4.0	21.0	1.0	0	270	<1.0
(*Stove Top* Micro)	130	4.0	20.0	3.5	0	450	<1.0
cornbread:							
(*Stove Top*)	110	3.0	21.0	1.0	0	510	1.0
(*Stove Top* Flexible Serving), ½ cup	110	3.0	19.0	2.5	0	500	1.0
homestyle (*Stove Top* Micro)	120	3.0	20.0	3.5	0	450	1.0
herb (*Stove Top* Flexi-ble Serve), 1 oz. ...	120	3.0	19.0	3.0	0	440	<1.0
herbs, savory (*Stove Top*)	110	4.0	20.0	1.0	0	510	<1.0
long grain/wild rice (*Stove Top*)	110	4.0	22.0	1.0	0	490	<1.0
mushroom/onion (*Stove Top*)	110	4.0	20.0	1.5	0	410	<1.0
for pork (*Stove Top*)	110	4.0	20.0	1.0	0	500	1.0
San Francisco style (*Stove Top*)	110	4.0	20.0	1.0	0	510	1.0
for turkey (*Stove Top*)	110	3.0	20.0	1.0	0	490	<1.0
Sturgeon, meat only:							
raw, 4 oz.	120	18.3	0	4.6	n.a.	n.a.	0
baked, broiled, or mi-crowaved, 4 oz. ...	153	23.5	0	5.9	n.a.	n.a.	0
smoked, 4 oz.	196	35.4	0	5.0	n.a.	n.a.	0

Food and Measure	cal.	prot. (gms)	carbo. (gms)	fat (gms)	chol. (mgs)	sod. (mgs)	fiber (gms)
Subway, 1 serving:							
sandwiches, 6":							
Classic Italian BMT:							
wheat	460	21.0	45.0	22.0	56	1664	3.0
white	445	21.0	39.0	21.0	56	1652	3.0
Cold Cut Trio:							
wheat	378	20.0	46.0	13.0	64	1412	3.0
white	362	19.0	39.0	13.0	64	1401	3.0
ham, wheat	302	19.0	45.0	5.0	28	1319	3.0
ham, white	287	18.0	39.0	5.0	28	1308	3.0
meatball, wheat	419	19.0	51.0	16.0	33	1046	3.0
meatball, white	404	18.0	44.0	16.0	33	1035	3.0
pizza sub, wheat	464	19.0	48.0	22.0	50	1621	3.0
pizza sub, white	448	19.0	41.0	22.0	50	1609	3.0
roast beef, wheat	303	20.0	45.0	5.0	20	939	3.0
roast beef, white	288	19.0	39.0	5.0	20	928	3.0
roast chicken breast:							
wheat	348	27.0	47.0	6.0	48	978	3.0
white	332	26.0	41.0	6.0	48	967	3.0
steak & cheese:							
wheat	398	30.0	47.0	10.0	70	1117	3.0
white	383	29.0	41.0	10.0	70	1106	3.0
Subway Club:							
wheat	312	21.0	46.0	5.0	26	1352	3.0
white	297	21.0	40.0	5.0	26	1341	3.0
Subway Melt:							
wheat	382	23.0	46.0	12.0	42	1746	3.0
white	366	22.0	40.0	12.0	42	1735	3.0
Subway Seafood & Crab, light mayo:							
wheat	347	20.0	45.0	10.0	32	884	3.0
white	332	19.0	39.0	10.0	32	8733	.0
tuna, light mayo:							
wheat	391	19.0	46.0	15.0	32	940	3.0
white	376	18.0	39.0	15.0	32	928	3.0
turkey, wheat	289	18.0	46.0	4.0	19	1403	3.0
turkey, white	273	17.0	40.0	4.0	19	1391	3.0
turkey & ham:							
wheat	295	18.0	46.0	5.0	24	1361	3.0
white	280	18.0	39.0	5.0	24	1350	3.0

Food and Measure	cal.	prot. (gms)	carbo. (gms)	fat (gms)	chol. (mgs)	sod. (mgs)	fiber (gms)
Veggie Delite :							
wheat	237	9.0	44.0	3.0	0	593	3.0
white	222	9.0	38.0	3.0	0	582	3.0
sandwiches, 6″ rounded, double meat:							
Classic Italian BMT	683	33.0	46.0	40.0	112	2734	3.0
Cold Cut Trio	518	30.0	48.0	23.0	128	2230	3.0
ham	367	28.0	46.0	8.0	57	2045	3.0
meatball	601	28.0	57.0	29.0	67	1499	3.0
pizza sub.........	690	29.0	51.0	41.0	101	2648	3.0
roast beef	369	30.0	47.07	.0	40	1285	3.0
roast chicken breast	458	44.0	50.0	9.0	96	1363	3.0
steak & cheese	560	50.0	51.0	17.0	141	1641	3.0
Subway Club	387	33.0	48.0	7.0	53	2111	3.0
Subway Melt	526	36.0	48.0	21.0	84	2899	3.0
Subway Seafood & Crab, light mayo	457	30.0	46.0	17.0	64	1175	3.0
tuna, light mayo ...	546	28.0	48.0	27.0	64	1286	3.0
turkey breast......	340	26.0	48.0	5.0	37	221	23.0
turkey & ham	354	27.0	47.0	7.0	47	2128	3.0
sandwiches, deli style:							
bologna	292	10.0	38.0	12.0	20	744	2.0
ham	234	11.0	37.0	4.0	14	773	2.0
roast beef	245	13.0	38.0	4.0	13	638	2.0
tuna, light mayo ...	279	11.0	38.0	9.0	16	583	2.0
turkey	235	12.0	38.0	4.0	12	944	2.0
sandwich fixins, optional:							
bacon, 2 slices	45	2.0	0	4.0	8	182	0
cheese, 2 triangles	41	2.0	0	3.0	10	201	0
mayo, 1 tsp.	37	0	0	4.0	3	27	0
mayo, light, 1 tsp.	18	0	0	2.0	2	33	0
mustard, 2 tsp. ...	8	1.0	1.0	0	0	0	0
oil, 1 tsp.	45	0	0	5.0	1	0	0
vinegar, 1 tsp.	1	0	0	0	0	0	0
salads:							
Classic Italian BMT	274	14.0	11.0	20.0	56	1379	1.0
Cold Cut Trio	191	13.0	11.0	11.0	64	1127	1.0
ham	116	12.0	11.0	3.0	28	1034	1.0
meatball	233	12.0	16.0	14.0	33	761	2.0

Food and Measure	cal.	prot. (gms)	carbo. (gms)	fat (gms)	chol. (mgs)	sod. (mgs)	fiber (gms)
Subway, salads (cont.)							
pizza	277	12.0	13.0	20.0	50	1336	2.0
roast beef	117	12.0	11.0	3.0	20	654	1.0
roast chicken breast	162	20.0	13.0	4.0	48	693	1.0
steak & cheese	212	22.0	13.0	8.0	70	832	1.0
Subway Club	126	14.0	12.0	3.0	26	1067	1.0
Subway Melt	195	16.0	12.0	10.0	42	1461	1.0
Subway Seafood & Crab	161	13.0	11.0	8.0	32	599	2.0
tuna, light mayo . . .	205	12.0	11.0	13.0	32	654	1.0
turkey breast	102	11.0	12.0	2.0	19	1117	1.0
turkey & ham	109	11.0	11.0	3.0	24	1076	1.0
Veggie Delite	51	2.0	10.0	1.0	0	308	1.0
cookies:							
Brazil nut	236	3.0	30.0	11.0	13	121	2.0
chocolate chip	234	3.0	33.0	10.0	10	148	1.0
chocolate chip, M&M's	228	2.0	34.0	9.0	10	156	1.0
chocolate chunk . . .	235	3.0	33.0	10.0	13	147	1.0
macadamia nut	248	2.0	31.0	13.0	12	147	1.0
oatmeal raisin	223	3.0	32.0	9.0	12	152	1.0
peanut butter	230	3.0	31.0	11.0	0	225	1.0
sugar	246	2.0	31.0	13.0	19	179	0
Succotash, 1/2 cup:							
fresh, boiled, drained	111	4.9	23.4	.8	0	16	n.a.
canned:							
kernel (Seneca)	90	3.0	18.0	.5	0	270	3.0
kernel (Stokely) . . .	100	3.0	14.0	1.0	0	340	2.0
cream-style corn . . .	102	3.5	23.4	.7	0	325	n.a.
frozen, boiled, drained	79	3.7	17.0	.8	0	38	4.6
Sucker, white, meat only:							
raw, 4 oz.	105	19.0	0	2.6	47	45	0
baked, broiled, or mi-crowaved, 4 oz. . . .	135	24.4	0	3.4	60	58	0
Sugar, beet or cane:							
brown:							
1 oz.	107	0	27.6	0	0	11	0
1 cup, not packed	546	0	141.0	0	0	57	0
1 cup, packed	828	0	214.0	0	0	86	0
granulated:							
1 oz.	110	0	28.3	0	0	<1	0

Food and Measure	cal.	prot. (gms)	carbo. (gms)	fat (gms)	chol. (mgs)	sod. (mgs)	fiber (gms)
1 cup	773	0	199.8	0	0	<1	0
1 tbsp.	46	0	12.0	0	0	<1	0
1 tsp.	15	0	4.0	0	0	<1	0
powdered or confectioners':							
1 cup, sifted	389	0	99.5	0	0	1	0
1 tbsp., unsifted	31	0	8.0	0	0	<1	0
Sugar, maple, 1 oz.	99	0	25.5	0	0	4	0
Sugar, substitute:							
(*Equal*), 1 pkt.	4	0	<1.0	0	0	0	0
(*NutraSweet*), 1 tsp.	2	0	<1.0	0	0	0	0
(*Sweet 'n Low*), 1 pkt.	4	0	1.0	0	0	0	0
Sugar apple:							
medium, 9.9 oz.	146	3.2	36.6	.5	0	15	6.8
½ cup	118	2.6	29.6	.4	0	12	5.5
Sugar snap peas, see "Peas, edible-podded"							
Summer sausage:							
(*Oscar Mayer*),							
2 slices, 1.6 oz.	140	7.0	0	13.0	40	650	0
beef (*Oscar Mayer*),							
2 slices, 1.6 oz.	140	7.0	1.0	12.0	35	640	0
smoked (*Old Smokehouse*), 2 oz.	200	2.0	2.0	18.0	55	970	0
Sun choke, see "Jerusalem artichoke"							
Sunfish, pumpkinseed, meat only:							
raw, 4 oz.	101	22.0	0	.8	76	91	0
baked, broiled, or microwaved, 4 oz.	129	28.2	0	1.0	98	117	0
Sunflower seed, 1 oz., except as noted:							
(*Frito-Lay*)	180	7.0	5.0	15.0	0	25	2.0
barbecued kernels (*Planters*), 1.7 oz.	290	11.0	10.0	25.0	0	180	6.0
dried, hulled (*Arrowhead Mills*), ¼ cup	180	8.0	6.0	15.0	0	10	2.0
dry-roasted:							
(*River Queen*), ¼ cup, 1.1 oz.	170	6.0	7.0	15.0	0	290	3.0

Food and Measure	cal.	prot. (gms)	carbo. (gms)	fat (gms)	chol. (mgs)	sod. (mgs)	fiber (gms)
Sunflower seed, dry-roasted *(cont.)*							
(*River Queen* Un-salted), ¼ cup, 1.2 oz.	200	7.0	8.0	17.0	0	0	3.0
dry-roasted, kernels:							
(*Planters*), ¼ cup	190	7.0	6.0	17.0	0	230	4.0
salted	165	5.5	6.8	14.1	0	221	2.6
honey-roasted, kernels							
(*Planters*), 1.7 oz.	280	10.0	15.0	22.0	0	105	6.0
oil-roasted, kernels							
(*Planters*), 2 oz. ...	340	13.0	11.0	29.0	0	310	8.0
salted kernels (*Plant-ers*)	170	7.0	5.0	14.0	0	140	4.0
Sunflower seed but-ter, 1 tbsp.	93	3.2	4.4	7.6	0	1	.8
Sunflower seed flour, partially defatted, 1 cup	261	38.5	28.7	1.3	0	2	4.2
Surimi, pollock, 4 oz.	112	17.2	7.8	1.0	34	162	0
Swamp cabbage:							
raw, .6-oz. shoot	2	.3	.4	<.1	0	15	.3
boiled, drained, chopped, ½ cup ...	10	1.0	1.8	.1	0	60	.9
Sweet dumpling squash (*Frieda's*), ¾ cup, 3 oz.	30	1.0	7.0	0	0	0	1.0
Sweet peas, see "Peas, green"							
Sweet potato:							
raw, 5″ x 2″ potato ...	136	2.1	31.6	.4	0	17	3.9
baked in skin:							
5″ x 2″ potato	118	2.0	27.7	.1	0	12	3.4
mashed, ½ cup	103	1.7	24.3	.1	0	10	3.0
boiled w/out skin:							
4 oz.	119	1.9	27.5	.3	0	15	2.8
mashed, ½ cup	172	2.7	39.8	.5	0	21	4.1
Sweet potato, canned, ½ cup, ex-cept as noted:							
in syrup, w/liquid	101	1.1	23.9	.2	0	50	2.1
in syrup, drained	106	1.3	24.9	.3	0	38	1.8

Food and Measure	cal.	prot. (gms)	carbo. (gms)	fat (gms)	chol. (mgs)	sod. (mgs)	fiber (gms)
whole (*Royal Prince/ Trappey's*), 4 pcs.	200	1.0	48.0	.5	0	40	4.0
halves (*Royal Prince*), 5.7 oz., 3 pcs.	190	1.0	46.0	.5	0	40	4.0
cut or pieces (*Allens/ Sugary Sam/ Princella* Yams), ²/₃ cup	160	0	40.0	.5	0	35	3.0
mashed (*Princella/ Sugary Sam*), ²/₃ cup	120	1.0	28.0	.5	0	30	3.0
candied (*Royal Prince*)	210	1.0	50.0	.5	0	30	2.0
orange-pineapple (*Royal Prince*)	210	1.0	43.0	.5	0	30	3.0
Sweet potato, frozen:							
baked, cubed, ½ cup	88	1.5	20.6	.1	0	7	2.6
patties (*McKenzie's Yam*), 2-oz. pc. . . .	60	<1.0	15.0	0	0	100	2.0
Sweet potato chips, 1 oz.:							
(*Terra*)	140	1.0	18.0	7.0	0	10	1.0
barbecue, mesquite (*Terra*)	140	1.0	18.0	7.0	0	65	1.0
jalapeño (*Terra*)	140	1.0	20.0	7.0	0	70	2.0
spiced:							
(*Terra*)	140	1.0	16.0	7.0	0	105	3.0
(*Wise* Mambo Mania)	160	2.0	15.0	10.0	0	180	1.0
Sweet potato leaf:							
raw, chopped, ½ cup	6	.7	1.1	.1	0	2	<1.0
steamed, ½ cup	11	.7	2.3	.1	0	4	.6
Sweet and sour drink mixer (*Mr & Mrs T*), 4 fl. oz.	100	0	23.0	0	0	50	0
Sweet and sour sauce, 2 tbsp., except as noted:							
(*Chun King*)	60	0	14.0	0	0	105	0
(*Contadina*)	40	0	8.0	1.0	0	110	0
(*4C*)	80	0	21.0	0	0	240	<1.0
(*Kikkoman*)	35	0	9.0	0	0	190	0
(*Kraft*)	80	0	19.0	.5	0	180	0

Food and Measure	cal.	prot. (gms)	carbo. (gms)	fat (gms)	chol. (mgs)	sod. (mgs)	fiber (gms)
Sweet and sour sauce *(cont.)*							
(*La Choy*)	60	0	14.0	0	0	120	0
(*Sauceworks*)	60	0	14.0	0	0	125	0
(*World Harbors Maui Mountain*)	60	0	14.0	0	0	250	0
chicken (*Gold's Dip'n Joy*), 1 tbsp.	30	0	7.0	0	0	125	0
concentrate (*House of Tsang*), 1 tsp.	10	0	3.0	0	0	15	0
duck sauce:							
(*Gold's*)	60	0	14.0	0	0	250	0
(*Ka•Me*)	80	0	20.0	0	0	0	0
(*La Choy*)	60	0	15.0	0	0	130	0
Sweetbreads, see "Pancreas" and "Thymus"							
Swiss chard, fresh:							
raw (*Frieda's*) 1 cup, 3 oz.	15	2.0	3.0	0	0	18	1.0
raw, chopped, ½ cup	3	.3	.7	<.1	0	38	.3
boiled, drained, chopped, ½ cup . . .	18	1.7	3.6	.1	0	158	1.8
Swiss steak gravy mix (*Durkee*), ¼ cup*	15	0	4.0	0	0	370	0
Swordfish, fresh, meat only:							
raw, 4 oz.	137	22.5	0	4.6	45	102	0
baked, broiled, or microwaved, 4 oz. . . .	176	28.8	0	5.8	57	130	0
Syrup, see "Pancake syrup" and specific syrup listings							
Szechuan sauce (see also "Stir-fry sauce"):							
(*Ka•Me*), 1 tbsp.	25	1.0	2.0	1.5	0	390	0
cooking (*Kylin* Chili & Tomato), ¼ cup . . .	50	1.0	11.0	1.0	0	810	0

T

Food and Measure	cal.	prot. (gms)	carbo. (gms)	fat (gms)	chol. (mgs)	sod. (mgs)	fiber (gms)
Tabouli:							
(*Frieda's*), 1/2 cup	152	3.0	17.0	9.0	0	265	5.0
salad (*Cedar's*),							
2 tbsp.	30	1.0	3.0	1.0	0	63	1.0
salad (*Yorgo*), 2 tbsp.	25	1.0	3.0	1.0	0	55	1.0
Tabouli mix:							
(*Casbah*), 1 1/4 oz.	120	3.0	24.0	.5	0	410	1.0
(*Fantastic Foods*),							
1/4 cup	120	4.0	26.0	.5	0	450	6.0
Taco Bell, 1 serving:							
breakfast items:							
Burrito, country ...	270	8.0	26.0	14.0	195	690	2.0
burrito, double ba-							
con and egg	480	18.0	39.0	27.0	400	1240	2.0
burrito, fiesta	280	9.0	25.0	16.0	25	580	2.0
burrito, grande	420	13.0	43.0	22.0	205	1050	3.0
hash brown nuggets	280	2.0	29.0	18.0	0	570	1.0
burritos:							
bean	380	13.0	55.0	12.0	10	1100	13.0
Big Beef Supreme	520	24.0	54.0	23.0	55	1520	11.0
Big Chicken Su-							
preme	500	27.0	51.0	20.0	70	1660	3.0
burrito supreme ...	440	17.0	51.0	19.0	35	1230	10.0
chili cheese	330	14.0	37.0	13.0	35	870	5
grilled chicken	400	19.0	50.0	14.0	40	1250	3.0
7-layer	530	16.0	66.0	23.0	25	1280	13.0
Fajita Wrap:							
chicken	460	19.0	51.0	20.0	45	1170	3.0
steak	470	20.0	50.0	21.0	40	1190	3.0
veggie	420	10.0	53.0	19.0	20	980	3.0
Fajita Wrap Supreme:							
chicken	520	18.0	53.0	26.0	70	1300	4.0
steak	510	21.0	52.0	25.0	50	1200	3.0

Food and Measure	cal.	prot. (gms)	carbo. (gms)	fat (gms)	chol. (mgs)	sod. (mgs)	fiber (gms)
Taco Bell, Fajita Wrap Supreme (cont.)							
veggie	510	20.0	53.0	24.0	55	1180	3.0
gorditas:							
Fiesta:							
beef	290	14.0	31.0	13.0	25	880	3.0
grilled chicken . . .	260	16.0	28.0	10.0	30	580	3.0
steak	270	17.0	27.0	10.0	25	600	3.0
Santa Fe:							
beef	380	14.0	33.0	20.0	35	440	4.0
grilled chicken . . .	370	17.0	30.0	20.0	40	610	3.0
steak	370	18.0	29.0	21.0	35	360	3.0
Supreme:							
beef	300	14.0	31.0	13.0	35	390	3.0
grilled chicken . . .	300	17.0	28.0	14.0	45	540	3.0
steak	310	17.0	27.0	14.0	35	550	3.0
tacos:							
regular	180	9.0	12.0	10.0	25	330	3.0
double decker	340	14.0	38.0	15.0	25	750	9.0
soft	220	11.0	21.0	10.0	25	580	3.0
soft, grilled chicken	200	14.0	21.0	7.0	35	540	2.0
soft, grilled steak	230	15.0	20.0	10.0	25	1020	2.0
Taco Supreme:							
regular	220	10.0	14.0	14.0	35	350	3.0
double decker	390	15.0	40.0	19.0	35	760	9.0
soft	260	12.0	23.0	14.0	35	590	3.0
soft, grilled steak	290	16.0	24.0	14.0	35.0	1040	3.0
specialties:							
Big Beef Mexi Melt	290	16.0	23.0	15.0	45	850	4.0
Mexican pizza	570	21.0	42.0	35.0	45	1040	8.0
taco salad, w/salsa	850	30.0	65.0	52.0	60	1780	16.0
taco salad, w/salsa, w/out shell	420	24.0	32.0	22.0	60	1520	15.0
tostada	300	10.0	31.0	15.0	15	650	12.0
quesadilla, cheese	350	16.0	32.0	18.0	50	860	2.0
quesadilla, chicken	410	25.0	33.0	19.0	75	1040	2.0
nachos and sides:							
Big Beef nacho su- preme	450	14.0	45.0	24.0	30	810	9.0
nachos	320	5.0	34.0	18.0	5	570	3.0
nachos *Bellgrande*	770	21.0	84.0	39.0	35	1310	17.0
Pintos 'n Cheese . . .	190	9.0	18.0	9.0	15	650	10.0

Food and Measure	cal.	prot. (gms)	carbo. (gms)	fat (gms)	chol. (mgs)	sod. (mgs)	fiber (gms)
rice, Mexican	190	5.0	23.0	9.0	15	760	1.0
twists, cinnamon	140	1.0	19.0	6.0	0	190	0
ice cream dessert:							
Choco Taco	310	3.0	37.0	17.0	20	100	1.0
Taco dinner mix (see also "Mexican dinner mix"), dry, except as noted:							
(*El Rio* Kit), ⅕ pkg.	130	3.0	18.0	5.0	0	510	1.0
(*Old El Paso* Kit), 2 pcs.*	330	17.0	20.0	20.0	55	950	2.0
(*Ortega* Kit), ⅙ pkg.	150	3.0	24.0	5.0	0	700	3.0
(*Pancho Villa* Kit), 2 pcs.*	360	20.0	20.0	22.0	65	890	2.0
soft:							
(*Chi-Chi's* Kit), seasoning, 2 shells	300	7.0	54.0	7.0	0	1290	2.0
(*Old El Paso* Kit), 2 pcs.*	400	22.0	33.0	20.0	65	1360	1.0
(*Ortega* Kit), ⅕ pkg.	240	4.0	47.0	5.0	0	1180	2.0
white or yellow (*ChiChi's* Kit), seasoning, 2 shells	200	4.0	29.0	8.0	0	860	3.0
Taco entree, frozen (*Kid Cuisine* Game Time Roll-up), 7.35-oz. pkg.	380	9.0	55.0	14.0	25	740	5.0
Taco John's, 1 serving:							
burritos:							
bean	387	15.3	56.6	11.1	18	866	n.a.
beef	449	23.3	44.0	20.0	52	863	n.a.
combination	418	19.3	50.3	15.6	35	865	n.a.
meat and potato . . .	503	16.9	53.0	24.4	25	1341	n.a.
ranch	447	17.6	43.8	22.7	74	804	n.a.
super	465	20.3	53.0	19.4	41	922	n.a.
fajitas, chicken:							
burrito	370	21.2	45.1	11.8	49	1536	n.a.
salad, no dressing	557	21.9	44.3	33.2	56	1541	n.a.
softshell	200	13.4	20.5	6.9	33	903	n.a.
kid's meal:							
w/crispy taco	579	12.8	53.8	33.9	35	789	n.a.

Food and Measure	cal.	prot. (gms)	carbo. (gms)	fat (gms)	chol. (mgs)	sod. (mgs)	fiber (gms)
Taco John's, kid's meal *(cont.)*							
w/softshell taco ...	617	15.3	63.7	32.7	35	1037	n.a.
platters:							
chimichanga	979	32.8	127.0	37.6	59	2341	n.a.
double enchilada ...	967	42.2	106.0	42.3	89	1921	n.a.
sampler	1406	60.9	156.0	60.5	126	2875	n.a.
smothered burrito	1031	39.3	132.0	40.0	70	2351	n.a.
special features:							
Mexi Rolls w/cheese	863	29.7	71.7	48.3	54	1392	n.a.
Potato Oles Bravo	579	10.7	47.2	37.7	7	1550	n.a.
Sierra chicken fillet							
sandwich.......	534	30.1	39.6	28.9	68	1406	n.a.
super nachos	919	26.1	72.1	56.4	48	1484	n.a.
taco salad, no							
dressing	584	19.7	42.8	37.8	46	766	n.a.
tacos:							
crispy	182	9.4	11.6	10.9	26	272	n.a.
soft shell.........	230	13.5	22.6	10.3	26	520	n.a.
Taco Bravo	346	15.1	38.9	14.4	28	677	n.a.
taco burger	280	15.0	27.5	12.0	32	576	n.a.
side orders/extras:							
beans, refried	357	17.7	52.6	8.6	17	1032	n.a.
chili.............	350	20.4	19.0	21.1	506	865	n.a.
Mexican rice	567	7.9	39.9	17.7	n.a.	1293	n.a.
nacho cheese	300	5.0	0	10.0	n.a.	600	0
nachos	333	6.8	26.6	20.6	n.a.	611	n.a.
Potato Oles	363	2.8	37.7	22.5	n.a.	964	n.a.
Potato Oles, large	484	3.7	50.3	30.1	n.a.	1285	n.a.
Potato Oles							
w/cheese	483	7.8	37.7	32.5	n.a.	1564	n.a.
sour cream	60	1.0	1.0	5.0	n.a.	15	0
desserts:							
apple flauta	84	1.0	18.8	1.1	0	72	n.a.
cherry flauta	143	2.1	26.7	3.6	0	110	n.a.
choco taco	320	3.0	38.0	17.0	20	100	n.a.
churro...........	147	2.0	17.4	7.8	4	160	n.a.
cream cheese flauta	181	2.5	26.5	7.9	10	135	n.a.
Italian ice	80	0	19.0	0	0	5	0
Taco mix, vegetarian							
(*Natural Touch*),							
3 tbsp.	60	8.0	5.0	1.0	0	590	3.0

Food and Measure	cal.	prot. (gms)	carbo. (gms)	fat (gms)	chol. (mgs)	sod. (mgs)	fiber (gms)
Taco sauce, 1 tbsp., except as noted:							
(*Chi-Chi's/ChiChi's* Thick & Chunky) . . .	10	0	1.0	0	0	75	0
(*El Rio*)	5	0	0	0	0	60	0
(*Lawry's* Chunky), 2 tbsp.	10	0	2.0	0	0	250	0
(*Lawry's* Sauce 'n Seasoner), 2 tbsp.	15	<1.0	3.0	0	0	320	<1.0
green (*La Victoria*) . . .	0	0	<1.0	0	0	95	0
hot (*Old El Paso*)	5	0	1.0	0	0	90	0
medium (*Old El Paso*)	5	0	1.0	0	0	70	0
mild (*Old El Paso*) . . .	5	0	1.0	0	0	85	0
mild or medium (*Old El Paso* Chunky) . . .	5	0	1.0	0	0	80	0
red (*La Victoria*)	5	0	1.0	0	0	105	0
Taco seasoning (*Tone's*), 2 tsp.	20	1.0	4.0	0	0	440	1.0
Taco seasoning mix:							
(*Lawry's*), 2 tsp.	15	0	3.0	0	0	300	0
(*Old El Paso*), 2 tsp.	20	0	5.0	0	0	550	0
(*Old El Paso* 40% Less Sodium), 2 tsp. . . .	15	0	4.0	0	0	330	0
(*Pancho Villa*), 2 tsp.	20	0	5.0	0	0	550	0
cheesy (*Old El Paso*), 1 tbsp.	15	0	3.0	.5	0	360	1.0
chicken (*Lawry's*), 2 tsp.	20	<1.0	5.0	0	0	450	0
mild (*Durkee* Pouch), 1/8 pkg.	15	.5	3.0	0	0	320	0
salad:							
(*Durkee* Pouch), 1/6 pkg.	20	.5	4.0	0	0	320	0
(*Lawry's*), 1 tsp.	15	0	3.0	0	0	210	0
Taco shell:							
(*Lawry's*), 2 pcs.	120	2.0	13.0	6.0	0	110	1.0
(*Lawry's* Super Size), 2 pcs.	180	2.0	22.0	10.0	0	180	1.0
(*Old El Paso*), 3 pcs.	150	2.0	19.0	7.0	0	135	2.0
(*Old El Paso* Super), 2 pcs.	170	2.0	22.0	8.0	0	150	2.0

Food and Measure	cal.	prot. (gms)	carbo. (gms)	fat (gms)	chol. (mgs)	sod. (mgs)	fiber (gms)
Taco shell *(cont.)*							
(*Pancho Villa*), 3 pcs.	160	2.0	21.	7.0	0	0	2.0
(*Rosarita*), 1 pc.	45	1.0	7.5	1.5	0	40	1.0
mini (*Old El Paso*),							
7 pcs.	150	2.0	19.0	7.0	0	130	2.0
soft, see "Tortilla"							
tostada:							
(*Lawry's*), 2 pcs.	110	1,0	13.0	6.0	0	110	1.0
(*Old El Paso*),							
3 pcs.	150	2.0	19.0	7.0	0	135	2.0
(*Rosarita*), 1 pc. ...	65	1.0	8.5	2.5	0	10	0
white corn (*Old El*							
Paso), 3 pcs.	150	2.0	19.0	7.0	0	135	2.0
white/yellow corn							
(*Chi-Chi's*), 2 pcs.	170	2.0	22.0	8.0	0	330	2.0
Tagliatelle, refriger-							
ated, spinach (*Con-*							
tadina), 1¼ cups ...	270	12.0	46.0	4.0	105	110	4.0
Tagliatelle entree,							
frozen (*The Budget*							
Gourmet Low Fat),							
8-oz. pkg.	260	8.0	42.0	6.0	5	500	3.0
Tahini, 2 tbsp.:							
(*Arrowhead Mills*) ...	190	6.0	5.0	19.0	0	5	3.0
(*Joyva*)	200	5.0	3.0	18.0	0	75	1.0
(*Krinos*)	260	9.0	5.0	23.0	0	0	n.a.
Tahini sauce mix							
(*Casbah*), 1.13 oz.,							
¼ cup*	200	4.0	10.0	13.0	0	160	.5
Tamale, canned,							
2 pcs., except as							
noted:							
(*Gebhardt*)	270	5.0	19.0	21.0	30	770	3.0
(*Gebhardt* Jumbo) ...	335	6.5	24.0	24.0	30	870	4.0
(*Just Rite*), 3 pcs. ...	255	7.0	21.0	17.0	20	1035	4.0
(*Nalley*), 3 pcs.	290	8.0	25.0	17.0	30	1000	1.0
(*Van Camp's*)	210	5.0	20.0	13.0	20	610	3.0
(*Wolf*)	210	6.0	23.0	12.0	20	450	4.0
beef:							
(*Hormel/Hormel*							
Hot-Spicy)	140	4.0	16.0	7.0	20	800	2.0

Food and Measure	cal.	prot. (gms)	carbo. (gms)	fat (gms)	chol. (mgs)	sod. (mgs)	fiber (gms)
chili sauce (*Nalley*), 3 pcs. w/sauce	290	8.0	25.0	17.0	30	1000	1.0
jumbo (*Hormel*) . . .	210	6.0	23.0	10.0	25	1120	3.0
chicken (*Hormel*)	130	3.0	15.0	7.0	30	660	1.0
in gravy (*Old El Paso*), 3 pcs.	320	7.0	31.0	19.0	30	590	5.0
Tamale pocket, frozen (*Amy's*), 1 pc.	250	8.0	39.0	7.0	10	580	3.0
Tamale pot pie, frozen, Mexican (*Amy's*), 8 oz.	220	10.0	41.0	3.0	0	480	11.0
Tamari, see "Soy sauce"							
Tamarillo, 2 pcs., 4.2 oz.:							
red (*Frieda's*)	40	2.0	9.0	0	0	0	4.0
yellow (*Frieda's*)	30	2.0	8.0	0	0	0	4.0
Tamarind:							
(*Frieda's* Tamarindo), 1 oz.	70	1.0	19.0	0	0	10	2.0
fruit, 3" x 1"	5	.1	1.3	<.1	0	1	.1
pulp, ½ cup	144	1.7	37.5	.4	0	17	3.1
Tandoori paste, (*Patak's*), 2 tbsp.	30	<1.0	3.0	1.0	0	1440	2.0
Tangerine, fresh:							
medium, 2⅜"	37	.5	9.4	.2	0	1	1.9
sections w/out membrane, ½ cup	43	.6	10.9	.2	0	2	2.2
Tangerine, canned, ½ cup:							
in juice	46	.8	11.9	<.1	0	7	.9
in light syrup:							
(*Del Monte* cup) . . .	70	0	17.0	0	0	10	<1.0
(*Sunfrost* Mandarin)	80	0	20.0	0	0	10	8.0
½ cup	76	.6	20.4	.1	0	8	.9
Tangerine drink, 8 fl. oz.:							
(*Fruitopia Tremendously Tangerine*)	109	0	29.0	0	0	58	0
(*Mandarin Magic*)	120	0	31.0	0	0	35	0
ruby red (*Veryfine Diet*)	15	0	3.0	0	0	10	0

Food and Measure	cal.	prot. (gms)	carbo. (gms)	fat (gms)	chol. (mgs)	sod. (mgs)	fiber (gms)
Tangerine juice, 8 fl. oz., except as noted:							
fresh, 6 fl. oz.	80	.9	18.7	.4	0	2	.4
blend:							
(*Dole* Mandarin) ...	140	1.0	35.0	0	0	30	0
(*Tropicana Pure Premium*)	110	2.0	25.0	0	0	0	0
frozen* (*Minute Maid* Beverage)	120	0	30.0	0	0	5	0
Tapenade, see "Tomato tapenade"							
Tapioca, dry (*Minute*), 1½ tsp.	20	0	5.0	0	0	5	0
Tapioca pudding, see "Pudding" and "Pudding and pie filling mix"							
Taramosalata, see "Caviar spread"							
Taro:							
raw, sliced, ½ cup ...	56	.8	13.8	.1	0	6	2.1
cooked:							
sliced, ½ cup	94	.3	22.8	.1	0	10	3.4
(*Frieda's*), 5 oz. ...	150	1.0	36.0	n.a.	0	10	4.0
Taro, Tahitian, ½ cup:							
raw, sliced	25	1.7	4.3	.6	0	31	n.a.
cooked, sliced	30	2.8	4.7	.5	0	37	n.a.
Taro chips:							
1 oz.	141	.7	19.3	7.1	0	97	n.a.
½ cup	57	.3	8.1	3.1	0	44	n.a.
spiced (*Terra*), 1 oz.	130	1.0	20.0	5.0	0	170	2.0
Taro leaf, ½ cup:							
raw................	6	.7	.9	.1	0	1	.5
steamed	18	2.0	3.0	.3	0	2	n.a.
Taro root, cooked (*Frieda's*), 5 oz.....	150	1.0	36.0	n.a.	0	10	4.0
Taro shoots, ½ cup:							
raw, sliced	5	.4	1.0	<.1	0	<1	n.a.
cooked, sliced	10	.5	2.2	.1	0	1	n.a.
Tarragon, ground, 1 tsp.	5	.4	.8	.1	0	1	.1

Food and Measure	cal.	prot. (gms)	carbo. (gms)	fat (gms)	chol. (mgs)	sod. (mgs)	fiber (gms)
Tart, snack, 1 pc.:							
all fruit varieties							
(*Health Valley*							
Healthy Tart)	150	3.0	35.0	0	0	40	3.0
chocolate fudge							
(*Healthy Valley*							
Healthy Tart)	150	3.0	35.0	0	0	50	3.0
Tart shell, see "Pastry shell"							
Tartar sauce, 2 tbsp.:							
(*Hellmann's/Best*							
Foods)	140	0	1.0	16.0	10	260	0
(*Hellmann's/Best*							
Foods Low Fat)	40	0	7.0	1.5	0	360	0
(*Kraft* Nonfat)	25	0	5.0	0	0	210	<1.0
(*Nalley*)	190	0	1.0	20.0	15	250	0
(*Sauceworks*)	100	0	4.0	10.0	10	180	0
lemon herb flavor							
(*Sauceworks*)	150	0	<1.0	16.0	15	170	0
Tartufo, frozen dessert							
(*Manzoni*), 3 oz.	200	3.0	30.0	9.0	5	40	2.0
TCBY, all flavors:							
hand-dipped, ½ cup:							
ice cream:							
regular	140	2.0	17.0	7.0	25	60	0
low fat, no sugar	100	3.0	19.0	2.5	10	60	0
nonfat	100	2.0	23.0	0	0	50	<1.0
yogurt, frozen:							
96% fat free	110	3.0	22.0	2.5	5	65	<1.0
nonfat	100	3.0	22.0	0	0	55	1.0
soft serve, ½ cup:							
sorbet	100	0	24.0	0	0	30	0
yogurt, frozen:							
96% fat free	140	4.0	23.0	3.0	15	60	0
nonfat	110	4.0	20.0	0	<5	60	0
nonfat, no sugar	80	4.0	20.0	0	<5	35	0
Tea (see also "Tea, iced"), 1 bag or 1 tsp.:							
plain, regular or instant, all varieties	0	0	0	0	0	0	0

Food and Measure	cal.	prot. (gms)	carbo. (gms)	fat (gms)	chol. (mgs)	sod. (mgs)	fiber (gms)
Tea *(cont.)*							
flavored, lemon, instant *(Lipton)*	0	0	1.0	0	0	0	0
Tea, iced, 8 fl. oz., except as noted:							
(Hood)	100	0	25.0	0	0	10	0
(Nestea)	63	0	17.0	0	0	0	0
(Nestea Cool)	82	0	22.0	0	0	46	0
(Nestea Unsweetened)	2	0	<1.0	0	0	0	0
(Schweppes)	90	0	22.0	0	0	60	0
(Snapple Just Plain)	70	0	18.0	0	0	10	0
(Snapple Just Plain Unsweetened)	0	0	0	0	0	10	0
all fruit flavors:							
(Apple & Eve)	100	0	25.0	0	0	5	0
(Lipton Chilled)	80	0	20.0	0	0	15	0
(Snapple Diet)	0	0	0	0	0	10	0
herbal *(R.W. Knudsen Coolers)*	90	0	23.0	0	0	40	0
all varieties *(Arizona Diet)*	0	0	0	0	0	20	0
ginseng:							
(Arizona)	60	0	15.0	0	0	20	0
(Snapple)	80	0	20.0	0	0	10	0
green tea:							
(Snapple)	100	0	25.0	0	0	10	0
ginseng *(After the Fall Green Tea Express)*	90	0	230	0	0	10	0
plum or w/ginseng and honey *(Arizona)*	70	0	18.0	0	0	20	0
herbal, w/honey *(Arizona)*	70	0	17.0	0	0	20	0
lemon:							
(Arizona)	90	0	25.0	0	0	20	0
(Nestea)	77	0	21.0	0	0	0	0
(Nestea Diet)	3	0	<1.0	0	0	0	0
(Snapple)	100	0	25.0	0	0	10	0
(Tropicana)	100	0	25.0	0	0	25	0
(Veryfine), 10 fl. oz.	120	0	29.0	0	0	10	0

Food and Measure	cal.	prot. (gms)	carbo. (gms)	fat (gms)	chol. (mgs)	sod. (mgs)	fiber (gms)
(*Veryfine* Chiller)...	90	0	23.0	0	0	10	0
(*Veryfine* Chiller),							
11.5 fl. oz.	130	0	33.0	0	0	15	0
(*Veryfine* Diet)	5	0	0	0	0	10	0
mint (*Snapple*)	110	0	27.0	0	0	10	0
orange jasmine herbal							
(*Snapple*)	80	0	20.0	0	0	10	0
peach:							
(*Arizona*).........	95	0	25.0	0	0	20	0
(*Nestea*).........	78	0	21.0	0	0	0	0
(*Snapple*)	100	0	26.0	0	0	10	0
(*Tropicana*), 11.5 fl.							
oz.	160	0	41.0	0	0	20	0
peach-kiwi (*Veryfine*							
Chiller)	80	0	18.0	0	0	5	0
raspberry:							
Arizona)	90	0	25.0	0	0	20	0
(*Nestea*), 8 fl oz.	78	0	21.0	0	0	0	0
(*Snapple*)	100	0	26.0	0	0	10	0
(*Tropicana*),							
11.5 fl. oz.	160	0	41.0	0	0	15	0
(*Veryfine* Chiller) ...	100	0	24.0	0	0	5	0
Tea, iced, mix:							
lemon flavor (*Lipton*),							
1⅔ tbsp..........	90	0	22.0	0	0	0	0
w/out lemon (*Lipton*),							
1⅔ tbsp..........	80	0	19.0	0	0	0	0
peach, raspberry, or							
tangerine (*Watkins*),							
4 tsp.	80	0	21.0	0	0	0	0
Teff seed or flour (*Arrowhead Mills*),							
2 oz.	200	7.0	41.0	1.0	0	6	7.7
Tempeh:							
1 oz.	56	5.4	4.8	2.2	0	2	n.a.
½ cup............	165	15.7	14.1	6.4	0	5	n.a.
Teriyaki entree (see also specific listings), frozen (*Lean Cuisine Lunch Express*), 9 oz.	260	15.0	39.0	5.0	30	550	4.0

Food and Measure	cal.	prot. (gms)	carbo. (gms)	fat (gms)	chol. (mgs)	sod. (mgs)	fiber (gms)
Teriyaki sauce, 1 tbsp., except as noted:							
(*Chun King*)	20	1.0	3.0	0	0	920	0
(*House of Tsang Korean*)	30	0	6.0	.5	0	460	0
(*La Choy*)	15	1.0	3.0	0	0	850	0
(*World Harbors Maui Mountain*), 2 tbsp.	70	0	17.0	0	0	270	0
barbecue (*Mary Rose* Sumi)	30	0	7.0	0	0	420	0
baste and glaze: (*Kikkoman*)	50	1.0	11.0	0	0	810	0
w/honey and pineapple (*Kikkoman*)	80	1.0	18.0	0	0	770	0
hot: (*Chun King*)	20	1.5	3.0	0	0	995	0
(*World Harbors Maui Mountain*), 2 tbsp.	70	0	17.0	0	0	300	0
marinade (*Lawry's*)	20	0	5.0	0	0	810	0
marinade and: (*Kikkoman*)	15	1.0	2.0	0	0	610	0
(*Kikkoman* Lite) . . .	15	<1.0	3.0	0	0	320	0
roasted garlic (*Kikkoman*)	25	1.0	5.0	0	0	730	0
Polynesian (*Trader Vic's*)	15	0	3.0	0	0	430	0
sesame and garlic (*Rice Road*)	15	0	4.0	0	0	300	0
tangy (*Watkins*)	15	1.0	2.0	0	0	600	0
Thai sauce (*World Harbors* Nong Khai Mountain), 2 tbsp.	40	0	8.0	0	0	350	0
Thuringer cervelat, see "Summer sausage"							
Thyme, ground, 1 tsp.	4	.1	.9	.1	0	1	.3
Thymus, 4 oz.:							
beef, braised	362	24.8	0	28.3	333	132	0
veal, braised	197	35.8	0	4.9	532	75	0

Food and Measure	cal.	prot. (gms)	carbo. (gms)	fat (gms)	chol. (mgs)	sod. (mgs)	fiber (gms)
Tikka sauce, see "Curry sauce, cooking"							
Tilefish, meat only:							
raw, 4 oz.	108	19.9	0	2.6	n.a.	60	0
baked, broiled, or microwaved, 4 oz.	167	27.8	0	5.3	n.a.	67	0
Tiramisu, see "Cake, frozen"							
Toaster muffins and pastries, 1 pc.:							
all fruit varieties (*Weight Watchers*)	190	2.0	38.0	3.0	0	180	2.0
apple:							
(*Toaster Strudel*) . . .	200	3.0	26.0	9.0	5	190	<1.0
cinnamon (*Pop-Tarts*)	210	2.0	37.0	6.0	0	180	1.0
cinnamon, frosted (*Pop-Tarts* Low Fat)	190	2.0	39.0	3.0	0	230	1.0
berry, wild:							
(*Toaster Strudel* Wildberry)	190	3.0	26.0	8.0	5	190	<1.0
frosted (*Pop-Tarts*)	210	2.0	39.0	5.0	0	170	1.0
blueberry:							
(*Natural Touch*)	180	6.0	33.0	2.0	0	65	6.0
(*Pop-Tarts*)	200	2.0	36.0	5.0	0	190	1.0
(*Pop-Tarts* Low Fat)	190	2.0	39.0	3.0	0	230	1.0
(*Toaster Strudel*) . . .	200	3.0	26.0	9.0	5	200	<1.0
frosted (*Barbara's Nature's Choice*)	190	3.0	42.0	2.0	0	40	3.0
frosted (*Pop-Tarts*)	200	2.0	37.0	5.0	0	170	1.0
brown sugar–cinnamon:							
(*Pop-Tarts*)	210	3.0	35.0	6.0	0	190	1.0
frosted (*Pop-Tarts*)	210	3.0	34.0	7.0	0	180	1.0
frosted (*Pop-Tarts* Low Fat)	190	2.0	39.0	3.0	0	230	1.0
cherry:							
(*Barbara's Nature's Choice* Wheat Free*)	180	3.0	36.0	3.0	0	30	3.0

Food and Measure	cal.	prot. (gms)	carbo. (gms)	fat (gms)	chol. (mgs)	sod. (mgs)	fiber (gms)
Toaster muffins and pastries, cherry *(cont.)*							
(*Pop-Tarts*)	200	2.0	37.0	5.0	0	180	1.0
(*Pop-Tarts* Low Fat)	190	2.0	39.0	3.0	0	230	1.0
(*Toaster Strudel*) . . .	190	3.0	26.0	8.0	5	200	<1.0
frosted (*Pop-Tarts*)	200	2.0	38.0	5.0	0	170	1.0
chocolate:							
frosted (*Barbara's Nature's Choice*)	200	3.0	42.0	2.5	0	45	3.0
fudge, frosted (*Pop-Tarts*)	200	3.0	37.0	5.0	0	220	1.0
fudge, frosted (*Pop-Tarts* Low Fat) . . .	190	3.0	39.0	3.0	0	270	2.0
graham (*Pop-Tarts*)	210	3.0	35.0	6.0	0	230	1.0
chocolate-vanilla creme, frosted (*Pop-Tarts*)	200	3.0	37.0	5.0	0	220	1.0
cinnamon:							
(*Barbara's Nature's Choice*)	190	3.0	42.0	2.0	0	40	3.0
(*Toaster Strudel*) . . .	190	3.0	26.0	8.0	5	230	<1.0
cream cheese:							
(*Toaster Strudel*) . . .	200	3.0	23.0	11.0	15	230	<1.0
and blueberry or strawberry (*Toaster Strudel*)	200	3.0	24.0	10.0	10	220	<1.0
date/walnut (*Natural Touch*)	200	6.0	36.0	3.0	0	50	8.0
grape, frosted (*Pop-Tarts*)	200	2.0	38.0	5.0	0	170	1.0
peach apricot (*Barbara's Nature's Choice* Wheat Free)	180	3.0	36.0	3.0	0	30	3.0
pizza, see "Pizza pocket"							
raspberry:							
(*Toaster Strudel*) . . .	190	3.0	26.0	8.0	5	200	0
frosted (*Pop-Tarts*)	210	2.0	37.0	5.0	0	170	1.0
S'mores (*Pop Tarts*)	200	3.0	36.0	6.0	0	200	1.0
strawberry:							
(*Pop-Tarts*)	200	2.0	37.0	5.0	0	190	1.0
(*Pop-Tarts* Low Fat)	190	2.0	39.0	3.0	0	230	1.0

Food and Measure	cal.	prot. (gms)	carbo. (gms)	fat (gms)	chol. (mgs)	sod. (mgs)	fiber (gms)
(*Toaster Strudel*) ...	200	3.0	26.0	9.0	5	190	<1.0
frosted (*Barbara's Nature's Choice*)	190	3./0	42.0	2.0	0	40	3.0
frosted (*Pop-Tarts*)	200	2.0	38.0	5.0	0	170	1.0
frosted (*Pop-Tarts* Low Fat)	190	2.0	39.0	3.0	0	210	1.0
watermelon, wild, frosted (*Pop-Tarts*)	210	2.0	39.0	5.0	0	170	1.0
Toffee baking bits (*Skor*), 1 tbsp.	60	0	7.0	4.0	10	75	0
Tofu:							
fresh:							
1 oz.	22	2.3	.5	1.4	0	2	.3
½ cup	94	10.0	2.3	5.9	0	9	1.5
extra firm (*Nasoya*), ⅕ of 1-lb. block	90	11.0	1.0	5.0	0	10	0
firm (*Frieda's*), 3 oz.	60	6.0	2.0	3.0	0	10	0
firm (*Nasoya*), ⅕ of 1-lb. block	80	9.0	2.0	4.0	0	10	0
firm, 1 oz.	41	4.5	1.2	2.5	0	4	.7
firm, ½ cup	183	19.9	5.4	11.0	0	17	2.9
silken (*Nasoya*), ⅕ of 1-lb. block	50	5.0	2.0	2.0	0	10	0
soft (*Nasoya*), ⅙ of 1-lb. block	60	7.0	2.0	3.0	0	5	0
flavored, ¼ block:							
5-spice (*Nasoya*)	70	8.0	0	4.0	0	70	0
French country (*Nasoya*)	70	8.0	0	4.0	0	130	0
salted and fermented (fuyu), 1 oz.	33	2.3	1.5	2.3	0	814	<1.0
Tofu seasoning mix, ¼ pkg., except as noted:							
breakfast scramble:							
(*Fantastic Foods Classics*), ½ tbsp.	60	3.0	12.0	.5	0	480	3.0
(*TofuMate*)	15	0	3.0	0	0	340	0

Food and Measure	cal.	prot. (gms)	carbo. (gms)	fat (gms)	chol. (mgs)	sod. (mgs)	fiber (gms)
Tofu seasoning mix *(cont.)*							
eggless salad (*Tofu-Mate*)	15	0	4.0	0	0	310	0
mandarin stir fry (*TofuMate*)	30	1.0	6.0	0	0	310	0
Mediterranean herb (*TofuMate*)	15	1.0	3.0	0	0	310	0
Szechwan stir-fry (*TofuMate*)	25	1.0	4.0	0	0	290	0
Texas taco (*TofuMate*)	15	1.0	3.0	0	0	380	0
Tom collins mixer, bottled (*Holland House*), 3 fl. oz. . . .	160	0	37.0	0	0	85	0
Tom and Jerry batter (*Trader Vic's*), 1 tbsp.	116	2.0	23.0	2.0	35	240	0
Tomatillo:							
(*Frieda's*), 3 oz.	25	1.0	5.0	1.0	0	0	2.0
(*La Victoria* Entero), 5 pcs., 4½ oz.	40	1.0	7.0	1.0	0	410	5.0
1 medium, 1⅝″ diam.	11	.3	2.0	.4	0	tr.	.6
chopped, ½ cup	21	.6	3.8	.7	0	1	1.3
crushed (*La Victoria*), 4½ oz.	45	2.0	8.0	.5	0	400	7.0
Tomato:							
raw:							
2⅗″ tomato	26	1.0	5.7	.4	0	11	1.4
chopped, ½ cup . . .	19	.8	4.2	.3	0	8	1.0
boiled, ½ cup	32	1.3	7.0	.5	0	13	1.2
dried, see "Tomato, dried"							
Tomato, canned (see also "Tomato sauce"), ½ cup, except as noted:							
(*Contadina* Pasta Ready)	40	1.0	5.0	2.0	0	620	1.0
(*Contadina* Recipe Ready)	25	1.0	5.0	0	0	200	1.0
whole:							
(*Del Monte*)	25	1.0	6.0	0	0	160	2.0

Food and Measure	cal.	prot. (gms)	carbo. (gms)	fat (gms)	chol. (mgs)	sod. (mgs)	fiber (gms)
Italian pear (*Contadina*)	25	1.0	4.0	0	0	220	1.0
peeled (*Contadina*)	25	1.0	4.0	0	0	20	1.0
peeled (*Hunt's*), 2 pcs.	20	1.5	4.0	0	0	375	<1.0
peeled (*Hunt's* No Salt), 2 pcs.	20	1.0	4.0	0	0	<5	<1.0
peeled (*Hunt's Pear*), 2 pcs.	20	1.5	4.0	0	0	360	<.0
peeled (*Progresso*)	25	1.0	5.0	0	0	220	1.0
peeled (*Progresso* Italian Style)	20	1.0	4.0	0	0	220	1.0
peeled, w/basil (*Muir Glen*)	30	1.0	5.0	0	0	260	1.0
w/cheeses, three (*Contadina* Pasta Ready)	70	1.0	8.0	4.0	<5	650	<1.0
chunky:							
chili style (*Del Monte*)	30	1.0	8.0	0	0	670	2.0
pasta style (*Del Monte*)	45	1.0	11.0	0	0	560	2.0
crushed:							
(*Contadina*), ¼ cup	20	<1.0	4,0	0	0	150	1.0
(*Del Monte* Original)	45	2.0	9.0	0	0	390	1.0
(*Del Monte* Italian)	45	2.0	9.0	0	0	390	1.0
(*Eden* Organic Roma)	20	1.0	3.0	0	0	0	1.0
(*Hunt's*)	30	1.0	7.0	0	0	285	1.5
(*Muir Glen*)	25	1.0	4.0	0	0	85	1.0
(*Progresso*)	20	1.0	4.0	0	0	95	1.0
w/garlic (*Del Monte*)	50	2.0	11.0	0	0	510	1.0
diced:							
(*Del Monte*)	25	1.0	6.0	0	0	250	2.0
(*Del Monte* No Salt)	25	1.0	6.0	0	0	50	2.0
(*Eden* Organic Roma)	30	1.0	6.0	0	0	5	2.0
(*Hunt's* Choice Cut)	25	1.0	6.0	0	0	395	1.0
(*Muir Glen*)	25	1.0	4.0	0	0	290	1.0
(*Muir Glen* No Salt)	25	1.0	4.0	0	0	45	1.0
in juice (*Muir Glen*)	25	1.0	4.0	0	0	190	1.0

Food and Measure	cal.	prot. (gms)	carbo. (gms)	fat (gms)	chol. (mgs)	sod. (mgs)	fiber (gms)
Tomato, canned, diced *(cont.)*							
in puree (*Hunt's*) . . .	25	1.0	5.0	0	0	305	1.0
w/basil, garlic, oregano (*Del Monte*)	50	2.0	11.0	0	0	650	<1.0
w/garlic and onion (*Del Monte*)	40	2.0	8.0	.5	0	610	<1.0
w/garlic and onion (*Muir Glen*)	25	1.0	4.0	0	0	290	1.0
w/green chilies (*Chi Chi's*), ¼ cup	20	0	4.0	0	0	290	0
w/green chilies (*Eden* Organic Roma)	30	2.0	5.0	0	0	35	2.0
w/green chilies (*Muir Glen*)	25	1.0	4.0	0	0	290	1.0
w/green chilies (*Ro*Tel*)	20	<1.0	4.0	0	0	370	1.0
w/green pepper, onion (*Del Monte*)	40	1.0	9.0	0	0	480	<2.0
Italian herb (*Hunt's* Choice Cut)	25	1.0	5.5	0	0	560	1.0
w/roasted garlic (*Hunt's* Choice Cut)	25	1.0	5.0	0	0	440	<1.0
w/green chilies (*Old El Paso*), ¼ cup	10	0	2.0	0	0	300	0
w/jalapeños (*Old El Paso*), ¼ cup	10	0	2.0	0	0	350	0
w/mushrooms (*Contadina* Pasta Ready)	50	1.0	9.0	1.5	0	640	1.0
w/olives (*Contadina* Pasta Ready)	60	1.0	8.0	3.0	0	640	1.0
paste, see "Tomato paste"							
primavera (*Contadina* Pasta Ready)	50	1.0	8.0	1.5	0	600	1.0
puree, see "Tomato puree"							
w/red pepper, crushed (*Contadina* Pasta Ready)	60	1.0	8.0	3.0	0	690	1.0

Food and Measure	cal.	prot. (gms)	carbo. (gms)	fat (gms)	chol. (mgs)	sod. (mgs)	fiber (gms)
stewed:							
(*Contadina*)	40	1.0	9.0	0	0	250	1.0
(*Del Monte*)	35	1.0	9.0	0	0	360	2.0
(*Del Monte* No Salt)	35	1.0	9.0	0	0	50	2.0
(*Green Giant* Classic)	35	1.0	7.0	0	0	360	2.0
(*Hunt's*)	30	<1.0	7.0	0	0	370	1.0
(*Hunt's* No Salt) . . .	35	1.0	7.0	0	0	30	1.5
Cajun (*Del Monte*)	35	1.0	9.0	0	0	460	2.0
Italian (*Contadina*)	40	1.0	8.0	0	0	260	1.0
Italian (*Del Monte*)	30	1.0	8.0	0	0	420	2.0
Italian (*Green Giant*)	30	1.0	7.0	0	0	360	2.0
Mexican (*Contadina*)	40	1.0	9.0	0	0	220	1.0
Mexican (*Del Monte*) . . . . : .	35	1.0	9.0	0	0	400	2.0
Mexican (*Green Giant*)	35	1.0	7.0	0	0	400	2.0
wedges (*Del Monte*)	35	1.0	9.0	0	0	380	2.0
Tomato, dried:							
(*Frieda's* No Salt), 1 oz.	86	3.7	21.2	.1	0	38	n.a.
1 oz.	73	4.0	15.8	.8	0	594	3.5
1 pc., 32 pcs. per cup	5	.3	1.1	.1	0	42	.3
½ cup	70	3.8	15.1	.8	0	566	3.3
bits (*Sonoma*), 2–3 tsp.	15	1.0	3.0	0	0	5	1.0
halves (*Sonoma*), 2 pcs.	15	1.0	2.0	0	0	5	1.0
julienne (*Sonoma*), 7–9 strips	15	1.0	3.0	0	0	5	1.0
in oil (*Christopher Ranch*), 1 oz., approx. 6 pcs.	80	2.0	7.0	4.0	0	10	2.0
in oil, drained (*Sonoma* Spice Medley), 1 tbsp.	50	1.0	3.0	4.0	0	200	1.0
seasoning (*Sonoma* Season It), 2–3 tsp.	20	1.0	3.0	0	0	25	1.0
Tomato, green, 2³/₅″ tomato	30	1.5	6.3	.3	0	16	1.8

Food and Measure	cal.	prot. (gms)	carbo. (gms)	fat (gms)	chol. (mgs)	sod. (mgs)	fiber (gms)
Tomato, pickled, 1 oz.:							
(*Claussen*)	5	0	1.0	0	0	320	<1.0
(*Hebrew National/ Shorr's*)	4	0	1.0	0	0	280	n.a.
Tomato, sun-dried, see "Tomato, dried"							
Tomato appetizer, 1 oz.:							
w/eggplant (*Sabra* Matbucha Salad) . . .	18	.3	1.6	1.1	0	116	.5
w/vegetables (*Sabra* Turkish Salad)	13	.5	2.5	0	0	150	.7
Tomato chutney, see "Chutney"							
Tomato dip mix, dry, 1 tsp.:							
bacon (*Watkins*)	10	1.0	2.0	0	0	170	0
horseradish (*Watkins*)	10	0	3..0	0	0	130	0
Tomato juice, 8 fl. oz., except as noted:							
(*Campbell's*)	50	2.0	9.0	0	0	860	1.0
(*Campbell's* Low Sodium)	50	2.0	10.0	0	0	140	1.0
(*Campbell's Healthy Request*)	50	1.0	12.0	0	0	480	1.0
(*Del Monte*)	50	2.0	10.0	0	0	760	1.0
(*Del Monte* Not from Concentrate)	40	3.0	7.0	0	0	550	0
(*Dole*), 12 fl. oz.	85	4.0	17.0	0	0	1000	2.0
(*Eden* Organic)	35	1.0	6.0	1.0	0	560	1.0
(*Hunt's* No Salt)	35	1.5	7.5	0	0	10	2.0
(*Muir Glen* From Concentrate)	40	3.0	7.0	0	0	620	1.0
(*Muir Glen* From Organic Concentrate)	60	2.0	12.0	0	0	620	6.0
(*R.W. Knudsen* Organic)	60	2.0	14.0	0	0	390	0
(*Sacramento*)	35	3.0	8.0	0	0	550	3.0
garlic (*R.W. Knudsen*)	60	2.0	13.0	0	0	620	0

Food and Measure	cal.	prot. (gms)	carbo. (gms)	fat (gms)	chol. (mgs)	sod. (mgs)	fiber (gms)
Tomato paste, 2 tbsp.:							
(*Contadina*)	30	2.0	6.0	0	0	20	1.0
(*Del Monte*)	30	1.0	7.0	0	0	25	2.0
(*Hunt's*)	25	1.0	5.5	0	0	95	1.5
(*Hunt's* No Salt)	30	1.0	6.0	0	0	<10	2.0
(*Muir Glen*)	30	2.0	6.0	0	0	20	1.0
(*Progresso*)	30	2.0	6.0	0	0	20	1.0
Italian (*Hunt's*)	25	1.0	6.0	0	0	265	2.0
Tomato powder (*Al-pineAire*), 2 oz. . . .	104	5.0	22.0	1.0	0	14	n.a.
Tomato preserve (*Smucker's*), 1 tbsp.	50	0	13.0	0	0	0	0
Tomato puree, ¼ cup, except as noted:							
(*Hunt's*), 2 tbsp.	10	.5	2.5	0	0	5	<1.0
(*Muir Glen*)	20	1.0	5.0	0	0	20	1.0
(*Progresso*)	25	1.0	5.0	0	0	15	1.0
thick (*Progresso*)	20	<1.0	5.0	0	0	15	1.0
Tomato sauce, **canned** (see also "Pasta sauce" and "Tomato, canned"), ¼ cup:							
(*Contadina*)	20	<1.0	4.0	0	0	280	<1.0
(*Del Monte*)	20	<1.0	4.0	0	0	340	<1.0
(*Del Monte* No Salt)	20	<1.0	4.0	0	0	20	<1.0
(*Goya*)	20	1.0	4.0	0	0	280	1.0
(*Hunt's*)	15	1.0	3.0	0	0	360	1.0
(*Hunt's* No Salt)	15	1.0	3.0	0	0	10	1.0
(*Hunt's* Special)	20	1.0	4.0	<1.0	0	145	1.0
(*Hunt's Ready Sauce* Chunky)	15	1.0	3.0	0	0	400	1.0
(*Muir Glen* Chunky)	20	<1.0	4.0	0	0	160	1.0
(*Muir Glen* No Salt)	20	<1.0	5.0	0	0	30	1.0
(*Muir Glen* Organic)	20	<1.0	5.0	0	0	190	1.0
(*Progresso*)	20	1.0	4.0	0	0	260	1.0
chili, chunky (*Hunt's Ready Sauce*)	20	1.0	4.0	0	0	320	1.0

Food and Measure	cal.	prot. (gms)	carbo. (gms)	fat (gms)	chol. (mgs)	sod. (mgs)	fiber (gms)
Tomato sauce, canned *(cont.)*							
garlic-herb (*Hunt's Ready Sauce*)	25	1.0	5.0	0	0	200	1.0
herb (*Hunt's*)	30	1.0	5.0	1.0	0	270	1.0
Italian:							
(*Contadina*).	15	<1.0	4.0	0	0	320	<1.0
(*Hunt's*)	30	1.0	5.0	1.0	0	210	1.0
chunky (*Hunt's Ready Sauce*) . . .	30	1.0	4.0	0	0	180	1.5
meatloaf (*Hunt's Ready Sauce Meatloaf Fixin's*) . . .	20	1.0	4.0	0	0	600	1.0
Mexican, chunky (*Hunt's Ready Sauce*)	20	1.0	4.0	0	0	390	1.0
salsa (*Hunt's Ready Sauce*)	20	1.0	3.0	0	0	360	1.0
seasoned, lightly (*Eden*).	25	1.0	5.0	0	0	45	1.0
Tomato tapenade, sun-dried (*Sonoma*), 1 tbsp.	70	1.0	4.0	6.0	0	5	1.0
Tomato-beef cocktail (*Beefamato*), 8 fl. oz.	80	1.0	20.0	0	0	780	1.0
Tomato-chile cocktail (*Snap-E-Tom*):							
6 fl. oz.	40	2.0	8.0	0	0	500	1.0
10 fl. oz.	60	3.0	13.0	0	0	840	2.0
Tomato-clam cocktail, 8 fl. oz.:							
(*Clamato*)	100	1.0	24.0	0	0	720	0
Caesar (*Clamato*)	100	0	24.0	0	0	780	0
Tongue, braised:							
beef, 4 oz.	321	25.1	.4	23.5	121	68	0
lamb, 4 oz.	312	24.5	0	23.0	214	76	0
pork, 4 oz.	307	27.3	0	21.1	166	124	0
veal, 4 oz.	229	29.3	0	11.5	n.a.	73	0
Tongue lunch meat, beef, corned (*Hebrew National*), 2 oz.	120	10.0	0	9.0	50	330	0

Food and Measure	cal.	prot. (gms)	carbo. (gms)	fat (gms)	chol. (mgs)	sod. (mgs)	fiber (gms)
Tortellini (see also "Tortelloni"), refrigerated, ¾ cup, except as noted:							
cheese:							
(*Contadina*)	250	11.0	39.0	6.0	50	350	2.0
(*Di Giorno*)	260	12.0	37.0	6.0	30	230	1.0
w/red pepper, hot (*Di Giorno*), 1 cup	310	16.0	41.0	9.0	40	310	3.0
3 (*Contadina*)	250	11.0	39.0	6.0	50	350	2.0
chicken and herb:							
(*Contadina*)	260	10.0	40.0	7.0	35	250	2.0
(*Di Giorno*), 1 cup	260	13.0	40.0	5.0	35	290	1.0
w/meat (*Di Giorno*) . . .	290	12.0	40.0	9.0	40	380	1.0
mozzarella-garlic (*Di Giorno*), 1 cup	300	15.0	40.0	9.0	45	440	1.0
mushroom (*Di Giorno*), 1 cup	290	14.0	42.0	7.0	30	510	2.0
spinach cheese (*Contadina*)	260	12.0	40.0	6.0	40	370	3.0
Tortellini entree, canned or packaged, 1 cup:							
cheese:							
(*Chef Boyardee*) . . .	230	9.0	46.0	1.0	15	770	4.0
(*Franco-American*)	240	6.0	44.0	4.0	25	1140	2.0
chicken (*Hormel Health Selections*)	180	8.0	34.0	1.0	10	450	2.0
meat:							
(*Chef Boyardee*) . . .	260	10.0	48.0	3.5	30	810	4.0
(*Franco-American*)	260	14.0	36.0	9.0	30	1140	2.0
Tortellini entree, frozen, 12-oz. pkg.:							
cheese, w/red bell pepper sauce (*Wolfgang Puck's*)	360	13.0	49.0	13.0	40	420	13.0
chicken, spicy (*Wolfgang Puck's*)	490	16.0	51.0	24.0	90	910	6.0
mushroom (*Wolfgang Puck's*)	430	14.0	54.0	18.0	40	660	6.0

Food and Measure	cal.	prot. (gms)	carbo. (gms)	fat (gms)	chol. (mgs)	sod. (mgs)	fiber (gms)
Tortelloni (see also "Tortellini"), refrigerated, 1 cup:							
cheese and herb (*Contadina*)	320	15.0	45.0	9.0	50	360	2.0
chicken and prosciutto (*Contadina*)	360	15.0	45.0	13.0	• 60	400	1.0
garlic and cheese (*Contadina* Light)	280	15.0	46.0	4.5	35	400	3.0
mushroom and cheese (*Contadina*)	290	12.0	46.0	6.0	30	340	3.0
tomato, sun-dried (*Contadina*)	320	11.0	46.0	10.0	30	350	3.0
Tortilla:							
(*Cedar's* Boston), 1.1-oz. pc.	100	4.0	18.0	2.0	0	210	1.0
(*Cedar's* Boston), 2.6-oz. pc.	200	8.0	35.0	3.5	0	395	2.0
corn:							
(*Azteca*), 2 pcs., 1.2 oz.	90	2.0	18.0	1.0	0	15	2.0
(*Tyson*), 3 pcs., 1.9 oz.	140	3.0	27.0	1.5	0	20	3.0
white (*Tyson*), 3 pcs., 1.9 oz. . . .	140	3.0	28.0	1.5	0	0	2.0
flour, 1 pc., except as noted:							
(*Azteca*), 2 pcs., 1.7 oz.	150	4.0	27.0	3.0	0	320	2.0
(*Azteca*), 1.4-oz. pc.	130	4.0	23.0	2.5	0	270	2.0
(*Azteca* Burrito Size), 1¾ oz. . . .	160	4.0	28.0	3.0	0	330	3.0
(*Azteca* Fat Free), 1.4-oz. pc.	110	3.0	24.0	0	0	340	1.0
(*Mesa* 6″)	80	2.0	15.0	1.5	0	210	<1.0
(*Old El Paso*)	130	3.0	21.0	3.5	0	290	0
(*Old El Paso* Refrigerated)	130	3.0	21.0	3.5	0	310	<1.0
(*Old El Paso* Refrigerated Low Fat)	110	3.0	22.0	1.5	0	280	<1.0
(*Tyson*), 1.4 oz. . . .	120	3.0	21.0	3.0	0	290	1.0

Food and Measure	cal.	prot. (gms)	carbo. (gms)	fat (gms)	chol. (mgs)	sod. (mgs)	fiber (gms)
(*Tyson*), 1.9 oz. . . .	170	4.0	30.0	4.0	0	410	2.0
(*Tyson*) heat pressed, 2 pcs., 1.9 oz.	170	4.0	30.0	4.0	0	410	2.0
jalapeño-cilantro (*Tumaro's* Burrito Size)	150	4.0	30.0	.5	0	230	1.0
sun-dried tomato (*Tumaro's* Burrito Size)	150	6.0	30.0	.5	0	200	1.0
whole wheat (*Tyson*), 1.4 oz.	120	4.0	20.0	3.0	0	240	3.0
soft taco:							
(*Old El Paso*), 2 pcs.	160	3.0	26.0	4.5	0	350	0
(*Old El Paso* Refrigerated), 1 pc. . . .	110	3.0	17.0	3.0	0	260	<1.0
Tortilla chips, see "Corn chips, puffs, and similar snacks"							
Tostada shell, see "Taco shell"							
Trail mix:							
(*Eden* Fruit & Nuts), 1 oz.	160	7.0	10.0	10.0	0	0	3.0
(*Sonoma*), 1/4 cup, 1.4 oz.	160	3.0	24.0	7.0	0	5	2.0
California:							
(*Dole*), 2 oz.	220	9.0	38.0	4.0	0	0	4.0
(*Eden* Harvest), 1 oz.	130	4.0	14.0	7.0	0	0	3.0
Hawaiian (*Dole*), 2 oz.	250	4.0	44.0	6.0	0	35	4.0
Tree fern, cooked, chopped, 1/2 cup . . .	28	.2	7.8	.1	0	3	2.6
Triticale, wholegrain, 1 cup	646	25.1	138.5	4.0	0	10	34.8
Triticale flour, wholegrain, 1 cup	440	17.1	95.1	2.4	0	3	19.0
Tropical punch, see "Fruit drink blend" and "Fruit juice blends"							

Food and Measure	cal.	prot. (gms)	carbo. (gms)	fat (gms)	chol. (mgs)	sod. (mgs)	fiber (gms)
Trout, meat only:							
mixed species:							
raw, 4 oz.	168	23.6	0	7.5	66	59	0
baked, broiled, or microwaved, 4 oz.	215	30.2	0	9.6	84	76	0
rainbow, farmed:							
raw, 4 oz.	156	23.7	0	6.1	67	40	0
baked, broiled, or microwaved, 4 oz.	192	27.5	0	8.2	77	48	0
rainbow, wild:							
raw, 4 oz.	135	23.2	0	3.9	67	35	0
baked, broiled, or microwaved, 4 oz.	170	26.0	0	6.6	78	64	0
sea, see "Sea trout"							
Trout, smoked, peppered, rainbow (*Spence & Co.*), 2 oz.	100	14.0	0	5.0	30	430	0
Tuna, meat only:							
bluefin:							
raw, 4 oz.	163	26.5	0	5.6	43	44	0
baked, broiled, or microwaved, 4 oz.	209	33.9	0	7.1	56	57	0
skipjack:							
raw, 4 oz.	117	25.0	0	1.2	53	42	0
baked, broiled, or microwaved, 4 oz.	150	32.0	0	1.5	68	53	0
yellowfin:							
raw, 4 oz.	123	26.5	0	1.1	51	42	0
baked, broiled, or microwaved, 4 oz.	158	34.0	0	1.4	66	53	0
Tuna, canned, drained, 2 oz. or ¼ cup:							
chunk light, oil: (*Bumble Bee*)	110	13.0	0	6.0	30	250	0

Food and Measure	cal.	prot. (gms)	carbo. (gms)	fat (gms)	chol. (mgs)	sod. (mgs)	fiber (gms)
(*Chicken of the Sea*)	110	13.0	0	6.0	30	250	0
(*Star-Kist*)	110	13.0	0	6.0	30	250	0
chunk light, water:							
(*Bumble Bee*)	60	13.0	0	.5	30	250	0
(*Star-Kist*)	60	13.0	0	.5	30	250	0
chunk white, water							
(*Star-Kist*)	60	13.0	0	1.0	25	250	0
solid, in olive oil							
(*Progresso*)	160	13.0	0	12.0	30	250	0
solid white, oil:							
(*Bumble Bee*)	90	14.0	0	3.0	25	250	0
(*Chicken of the Sea*)	90	14.0	0	3.0	25	250	0
(*Star-Kist*)	90	15.0	0	3.0	25	250	0
solid white, water:							
(*Bumble Bee*)	70	15.0	0	1.0	25	250	0
(*Star-Kist*)	70	15.0	0	1.0	25	250	0
Tuna, freeze-dried, Albacore (*AlpineAire*), 1 oz. . . .	110	26.0	0	.5	0	0	0
Tuna, frozen, yellowtail (*Peter Pan*), 4 oz.	110	26.0	0	.5	35	35	0
"Tuna," vegetarian, drained:							
canned (*Worthington Tuno*), 1/3 cup	80	7.0	4.0	4.0	0	380	1.0
frozen (*Worthington Tuno*), 1/2 cup	80	6.0	2.0	6.0	0	290	1.0
Tuna burger, frozen (*Ocean Beauty*), 3.2-oz. pc.	90	17.0	3.0	1.0	40	350	0
Tuna entree, dried, w/noodles, cheese (*AlpineAire*), 1 1/2 cups	310	18.0	40.0	9.0	20	670	4.0
Tuna entree, frozen, 1 pkg., except as noted:							
grilled, fillet, 1 pc.:							
barbecue (*Mrs. Paul's/Van de Kamp's*)	100	19.0	5.0	.5	30	180	0

Food and Measure	cal.	prot. (gms)	carbo. (gms)	fat (gms)	chol. (mgs)	sod. (mgs)	fiber (gms)
Tuna entree, frozen, grilled, fillet *(cont.)*							
sesame teriyaki							
(*Mrs. Paul's/Van de Kamp's*)	110	19.0	4.0	1.5	30	330	0
and noodle:							
(*Smart Ones* Casserole), 9½ oz.	270	13.0	38.0	7.0	45	670	4.0
(*Stouffer's* Casserole), 10 oz.	320	20.0	37.0	10.0	40	1130	0
chunky (*Marie Callender's*), 12 oz.	960	18.0	143.0	35.0	55	1670	6.0
Tuna entree mix (*Tuna Helper*):							
au gratin:							
1 cup*	300	13.0	37.0	11.0	20	890	1.0
less fat, 1 cup*	240	13.0	37.0	5.0	15	840	1.0
broccoli, cheesy:							
1 cup*	290	15.0	38.0	9.0	20	860	1.0
less fat, 1 cup*	240	15.0	38.0	5.0	15	820	1.0
broccoli, creamy:							
1 cup*	310	14.0	35.0	12.0	20	880	1.0
less fat, 1 cup*	240	14.0	35.0	5.0	15	820	1.0
cheddar, garden:							
1 cup*	290	13.0	36.0	11.0	20	1030	1.0
less fat, 1 cup*	240	13.0	36.0	5.0	15	980	1.0
fettuccine Alfredo:							
1 cup*	310	14.0	32.0	14.0	15	950	1.0
less fat, 1 cup*	240	14.0	32.0	6.0	15	870	1.0
pasta, cheesy:							
1 cup*	280	14.0	32.0	11.0	20	890	<1.0
less fat, 1 cup*	230	14.0	32.0	5.0	15	850	<1.0
pasta, creamy:							
1 cup*	300	14.0	31.0	13.0	20	910	1.0
less fat, 1 cup*	230	14.0	31.0	6.0	15	840	1.0
pasta salad:							
⅔ cup*	380	10.0	26.0	27.0	10	730	1.0
less fat, ⅔ cup*	230	10.0	26.0	1.5	10	790	1.0
pot pie, 1 cup*	440	18.0	40.0	24.0	110	1080	1.0
Romanoff:							
1 cup*	280	15.0	38.0	8.0	20	800	1.0
less fat, 1 cup*	240	15.0	38.0	3.0	20	740	1.0

Food and Measure	cal.	prot. (gms)	carbo. (gms)	fat (gms)	chol. (mgs)	sod. (mgs)	fiber (gms)
tetrazzini:							
1 cup*	300	14.0	34.0	12.0	20	1040	1.0
less fat, 1 cup*	230	14.0	34.0	5.0	20	980	1.0
tuna melt:							
1 cup*	300	12.0	34.0	13.0	20	900	1.0
less fat, 1 cup*	240	12.0	34.0	6.0	15	850	1.0
Tuna salad, ⅓ cup:							
(*Wampler*)	180	6.0	9.0	12.0	20	450	1.0
chunky (*Wampler*) . . .	180	8.0	8.0	13.0	20	380	1.0
Tuna spread (*Underwood*), ¼ cup, 2 oz.	50	9.0	2.0	1.0	30	480	0
Turban squash (*Frieda's*), ¾ cup, 3 oz.	30	1.0	7.0	0	0	0	1.0
Turbot, European, meat only:							
raw, 4 oz.	108	18.2	0	3.4	n.a.	170	0
baked, broiled, or microwaved, 4 oz. . . .	138	23.3	0	4.3	n.a.	218	0
Turkey (see also "Turkey, frozen and refrigerated"), fresh, all classes, roasted:							
meat w/skin, 4 oz. . . .	236	31.9	0	11.0	93	77	0
meat only:							
4 oz.	193	3.2	0	5.6	86	79	0
diced, 1 cup	238	41.0	0	7.0	107	99	0
skin only, 1 oz.	125	5.6	0	11.2	32	15	0
dark meat:							
w/skin, 4 oz.	251	31.2	0	13.1	101	86	0
meat only, 4 oz. . . .	212	32.4	0	8.2	96	90	0
meat only, diced, 1 cup	262	40.0	0	10.1	119	110	0
light meat:							
w/skin, 4 oz.	223	32.4	0	9.4	86	71	0
meat only, 4 oz. . . .	178	33.9	0	3.7	78	73	0
meat only, diced, 1 cup	219	41.9	0	4.5	97	89	0
breast, meat w/skin:							
½ breast, 1.9 lbs., (4.2 lbs. raw w/bone)	1637	248.1	0	64.1	643	541	0

Food and Measure	cal.	prot. (gms)	carbo. (gms)	fat (gms)	chol. (mgs)	sod. (mgs)	fiber (gms)
Turkey, breast, meat w/skin *(cont.)*							
4 oz.	214	32.6	0	8.4	84	71	0
ground, see "Turkey, ground"							
leg, meat w/skin:							
1.2 lbs. (1.5 lbs. raw w/bone)	1133	152.2	0	53.6	466	420	0
4 oz.	236	31.6	0	11.1	96	87	0
wing, meat w/skin:							
6.6 oz. (9.9 oz. raw w/bone)	426	50.9	0	23.1	150	114	0
4 oz.	260	31.0	0	14.1	92	69	0
Turkey, canned,							
2 oz., ¼ cup:							
(*Hormel*)	70	11.0	0	3.0	35	340	0
(*Swanson* Premium)	100	6.0	2.0	4.0	50	230	0
white:							
(*Hormel*)	60	13.0	0	1.0	25	320	0
(*Swanson* Premium)	90	3.0	4.0	2.0	35	220	1.0
Turkey, freeze-dried,							
diced (*AlpineAire*), ½ oz.	60	12.0	0	1.5	45	25	0
Turkey, frozen or re-frigerated, raw,							
4 oz., except as noted:							
whole:							
(*Butterball Li'l Butterball*)	170	23.0	1.0	8.0	75	150	0
(*Shady Brook Farms*)	180	23.0	0	9.0	75	75	0
whole, young:							
(*Butterball* Fresh)	170	24.0	0	8.0	80	70	0
(*Butterball Fresh Li'l Butterball*)	140	24.0	0	4.0	80	70	0
(*Norbest* Family Tradition, 8-16 lbs.)	190	23.0	0	10.0	70	70	0
(*Norbest* Family Tradition, 16-24 lbs.)	170	23.0	0	8.5	80	80	0
basted (*Norbest,* 8-16 lbs.)	180	21.0	0	9.5	65	180	0

Food and Measure	cal.	prot. (gms)	carbo. (gms)	fat (gms)	chol. (mgs)	sod. (mgs)	fiber (gms)
basted (*Norbest*, 16-24 lbs.)	165	22.0	0	8.0	75	190	0
boneless (*Butterball*)	160	20.0	0	9.0	80	600	0
boneless (*Norbest*)	135	20.0	0	6.0	60	490	0
stuffed (*Butterball*), w/out stuffing ...	180	23.0	0	10.0	75	150	0
boneless roast (*Norbest*)	135	18.0	0	7.0	65	490	0
breast:							
(*Butterball* Young)	170	22.0	0	8.0	65	160	0
basted (*Norbest*)...	170	22.0	0	8.5	60	270	0
boneless (*Butterball* Young)	130	21.0	0	5.0	50	600	0
boneless (*Perdue*)	130	29.0	0	1.0	60	60	0
cutlet, thin sliced (*Perdue Fit 'n Easy*), 3½ oz.	100	23.0	0	1.0	50	45	0
fillet (*Perdue*)	130	29.0	0	1.0	60	55	0
roast (*Shady Brook Farms*)	130	28.0	0	.5	70	55	0
whole or split (*Shady Brook Farms*)	190	24.0	0	9.0	70	60	0
cured, dark (*Wampler*), 2 oz.	80	8.0	2.0	4.5	30	600	0
cutlet:							
(*Shady Brook Farms*)	130	28.0	0	.5	70	55	0
thin sliced (*Perdue*), 3½ oz.	100	23.0	0	1.5	60	40	0
drummette (*Shady Brook Farms*)	170	24.0	0	9.0	70	105	0
drumstick (*Shady Brook Farms*)	170	22.0	0	9.0	70	60	0
ground, see "Turkey, ground"							
leg quarter (*Shady Brook Farms*)	200	21.0	0	12.0	75	75	0
neck (*Shady Brook Farms*)	150	23.0	0	6.0	90	105	0

Food and Measure	cal.	prot. (gms)	carbo. (gms)	fat (gms)	chol. (mgs)	sod. (mgs)	fiber (gms)
Turkey, frozen or refrigerated, raw *(cont.)*							
steak, cubed *(Perdue)*	110	23.0	0	2.0	90	95	0
tenderloin:							
(Perdue)	120	26.0	0	1.0	60	60	0
(Shady Brook Farms)	130	28.0	0	.5	70	55	0
lemon pepper *(Shady Brook Farms)*	120	24.0	0	1.5	60	250	0
mesquite *(Shady Brook Farms)* . . .	110	23.0	0	.5	50	360	0
teriyaki *(Shady Brook Farms)* . . .	120	24.0	0	.5	50	460	0
thigh *(Shady Brook Farms)*	220	21.0	0	15.0	75	75	0
wing:							
(Shady Brook Farms)	220	23.0	0	14.0	80	60	0
portion *(Shady Brook Farms*	210	24.0	0	12.0	110	70	0
Turkey, frozen or re-frigerated, cooked, 3 oz., except as noted:							
whole:							
dark meat *(Perdue)*	200	19.0	0	14.0	95	55	0
white meat *(Perdue)*	170	22.0	0	9.0	70	35	0
baked *(Butterball Young)*	160	19.0	1.0	9.0	65	300	0
oven-roasted *(Shady Brook Farm)*, 2 oz.	90	11.0	0	4.0	30	760	0
smoked *(Butterball Young)*	160	19.0	1.0	9.0	65	390	0
smoked, honey roasted *(Butterball Young)*	140	19.0	1.0	7.0	65	300	0
breast:							
(Mosey's Time for Dinner), 5 oz. . . .	140	25.0	6.0	2.0	110	870	0
(Perdue Whole) . . .	160	23.0	0	8.0	60	30	0

Food and Measure	cal.	prot. (gms)	carbo. (gms)	fat (gms)	chol. (mgs)	sod. (mgs)	fiber (gms)
(*Perdue* Half)	160	23.0	0	7.0	65	35	0
boneless (*Perdue*)	110	26.0	0	1.0	55	35	0
cutlet, thin sliced (*Perdue*), 2½ oz.	100	22.0	0	1.0	50	35	0
cutlet, thin sliced (*Perdue Fit 'n Easy*), 2.4 oz.	90	20.0	0	.5	45	30	0
fillet (*Perdue*)	120	27.0	0	1.0	60	40	0
fillet (*Perdue Fit 'n Easy*)	110	26.0	0	.5	60	40	0
honey-roasted (*Shady Brook Farms*), 2 oz. ...	60	11.0	n.a.	.5	30	400	0
hickory, smoked(*Norbest*)	145	16.0	0	9.0	50	720	0
hickory smoked (*Shady Brook Farms*), 2 oz. ...	50	11.0	0	0	25	470	0
Italian seasoned (*Shady Brook Farms* Carved), 2 oz.	60	12.0	n.a.	0	20	490	0
oven-roasted (*Shady Brook Farms*), 2 oz. ...	90	12.0	0	3.5	25	360	0
tenderloin (*Perdue*)	110	26.0	0	1.0	55	35	0
tenderloin (*Perdue Fit 'n Easy*)	110	26.0	0	1.0	55	45	0
breast, smoked:							
(*Butterball*)	130	19.0	1.0	6.0	50	390	0
(*Hebrew National*), 2 oz.	60	12.0	0	.5	25	330	0
(*Hormel Light & Lean* 97)	80	17.0	1.0	1.0	35	780	0
(*Shady Brook Farms*)	130	17.0	0	1.5	50	760	0
drumstick:							
(*Perdue*)	150	22.0	0	7.0	95	70	0
smoked (*Shady Brook Farms*) ...	180	22.0	0	8.0	70	620	0

Food and Measure	cal.	prot. (gms)	carbo. (gms)	fat (gms)	chol. (mgs)	sod. (mgs)	fiber (gms)
Turkey, frozen or, drumstick *(cont.)*							
maple glaze (*Boar's Head Honey Coat*)	100	21.0	3.0	1.0	45	660	0
meatballs, Italian (*Shady Brook Farms*)	130	12.0	n.a.	7.0	45	350	n.a.
neck, smoked (*Shady Brook Farms*)	150	22.0	0	6.0	65	700	0
thigh (*Perdue*)	180	20.0	0	11.0	100	55	0
wing:							
(*Perdue* Tom)	160	23.0	0	8.0	85	65	0
portion (*Perdue*), 2½ oz.	140	17.0	0	8.0	75	45	0
roasted (*Perdue*) . . .	180	22.0	0	10.0	95	60	0
roasted (*Perdue* Drummettes), 3½-oz. pc.	180	24.0	0	9.0	95	65	0
wing, smoked (*Shady Brook Farms*)	200	22.0	0	10.0	65	680	0
Turkey, ground:							
raw, 4 oz.:							
(*Norbest*)	170	21.0	0	10.0	75	75	0
(*Perdue*)	160	23.0	0	8.0	110	80	0
(*Shady Brook Farm* 85% Turkey)	220	21.0	0	15.0	75	75	0
(*Wampler*)	210	18.0	0	15.0	100	30	0
breast (*Perdue*)	130	28.0	0	1.5	60	75	0
breast (*Shady Brook Farms*)	120	28.0	0	1.0	70	55	0
burger (*Wampler*) . . .	210	18.0	0	15.0	100	30	0
burger, barbecue (*Wampler*)	220	10.0	3.0	15.0	100	260	0
burger, specially seasoned (*Wampler*)	180	21.0	1.0	11.0	75	400	0
lean or burgers (*Shady Brook Farms*)	170	20.0	0	9.0	90	105	0
meatloaf (*Shady Brook Farms*) . . .	150	18.0	n.a.	7.0	95	400	0

Food and Measure	cal.	prot. (gms)	carbo. (gms)	fat (gms)	chol. (mgs)	sod. (mgs)	fiber (gms)
cooked, 3 oz.:							
(*Perdue*)	170	21.0	0	9.0	110	65	0
breast (*Perdue*)	110	24.0	0	1.0	55	45	0
"Turkey," vegetarian:							
canned (*Worthington* Turkee), 3 slices . . .	170	13.0	3.0	12.0	0	580	2.0
frozen, smoked, sliced (*Worthington*), 3 slices	140	10.0	3.0	10.0	0	620	2.0
Turkey bacon, 1/2-oz. slice:							
(*Jennie-O* Fat Free) . . .	20	3.0	0	0	15	130	0
(*Louis Rich*)	35	2.0	0	2.5	15	180	0
Turkey bologna:							
(*Norbest*), 2 oz.	130	7.0	0	11.0	45	640	0
(*Wampler*), 2 oz.	100	8.0	1.0	8.0	40	240	0
Turkey dinner, frozen, 1 pkg.:							
(*Swanson*), 11¾ oz.	310	22.0	40.0	8.5	30	890	5.0
(*Swanson Hungry Man*), 16¾ oz.	500	30.0	61.0	15.0	50	1550	7.0
Turkey entree, canned or packaged:							
chili, see "Chili, canned or packaged"							
and dressing (*Dinty Moore American Classics*), 1 bowl	290	22.0	32.0	8.0	45	1120	3.0
w/potatoes (*Dinty Moore American Classics*), 1 bowl	250	19.0	27.0	7.0	25	1040	3.0
stew 1 cup:							
(*Dinty Moore* Can)	140	10.0	19.0	3.0	20	910	2.0
(*Dinty Moore* Microwave Cup)	130	9.0	16.0	2.5	10	760	2.0
Turkey entree, dried, 1 serving:							
mashed potato and gravy w/ (*AlpineAire*)	270	12.0	52.0	1.5	35	700	1.0

Food and Measure	cal.	prot. (gms)	carbo. (gms)	fat (gms)	chol. (mgs)	sod. (mgs)	fiber (gms)
Turkey entree, dried *(cont.)*							
Romanoff (*AlpineAire*)	320	24.0	33.0	11.0	70	640	1.0
teriyaki (*AlpineAire*)	270	16.0	46.0	2.0	40	400	1.0
tetrazzini (*Mountain House*)	210	14.0	20.0	8.0	45	1060	1.0
wild thyme (*AlpineAire*)	380	21.0	49.0	11.0	55	620	6.0
Turkey entree, frozen, 1 pkg., except as noted:							
(*Lean Cuisine* Homestyle), 9 oz.	230	17.0	30.0	5.0	40	590	3.0
breast:							
(*Healthy Choice* Traditional), 10½ oz.	290	22.0	40.0	4.5	45	460	5.0
w/rice pilaf (*Marie Callender's*), 11¾ oz.	320	22.0	34.0	10.0	35	940	4.0
slow roasted (*Weight Watchers*), 10 oz.	220	18.0	20.0	7.0	25	660	2.0
stuffed (*Weight Watchers Main Street Bistro*), 10 oz.	270	13.0	37.0	7.0	30	720	5.0
chili, see "Chili entree"							
croquettes, gravy and (*Freezer Queen* Family), 1 patty w/gravy	150	9.0	16.0	5.0	25	590	1.0
glazed:							
(*The Budget Gourmet* Low Fat), 8½ oz.	260	11.0	39.0	5.0	15	660	1.0
tenderloins (*Lean Cuisine Cafe Classics*), 9 oz.	240	14.0	37.0	5.0	30	590	5.0
gravy, and:							
dressing (*Banquet Extra Helping*), 17 oz.	630	28.0	57.0	32.0	80	2250	10.0

Food and Measure	cal.	prot. (gms)	carbo. (gms)	fat (gms)	chol. (mgs)	sod. (mgs)	fiber (gms)
dressing (*Marie Callender's*), 14 oz.	500	31.0	52.0	19.0	80	2040	4.0
dressing, mashed potato (*Freezer Queen* Homestyle), 8½ oz. . . .	210	10.0	31.0	5.0	20	620	3.0
dressing, mashed potato, corn (*Freezer Queen* Meal), 9¼ oz. . . .	220	14.0	31.0	4.5	65	1030	3.0
dressing, rolls (*Freezer Queen Deluxe Family*), 7-oz. roll	170	12.0	33.0	4.0	35	820	3.0
mashed potato (*Marie Callender's*), 2 slices, ½ cup potato	290	25.0	25.0	10.0	70	1080	2.0
pie or pot pie:							
(*Banquet*), 7 oz. . . .	370	10.0	38.0	20.0	45	850	3.0
(*Marie Callender's*), 9½ oz.	610	15.0	57.0	36.0	15	1070	3.0
(*Marie Callender's* 16½ oz.), 1 cup	320	15.0	56.0	36.0	15	1320	3.0
(*Stouffer's*), 10 oz.	530	21.0	36.0	33.0	65	1040	3.0
(*Swanson*), 7 oz.	400	10.0	42.0	21.0	25	700	3.0
(*Swanson Hungry Man*), 14 oz.	690	20.0	66.0	38.0	45	1430	6.0
roast:							
(*Healthy Choice* Country Inn), 10 oz.	250	20.0	28.0	6.0	40	530	4.0
(*Lean Cuisine Skillet Sensations*), ½ of 24-oz. pkg.	220	14.0	37.0	2.0	25	790	6.0
(*Stouffer's* Homestyle), 9⅝ oz. . . .	310	22.0	27.0	13.0	50	930	3.0
breast (*Lean Cuisine American Favorites*), 9¾ oz.	270	13.0	49.0	3.0	20	590	5.0

Food and Measure	cal.	prot. (gms)	carbo. (gms)	fat (gms)	chol. (mgs)	sod. (mgs)	fiber (gms)
Turkey entree, frozen, roast *(cont.)*							
breast (*Lean Cuisine Hearty Portions*), 14 oz.	350	24.0	49.0	6.0	25	840	8.0
breast (*Stouffer's Hearty Portions*), 16 oz.	490	25.0	52.0	20.0	35	1880	6.0
honey, breast (*Banquet*), 9 oz.	270	11.0	29.0	12.0	30	1310	4.0
medallions and mushrooms (*Smart Ones*), 9 oz.	200	12.0	33.0	2.0	20	550	2.0
w/mushrooms (*Healthy Choice* Country), 8½ oz.	220	19.0	28.0	4.0	25	440	3.0
sausage, w/peppers and onions (*Wampler*), 1 cup or ⅑ pkg.	210	17.0	14.0	11.0	70	1120	3.0
sliced:							
gravy and (*Banquet* Family), 2 slices w/gravy	150	8.0	5.0	11.0	35	670	1.0
gravy and (*Freezer Queen* Cook-in-Pouch), 5 oz. . . .	70	7.0	6.0	2.0	15	750	1.0
gravy and (*Freezer Queen* Family), 4½ oz.	60	4.0	6.0	2.0	15	560	<1.0
tetrazzini (*Stouffer's*), 10 oz.	360	19.0	33.0	17.0	55	1060	1.0
w/vegetables (*Healthy Choice Hearty Handfuls*), 6.1 oz.	320	18.0	51.0	5.0	20	590	5.0
white meat, mostly (*Banquet* Meal), 9¼ oz.	280	14.0	34.0	10.0	55	1060	3.0
Turkey fat, 1 tbsp. . . .	115	0	0	12.8	13	0	0
Turkey frankfurter, see "Frankfurter"							

Food and Measure	cal.	prot. (gms)	carbo. (gms)	fat (gms)	chol. (mgs)	sod. (mgs)	fiber (gms)
Turkey giblets:							
simmered, 4 oz.	189	30.1	2.4	5.8	474	67	0
simmered, diced,							
1 cup	243	38.5	3.0	7.4	606	85	0
Turkey gravy, 1/4 cup:							
(*Franco-American*) ...	25	1.0	3.0	1.0	<5	290	0
(*Franco-American* Fat							
Free)	20	1.0	4.0	0	0	280	0
(*Franco-American*							
Slow Roasted)	30	1.0	4.0	1.0	<5	330	0
(*Franco-American*							
Slow Roasted Fat							
Free)	30	1.0	6.0	0	<5	370	0
(*Heinz* Home Style							
Roasted)	20	1.0	3.0	.5	0	340	0
Turkey gravy mix,							
roasted (*Knorr*),							
1 tbsp.	25	2.0	4.0	.5	<5	300	0
Turkey ham:							
(*Healthy Deli*), 2 oz.	80	10.0	2.0	2.5	30	470	0
(*Norbest* 15% Water),							
3 oz.	95	14.0	0	4.0	45	920	0
(*Norbest* 25% Water),							
3 oz.	90	13.0	2.0	3.0	45	990	0
(*Wampler*), 2 oz.	50	8.0	1.0	2.0	30	630	0
Black Forest:							
(*Shady Brook*							
Farms), 2 oz. ...	70	10.0	0	2.5	30	470	0
(*Wampler*), 2 oz.	60	10.0	2.0	1.5	25	650	0
canned (*Hormel*),							
2 oz.	70	9.0	0	4.0	40	600	0
smoked (*Wampler*),							
2 oz.	60	10.0	0	2.5	40	590	0
Turkey ham salad							
(*Wampler*), 1/3 cup	150	7.0	9.0	10.0	30	500	1.0
Turkey hash, roast							
(*Mary Kitchen*),							
1 cup	210	23.0	23.0	3.0	60	950	2.0 d
Turkey liver, see							
"Liver"							

Food and Measure	cal.	prot. (gms)	carbo. (gms)	fat (gms)	chol. (mgs)	sod. (mgs)	fiber (gms)
Turkey lunch meat (see also "Turkey ham," etc.), 2 oz. breast, except as noted:							
(*Boar's Head* Premium Lower Sodium)	60	11.0	<1.0	2.0	25	310	0
(*Boar's Head* Premium Lower Sodium Skinless)	60	12.0	<1.0	.5	25	340	0
(*Boar's Head Ovengold*)	60	12.0	1.0	1.5	35	360	0
(*Boar's Head Ovengold* Skinless)	60	13.0	0	1.0	20	350	0
(*Boar's Head Salsalito*)	60	13.0	1.0	.5	25	460	0
(*Hansel 'n Gretel*)	50	7.0	3.0	1.0	15	550	0
(*Healthy Choice* Variety Pack), 1-oz. slice	30	5.0	3.0	1.0	15	240	0
(*Hormel Light & Lean* 97), 1-oz. slice	30	5.0	0	1.0	15	380	0
(*Norbest* Bronze Label Deli)	60	7.0	2.0	2.0	20	560	0
(*Norbest* Gold Label Deli)	55	10.0	0	1.5	25	500	0
(*Norbest* Silver Label Deli)	55	8.0	2.0	2.0	25	500	0
(*Wampler* 5 Diamond)	50	13.0	0	0	30	240	0
(*Wampler* 5 Diamond Skin On)	70	12.0	0	2.5	35	240	0
(*Wampler* 4 Diamond Skinless)	60	11.0	0	1.5	20	400	0
(*Wampler* 3 Diamond Fat Free)	45	9.0	1.0	0	20	440	0
browned:							
(*Healthy Choice*) ...	50	11.0	0	1.0	20	360	0
golden (*Norbest* Gold Label Deli)	60	10.0	0	1.5	30	500	0
cured (*Norbest* Gourmet)	70	7.0	0	4.5	35	620	0
honey cured, Champagne glazed (*Black Bear*)	70	11.0	3.0	1.0	20	400	0

Food and Measure	cal.	prot. (gms)	carbo. (gms)	fat (gms)	chol. (mgs)	sod. (mgs)	fiber (gms)
honey roasted:							
(*Healthy Deli*)	60	10.0	3.0	.5	20	480	0
w/cracked pepper (*Shady Brook Farms*)	60	11.0	0	0	25	470	0
smoked (*Healthy Choice*)	60	11.0	2.0	0	25	420	0
smoked (*Healthy Choice*), 1-oz. slice	35	5.0	2.0	1.0	15	240	0
smoked (*Healthy Choice* Deli-Thin Savory Selections), 6 slices, 1.9 oz.	60	10.0	4.0	1.5	25	470	0
maple honey:							
(*Boar's Head Maple Glazed Honey Coat*)	70	14.0	2.0	.5	30	440	0
(*Healthy Deli* Fat Free*)	70	11.0	4.0	0	20	480	0
natural-roasted (*Shady Brook Farms Carved*)	60	12.0	n.a.	0	20	470	0
oil browned:							
(*Wampler* 5 Diamond Skin On)	70	11.0	3.0	1.0	15	39	0
(*Wampler* 5 Diamond Skinless)	45	9.0	1.0	.5	20	530	0
(*Wampler* 4 Diamond)	60	10.0	1.0	1.5	25	490	0
(*Wampler* 3 Diamond)	50	12.0	1.0	1.5	20	360	0
(*Wampler* 3 Diamond Skinless)	45	9.0	1.0	.5	20	530	0
orange flavor (*Healthy Deli*)	65	11.0	2.0	.5	20	360	0
oven browned (*Wampler* 4 Diamond) ...	50	9.0	1.0	1.0	20	540	0
oven roasted:							
(*Black Bear*)	50	11.0	1.0	1.0	20	280	0

Food and Measure	cal.	prot. (gms)	carbo. (gms)	fat (gms)	chol. (mgs)	sod. (mgs)	fiber (gms)
Turkey lunch meat, oven roasted *(cont.)*							
(*Boar's Head Golden*)	60	11.0	0	2.0	25	340	0
(*Boar's Head* Golden Skinless)	60	13.0	<1.0	.5	25	350	0
(*Empire*), 3 slices	50	10.0	1.0	.5	15	200	0
(*Healthy Choice*) . . .	45	10.0	1.0	0	20	360	0
(*Healthy Deli* Gourmet)	60	11.0	1.0	0	20	440	0
(*Hebrew National* Thin Sliced)	50	11.0	1.0	.5	20	430	0
(*Oscar Mayer Free*), 4 slices, 1.8 oz.	45	8.0	2.0	0	15	670	0
(*Wampler* 3 Diamond)	50	9.0	1.0	1.0	15	390	0
(*Wampler* 2 Diamond)	50	8.0	1.0	1.5	10	430	0
(*Wampler* 1 Diamond)	60	7.0	1.0	2.0	20	490	0
browned (*Shady Brook Farms* Homestyle)	60	11.0	0	1.0	20	400	0
glazed (*Healthy Deli* Gourmet)	60	11.0	1.0	.5	20	440	0
Italian (*Healthy Deli*)	70	10.0	4.0	.5	20	490	0
white (*Oscar Mayer*), 1-oz. slice	30	4.0	1.0	1.0	10	300	0
and white (*Healthy Choice*), 1-oz. slice	30	5.0	2.0	1.0	15	240	0
and white (*Healthy Choice* Deli-Thin), 6 slices, 1.9 oz.	60	9.0	2.0	1.5	20	470	0
and white (*Oscar Mayer Deli-Thin*), 4 slices, 1.8 oz.	50	8.0	2.0	1.0	20	610	0
pan-roasted:							
(*Wampler*)	50	12.0	1.0	0	20	400	0
(*Wampler* All Natural)	50	12.0	0	1.0	25	250	0

Food and Measure	cal.	prot. (gms)	carbo. (gms)	fat (gms)	chol. (mgs)	sod. (mgs)	fiber (gms)
peppered:							
(*Shady Brook Farms* Carved)	60	12.0	n.a.	0	20	450	0
(*Wampler*)	40	8.0	1.0	0	20	520	0
roasted (*Healthy Choice* Hearty Deli)	60	11.0	1.0	.5	25	480	0
rotisserie:							
(*Healthy Choice* Deli-Thin), 6 slices, 1.9 oz.	60	9.0	4.0	1.5	20	470	0
(*Wampler*)	50	9.0	1.0	1.5	20	500	0
salsa (*Healthy Choice*) .	60	11.0	1.0	1.0	20	360	0
slow-roasted, browned (*Shady Brook Farms*)	60	11.0	0	0	20	400	0
smoked:							
Boar's Head Cracked Pepper Mill)	60	13.0	0	.5	30	460	0
(*Empire*), 3 slices	40	8.0	0	0	15	350	0
(*Healthy Deli*)	60	11.0	1.0	0	20	470	0
(*Norbest* Deli Gold Label)	60	10.0	0	1.5	30	510	0
(*Wampler* 5 Diamond Skin On)	70	12.0	0	2.5	20	420	0
(*Wampler* 4 Diamond)	60	11.0	2.0	2.0	20	490	0
(*Wampler* 3 Diamond)	45	8.0	1.0	1.0	15	430	0
(*Wampler* 2 Diamond)	60	8.0	2.0	2/5	20	380	0
(*Wampler* 1 Diamond)	50	8.0	1.0	1.5	20	520	0
hickory (*Boar's Head*)	70	12.0	<1.0	2.0	25	340	0
hickory (*Hebrew National* Sliced)	50	12.0	0	.5	25	420	0
honey cured (*Wampler* 4 Diamond)	70	9.0	4.0	2.0	25	560	0
honey cured (Wampler 4 Diamond Petite)	50	9.0	4.0	0	25	380	0

Food and Measure	cal.	prot. (gms)	carbo. (gms)	fat (gms)	chol. (mgs)	sod. (mgs)	fiber (gms)
Turkey lunch meat, smoked *(cont.)*							
honey pepper (*Norbest* Gold Label)	50	10.0	3.0	0	25	490	0
honey-roasted (*JOscar Mayer Deli-Thin*), 4 slices, 1.8 oz.	50	9.0	2.0	1.0	20	500	0
mesquite (*Boar's Head Mesquite Wood Smoked*)	60	12.0	0	1.0	25	440	0
mesquite (*Boar's Head Mesquite Wood Smoked Skinless*)	60	13.0	0	.5	25	440	0
mesquite (*Healthy Choice* Deli-Thin Savory Selections), 6 slices, 1.9 oz.	60	9.0	3.0	1.5	20	470	0
mesquite (*Healthy Deli*)	60	11.0	1.0	0	20	480	0
mesquite (*Hormel Light & Lean* 97), 1 oz.	30	5.0	0	1.0	15	380	0
mesquite, honey (*Norbest* Gold Label)	50	9.0	3.0	0	25	500	0
mesquite, honey cured (*Wampler* 4 Diamond)	50	9.0	4.0	0	25	380	0
skinless (*Healthy Choice*)	50	10.0	1.0	0	25	400	0
white (*Norbest*)	70	7.0	2.0	3.0	25	540	0
and white (*Healthy Choice*), 1-oz. slice	30	5.0	2.0	1.0	15	240	0
Southwest grill (*Healthy Choice*) . . .	60	11.0	1.0	1.0	20	360	0
spiced (*Wampler* Classic)	70	16.0	1.0	.5	25	380	0

Food and Measure	cal.	prot. (gms)	carbo. (gms)	fat (gms)	chol. (mgs)	sod. (mgs)	fiber (gms)
Tex-Mex (*Black Bear*)	60	12.0	1.0	.5	20	460	0
Turkey pastrami, 2 oz.:							
(*Boar's Head*)	60	14.0	0	.5	30	390	0
(*Healthy Deli*)	70	10.0	2.0	2.5	30	480	0
(*Hebrew National*) ...	60	10.0	0	2.5	45	560	0
(*Norbest*)	70	10.0	0	3.0	30	570	0
(*Wampler*)	80	11.0	1.0	4.0	40	290	0
Turkey pepperoni (*Hormel Pillow Pack*), 17 slices, 1.1 oz.	80	9.0	0	4.0	40	550	0
Turkey pie, see "Turkey entree"							
Turkey pocket, frozen, 4½-oz. pc.:							
broccoli and cheese (*Lean Pockets*)	250	12.0	35.0	7.0	35	540	4.0
and ham, w/cheese: (*Hot Pockets*)	300	14.0	35.0	11.0	40	600	4.0
cheddar (*Lean Pockets*)	270	14.0	41.0	7.0	35	700	1.0
Swiss (*Croissant Pockets*)	290	14.0	37.0	10.0	40	730	2.0
Turkey salad spread (*Libby's Spreadables*), ⅓ cup	150	7.0	6.0	10.0	25	310	2.0
Turkey salami:							
(*Empire*), 3 slices	70	9.0	1.0	3.5	35	350	0
(*Norbest*), 2 oz.	85	9.0	2.0	5.0	30	510	0
(*Wampler*), 2 oz.	90	9.0	1.0	6.0	55	560	0
cooked, 1 oz.	56	4.6	.2	3.9	23	285	0
Turkey sandwich, see "Turkey pocket"							
Turkey sausage, see "Sausage"							
Turmeric, ground, 1 tsp.	8	.2	1.4	.2	0	1	.5
Turnip, ½ cup, except as noted:							
fresh or stored: raw, cubed	18	.6	4.1	.1	0	44	1.2

Food and Measure	cal.	prot. (gms)	carbo. (gms)	fat (gms)	chol. (mgs)	sod. (mgs)	fiber (gms)
Turnip, fresh or stored *(cont.)*							
boiled, cubed	14	.6	3.8	.1	0	39	1.6
boiled, mashed	21	.8	5.6	.1	0	58	2.3
frozen, boiled, drained,							
4 oz.	26	1.7	4.9	.3	0	41	n.a.
Turnip greens, fresh:							
raw, untrimmed, 1 lb.	85	4.8	18.2	1.0	0	126	7.6
raw, chopped, ½ cup	7	.4	1.6	.1	0	11	.7
boiled, chopped,							
½ cup	15	.8	3.1	.2	0	21	2.2
Turnip greens,							
canned, ½ cup:							
(*Allens/Sunshine*)	25	2.0	3.0	.5	0	15	2.0
(*Stubb's*)	25	2.0	3.0	.5	0	15	2.0
chopped:							
(*Bush's Best*)	25	2.0	3.0	0	0	300	2.0
w/diced turnips (*Allens/Sunshine*)	30	1.0	5.0	.5	0	20	3.0
w/diced turnips							
(*Bush's Best*) . . .	30	1.0	5.0	0	0	380	2.0
w/liquid	17	1.6	2.8	.4	0	325	1.5
Turnip greens, frozen,							
w/diced turnips:							
(*Birds Eye*), 1 cup	25	2.0	2.0	0	0	20	2.0
(*McKenzie's*), 1 cup	25	2.0	2.0	0	0	20	2.0
boiled, drained, 4 oz.	19	2.4	3.3	.2	0	17	3.5
Turnover, frozen or refrigerated, 1 pc.:							
apple:							
(*Pepperidge Farm*)	330	4.0	48.0	14.0	0	180	6.0
(*Pillsbury*), 2-oz.							
pc.	170	2.0	23.0	8.0	0	310	<1.0
iced (*Pepperidge Farm*)	360	4.0	53.0	14.0	0	190	2.0
mini (*Pepperidge Farm*)	140	2.0	15.0	8.0	0	80	1.0
blueberry (*Pepperidge Farm*)	340	4.0	45.0	16.0	0	200	6.0
cherry:							
(*Pepperidge Farm*)	320	4.0	46.0	13.0	0	190	6.0

Food and Measure	cal.	prot. (gms)	carbo. (gms)	fat (gms)	chol. (mgs)	sod. (mgs)	fiber (gms)
(*Pillsbury*), 2-oz. pc.	180	2.0	24.0	8.0	0	310	0
iced (*Pepperidge Farm*)	340	4.0	51.0	13.0	0	200	3.0
mini (*Pepperidge Farm*)	140	2.0	16.0	8.0	0	70	1.0
peach:							
(*Pepperidge Farm*)	340	4.0	47.0	15.0	0	180	6.0
cobbler, mini (*Pepperidge Farm*) ...	160	2.0	21.0	8.0	0	45	<1.0
raspberry:							
(*Pepperidge Farm*)	330	4.0	47.0	14.0	0	190	6.0
iced (*Pepperidge Farm*)	360	4.0	53.0	14.0	0	190	3.0
strawberry, mini (*Pepperidge Farm*)	140	2.0	18.0	7.0	0	100	<1.0
Twists, pasta, mix:							
w/creamy tomato sauce (*Knorr* Cup), 1 cont.	230	7.0	41.0	4.5	10	890	2.0
Tzatziki (*Western Creamy*), 2 tbsp.	60	3.0	1.0	5.0	5	115	0

V

Food and Measure	cal.	prot. (gms)	carbo. (gms)	fat (gms)	chol. (mgs)	sod. (mgs)	fiber (gms)
Vanilla syrup:							
(*Ferrara*), 2 oz.	130	0	32.0	0	0	12	0
(*Fox's U-Bet*), 2 tbsp.	80	0	21.0	0	0	10	0
(*Watkins*), 1 tbsp. . . .	40	0	18.0	0	0	0	0
Veal, meat only, 4 oz.:							
cubed, lean only,							
braised or stewed	213	39.6	0	4.9	164	105	0
ground, broiled	195	27.6	0	8.6	117	94	0
leg:							
braised, lean w/fat	239	41.0	0	7.2	152	76	0
braised, lean only	230	41.6	0	5.8	159	76	0
roasted, lean w/fat	181	31.4	0	5.3	117	77	0
roasted, lean only	170	31.8	0	3.8	117	77	0
loin:							
raised, lean w/fat	322	34.2	0	19.5	134	91	0
braised, lean only	256	38.1	0	10.4	142	95	0
roasted, lean w/fat	246	28.1	0	14.0	117	105	0
roasted, lean only	198	29.8	0	7.9	120	109	0
rib:							
braised, lean w/fat	285	36.8	0	14.2	158	108	0
braised, lean only	247	39.1	0	8.9	163	112	0
roasted, lean w/fat	259	27.2	0	15.8	125	104	0
roasted, lean only	201	29.2	0	8.4	130	110	0
shoulder, whole:							
braised, lean w/fat	259	36.4	0	11.5	143	108	0
braised, lean only	226	38.2	0	6.9	147	110	0
roasted, lean w/fat	209	28.7	0	9.5	128	109	0
roasted, lean only	193	29.3	0	7.5	129	110	0
shoulder, arm:							
raised, lean w/fat	268	38.1	0	11.6	168	99	0
braised, lean only	228	40.5	0	6.0	176	102	0
roasted, lean w/fat	208	28.9	0	9.4	122	102	0
roasted, lean only	186	29.6	0	6.6	124	103	0

Food and Measure	cal.	prot. (gms)	carbo. (gms)	fat (gms)	chol. (mgs)	sod. (mgs)	fiber (gms)
shoulder, blade:							
raised, lean w/fat	255	35.4	0	11.4	174	111	0
braised, lean only	224	37.0	0	7.3	179	115	0
roasted, lean w/fat	211	28.5	0	9.8	133	113	0
roasted, lean only	194	29.1	0	7.8	135	116	0
sirloin:							
braised, lean w/fat	286	35.4	0	14.9	122	90	0
braised, lean only	231	38.5	0	7.4	128	92	0
roasted, lean w/fat	229	28.5	0	11.9	116	94	0
roasted, lean only	191	29.8	0	7.1	118	96	0
"Veal," vegetarian, frozen (*Worthington Veelets*), 1 patty . . .	180	14.0	10.0	9.0	0	390	5.0
Veal dinner, frozen, parmigiana, 1 pkg.:							
(*Swanson*), 11¼ oz.	390	19.0	40.0	18.0	85	1060	5.0
(*Swanson Hungry Man*), 18¼ oz.	630	34.0	71.0	23.0	90	1870	4.0
Veal entree, frozen, parmigiana, 1 pkg.:							
(*Banquet*), 9 oz.	360	13.0	35.0	19.0	25	960	7.0
(*Banquet* Family), 1 patty w/sauce	230	9.0	19.0	14.0	20	740	2.0
(*Freezer Queen* Cook-in-Pouch), 5 oz. . . .	190	10.0	17.0	8.0	60	480	2.0
(*Freezer Queen* Family), 1 patty	170	10.0	15.0	8.0	20	600	4.0
(*Freezer Queen* Meal), 9 oz.	320	20.0	40.0	9.0	100	690	3.0
(*Stouffer's* Home-style), 11⅞ oz.	430	21.0	49.0	17.0	80	1120	6.0
(*Stouffer's Hearty Portions*), 17½ oz. .	630	32.0	68.0	26.0	75	1610	6.0
Veal seasoning, see "Pork and veal seasoning"							
Vegetable burger, see "Burger, vegetarian"							
Vegetable chips:							
(*Eden*), 1.1 oz.	130	<1.0	24.0	4.0	0	260	0
assorted (*Terra*), 1 oz.	190	1.0	18.0	7.0	0	70	3.0
sea (*Eden*), 1.1 oz. . . .	140	<1.0	23.0	5.0	0	220	0

Food and Measure	cal.	prot. (gms)	carbo. (gms)	fat (gms)	chol. (mgs)	sod. (mgs)	fiber (gms)
Vegetable dinner, frozen, 1 pkg.:							
(*Amy's* Country), 11 oz.	380	11.0	60.0	12.0	15	570	9.0
veggie loaf (*Amy's*), 10 oz.	260	8.0	47.0	5.0	0	690	7.0
Vegetable dip (see also specific listings) (*Heluva* Good), 2 tbsp.	60	1.0	3.0	5.0	20	240	0
Vegetable dip mix:							
(*Watkins* Garden), 1 tsp.	10	0	2.0	0	0	110	0
garden (*Hidden Valley*), 2 tbsp.*	70	<1.0	2.0	6.0	15	150	0
Vegetable dishes, canned, ½ cup:							
curry (*Patak's*)	180	6.0	18.0	10.0	10	580	3.0
hot and spicy (*House of Tsang*Szechuan)	70	1.0	14.0	1.0	0	1130	1.0
sweet and sour (*House of Tsang* Hong Kong)	160	0	40.0	0	0	580	0
teriyaki (*House of Tsang* Tokyo)	100	1.0	23.0	0	0	1240	1.0
Vegetable dishes, frozen (see also "Vegetable entree mix, frozen," "Vegetables, mixed, frozen," and specific listings):							
au gratin (*Cascadian Farm Veggie Bowl*), 9 oz.	170	9.0	24.0	6.0	10	630	4.0
Bavarian style (*Birds Eye Side Orders*), 1 cup	150	5.0	15.0	8.0	30	460	3.0
California style (*Birds Eye Side Orders*), ½ cup	100	3.0	9.0	5.0	10	240	3.0
French country style (*Birds Eye Side Orders*), ⅔ cup	110	2.0	10.0	6.0	10	290	2.0

Food and Measure	cal.	prot. (gms)	carbo. (gms)	fat (gms)	chol. (mgs)	sod. (mgs)	fiber (gms)
Italian style (*Birds Eye Side Orders*), 1 cup	150	3.0	12.0	10.0	15	380	3.0
New England recipe (*The Budget Gourmet* Side Dish), 5 oz.	210	4.0	19.0	13.0	20	380	2.0
New England style (*Birds Eye Side Orders*), 9-oz. pkg.	260	6.0	29.0	14.0	15	480	3.0
Oriental style (*Birds Eye Side Orders*), ½ cup	60	2.0	4.0	4.0	10	260	2.0
w/pasta, see "Pasta dishes, frozen"							
stir-fry style (*Birds Eye Side Orders*), ½ cup	60	2.0	5.0	4.0	10	270	1.0
Vegetable entree, frozen (see also "Vegetarian entree"), 1 pkg.:							
Chinese style, w/chicken (*The Budget Gourmet Value Classics* Low Fat), 8 oz.	250	8.0	39.0	6.0	15	640	3.0
chow mein (*La Choy*), 1 cup	110	3.0	20.0	2.0	0	1135	5.0
Italian style, w/white chicken (*The Budget Gourmet Value Classics* Low Fat), 8 oz.	250	7.0	39.0	7.0	25	540	2.0
oven roasted primavera (*Weight Watchers Main Street Bistro*), 10 oz.	300	6.0	46.0	8.0	10	790	2.0
pie/pot pie: (*Amy's*), 7½ oz. . . .	360	7.0	44.0	18.0	45	540	4.0
(*Amy's* Country), 7½ oz.	370	12.0	47.0	16.0	40	580	4.0
(*Amy's* Nondairy), 7½ oz.	320	9.0	50.0	9.0	0	590	4.0
cheese (*Banquet*), 7 oz.	340	6.0	39.0	17.0	10	920	1.0

Food and Measure	cal.	prot. (gms)	carbo. (gms)	fat (gms)	chol. (mgs)	sod. (mgs)	fiber (gms)
Vegetable entree, frozen *(cont.)*							
Szechuan style, spicy (*The Budget Gourmet Value Classics*), 8 oz.	290	10.0	41.0	9.0	15	890	3.0
Vegetable entree, packaged, 1 pkg.:							
creamy, w/pistachios, raisins, rice (*Tamarind Tree* Navratan Korma)	430	12.0	60.0	16.0	5	700	7.0
curry sauce w/:							
hot (*House*)	190	5.0	23.0	9.0	5	1130	6.0
medium hot (*House*)	190	5.0	22.0	10.0	<5	1090	5.0
mild (*House*)	200	5.0	23.0	10.0	5	1050	5.0
peas, mushrooms, rice (*Tamarind Tree* Dhingri Mutter)	290	8.0	53.0	5.0	0	680	7.0
spicy garden, rice (*Tamarind Treef* Jalfrazzi)	310	8.0	57.0	6.0	0	600	7.0
stew, w/beef (*Hormel Health Selections*), 1 cup	140	8.0	18.0	2.5	15	590	1.0
Vegetable entree mix, frozen, prepared[1], except as noted:							
Alfredo, creamy (*Green Giant Create a Meal!*), 1⅓ cups*	380	34.0	33.0	12.0	75	990	3.0
Alfredo tortellini (*Freshlike Meal Starter*), 1 cup* . . .	280	23.0	16.0	13.0	90	450	3.0
Asian, spicy (*Birds Eye Easy Recipe Meal Starter*), 2¼ cups	230	8.0	15.0	1.5	0	2160	3.0
beefy noodle (*Green Giant Create a Meal! Ground Beef*), 1¼ cups*	350	26.0	31.0	14.0	70	1130	3.0

[1] *Frozen vegetables prepared with oil and meat, except as noted.*

Food and Measure	cal.	prot. (gms)	carbo. (gms)	fat (gms)	chol. (mgs)	sod. (mgs)	fiber (gms)
broccoli stir fry (*Green Giant Create a Meal!*), 1⅓ cups*	290	27.0	16.0	13.0	60	1160	4.0
cacciatore (*Birds Eye Easy Recipe Meal Starter*), 2 cups	180	6.0	7.0	2.5	0	690	1.0
cashew stir fry (*Freshlike Meal Starter*), 1 cup* ...	230	21.0	20.0	7.0	55	660	2.0
cheddar, creamy (*Green Giant Create a Meal!*), 1½ cups*	280	20.0	28.0	10.0	45	1470	3.0
(*Freshlike Meal-Starter*), 1 cup* ...	270	23.0	20.0	11.0	55	720	2.0
cheese/herb primavera (*Green Giant Create a Meal!*), 1¼ cups*	330	30.0	27.0	11.0	65	920	4.0
cheesy cheese: (*Birds Eye Easy Recipe Meal Starter*), 1¾ cups	230	9.0	25.0	11.0	15	1080	2.0
cheesy pasta-vegetable (*Green Giant Create a Meal!* Ground Beef), 1¼ cups*	440	31.0	27.0	23.0	100	1220	2.0
chicken Alfredo (*Birds Eye Easy Recipe Meal Starter*), 2½ cups	250	8.0	25.0	14.0	35	620	2.0
chicken noodle, creamy (*Green Giant Create a Meal!*), 1¼ cups*	340	28.0	31.0	11.0	650	960	3.0
chicken primavera (*Birds Eye Easy Recipe Meal Starter*), 1¾ cups	180	6.0	27.0	5.0	0	610	3.0
curry, South Indian (*Cascadian Farm Quickstart*), 2¼ cups* w/tofu ...	300	11.0	39.0	13.0	0	620	3.0

Food and Measure	cal.	prot. (gms)	carbo. (gms)	fat (gms)	chol. (mgs)	sod. (mgs)	fiber (gms)
Vegetable entree mix, frozen *(cont.)*							
fajita style (*Green Giant Create a Meal!*), 1⅓ cups*	430	32.0	40.0	16.0	70	1300	4.0
garlic herb (*Green Giant Create a Meal!*), 1¼ cups*	330	24.0	27.0	14.0	145	660	3.0
garlic herb (*Green Giant Create a Meal! Oven Roasted*), 1¾ cups*	360	32.0	37.0	14.0	70	760	6.0
lasagna, skillet (*Green Giant Create a Meal! Ground Beef*), 1¼ cups*	350	26.0	33.0	13.0	70	830	3.0
lemon herb (*Green Giant Create a Meal!*), 1½ cups*	360	28.0	37.0	11.0	65	830	3.0
lo mein stir-fry (*Green Giant Create a Meal!*), 1¼ cups*	320	30.0	35.0	7.0	60	980	4.0
mushroom-wine saute (*Green Giant Create a Meal!*), 1¼ cups*	390	28.0	31.0	16.0	75	910	3.0
onion, savory (*Green Giant Create a Meal! Oven Roasted*), 1¾ cups*	340	28.0	28.0	11.0	70	1130	5.0
orange glaze chicken (*Birds Eye Easy Recipe Meal Starter*), 2½ cups	200	6.0	13.0	2.0	0	440	3.0
Oriental stir-fry (*Birds Eye Easy Recipe Meal Starter*), 2¼ cups	210	8.0	33.0	4.0	0	1400	2.0
Parmesan, creamy (*Freshlike Meal Starter*), 1 cup* ...	300	22.0	21.0	14.0	65	800	2.0
Parmesan herb (*Green Giant Create a Meal! Oven Roasted*), 1¾ cups*	330	31.0	27.0	11.0	75	1080	5.0

Food and Measure	cal.	prot. (gms)	carbo. (gms)	fat (gms)	chol. (mgs)	sod. (mgs)	fiber (gms)
pot roast, homestyle (*Green Giant Create a Meal!* Oven Roasted), 2 cups*	370	29.0	33.0	13.0	70	860	5.0
Southwest skillet (*Cascadian Farm Quickstart*), 2¼ cups* w/tofu	290	13.0	42.0	10.0	0	640	5.0
Southwestern (*Birds Eye Easy Recipe Meal Starter*), 1¾ cups	200	7.0	32.0	6.0	0	730	3.0
stew, homestyle (*Green Giant Create a Meal!* Ground Beef), 1 cup*	340	24.0	25.0	16.0	70	1310	4.0
sweet/sour (*Birds Eye Easy Recipe Meal Starter*), 2 cups	210	4.0	43.0	1.0	0	270	3.0
sweet/sour blend (*Freshlike Meal Starter*), 1 cup* . . .	270	21.0	12.0	4.5	60	280	2.0
sweet/sour stir-fry: (*Green Giant Create a Meal!*), 1¼ cups*	290	27.0	29.0	7.0	60	460	5.0
Szechuan, spicy (*Freshlike Meal Starter*), 1 cup* . . .	270	23.0	32.0	4.0	65	1140	2.0
Szechuan stir-fry (*Green Giant Create a Meal!*), 1¼ cups*	310	26.0	20.0	14.0	60	1390	4.0
teriyaki blend (*Freshlike Meal Starter*), 1 cup* . . .	230	22.0	26.0	5.0	30	860	2.0
teriyaki stir-fry: (*Birds Eye Easy Recipe Meal Starter*), 2 cups	210	8.0	13.0	2.5	0	1680	2.0
(*Green Giant Create a Meal!*), 1¼ cups*	230	27.0	18.0	9.0	55	920	4.0

Food and Measure	cal.	prot. (gms)	carbo. (gms)	fat (gms)	chol. (mgs)	sod. (mgs)	fiber (gms)
Vegetable entree mix, frozen *(cont.)*							
teriyaki veggies/rice (*Cascadian Farm Quickstart*), 2¼ cups* w/tofu...	330	11.0	40.0	15.0	0	650	4.0
Thai veggies/rice (*Cascadian Farm Quickstart*), 2¼ cups* w/tofu...........	310	12.0	41.0	12.0	0	470	3.0
vegetable almond stir-fry (*Green Giant Create a Meal!*), 1¼ cups*........	320	32.0	20.0	12.0	65	1070	5.0
vegetable stew, hearty (*Green Giant Create a Meal!*), 1¼ cups*	280	23.0	25.0	9.0	55	1000	3.0
Vegetable juice, 8 fl. oz., except as noted:							
(*Dole*), 12 fl. oz.	90	4.0	19.0	0	0	820	0
(*Muir Glen*)	70	2.0	15.0	0	0	620	3.0
(*Muir Glen* Reduced Sodium)	70	2.0	15.0	0	0	465	3.0
(*R.W. Knudsen Very Veggie* Original/Organic/Spicy)	50	3.0	10.0	1.0	0	610	0
(*R.W. Knudsen Very Veggie* Low Salt) ...	50	3.0	10.0	1.0	0	32	0
(*V8*)	50	1.0	10.0	0	0	620	1.0
(*V8* Low Sodium)	60	2.0	11.0	0	0	140	2.0
(*V8 Healthy Request*)	50	1.0	12.0	0	0	460	1.0
picante (*V8*)	50	2.0	10.0	0	0	680	1.0
spicy (*Muir Glen*)	70	2.0	15.0	0	0	620	3.0
spicy blend (*Dole*), 12 fl. oz.	80	3.0	16.0	0	0	950	0
spicy hot (*V8*)........	50	2.0	10.0	0	0	780	1.0
tangy, lightly (*V8*)	60	2.0	11.0	0	0	630	1.0
Vegetable oyster, see "Salsify"							
Vegetable pie, see "Vegetable entree, frozen"							

Food and Measure	cal.	prot. (gms)	carbo. (gms)	fat (gms)	chol. (mgs)	sod. (mgs)	fiber (gms)
Vegetable pocket (see also specific listings), frozen, 1 pc.:							
Bar-B-Q (*Ken & Robert's Veggie Pockets*)	290	10.0	45.0	8.0	0	490	5.0
Greek (*Ken & Robert's Veggie Pockets*)	250	10.0	37.0	8.0	0	490	4.0
Indian (*Ken & Robert's Veggie Pockets*)	260	8.0	40.0	8.0	0	490	5.0
Mediterranean (*Amy's*)	220	9.0	33.0	7.0	15	540	3.0
Oriental (*Ken & Robert's Veggie Pockets*)	250	8.0	40.0	8.0	0	490	5.0
pot pie:							
(*Amy's*)	230	7.0	37.0	6.0	0	420	2.0
(*Ken & Robert's Veggie Pockets*)	250	6.0	38.0	9.0	0	410	2.0
roasted vegetables (*Amy's*)	220	6.0	35.0	8.0	0	480	4.0
Santa Fe (*Ken & Robert's Veggie Pockets*)	250	8.0	39.0	8.0	0	550	5.0
Tex-Mex (*Ken & Robert's Veggie Pockets*)	280	9.0	46.0	8.0	0	490	6.0
Vegetable seasoning (*Chef Paul Prudhomme's Magic Seasoning Blends*), 1/4 tsp.	0	0	0	0	0	135	0
Vegetables, see specific listings							
Vegetables, mixed, fresh, Asian stir-fry (*Frieda's*), 3 oz.	15	1.0	3.0	0	0	35	1.0
Vegetables, mixed, canned, 1/2 cup, except as noted:							
(*Del Monte*)	40	2.0	8.0	0	0	360	2.0
(*Del Monte* No Salt)	40	2.0	8.0	0	0	25	2.0
(*Green Giant*)	60	2.0	12.0	0	0	460	2.0

Food and Measure	cal.	prot. (gms)	carbo. (gms)	fat (gms)	chol. (mgs)	sod. (mgs)	fiber (gms)
Vegetables, mixed, canned *(cont.)*							
(*Green Giant Garden*							
Medley)	40	1.0	9.0	0	0	360	2.0
(*Seneca*)	45	1.0	9.0	0	0	300	2.0
(*Seneca* No Salt)	45	1.0	9.0	0	0	10	2.0
Chinese, mixed (*La*							
Choy)	10	1.0	1.0	0	0	25	1.0
chop suey:							
(*Chun King*), ²/₃ cup	15	1.0	3.0	0	0	n.a.	1.0
(*La Choy*)	10	1.0	2.0	0	0	240	1.0
and sauce:							
hot and spicy							
(*House of Tsang*							
Szechuan)	70	1.0	14.0	1.0	0	1130	1.0
sweet and sour							
(*House of Tsang*							
Hong Kong)	160	0	40.0	0	0	580	0
teriyaki (*House of*							
Tsang Tokyo)	100	1.0	23.0	0	0	1240	1.0
stew (*Seneca*)	45	1.0	9.0	0	0	300	2.0
stir-fry (*La Choy*)	15	<1.0	4.5	0	0	200	3.0
Vegetables, mixed,							
freeze-dried, ¹/₂ cup:							
(*AlpineAire*)	71	3.0	16.0	.4	0	65	n.a.
garden (*AlpineAire*)	79	4.0	17.0	.5	0	20	n.a.
Vegetables, mixed,							
frozen (see also							
"Vegetable dishes,							
frozen"):							
(*Birds Eye*), ¹/₃ cup . . .	50	2.0	12.0	0	0	35	3.0
(*Birds Eye* Medley),							
1 cup, 3 oz.	30	2.0	6.0	0	0	35	2.0
(*Freshlike*), ²/₃ cup . . .	60	3.0	11.0	0	0	50	2.0
(*Green Giant*), ³/₄ cup	50	2.0	11.0	0	0	35	3.0
(*Green Giant Harvest*							
Fresh), ²/₃ cup	50	2.0	10.0	0	0	125	3.0
(*McKenzie's*), ²/₃ cup	60	3.0	12.0	.5	0	40	3.0
(*Seneca*), ²/₃ cup	60	3.0	11.0	0	0	35	4.0
Alfredo (*Green Giant*),							
³/₄ cup	80	4.0	9.0	3.0	5	450	3.0
in butter sauce (*Green*							
Giant), ³/₄ cup	70	2.0	11.0	2.0	<5	240	3.0

Food and Measure	cal.	prot. (gms)	carbo. (gms)	fat (gms)	chol. (mgs)	sod. (mgs)	fiber (gms)
California:							
(*Cascadian Farm*), ⅔ cup	20	1.0	4.0	0	0	20	0
(*Freshlike*), 1 cup	30	2.0	5.0	0	0	30	2.0
in cheese sauce (*Cascadian Farm* Medley), ⅔ cup	80	4.0	11.0	2.5	5	280	2.0
Chinese stir-fry (*Cascadian Farm*), 1 cup	25	2.0	6.0	0	0	15	2.0
country mix (*Freshlike*), ⅔ cup	45	1.0	10.0	0	0	20	1.0
gardener's blend (*Cascadian Farm*), ¾ cup	57	2.0	12.0	0	0	28	4.0
gumbo blend:							
(*Birds Eye*), ¾ cup	40	2.0	10.0	0	0	30	2.0
(*McKenzie's*), ⅔ cup	35	1.0	8.0	0	0	30	2.0
Italian (*Seneca*), ¾ cup	30	1.0	6.0	0	0	10	2.0
Midwestern (*Freshlike*), ¾ cup	25	1.0	5.0	0	0	30	2.0
Oriental stir-fry:							
(*Freshlike*), 1 cup	30	2.0	5.0	0	0	25	2.0
(*Seneca*), ¾ cup ...	25	1.0	5.0	0	0	5	2.0
Santa Fe blend (*Cascadian Farm*), ¾ cup	60	3.0	12.0	.5	0	65	3.0
Scandinavian blend (*Seneca*), ¾ cup ...	40	2.0	7.0	0	0	25	3.0
soup mix:							
(*Birds Eye*), ⅔ cup	45	1.0	9.0	0	0	45	2.0
(*Freshlike*), ⅔ cup	45	1.0	9.0	0	0	45	2.0
(*McKenzie's*), ⅔ cup	50	2.0	10.0	0	0	40	2.0
(*Seneca*), ¾ cup ...	40	1.0	9.0	0	0	20	2.0
stew mix:							
(*Birds Eye*), ¾ cup	40	1.0	9.0	0	0	40	1.0
(*Freshlike*), ⅔ cup	45	1.0	10.0	0	0	40	1.0
hearty (*Cascadian Farm*), ⅔ cup ...	45	1.0	10.0	0	0	40	2.0
stir-fry (*Birds Eye*), 1 cup, 3 oz.	30	2.0	5.0	0	0	40	2.0
teriyaki (*Green Giant*), 1¼ cups	100	2.0	7.0	7.0	0	510	2.0

Food and Measure	cal.	prot. (gms)	carbo. (gms)	fat (gms)	chol. (mgs)	sod. (mgs)	fiber (gms)
Vegetables, mixed, frozen *(cont.)*							
Thai stir-fry (*Cascadian Farm*), ¾ cup	25	2.0	6.0	0	0	15	2.0
winter blend:							
(*Freshlike*), 1 cup	25	2.0	4.0	0	0	25	2.0
(*Seneca*), ¾ cup ...	25	1.0	4.0	0	0	10	2.0
Vegetables, mixed, pickled							
(Giardiniera):							
(*Krinos*), 3 oz.	0	0	0	0	0	900	2.0
(*Perfecta*), 5.3 oz. ...	0	0	0	0	0	900	0
(*Zorba*), ½ cup	20	<1.0	2.0	1.0	0	850	0
Vegetarian burger, see "Burger, vegetarian"							
Vegetarian dishes (see also "Vegetarian entree" and specific listings):							
canned:							
(*Loma Linda Nuteena*), ⅜" slice	160	6.0	6.0	13.0	0	120	2.0
(*Loma Linda Swiss Stake*), 1 pc.	120	9.0	8.0	6.0	0	430	4.0
(*Worthington Numete*), ⅜" slice	130	6.0	5.0	10.0	0	270	3.0
(*Worthington Protose*), ⅜" slice	130	13.0	5.0	7.0	0	280	3.0
choplet (*Worthington*), 2 pcs.	90	17.0	3.0	1.5	0	500	2.0
cuts, dinner (*Loma Linda*), 2 pcs. ...	90	17.0	3.0	1.5	0	500	2.0
canned, cutlet:							
(*Worthington*), 1 pc.	70	11.0	3.0	1.0	0	340	2.0
multigrain (*Worthington* 20 oz.), 2 pcs.	100	15.0	5.0	2.0	0	390	4.0
frozen:							
(*Worthington FriPats*), 1 patty	130	14.0	4.0	6.0	0	320	3.0

Food and Measure	cal.	prot. (gms)	carbo. (gms)	fat (gms)	chol. (mgs)	sod. (mgs)	fiber (gms)
(*Worthington Stakelets*), 1 pc.	140	12.0	6.0	8.0	0	480	2.0
croquettes (*Worthington* Golden), 4 pcs.	210	14.0	14.0	10.0	0	600	3.0
entree, dinner (*Natural Touch*), 3-oz. patty	220	19.0	2.0	15.0	0	380	2.0
nuggets, w/rice (*Hain* Hawaiian), 10 oz.	310	13.0	55.0	5.0	0	495	6.0
roast, dinner (*Worthington*), 3/4″ slice	180	12.0	5.0	12.0	<5	580	3.0
mix, dry, 1/3 cup:							
loaf, dinner (*Loma Linda*)	90	14.0	7.0	1.5	0	560	5.0
patty (*Loma Linda*)	90	14.0	7.0	1.0	0	480	5.0
Vegetarian entree, frozen (see also "Vegetable entree mix, frozen" and specific listings):							
Aztec (*Cascadian Farm Meals for a Small Planet*), 1/2 bag	230	10.0	44.0	3.0	0	339	10.0
Cajun (*Cascadian Farm Meals for a Small Planet*), 1/2 bag	230	10.0	46.0	2.0	0	368	10.0
curry (*Thai Chef* Massaman), 12 oz.	390	9.0	71.0	9.0	0	260	5.0
Indian (*Cascadian Farm Meals for a Small Planet*), 1/2 bag	250	9.0	46.0	4.0	0	550	7.0
Mediterranean (*Cascadian Farm Meals for a Small Planet*), 1/2 bag	215	8.0	35.0	6.0	0	480	6.0
mu shu (*Fantastic Wrap Stuffers*), 16 oz.	220	5.0	35.0	3.0	0	470	3.0

Food and Measure	cal.	prot. (gms)	carbo. (gms)	fat (gms)	chol. (mgs)	sod. (mgs)	fiber (gms)
Vegetarian entree, frozen *(cont.)*							
Oriental (*Cascadian Farm Meals for a Small Planet*), ½ bag	260	13.0	40.0	7.0	0	732	10.0
pot pie, see "Vegetable entree, frozen"							
Santa Fe (*Fantastic Wrap Stuffers*), 16 oz.	240	9.0	45.0	4.0	0	570	9.0
shepherd's pie (*Amy's* Nondairy), 8 oz. . . .	160	5.0	27.0	4.0	0	490	5.0
Spanish (*Fantastic Wrap Stuffers*), 16 oz.	220	7.0	39.0	5.0	0	690	6.0
sweet and sour, Thai (*Thai Chef*), 12 oz.	340	6.0	70.0	5.0	0	490	4.0
teriyaki (*Fantastic Wrap Stuffers*), 16 oz.	230	6.0	41.0	4.0	0	590	3.0
Vegetarian foods, see specific listings							
Venison, meat only, roasted, 4 oz.	179	34.3	0	3.6	127	61	0
Vermicelli pasta mix, w/garlic and olive oil (*Pasta Roni*), 1 cup*	360	9.0	48.0	16.0	0	1010	2.0
Vienna sausage, see "Sausage, canned"							
Vindaloo sauce, see "Curry sauce"							
Vine spinach, raw, untrimmed, 1 lb.	86	8.2	15.4	1.4	0	n.a.	4.0
Vinegar, 1 tbsp.:							
all varieties: (*Regina*)	0	0	0	0	0	0	0
except balsamic (*Progresso*)	0	0	0	0	0	0	0
apple cider or red wine (*Eden* Organic)	0	0	0	0	0	0	0
balsamic: (*Pastorelli Italian Chef*)	5	0	2.0	0	0	0	0

Food and Measure	cal.	prot. (gms)	carbo. (gms)	fat (gms)	chol. (mgs)	sod. (mgs)	fiber (gms)
(*Pompeian*)	5	0	2.0	0	0	0	0
(*Progresso*)	10	0	1.0	0	0	0	0
plum or brown rice							
(*Eden* Organic)	2	0	0	0	0	0	0
red wine:							
(*Pastorelli Italian*							
Chef)	2	0	0	0	0	0	0
(*Pompeian*)	2	0	0	0	0	0	0

W

Food and Measure	cal.	prot. (gms)	carbo. (gms)	fat (gms)	chol. (mgs)	sod. (mgs)	fiber (gms)
Waffle, frozen, 2 pcs., except as noted:							
(*Aunt Jemima* Homestyle)	200	5.0	32.0	6.0	<5	440	1.0
(*Aunt Jemima* Lowfat)	160	5.0	32.0	1.5	0	540	1.0
(*Belgian Chef*), 2.6 oz.	180	6.0	34.0	2.0	0	450	0
(*Eggo* Homestyle) . . .	220	5.0	32.0	8.0	25	480	1.0
(*Eggo* Homestyle Low Fat)	180	6.0	34.0	2.5	20	340	1.0
(*Eggo Minis* Homestyle), 3 sets of 4 pcs.	260	7.0	38.0	9.0	25	600	2.0
(*Eggo Nutri-Grain*) . . .	190	5.0	30.0	6.0	0	450	4.0
(*Eggo Nutri-Grain* Low Fat)	160	5.0	31.0	2.5	0	480	3.0
(*Eggo Special K*)	120	6.0	26.0	0	0	280	1.0
(*Hungry Jack* Homestyle)	180	3.0	29.0	6.0	0	540	<1.0
(*Hungry Jack* Homestyle Low Fat)	170	4.0	34.0	2.0	0	350	1.0
apple cinnamon:							
(*Eggo*)	220	5.0	33.0	8.0	20	450	0
(*Hungry Jack*)	200	4.0	33.0	6.0	0	540	<1.0
banana bread (*Eggo*)	200	5.0	32.0	7.0	0	280	2.0
blueberry:							
Aunt Jemima)	210	5.0	34.0	6.0	<5	470	1.0
(*Eggo*)	220	5.0	32.0	9.0	20	460	1.0
(*Eggo Nutri-Grain* Low Fat)	160	5.0	33.0	2.0	0	460	3.0
(*Hungry Jack*)	210	3.0	33.0	7.0	0	540	<1.0
buttermilk:							
(*Aunt Jemima*)	200	5.0	34.0	6.0	<5	470	1.0

Food and Measure	cal.	prot. (gms)	carbo. (gms)	fat (gms)	chol. (mgs)	sod. (mgs)	fiber (gms)
(*Eggo*)	220	5.0	31.0	8.0	25	460	1.0
(*Hungry Jack*)	180	4.0	29.0	6.0	0	530	<1.0
cinnamon toast (*Eggo*), 3 sets of 4 pcs.	290	5.0	45.0	10.0	25	470	2.0
multi bran (*Eggo Nutri-Grain*)	180	5.0	32.0	6.0	0	410	6.0
multigrain (*Hungry Jack*)	180	5.0	28.0	6.0	0	470	3.0
nut and honey (*Eggo*)	240	6.0	31.0	10.0	25	450	2.0
oat, golden (*Eggo*) ...	150	6.0	29.0	2.5	0	340	3.0
raisin and bran (*Eggo Nutri-Grain*)	210	5.0	36.0	6.0	0	430	5.0
strawberry (*Eggo*) ...	220	5.0	32.0	8.0	20	460	1.0
wildberry (*Hungry Jack*)	200	3.0	33.0	6.0	0	540	<1.0
Waffle mix, see "Pancake mix"							
Waffle sticks, frozen (*Kid Cuisine* Wave Rider), 6.6-oz. pkg.	380	3.0	75.0	8.0	15	580	3.0
Wakame, see "Seaweed"							
Walnut, dried:							
(*Paradise/Wild Swan*), ¼ cup, 1 oz.	190	4.0	3.0	18.0	0	0	3.0
black:							
(*Planters*), 2-oz. pkg.	340	14.0	8.0	31.0	0	0	3.0
shelled, 1 oz.	172	6.9	3.4	16.1	0	<1	1.4
chopped, 1 cup	759	30.4	15.1	70.7	0	2	6.3
English or Persian:							
shelled, 1 oz.	182	4.1	5.2	17.6	0	3	1.4
halves, 1 cup	642	14.3	18.3	61.9	0	10	4.8
pcs., 1 cup	770	17.2	22.0	74.2	0	12	5.8
halves (*Planters*), ⅓ cup	220	5.0	5.0	22.0	0	0	1.0
pieces (*Planters*), ¼ cup	190	4.0	4.0	20.0	0	0	1.0
Walnut topping, in syrup (*Smucker's*), 2 tbsp.	170	2.0	20.0	9.0	0	0	0

Food and Measure	cal.	prot. (gms)	carbo. (gms)	fat (gms)	chol. (mgs)	sod. (mgs)	fiber (gms)
Wasabi chips (*Eden*), 50 pcs., 1.1 oz. . . .	130	<1.0	24.0	4.0	0	260	0
Water chestnuts, Chinese, fresh:							
(*Frieda's*), 1 tbsp. . . .	30	0	7.0	0	0	0	1.0
4 medium, 2″ diam.	38	.5	8.6	<.1	0	5	1.1
sliced, ½ cup	66	.9	14.8	.1	0	9	1.9
Water chestnuts, canned:							
whole:							
(*Chun King/La Choy*), 2 pcs. . . .	10	0	2.0	0	0	0	1.0
4 medium or 1 oz.	14	.3	3.5	<.1	0	2	.7
sliced:							
(*Chun King/La Choy*), 2 tbsp. . . .	10	0	3.0	0	0	0	1.0
(*Sun Luck*), ¼ cup	15	0	4.0	0	0	0	1.0
w/liquid, ½ cup	35	.6	8.7	<.1	0	6	1.8
Watercress:							
(*Frieda's*), 1 cup, 3 oz.	10	2.0	1.0	0	0	35	2.0
10 sprigs, 11¼″	3	.6	.3	<.1	0	10	.6
chopped, ½ cup	2	.4	.2	<.1	0	7	.4
Watermelon:							
1″ slice, 10″ diam. . . .	152	3.0	34.6	2.0	0	10	2.4
diced, ½ cup	25	.5	5.7	.3	0	2	.4
yellow, seedless (*Frieda's*), 2 cups, 9.9 oz.	90	1.0	23.0	0	0	10	1.0
Watermelon drink (*R.W. Knudsen* Cooler), 8 fl. oz. . . .	120	0	29.0	0	0	10	0
Watermelon juice (*After the Fall*), 8 fl. oz.	90	1.0	22.0	0	0	15	0
Watermelon seed, dried, 1 oz.	158	8.1	4.4	13.5	0	28	n.a.
Watermelon-cherry drink mix*, 8 fl. oz.:							
(*Kool-Aid Pink Swimmingo*)	100	0	25.0	0	0	15	0
(*Kool-Aid Pink Swimmingo* Presweetened)	60	0	16.0	0	0	0	0

Food and Measure	cal.	prot. (gms)	carbo. (gms)	fat (gms)	chol. (mgs)	sod. (mgs)	fiber (gms)
Wax beans:							
fresh, see "Green beans"							
canned, cut, 1/2 cup:							
(*Del Monte*)	20	1.0	4.0	0	0	360	2.0
(*Seneca*)	25	<1.0	5.0	0	0	380	2.0
(*Seneca* No Salt) . . .	25	<1.0	5.0	0	0	10	2.0
golden (*Del Monte*)	20	1.0	4.0	0	0	360	2.0
frozen (*Seabrook*),							
2/3 cup	25	1.0	4.0	0	0	10	2.0
Wax gourd, boiled,							
cubed, 1/2 cup	11	.4	2.6	.2	0	93	.9
Welsh rarebit, frozen							
(*Stouffer's* Side							
Dish), 1/4 cup	110	5.0	6.0	7.0	20	270	1.0
Wendy's, 1 serving:							
sandwiches:							
bacon cheese-							
burger, Jr.	380	20.0	34.0	19.0	60	850	2.0
Big Bacon Classic	580	34.0	46.0	30.0	100	1460	3.0
cheeseburger:							
Jr.	320	17.0	34.0	13.0	45	830	2.0
Jr, deluxe	360	18.0	36.0	17.0	50	890	3.0
Kid's Meal	320	17.0	33.0	13.0	45	830	2.0
chicken, breaded	440	28.0	44.0	18.0	60	840	2.0
chicken, grilled	310	27.0	35.0	8.0	65	790	2.0
chicken, spicy	410	28.0	43.0	15.0	65	1280	2.0
chicken club	470	31.0	44.0	20.0	70	970	2.0
hamburger:							
Jr.	270	15.0	34.0	10.0	30	610	2.0
Kid's Meal	270	15.0	33.0	10.0	30	610	2.0
single, plain	360	24.0	31.0	16.0	65	580	2.0
single,							
w/everything	420	25.0	37.0	20.0	70	920	3.0
sandwich condiments:							
American cheese	70	3.0	1.0	5.0	15	320	0
American cheese							
Jr.	45	2.0	0	3.5	10	220	0
bacon, 1 slice	20	2.0	0	1.5	5	65	0
honey mustard, re-							
duced cal, 1 tsp.	25	0	2.0	1.5	0	45	0
ketchup, 1 tsp.	10	0	2.0	0	0	75	0

Food and Measure	cal.	prot. (gms)	carbo. (gms)	fat (gms)	chol. (mgs)	sod. (mgs)	fiber (gms)
Wendy's, sandwich condiments *(cont.)*							
mayonnaise,							
1½ tsp.	30	0	1.0	3.0	5	60	0
mustard, ½ tsp. . . .	0	0	0	0	0	50	0
onion, 4 rings	5	0	1.0	0	0	0	0
pickles, 4 slices . . .	0	0	0	0	0	140	0
tomatoes, 1 slice	5	0	1.0	0	0	0	0
Fresh Stuffed Pitas,							
w/dressing:							
chicken Caesar	490	34.0	48.0	18.0	65	1320	4.0
classic Greek	440	15.0	50.0	20.0	35	1050	4.0
garden ranch chic-							
ken	480	30.0	51.0	18.0	70	1180	5.0
garden veggie	400	11.0	52.0	17.0	20	760	5.0
pita dressings:							
Caesar vinaigrette	70	0	1.0	7.0	0	170	0
garden ranch	50	0	1.0	4.5	10	125	0
chicken nuggets:							
5 pcs.	230	11.0	11.0	16.0	30	470	0
4 pcs., kid's meal	190	9.0	9.0	13.0	25	380	0
nuggets sauce, 1 pkt.:							
barbecue	45	1.0	10.0	0	0	160	0
honey mustard	130	0	6.0	12.0	0	220	0
sweet and sour	50	0	12.0	0	0	120	0
chili:							
small, 8 oz.	210	15.0	21.0	7.0	30	800	5.0
large, 12 oz.	310	23.0	32.0	10.0	45	1190	7.0
cheddar cheese,							
shredded, 2 tbsp.	70	4.0	1.0	6.0	15	110	0
saltines, 2	25	1.0	4.0	.5	0	80	0
baked potato:							
plain, 10 oz.	310	7.0	71.0	0	0	25	7.0
bacon and cheese	530	17.0	78.0	18.0	20	1390	7.0
broccoli and cheese	470	9.0	80.0	14.0	5	470	9.0
cheese	570	14.0	78.0	23.0	30	640	7.0
chili and cheese . . .	630	20.0	83.0	24.0	40	770	9.0
margarine pkt.	600	0	0	7.0	0	115	0
sour cream & chives	380	8.0	74.0	6.0	15	40	8.0
sour cream pkt. . . .	60	1.0	1.0	6.0	10	15	0
french fries:							
small	270	4.0	35.0	13.0	0	85	3.0
medium	390	5.0	50.0	19.0	0	120	5.0
Biggie	470	7.0	61.0	23.0	0	150	6.0

Food and Measure	cal.	prot. (gms)	carbo. (gms)	fat (gms)	chol. (mgs)	sod. (mgs)	fiber (gms)
Great Biggie	570	8.0	73.0	27.0	0	180	7.0
salads-to-go, fresh, w/out dressing:							
Caesar side salad	110	10.0	7.0	5.0	15	650	1.0
deluxe garden	110	7.0	9.0	6.0	0	350	3.0
grilled chicken	200	25.0	9.0	8.0	50	720	3.0
side salad	60	4.0	5.0	3.0	0	180	2.0
taco salad	380	26.0	28.0	19.0	65	1040	7.0
taco chips, 15 pcs.	100	3.0	24.0	11.0	0	180	2.0
soft breadstick, 1 pc.	130	4.0	23.0	3.0	5	250	1.0
dressing, 2 tbsp., except as noted:							
blue cheese	180	1.0	0	19.0	15	180	0
French	120	0	6.0	10.0	0	330	0
French, fat free	35	0	8.0	0	0	150	0
Italian, reduced fat/ cal.	40	0	2.0	3.0	0	340	0
Italian Caesar	150	1.0	1.0	16.0	20	240	0
ranch, *Hidden Valley*	100	1.0	1.0	10.0	10	220	0
ranch, *Hidden Valley,* reduced fat/ cal.	60	1.0	2.0	5.0	10	240	0
salad oil, 1 tbsp.	120	0	0	14.0	0	0	0
Thousand Island . . .	90	0	2.0	8.0	10	125	0
wine vinegar, 1 tbsp.	0	0	0	0	0	0	0
desserts:							
chocolate chip cookie	270	3.0	36.0	13.0	30	120	3.0
Frosty, small	330	8.0	56.0	8.0	35	200	0
Frosty, medium . . .	440	11.0	73.0	11.0	50	260	0
Frosty, large	540	14.0	91.0	14.0	60	320	0
Wheat, whole-grain:							
durum, 1 cup	650	26.3	136.6	4.7	0	3	n.a.
hard red:							
spring, 1 cup	631	29.6	130.6	3.7	0	4	24.2
winter, 1 cup	628	24.2	136.7	3.0	0	4	24.2
winter (*Arrowhead Mills*), ¼ cup	160	6.0	34.0	1.0	0	0	7.0
soft red winter, 1 cup	556	17.4	124.7	2.6	0	4	n.a.
hard white, 1 cup	656	21.7	145.7	3.3	0	n.a.	n.a.
soft white, 1 cup	571	18.0	126.6	3.3	0	n.a.	n.a.

Food and Measure	cal.	prot. (gms)	carbo. (gms)	fat (gms)	chol. (mgs)	sod. (mgs)	fiber (gms)
Wheat, parboiled, see "Bulgur"							
Wheat, sprouted, 1 cup	214	8.1	45.9	1.4	0	18	n.a.
Wheat bran (see also "Cereal, ready-to-eat"), ¼ cup, except as noted:							
(*Arrowhead Mills*) . . .	35	2.0	10.0	1.0	0	0	6.0
crude, 2 tbsp.	15	1.1	4.5	.3	0	<1	3.0
toasted (*Kretschmer*)	30	3.0	10.0	1.0	0	210	7.0
unprocessed (*Quaker*), ⅓ cup	30	3.0	11.0	0	0	0	8.0
Wheat flakes, rolled (*Arrowhead Mills*), ⅓ cup	110	4.0	24.0	.5	0	0	5.0
Wheat flour, ¼ cup, except as noted:							
(*All Trump*)	100	4.0	22.0	0	0	0	<1.0
(*La Pina*)	100	2.0	23.0	0	0	0	<1.0
all-purpose, white:							
(*Gold Medal/Gold Medal* Organic)	100	3.0	22.0	0	0	0	<1.0
(*Red Band*)	100	2.0	23.0	0	0	0	<1.0
(*Robin Hood*)	100	3.0	22.0	0	0	0	<1.0
1 cup	455	12.9	95.4	1.2	0	2	3.4
bleached (*Martha White/Omega*) . . .	110	3.0	23.0	.5	0	0	<1.0
bleached (*Pillsbury*)	100	3.0	23.0	0	0	0	<1.0
unbleached (*Arrowhead Mills*), ⅓ cup	160	5.0	33.0	.5	0	0	0
unbleached (*Pillsbury*)	100	3.0	21.0	0	0	0	<1.0
bread:							
(*Gold Medal/Red Band* Better for Bread)	100	4.0	22.0	0	0	0	<1.0
(*Red Band*)	100	4.0	22.0	0	0	0	<1.0
wheat (*Gold Medal* Better for Bread)	110	4.0	21.0	.5	0	0	1.0
white (*Pillsbury*) . . .	100	4.0	22.0	0	0	0	<1.0

Food and Measure	cal.	prot. (gms)	carbo. (gms)	fat (gms)	chol. (mgs)	sod. (mgs)	fiber (gms)
cake, white:							
(*Betty Crocker Softasilk*)	100	2.0	23.0	0	0	0	<1.0
(*Martha White*)	100	2.0	23.0	.5	0	0	<1.0
(*Swan's Down*)	100	2.0	22.0	0	0	0	0
1 cup	395	8.9	85.1	.9	0	2	1.8
gluten:							
(*Arrowhead Mills*), 3 tbsp.	35	5.0	3.0	0	0	0	0
(*General Mills* Supreme Hygluten)	100	4.0	22.0	0	0	0	<1.0
pastry (*Arrowhead Mills*)	110	4.0	23.0	.5	0	0	3.0
presifted:							
(*Pillsbury* Shake & Blend)	100	3.0	23.0	0	0	0	<1.0
(*Wondra*)	100	3.0	23.0	0	0	0	<1.0
self-rising, white:							
(*Gold Medal/Robin Hood*)	100	3.0	22.0	0	0	400	<1.0
(*Red Band*)	100	2.0	22.0	0	0	400	<1.0
1 cup	442	12.4	92.8	1.2	0	1587	4.0
bleached (*Martha White/Mother's Best*)	110	3.0	23.0	.5	0	380	<1.0
bleached/unbleached (*Pillsbury*)	100	3.0	22.0	0	0	360	<1.0
tortilla mix	449	10.7	74.5	11.8	0	751	n.a.
unbleached (*Gold Medal/Robin Hood*)	100	3.0	22.0	0	0	0	<1.0
whole-grain, 1 cup . . .	407	16.4	87.1	2.2	0	1	15.1
whole wheat:							
(*Martha White*)	120	5.0	24.0	.5	0	0	4.0
(*Pillsbury*)	120	5.0	22.0	1.0	0	0	4.0
stone ground (*Arrowhead Mills*)	130	5.0	25.0	.5	0	0	4.0
Wheat germ:							
(*Kretschmer*), 2 tbsp.	50	4.0	6.0	1.0	0	140	2.0
crude, 1 oz.	102	6.6	14.7	2.8	0	3	3.7

Food and Measure	cal.	prot. (gms)	carbo. (gms)	fat (gms)	chol. (mgs)	sod. (mgs)	fiber (gms)
Wheat germ *(cont.)*							
honey crunch (*Kret-schmer*), 1⅔ tbsp.	50	4.0	8.0	1.0	0	135	1.0
raw (*Arrowhead Mills*), 3 tbsp.	50	4.0	10.0	1.5	0	0	2.0
toasted, 1 oz.	108	8.3	14.1	3.0	0	1	3.7
Wheat malt syrup (*Eden* Organic), 1 tbsp.	60	1.0	14.0	0	0	5	0
Wheat pilaf mix (*Near East*), 2 oz.	180	6.0	42.0	1.0	0	645	5.0
Whelk, meat only, raw, 4 oz.	156	27.0	8.8	.5	74	234	0
Whey, fluid:							
acid, 1 cup	59	1.9	12.6	.2	0	118	0
sweet, 1 cup	66	2.1	12.6	.9	5	132	0
Whipped topping, see "Cream topping"							
Whiskey, see "Liquor"							
White beans, dry, ½ cup:							
boiled	125	8.6	22.6	.3	0	6	5.7
small, boiled	127	8.1	23.2	.6	0	2	3.7
White beans, canned:							
w/liquid, ½ cup	153	9.5	28.7	.4	0	595	6.3
small (*S&W*), ½ cup	80	7.0	19.0	.5	0	440	6.0
Spanish style (*Goya*), 7.5 oz.	130	13.0	29.0	1.0	0	990	12.0
White bean dishes, mix, and gemell, dry (*Marrakesh Express* Terrazza Tuscan), ⅓ cup	220	10.0	44.0	1.0	<5	450	3.0
White Castle, 1 serving:							
sandwiches:							
breakfast	340	14.0	17.0	25.0	130	900	0
cheeseburger	160	7.0	11.0	9.0	15	250	2.0
cheeseburger, bacon	200	10.0	12.0	13.0	25	400	3.0
cheeseburger, double	285	14.0	16.0	18.0	30	430	5.0
chicken ring	170	5.0	5.0	7.0	24	210	0
fish	160	8.0	18.0	6.0	15	220	0

Food and Measure	cal.	prot. (gms)	carbo. (gms)	fat (gms)	chol. (mgs)	sod. (mgs)	fiber (gms)
hamburger	135	6.0	11.0	7.0	10	135	2.0
hamburger, double	235	11.0	16.0	14.0	10	200	2.0
chicken rings, 6 pcs.	310	16.0	14.0	21.0	70	620	0
sides:							
cheese sticks,							
5 pcs.	491	25.0	32.0	28.0	0	1216	0
french fries, small	115	0	15.0	6.0	0	15	2.0
onion rings, 8 pcs.	460	12.0	56.0	27.0	0	550	0
shakes, 14 oz.:							
chocolate	220	8.0	32.0	7.0	25	140	0
vanilla	230	8.0	35.0	7.0	25	150	0
White sauce mix:							
(*Knorr*), 2 tsp.	25	0	4.0	1.0	0	220	0
1¾-oz. pkt.	230	5.4	25.1	13.2	tr.	1691	<1.0
Whitefish, meat only:							
raw, 4 oz.	153	21.7	0	6.7	68	58	0
baked, broiled, or mi-							
crowaved, 4 oz. ...	195	27.7	0	8.5	87	74	0
Whitefish, smoked:							
(*Ducktrap River*),							
2 oz.	70	12.0	0	2.0	5	730	0
4 oz.	122	26.5	0	1.1	37	1156	0
Whiting, meat only:							
raw, 4 oz.	102	20.8	0	1.5	76	82	0
baked, broiled, or mi-							
crowaved, 4 oz. ...	130	26.6	0	1.9	95	150	0
Wiener, see "Frank-							
furter"							
Wild rice:							
raw:							
(*Fantastic Foods*),							
¼ cup	140	6.0	28.0	0	0	0	2.0
(*Frieda's*), ¼ cup	120	5.0	26.0	0	0	0	2.0
1 oz.	101	4.2	21.2	.3	0	2	1.7
cooked, 1 cup	166	6.5	35.0	.6	0	6	1.5
blends, see "Rice"							
Wild rice dishes, see							
"Rice dishes"							
Wine, 1 fl. oz.:							
dessert or aperitif[1] ...	41	tr.	2.3	0	0	1	0

[1] *Includes fortified wines containing more than 15% alcohol, such as port, sherry, and vermouth.*

Food and Measure	cal.	prot. (gms)	carbo. (gms)	fat (gms)	chol. (mgs)	sod. (mgs)	fiber (gms)
Wine *(cont.)*							
dry or table[2]	25	tr.	1.2	0	0	1	0
Wine cooler (*Bartles & Jaymes*), 12 fl. oz.:							
berry	220	0	34.0	0	0	0	0
berry, Brazilian mist	210	0	32.0	0	0	0	0
Fuzzy Navel	250	0	43.0	0	0	0	0
kiwi strawberry	230	0	37.0	0	0	0	0
Margarita	270	0	46.0	0	0	35	0
Oriental dragon fruit	250	0	32.0	0	0	0	0
original	200	0	29.0	0	0	0	0
strawberry daiquiri . . .	230	0	38.0	0	0	0	0
tropical	240	0	39.0	0	0	0	0
Winged beans, ½ cup:							
fresh:							
raw, sliced	11	1.5	1.0	.2	0	1	n.a.
boiled, drained	12	1.6	1.0	.2	0	1	n.a.
dried:							
raw	372	27.0	38.0	14.9	0	35	14.1
boiled	126	9.1	12.8	5.0	0	11	n.a.
Winged bean leaves, trimmed, 1 oz.	21	1.7	4.0	.3	0	n.a.	n.a.
Winged bean tuber, trimmed, 1 oz.	45	3.3	8.0	.3	0	n.a.	n.a.
Wolffish, Atlantic, meat only:							
raw, 4 oz.	109	19.9	0	2.7	52	97	0
baked, broiled, or microwaved, 4 oz. . . .	139	25.4	0	3.5	67	124	0
Wonton wrapper:							
(*Frieda's*), 4 pcs.	80	3.0	17.0	0	0	160	1.0
(*Nasoya*), 5 pcs.	90	3.0	18.0	0	5	230	0
Worcestershire sauce, 1 tsp.:							
(*Crosse & Blackwell*)	5	0	1.0	0	0	65	0
(*French's*)	0	0	<1.0	0	0	55	0
(*Lea & Perrins*)	5	0	1.0	0	0	65	0
white wine (*Lea & Perrins*)	0	0	0	0	0	50	0

[2] *Includes wines containing less than 15% alcohol, such as burgundy, Chablis, and champagne.*

Y

Food and Measure	cal.	prot. (gms)	carbo. (gms)	fat (gms)	chol. (mgs)	sod. (mgs)	fiber (gms)
Yam, 1/2 cup:							
baked or boiled	79	1.0	18.8	.1	0	6	2.7
canned or frozen, see "Sweet potato"							
Yam, mountain, Hawaiian, 1/2 cup:							
raw, cubed	46	.9	11.1	.1	0	9	n.a.
steamed, cubed	59	1.2	14.4	.1	0	9	n.a.
Yam bean tuber:							
raw:							
(*Frieda's* Jicama), 3/4 cup, 3 oz.	35	1.0	7.0	0	0	5	1.0
sliced, 1/2 cup	23	.4	5.3	.1	0	3	n.a.
boiled, drained, 4 oz.	43	.8	10.0	.1	0	5	n.a.
Yam patties, see "Sweet potato, frozen"							
Yard-long beans:							
fresh, sliced, 1/2 cup:							
raw	22	1.3	3.8	.2	0	2	n.a.
boiled, drained	25	1.3	4.8	.1	0	2	n.a.
dried, 1/2 cup:							
raw	292	20.4	52.0	1.1	0	14	4.0
boiled	102	7.1	18.1	.4	0	4	1.4
Yeast, baker's, all varieties (*Fleischmann's*), 1/4 tsp. . . .	0	0	0	0	0	0	0
Yellow beans, dried, boiled, 1/2 cup	126	8.1	22.2	1.0	0	4	n.a.
Yellow-eye beans, dry (*Frieda's*), 1/2 cup	120	7.0	22.0	0	0	0	9.0

Food and Measure	cal.	prot. (gms)	carbo. (gms)	fat (gms)	chol. (mgs)	sod. (mgs)	fiber (gms)
Yellow squash:							
fresh, see "Crookneck squash"							
canned (*Allens/Sunshine*), 1/2 cup	25	0	5.0	0	0	160	2.0
frozen (*McKenzie's*), 2/3 cup	15	1.0	2.0	0	0	15	1.0
Yellowtail, meat only:							
raw, 4 oz.	166	26.3	0	6.0	n.a.	44	0
baked, broiled, or microwaved, 4 oz. . . .	212	33.6	0	7.6	n.a.	57	0
Yogurt, 8 oz., except as noted:							
plain:							
(*Breyers* 1.5% Fat)	130	11.0	15.0	3.0	20	150	0
(*Columbo* Fat Free)	110	9.0	17.0	0	5	150	0
(*Dannon* Fat Free)	110	12.0	16.0	0	5	150	0
(*Dannon* Lowfat) . . .	150	11.0	18.0	3.5	20	170	0
(*Dannon* Organic)	150	8.0	12.0	8.0	35	120	0
(*Friendship*)	150	12.0	18.0	3.0	15	190	0
all flavors (*Columbo* Light)	100	7.0	17.0	0	<5	110	0
all fruit flavors:							
(*Yoplait*), 6 oz.	180	6.0	34.0	1.5	10	80	0
(*Yoplait* Custard Style), 6 oz.	190	7.0	32.0	3.5	15	100	0
(*Yoplait* Custard Style Multi-Pack), 4 oz.	120	5.0	21.0	2.0	10	70	0
(*Yoplait* Light), 6 oz.	90	5.0	16.0	0	5	75	0
(*Yoplait* 99% Fat Free), 4 oz.	120	4.0	23.0	1.0	5	55	0
(*Yoplait Trix*), 6 oz.	190	6.0	36.0	2.0	10	85	0
(*Yoplait Trix* Multi-Pack), 4 oz.	130	4.0	24.0	1.5	5	55	0
except banana/ strawberry (*Columbo* Fat Free)	200	7.0	43.0	0	5	110	0

Food and Measure	cal.	prot. (gms)	carbo. (gms)	fat (gms)	chol. (mgs)	sod. (mgs)	fiber (gms)
apple cinnamon:							
(*Dannon* Fruit on the Bottom)	240	9.0	46.0	1.5	15	140	1.0
(*Dannon Chunky Fruit*), 6 oz.	160	7.0	33.0	0	5	100	0
banana berry (*Light n' Lively* Kidpack), 4.4 oz.	130	5.0	24.0	1.0	10	65	0
banana cream:							
(*Yoplait* Light), 6 oz.	90	6.0	16.0	0	0	95	0
pie (*Dannon Light*)	100	8.0	16.0	0	5	120	0
banana/strawberry (*Columbo* Fat Free)	220	7.0	47.0	0	5	120	0
berries, mixed:							
(*Breyers* 1% Fat) . . .	250	8.0	48.0	2.5	15	110	0
(*Dannon* Fruit on the Bottom)	240	9.0	45.0	3.0	15	150	1.0
(*Dannon* Fruit on the Bottom), 4 oz.	120	5.0	22.0	1.5	5	70	<1.0
(*Knudsen Free*), 6 oz.	170	8.0	33.0	0	0	105	0
(*Light n' Lively Free*), 6 oz.	170	8.0	34.0	0	5	105	0
berry:							
blue (*Light n' Lively* Kidpack), 4.4 oz.	150	5.0	30.0	1.0	10	65	0
ild (*Light n' Lively* Kidpack), 4.4 oz.	140	5.0	27.0	1.0	10	65	0
blueberry:							
(*Breyers* 1% Fat) . . .	250	8.0	48.0	2.5	15	110	0
(*Dannon* Fruit on the Bottom)	240	9.0	46.0	3.0	15	140	1.0
(*Dannon Chunky Fruit*), 6 oz.	160	7.0	32.0	0	5	110	0
(*Dannon Light*)	100	8.0	17.0	0	5	115	0
(*Knudsen Cal 70*), 6 oz.	70	7.0	12.0	0	5	80	0
(*Light n' Lively* 1% Milkfat), 4.4 oz.	140	5.0	27.0	1.0	10	65	0
(*Light n' Lively Free*), 6 oz.	190	8.0	38.0	0	5	105	0

Food and Measure	cal.	prot. (gms)	carbo. (gms)	fat (gms)	chol. (mgs)	sod. (mgs)	fiber (gms)
Yogurt, blueberry *(cont.)*							
(Light n' Lively Free 50 Cal), 4.4 oz.	50	5.0	8.0	0	<5	60	0
(Light n' Lively Free 70 Cal), 6 oz. ...	70	7.0	11.0	0	<5	80	0
Boston cream pie *(Yoplait* Light), 6 oz.	90	6.0	16.0	0	0	95	0
boysenberry *(Dannon* Fruit on the Bottom)	240	9.0	45.0	3.0	15	150	1.0
café au lait *(Yoplait)*, 6 oz.	170	6.0	31.0	2.0	10	80	0
cappuccino:							
(Columbo Fat Free)	170	8.0	34.0	0	5	130	0
(Dannon Light)	100	8.0	16.0	0	5	120	0
caramel apple *(Yoplait* Light), 6 oz.	90	6.0	16.0	0	0	95	0
cheesecake:							
amaretto *(Yoplait* Light), 6 oz.	90	6.0	16.0	0	5	95	0
cherry *(Dannon Double Delights)*, 6 oz.	170	7.0	34.0	1.0	10	100	0
strawberry *(Dannon Double Delights)*, 6 oz.	170	7.0	33.0	1.0	10	100	0
cherry:							
(Dannon Fruit on the Bottom)	240	9.0	45.0	3.0	15	140	<1.0
(Light n' Lively Kidpack), 4.4 oz.	140	5.0	27.0	1.0	10	65	0
black *(Breyers* 1% Fat)	260	8.0	50.0	2.5	15	110	0
black *(Knudsen Cal 70)*, 6 oz.	70	7.0	12.0	0	5	85	0
black *(Light n' Lively Free 70 Cal)*, 6 oz.	70	7.0	11.0	0	<5	85	0
cherry vanilla:							
(Dannon Chunky Fruit), 6 oz.	160	7.0	31.0	0	5	100	0
(Dannon Light)	100	8.0	18.0	0	5	115	0

Food and Measure	cal.	prot. (gms)	carbo. (gms)	fat (gms)	chol. (mgs)	sod. (mgs)	fiber (gms)
(*Dannon Sprinkl'ins*), 4.1 oz.	130	5.0	24.0	1.5	5	85	0
chocolate cheesecake (*Dannon Double Delights*), 6 oz.	220	8.0	45.0	1.0	10	150	0
coconut cream pie:							
(*Dannon Light*)	100	8.0	15.0	0	5	120	0
(*Yoplait*), 6 oz.	200	6.0	35.0	3.5	10	80	0
coffee:							
(*Breyers* 1.5% Fat)	220	10.0	38.0	3.0	20	135	0
(*Dannon*)	210	10.0	36.0	3.0	15	160	0
cranberry-raspberry (*Dannon*)	210	10.0	36.0	3.0	15	160	0
creme caramel (*Dannon Light*)	100	8.0	15.0	0	5	120	0
French roast (*Columbo Fat Free*)	170	8.0	34.0	0	5	130	0
grape (*Light n' Lively* Kidpack), 4.4 oz.	130	5.0	24.0	1.0	10	65	0
lemon:							
(*Columbo Fat Free*)	170	8.0	34.0	0	5	130	0
(*Dannon*)	210	10.0	36.0	3.0	15	160	0
(*Knudsen Cal 70*), 6 oz.	70	7.0	11.0	0	5	100	<1.0
(*Knudsen Free*), 6 oz.	160	8.0	33.0	0	5	105	0
(*Light n' Lively Free*), 6 oz.	170	8.0	35.0	0	5	105	0
(*Light n' Lively Free 70 Cal*), 6 oz. ...	.70	7.0	12.0	0	<5	120	0
chiffon (*Dannon Light*)	100	8.0	15.0	0	5	120	0
cream pie (*Yoplait Light*), 6 oz.	90	6.0	16.0	0	0	95	0
creamy (*Breyers* 1.5% Fat)	220	10.0	38.0	3.0	20	140	0
meringue pie (*Dannon Double Delights*), 6 oz.	180	6.0	37.0	1.0	10	170	0

Food and Measure	cal.	prot. (gms)	carbo. (gms)	fat (gms)	chol. (mgs)	sod. (mgs)	fiber (gms)
Yogurt *(cont.)*							
lime pie, Key (*Yoplait Light*), 6 oz.	90	6.0	16.0	0	0	95	0
orange (*Light n' Lively Kidpack*), 4.4 oz.	150	5.0	29.0	1.0	10	65	0
peach:							
(*Breyers* 1% Fat) ...	250	8.0	48.0	2.5	15	110	0
(*Dannon* Fruit on the Bottom)	240	9.0	45.0	3.0	15	140	1.0
(*Dannon Chunky Fruit*), 6 oz.	160	7.0	33.0	0	5	100	0
(*Dannon Light*)	100	8.0	16.0	0	5	120	0
(*Knudsen Cal 70*), 6 oz.	70	7.0	11.0	0	5	80	<1.0
(*Knudsen Free*), 6 oz.	170	8.0	33.0	0	5	105	0
(*Light n' Lively* 1% Fat), 4.4 oz.	140	5.0	27.0	1.0	10	65	0
(*Light n' Lively Free*), 6 oz.	170	8.0	35.0	0	5	105	0
(*Light n' Lively Free 50 Cal*), 4.4 oz.	50	5.0	9.0	0	<5	60	0
(*Light n' Lively Free 70 Cal*), 6 oz. ...	70	6.0	12.0	0	<5	80	0
piña colada (*Dannon Chunky Fruit*), 6 oz.	160	7.0	32.0	0	5	110	0
pineapple:							
(*Breyers* 1% Fat) ...	250	8.0	49.0	2.5	15	110	0
(*Knudsen Cal 70*), 6 oz.	70	7.0	11.0	0	5	80	0
(*Light n' Lively* 1% Fat), 4.4 oz.	140	5.0	27.0	1.0	5	60	0
raspberry:							
(*Dannon* Blended), 6 oz.	110	5.0	24.0	0	5	75	0
(*Dannon* Fruit on the Bottom)	240	9.0	45.0	3.0	15	140	1.0
(*Dannon Light*)	100	8.0	16.0	0	5	130	0
red (*Breyers* 1% Fat)	250	8.0	48.0	2.5	15	110	2.0
red (*Knudsen Cal 70*), 6 oz.	70	7.0	11.0	0	5	75	0

Food and Measure	cal.	prot. (gms)	carbo. (gms)	fat (gms)	chol. (mgs)	sod. (mgs)	fiber (gms)
red (*Knudsen Free*), 6 oz.	160	8.0	31.0	0	5	105	0
red (*Light n' Lively 1% Fat*), 4.4 oz.	130	5.0	24.0	1.0	10	65	0
red (*Light n' Lively Free*), 6 oz.	180	8.0	36.0	0	5	105	0
red (*Light n' Lively Free 50 Cal*), 4.4 oz.	50	5.0	8.0	0	<5	60	0
red (*Light n' Lively Free 70 Cal*), 6 oz.	70	7.0	11.0	0	<5	80	0
raspberry Bavarian creme (*Dannon Double Delights*), 6 oz.	170	7.0	34.0	1.0	10	125	0
strawberry:							
(*Breyers 1% Fat*) . . .	250	8.0	47.0	2.5	15	110	0
(*Dannon Blended*), 4 oz.	110	5.0	23.0	0	5	80	0
(*Dannon Fruit on the Bottom*)	240	9.0	45.0	3.0	15	140	<1.0
(*Dannon Fruit on the Bottom*), 4 oz.	120	5.0	22.0	1.5	5	70	<1.0
(*Dannon Chunky Fruit*), 6 oz.	160	7.0	32.0	0	5	115	0
(*Dannon Light*)	100	8.0	16.0	0	5	120	0
(*Dannon Sprinkl'ins*), 4.1 oz.	130	5.0	24.0	1.5	5	85	0
(*Knudsen Cal 70*), 6 oz.	70	7.0	11.0	0	5	85	0
(*Knudsen Free*), 6 oz.	160	8.0	32.0	0	5	105	0
(*Light n' Lively 1% Fat*), 4.4 oz.	140	5.0	26.0	1.0	10	65	0
(*Light n' Lively Free*), 6 oz.	180	8.0	36.0	0	5	105	0
(*Light n' Lively Free 50 Cal*), 4.4 oz.	50	5.0	8.0	0	<5	60	0
(*Light n' Lively Free 70 Cal*), 6 oz. . . .	70	7.0	11.0	0	<5	85	0

Food and Measure	cal.	prot. (gms)	carbo. (gms)	fat (gms)	chol. (mgs)	sod. (mgs)	fiber (gms)
Yogurt, strawberry (cont.)							
fruit basket (Knudsen Cal 70), 6 oz.	70	7.0	11.0	0	5	90	0
fruit cup (Light n' Lively 1% Fat), 4.4 oz.	140	5.0	27.0	1.0	10	60	0
fruit cup (Light n' Lively Free), 6 oz.	170	8.0	35.0	0	5	105	0
fruit cup (Light n' Lively Free 50 Cal), 4.4 oz.	50	5.0	8.0	0	<5	60	0
fruit cup (Light n' Lively Free 70 Cal), 6 oz.	70	7.0	11.0	0	<5	80	0
wild (Light n' Lively Kidpack), 4.4 oz.	140	5.0	28.0	1.0	10	65	0
strawberry banana:							
(Breyers 1% Fat) ...	250	9.0	50.0	2.5	15	115	<1.0
(Dannon Blended), 4 oz.	110	5.0	23.0	0	5	75	0
(Dannon Fruit on the Bottom)	240	9.0	43.0	3.0	15	140	1.0
(Dannon Chunky Fruit), 6 oz.	160	7.0	32.0	0	5	105	0
(Dannon Light)	100	8.0	16.0	0	5	120	0
(Dannon Sprinkl'ins), 4.1 oz.	130	5.0	24.0	1.5	5	80	0
(Knudsen Cal 70), 6 oz.	70	7.0	11.0	0	5	85	0
(Light n' Lively 1% Fat), 4.4 oz.	140	5.0	28.0	1.0	10	60	0
(Light n' Lively Free 50 Cal), 4.4 oz.	50	5.0	8.0	0	<5	60	0
(Light n' Lively Free 70 Cal), 6 oz. ...	70	7.0	11.0	0	<5	85	0
tangerine chiffon (Dannon Light)	100	8.0	16.0	0	5	120	0
tropical punch (Light n' Lively Kidpack), 4.4 oz.	140	5.0	28.0	1.0	10	65	0

Food and Measure	cal.	prot. (gms)	carbo. (gms)	fat (gms)	chol. (mgs)	sod. (mgs)	fiber (gms)
vanilla:							
(*Breyers* 1.5% Fat)	220	10.0	38.0	3.0	20	135	0
(*Columbo* Fat Free)	170	8.0	34.0	0	5	130	0
(*Dannon*)	210	10.0	36.0	3.0	15	160	0
(*Dannon Light*)	100	8.0	15.0	0	5	120	0
(*Knudsen Cal 70*),							
6 oz.	70	7.0	11.0	0	5	80	0
(*Knudsen Free*),							
6 oz.	170	8.0	32.0	0	5	100	0
(*Light n' Lively*							
Free), 6 oz.	160	8.0	32.0	0	5	105	0
(*Yoplait* Custard							
Style), 6 oz.	190	8.0	32.0	3.5	15	95	0
w/cherry or orange							
crystals (*Dannon*							
Sprinkl'ins),							
4.1 oz.	110	5.0	21.0	.5	5	85	0
French (*Yoplait*),							
6 oz.	180	6.0	34.0	1.5	10	90	0
vanilla caramel sundae							
(*Columbo* Fat Free)	220	7.0	47.0	0	5	120	0
Yogurt, frozen, 1/2 cup:							
all fruit flavors:							
(*Columbo* Nonfat)	100	3.0	20.0	0	<5	55	0
(*Columbo* Slender							
Sensations)	60	4.0	11.0	0	<5	60	0
banana split (*Blue Bell*							
Nonfat)	110	4.0	24.0	0	0	75	0
(*Ben & Jerry's* Cherry							
Garcia)	170	4.0	32.0	3.0	20	80	0
(*Ben & Jerry's* Choco-							
late Cherry Garcia)	190	5.0	35.0	4.0	15	65	1.0
blueberry pie (*Dannon*							
Fat Free)	100	3.0	21.0	0	0	55	0
butter pecan or butter							
nut toffee (*Columbo*							
Nonfat)	100	3.0	20.0	0	<5	140	0
cappuccino:							
(*Columbo* Nonfat)	100	3.0	20.0	0	<5	55	0
(*Dannon* Fat Free)	100	3.0	20.0	0	0	55	0

Food and Measure	cal.	prot. (gms)	carbo. (gms)	fat (gms)	chol. (mgs)	sod. (mgs)	fiber (gms)
Yogurt, frozen *(cont.)*							
caramel praline crunch (*Edy's/Dreyer's* Fat Free)	100	3.0	21.0	0	0	70	0
cheesecake:							
(*Columbo* Nonfat)	100	3.0	20.0	0	<5	55	0
(*Dannon* NY Fat Free)	100	3.0	20.0	0	0	55	0
cherry, black, vanilla swirl (*Edy's/Dreyer's* Fat Free)	80	3.0	18.0	0	0	65	0
cherry chocolate chunk (*Edy's/ Dreyer's*)	110	2.0	18.0	3.0	10	25	0
cherry vanilla (*Häagen-Dazs*)	140	6.0	30.0	0	<5	40	0
chocolate:							
(*Breyers*)	130	n.a.	23.0	3.0	10	45	0
(*Columbo* Slender Sensations)	70	4.0	11.0	0	<5	70	0
(*Dannon* Fat Free)	100	3.0	22.0	0	0	50	0
(*Dannon* Fat Free Light)	70	4.0	16.0	0	0	65	0
(*Dannon* Lowfat) . . .	120	3.0	22.0	2.0	5	55	1.0
(*Häagen-Dazs*)	140	6.0	28.0	0	<5	45	<1.0
brownie chunk (*Edy's/Dreyer's*)	120	3.0	17.0	4.0	10	35	0
chip cookie dough (*Ben & Jerry's*)	200	4.0	35.0	4.5	10	120	1.0
Dutch, double (*Columbo* Nonfat)	100	3.0	22.0	0	<5	65	1.0
old world (*Columbo* Lowfat)	110	3.0	22.0	2.0	10	65	1.0
silk mousse (*Edy's/ Dreyer's* Fat Free)	90	3.0	19.0	0	0	60	0
chocolate almond, Swiss (*Columbo* Nonfat)	100	3.0	22.0	0	<5	65	1.0
chocolate fudge:							
(*Edy's/Dreyer's* Fat Free)	100	3.0	21.0	0	0	70	0

Food and Measure	cal.	prot. (gms)	carbo. (gms)	fat (gms)	chol. (mgs)	sod. (mgs)	fiber (gms)
brownie (*Ben & Jerry's*)	190	5.0	36.0	2.5	5	105	1.0
German (*Columbo Nonfat*)	110	4.0	23.0	0	<5	60	1.0
chocolate mousse, white:							
(*Columbo* Nonfat)	100	3.0	20.0	0	<5	55	0
(*Dannon* Fat Free)	100	3.0	20.0	0	0	55	0
coconut (*Columbo Nonfat Cooler*)	100	3.0	20.0	0	<5	55	0
coffee:							
(*Häagen-Dazs*)	140	6.0	29.0	0	<5	45	0
fudge sundae (*Edy's/Dreyer's* Fat Free)	100	3.0	21.0	0	0	75	0
cookie dough (*Edy's/ Dreyer's*)	130	2.0	22.0	4.0	10	70	0
cookies and cream:							
(*Columbo* Nonfat)	120	4.0	25.0	0	<5	85	0
(*Edy's/Dreyer's*) ...	110	2.0	19.0	3.0	10	45	0
cookies in cream (*Breyers* Fat Free)	110	n.a.	25.0	0	0	75	0
eggnog (*Columbo Nonfat*)	100	3.0	20.0	0	<5	55	0
honey almond (*Columbo* Nonfat)	100	3.0	21.0	0	<5	60	0
Irish creme (*Columbo Nonfat*)	100	3.0	20.0	0	<5	55	0
marble fudge (*Edy's/ Dreyer's* Fat Free)	100	3.0	21.0	0	0	75	0
mint chocolate, frango (*Columbo* Nonfat)	100	3.0	22.0	0	<5	65	1.0
mocha madness (*Columbo* Nonfat)	100	3.0	20.0	0	<5	55	0
orange blossom (*Dannon* Fat Free)	100	3.0	20.0	0	0	55	0
peach:							
passion (*Dannon* Fat Free)	100	3.0	20.0	0	0	55	0
raspberry trifle (*Ben & Jerry's*)	180	7.0	32.0	2.5	5	105	0

Food and Measure	cal.	prot. (gms)	carbo. (gms)	fat (gms)	chol. (mgs)	sod. (mgs)	fiber (gms)
Yogurt, frozen *(cont.)*							
peanut butter:							
(*Columbo* Lowfat)	120	4.0	20.0	2.5	<5	75	0
(*Dannon* Lowfat) . . .	120	3.0	19.0	3.0	10	65	0
peppermint stick							
(*Columbo* Nonfat)	100	3.0	20.0	0	<5	55	0
praline pecan (*Dannon*							
Fat Free)	100	3.0	20.0	0	0	55	0
raspberry, red (*Dan-*							
non Fat Free)	100	3.0	20.0	0	0	55	0
strawberry:							
(*Blue Bell* Nonfat)	120	4.0	25.0	0	0	80	0
(*Breyers* Fat Free)	100	n.a.	22.0	0	0	40	0
(*Columbo* Lowfat)	110	3.0	21.0	1.5	10	55	0
(*Dannon* Fat Free)	100	3.0	20.0	0	0	60	0
strawberry cheesecake							
(*Blue Bell* Lowfat)	130	4.0	25.0	1.0	5	150	0
toffee crunch:							
(*Edy's/Dreyer's*							
Heath)	120	2.0	18.0	4.0	10	50	0
vanilla (*Ben &*							
Jerry's Vanilla							
Heath)	210	5.0	34.0	6.0	10	120	0
vanilla:							
(*Blue Bell* Country							
Lowfat)	120	4.0	23.0	1.0	10	90	0
(*Breyers*)	120	n.a.	22.0	3.0	10	40	0
(*Breyers* Fat Free)	100	n.a.	23.0	0	0	50	0
(*Columbo* Slender							
Sensations)	60	4.0	11.0	0	<5	60	0
(*Dannon* Fat Free)	100	3.0	20.0	0	0	60	0
(*Dannon* Fat Free							
Light)	70	4.0	16.0	0	0	75	0
(*Dannon* Lowfat) . . .	110	3.0	19.0	2.0	10	60	0
(*Edy's/Dreyer's*) . . .	100	2.0	17.0	2.5	10	30	0
(*Edy's/Dreyer's* Fat							
Free)	80	3.0	18.0	0	0	65	0
(*Häagen-Dazs*)	140	6.0	29.0	0	<5	45	0
all varieties							
(*Columbo* Nonfat)	100	3.0	21.0	0	<5	60	0

Food and Measure	cal.	prot. (gms)	carbo. (gms)	fat (gms)	chol. (mgs)	sod. (mgs)	fiber (gms)
bean (*Blue Bell* Nonfat)	110	4.0	24.0	0	0	90	0
French (*Dannon* Fat Free)	100	3.0	20.0	0	0	60	0
French or simply (*Columbo* Lowfat)	110	3.0	21.0	1.5	10	55	0
vanilla chocolate: (*Breyers* Fat Free Take Two)	100	n.a.	23.0	0	0	45	0
swirl (*Edy's/Dreyer's* Fat Free)	80	3.0	18.0	0	0	65	0
vanilla chocolate strawberry (*Breyers*)	120	n.a.	22.0	2.5	10	40	0
vanilla fudge: (*Häagen-Dazs*)	160	6.0	34.0	0	<5	100	0
twirl (*Breyers* Fat Free)	110	n.a.	25.0	0	0	45	0
vanilla raspberry swirl (*Häagen-Dazs*)	130	4.0	28.0	0	<5	30	0
Yogurt bar, frozen, 1 pc.:							
all flavors (*Starburst*)	70	2.0	13.0	1.0	<5	25	0
banana and strawberry (*Häagen-Dazs*)	90	2.0	20.0	0	0	15	0
cherry chocolate chip (*Ben & Jerry's Cherry Garcia*)	260	5.0	31.0	14.0	15	70	2.0
chocolate almond (*Frozfruit*)	130	4.0	23.0	4.0	0	10	0
chocolate banana, chocolate, cherry, or raspberry (*SnackWell's*)	120	4.0	22.0	2.0	10	55	1.0
chocolate and cherry (*Häagen-Dazs*)	100	3.0	21.0	0	0	40	<1.0
chocolate fudge (*Edy's*)	240	4.0	26.0	15.0	10	45	0
chocolate and vanilla (*Häagen-Dazs*)	90	3.0	20.0	0	0	45	<1.0
peach (*Frozfruit*).....	100	3.0	22.0	0	0	95	0

Food and Measure	cal.	prot. (gms)	carbo. (gms)	fat (gms)	chol. (mgs)	sod. (mgs)	fiber (gms)
Yogurt bar *(cont.)*							
raspberry and vanilla (*Häagen-Dazs*)	90	2.0	20.0	0	0	15	0
strawberry/strawberry banana (*Frozfruit*)	100	3.0	22.0	0	0	85	0
Strawberry Cheese-cake Craze (*Häagen-Dazs Exträas*)	220	7.0	31.0	8.0	65	140	0
strawberry daiquiri (*Häagen-Dazs*)	90	2.0	18.0	1.0	15	20	0
toffee crunch (*Edy's*)	250	3.0	31.0	14.0	15	75	0
Tropical Orange Pas-sion (*Häagen-Dazs*)	100	2.0	20.0	1.0	15	20	0
vanilla almond (*Edy's*)	230	4.0	24.0	15.0	10	40	0
Yow choy sum (*Frieda's*), 1 cup, 3 oz.	20	2.0	3.0	0	0	20	0
Yuca root (*Frieda's*), 3 oz.	100	3.0	23.0	0	0	5	1.0

Z

Food and Measure	cal.	prot. (gms)	carbo. (gms)	fat (gms)	chol. (mgs)	sod. (mgs)	fiber (gms)
Zabaglione, see "Cake, frozen"							
Ziti entree, frozen, 1 pkg.:							
mozzarella (*Smart Ones*), 9 oz.	290	11.0	47.0	7.0	5	600	5.0
Parmesano (*The Budget Gourmet Value Classics* Low Fat), 8 oz.	280	11.0	39.0	9.0	10	550	4.0
Zucchini, fresh, ½ cup, except as noted:							
raw:							
sliced	9	.8	1.9	.1	0	2	.8
baby, 1 large, 3⅛"	3	.4	.5	.1	0	tr.	n.a.
boiled, drained:							
sliced	14	.6	3.5	.1	0	2	1.3
mashed	19	.8	4.7	.1	0	3	1.7
Zucchini, canned, Italian style, ½ cup:							
(*Del Monte*)	30	1.0	7.0	0	0	490	1.0
(*Progresso*)	50	2.0	7.0	2.0	0	400	2.0
w/tomato juice	33	1.2	7.8	.1	0	424	1.0
Zucchini, frozen:							
(*Seneca*), ⅔ cup	15	4.0	3.0	0	0	0	1.0
breaded (*Empire*), 1 pc.	100	5.0	18.0	0	0	280	1.0
Zucchini, marinated, sun-dried, in jars (*Antica Italia*), 1 oz.	160	0	2.0	17.0	0	15	1.0
Zucchini soufflé, frozen (*Melrose*), ½ cup	90	3.0	19.0	0	0	160	3.0